Long-term Potentiation

Long-term Potentiation: Enhancing Neuroscience for 30 years

Compiled and edited by

T. V. P. BLISS,
G. L. COLLINGRIDGE,
AND
R. G. M. MORRIS

Originating from a Theme Issue first published in the
Philosophical Transactions of the Royal Society, Series B

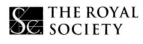
THE ROYAL SOCIETY

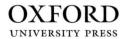
OXFORD
UNIVERSITY PRESS

OXFORD
UNIVERSITY PRESS

Great Clarendon Street, Oxford OX2 6DP

Oxford University Press is a department of the University of Oxford.
It furthers the University's objective of excellence in research, scholarship,
and education by publishing worldwide in

Oxford New York

Auckland Bangkok Buenos Aires Cape Town Chennai
Dar es Salaam Delhi Hong Kong Istanbul Karachi Kolkata
Kuala Lumpur Madrid Melbourne Mexico City Mumbai Nairobi
São Paulo Shanghai Taipei Tokyo Toronto

Oxford is a registered trade mark of Oxford University Press
in the UK and in certain other countries

Published in the United States
by Oxford University Press Inc., New York

First published by the Royal Society 2003
First published by Oxford University Press 2004

A catalogue record for this title is available from the British Library

ISBN 0 19 853030 7 (Hbk)

10 9 8 7 6 5 4 3 2 1

Typeset by Newgen Imaging Systems (P) Ltd., Chennai, India
Printed in Great Britain
on acid-free paper by
Biddles Ltd, King's Lynn

Foreword

The ability to capture information from the outside world and from personal experiences, and to incorporate that information in the subsequent control of behaviour, is a fundamental characteristic of advanced animals. Call it learning or memory or adaptation, it all adds up to one thing – the capacity to transcend the limitations of the information inherited in the genes and to modify behaviour on the basis of individual experience.

Memory is central to being a person. What would life be without being able to recognize friends, to know the rules of language or social behaviour, to reminisce about the tapestry of recollections that makes up a life?

But how does experience write its impressions on our minds? That question has puzzled philosophers and scientists – from John Locke and his wax tablet analogy to the one protein-one memory hypothesis of the 1960s.

This book, consisting of papers presented at a meeting at the Royal Society in London, commemorates the 30th anniversary of the discovery of Long-Term Potentiation (LTP). This remarkable physiological phenomenon, which has entered the folklore of neuroscience and the contemporary textbooks, is widely regarded as a likely basis of memory. We are still far from understanding the complete nature of the internal representations that create the subjective recollections of personal experience, but LTP, operating at synaptic connections, especially in the hippocampus and the cerebral cortex, is thought to be essential to the process.

The first detailed description of LTP appeared in 1973. It described simple experiments done at the University of Oslo by Terje Lømo and by Tim Bliss, who was visiting from the Medical Research Council's National Institute for Medical Research in London. They recorded electrical responses from neurons in the hippocampus of anaesthetized rabbits. The hippocampus, an evolutionarily ancient part of the forebrain, tucked under the temporal lobe, had been implicated in human memory by the devastating loss of personal memory suffered by a patient, HM, who had undergone surgical removal of the hippocampus, on both sides, in an attempt to treat intractable epilepsy. HM's amnesia was studied by Brenda Milner, a psychologist from McGill University in Montreal, where Tim Bliss studied for his PhD in the sixties. McGill was also home to Donald Hebb, author of that remarkable book *Organization of Behavior*, in which Hebb postulated that associative learning depends on modification in the efficiency of connections between nerve cells.

Tim, working with Ben Delisle Burns, spent his PhD searching for long-lasting changes in the responsiveness of cortical neurons as a result of repetitive stimulation of input axons. The results were complicated and generally rather unconvincing. The hippocampus offered a structure simpler and more orderly than that of the cerebral cortex, and one in which extracellular electrodes could be used to record field potentials reflecting the activity of large numbers of similar nerve cells. In the autumn of 1968, Lømo and Bliss, studying the hippocampus in anaesthetized rabbits, reproduced a phenomenon first described by Lømo in an abstract in 1966. After briefly, but rapidly, stimulating the nerve fibres connecting to the cell layers of the hippocampus, they found that the size of the response produced by a single pulse to the same fibres was much enhanced. To their amazement, this effect persisted for at least several hours.

They realized at once the possible significance of this finding but were tormented by the possibility that their "long-lasting potentiation", as they first called it, was an artifactual result of changes in physical properties of the stimulating electrode – perhaps polarized in some way by the repetitive, "tetanic" stimulation – rather than a genuine property of the synaptic connections on to hippocampal neurons. But when they saw the same potentiation with two different stimulating electrodes, one for test stimulation, the other for the tetanic stimulation, this convinced them that the phenomenon was real. LTP was launched.

Whether LTP actually underlies learning and memory remains unproven, although the weight of circumstantial evidence leads Bliss, in his own chapter in this volume, to say "surely it must". The phenomenon itself has been demonstrated beyond doubt and it has spawned an enormous range of elegant research, ranging from genes to cognition.

LTP has been a major driver for research into synaptic function, leading or adding to such novel ideas as multiple receptors for a single transmitter, "neuromodulation", transmitter spillover, retrograde messengers, and receptor trafficking. It stimulated some sophisticated applications of mathematics in neuroscience, and has led to a search for new treatments for memory disorders.

This book provides a definitive overview of the development of ideas about synaptic plasticity and about the wide range of current research in this fascinating field. The historical chapters at the beginning offer an enthralling insight into the development of this field of science and provide a wonderful example of the speed with which the sophistication of scientific enquiry can develop. Thirty years ago, LTP was an intriguing physiological phenomenon. Today we recognize a clear distinction between the induction, expression, and maintenance of LTP, and the organization of the subsequent chapters reflects the types of research conducted on each of these distinct facets. The techniques involved reflect the full ingenuity of modern brain research.

LTP was and is still the dominant model of the "Hebb synapse". While the idea that information might be stored at synapses goes back much further, at least to the great Spanish anatomist Ramón y Cajal, Donald Hebb was the first to specify physiological conditions that should be met for synapses to change in strength to explain behavioural observations. The concept of activity-dependent plasticity has also been applied in many other systems – the fine-tuning during development of the visual system and the sensorimotor timing machine of the cerebellum.

LTP has even brought insights into the nature of memory disorders and the possibility of clinical translation. Research into the mechanisms of LTP has already led to the development of potentially useful cognitive enhancing drugs for treatment of memory dysfunction, including Gary Lynch's "ampakines". Drugs targeting the mechanisms responsible for the maintenance of LTP are a current focus for improving memory function in the elderly and those afflicted by neurodegenerative diseases.

It gives me particular pleasure to write the Foreword for this book because LTP has been a focus of researchers in the United Kingdom supported by the Medical Research Council, of which I now serve as Chief Executive.

The editors of this book, all supported by the MRC, have contributed major milestones to this subject. Tim Bliss, of course, was involved in the initial description of the phenomenon in 1973. Graham Collingridge provided the first evidence, in 1983, that the NMDA glutamate receptor plays an important role in mediating LTP. And in 1986, Richard Morris demonstrated that activation of the NMDA receptor is required for spatial learning in the rat.

My predecessor as Chief Executive of the MRC, Sir George Radda, was responsible for the establishment of the MRC Centre for Synaptic Plasticity in Bristol – the first MRC centre to be opened, testifying to MRC's continuing commitment to this exciting field of research.

Colin Blakemore
Chief Executive
Medical Research Council
London

This book was originally published as an issue of the Philosophical Transactions of the Royal Society, Series B (*Phil. Trans. R. Soc. Lond.* B (2003) **358**, 607–842) but has been materially changed and updated.

Contents

Contributors

Wickliffe Abraham Department of Psychology, Box 56, University of Otago, Dunedin, New Zealand

Per Andersen Department of Physiology, Institute of Medical Sciences, University of Oslo, PO Box 1103, Blindern, 0317 Oslo, Norway

Roger Anwyl Department of Physiology, Trinity College Institute of Neuroscience, Trinity College, Dublin 2, Ireland

Carol Barnes Departments of Psychology and Neurology, and ARL Division of Neural Systems, Memory and Aging, University of Arizona, Tucson, AZ 85724, USA

Mark Bear Howard Hughes Medical Institute, Department of Neuroscience, Brown University, Providence, RI 02912, USA

Tim Bliss Division of Neurophysiology, National Institute for Medical Research, Mill Hill, London NW7 1AA, UK

Zuner Bortolotto, MRC Centre for Synaptic Plasticity, Department of Anatomy, School of Medical Sciences, University Walk, Bristol BS8 1TD, UK

Bruno Bozon Laboratoire de Neurobiologie de l'Apprentissage, de la Mémoire et de la Communication, CNRS UMR 8620, Université Paris-Sud, 91405 Orsay, France

Sukwoo Choi Department of Neuroscience, Ewha Institute for Neuroscience (EIN), School of Medicine, Ewha Womans University, Seoul 110-783, South Korea

Brian Christie Department of Psychology, University of British Columbia, Vancouver, British Columbia, V6T 1Z4, Canada

Graham Collingridge MRC Centre for Synaptic Plasticity, Department of Anatomy, School of Medical Sciences, University Walk, Bristol BS8 1TD, UK

William Cullen Department of Pharmacology and Therapeutics, Trinity College Institute of Neuroscience, Trinity College, Dublin 2, Ireland

Sabrina Davis Laboratoire de Neurobiologie de l'Apprentissage, de la Mémoire et de la Communication, CNRS UMR 8620, Université Paris-Sud, 91405 Orsay, France

Michael Daw MRC Centre for Synaptic Plasticity, Department of Anatomy, School of Medical Sciences, University Walk, Bristol BS8 1TD, UK

M. Day Centre and Division of Neuroscience, College of Medicine and Veterinary Medicine, The University of Edinburgh, 1 George Square, Edinburgh EH8 9JZ, UK and GSK Neurology Centre of Excellence for Drug Discovery, New Frontiers Science Park (North), Harlow, Essex CM19 5AW, UK

Fabrice Duprat Institut de Pharmacologie Moléculaire et Cellulaire, 06560 Valbonne, France

Mick Errington Division of Neurophysiology, National Institute for Medical Research, Mill Hill, London NW7 1AA, UK

John Fiala Department of Biology and Program in Neuoscience, Boston University, 44 Cummington Street, Boston, MA 02215, USA

Alan Fine Division of Neurophysiology, National Institute for Medical Research, Mill Hill, London NW7 1AA, UK and Dalhousie University Faculty of Medicine, Halifax, Nova Scotia B3H 4H7, Canada

Andreas Frick Division of Neuroscience, Baylor College of Medicine, One Baylor Plaza, Houston, TX 77030, USA

Peter Galley Division of Neurophysiology, National Institute for Medical Research, Mill Hill, London NW7 1AA, UK

Richard Gray Division of Neuroscience, Baylor College of Medicine, One Baylor Plaza, Houston, TX 77030, USA

Kristen Harris Synapses and Cell Signaling Program, Medical College of Georgia, Institute of Molecular Medicine and Genetics, 1120 15th Street, CB-2803, Augusta, GA 30912-2630, USA

Gaël Hédou Institute of Cell Biology, Swiss Federal Institute of Technology, ETH Hönggerberg CH-8093, Zürich, Switzerland

Dax Hoffman Building 49, Room 5A64, NICHD-LCSN, Bethesda, MD 20892, USA

Toshiyuki Hosokawa Center for Research and Development in Higher Education, Hokkaido University, Sapporo 060-0809, Japan

John Isaac MRC Centre for Synaptic Plasticity, Department of Anatomy, School of Medical Sciences, University Walk, Bristol BS8 1TD, UK

Daniel Johnston Division of Neuroscience, Baylor College of Medicine, One Baylor Plaza, Houston, TX 77030, USA

Sheena Josselyn Departments of Neurobiology, Psychiatry, Psychology and Brain Research Institute, University of California Los Angeles, Los Angeles, CA 90095, USA

Eric Kandel Center for Neurobiology and Behavior, Howard Hughes Medical Institute, Columbia University College of Physicians and Surgeons, 1051 Riverside Drive, New York, NY 10032, USA

Áine Kelly Department of Physiology, Trinity College, Dublin 2, Ireland

Jürgen Klingauf Max Planck Institute for Biophysical Chemistry, Department of Membrane Biopsychics, Am Fassberg 11, D-37007 Göttingen, Germany

Igor Klyubin Department of Pharmacology and Therapeutics, Trinity College Institute of Neuroscience, Trinity College, Dublin 2, Ireland

Dimitri Kullmann Institute of Neurology, University College London, Queen Square, London WC1N 3BG, UK

Serge Laroche Laboratoire de Neurobiologie de l'Apprentissage, de la Mémoire et de la Communication, CNRS UMR 8620, Université Paris-Sud, 91405 Orsay, France

Sari Lauri MRC Centre for Synaptic Plasticity, Department of Anatomy, School of Medical Sciences, University Walk, Bristol BS8 1TD, UK

Wonil Lim MRC Centre for Synaptic Plasticity, Department of Anatomy, School of Medical Sciences, University Walk, Bristol BS8 1TD, UK

John Lisman Department of Biology and Volen Center for Complex Systems, MS 008, 415 South Street, Waltham, MA 02454, USA

Terje Lømo Department of Physiology, Institute of Medical Sciences, University of Oslo, PO Box 1103, Blindern, 0317 Oslo, Norway

Gary Lynch Department of Psychiatry and Human Behavior, University of California, Irvine, CA 92616, USA

Robert Malenka Nancy Friend Pritzker Laboratory, Department of Psychiatry and Behavioral Sciences, Stanford University School of Medicine, Palo Alto, CA 94304, USA

Roberto Malinow Cold Spring Harbor Laboratory, Cold Spring Harbor, NY 11724, USA

Isabelle Mansuy Institute of Cell Biology, Swiss Federal Institute of Technology, ETH Hönggerberg CH-8093, Zürich, Switzerland

S. J. Martin Centre and Division of Neuroscience, College of Medicine and Veterinary Medicine, The University of Edinburgh, 1 George Square, Edinburgh EH8 9JZ, UK

Bruce McNaughton Room 384, Life Sciences North Building, University of Arizona, Tucson, AZ 85724, USA

Richard Morris Centre and Division of Neuroscience, College of Medicine and Veterinary Medicine, The University of Edinburgh, 1 George Square, Edinburgh EH8 9JZ, UK

Edvard Moser Centre for the Biology of Memory, NTNU, 7489 Trondheim, Norway

Sachiko Murase Caltech/Howard Hughes Medical Institute, Division of Biology, 114-96, Pasadena, CA 91125, USA

Kazu Nakazawa Picower Center for Learning and Memory and RIKEN-MIT Neuroscience Research Center, Massachusetts Institute of Technology, Cambridge, MA 02139, USA

Roger Nicoll Departments of Cellular and Molecular Pharmacology and Physiology, University of California San Francisco, San Francisco, CA 94143, USA

C. O'Carroll Centre and Division of Neuroscience, College of Medicine and Veterinary Medicine, The University of Edinburgh, 1 George Square, Edinburgh EH8 9JZ, UK

Masaki Ohta Department of Hygiene and Preventive Medicine, Hokkaido University School of Medicine, Sapporo 060-8638, Japan

Linnaea Ostroff Program in Neuoscience, Boston University, 44 Cummington Street, Boston, MA 02215, USA

Christopher Pittenger Center for Neurobiology and Behavior, Howard Hughes Medical Institute, Columbia University College of Physicians and Surgeons, 1051 Riverside Drive, New York, NY 10032, USA

Gernot Riedel Department of Biomedical Sciences, University of Aberdeen, Foresterhill, Aberdeen AB25 2ZD, UK

Michael Rowan Department of Pharmacology and Therapeutics, Trinity College Institute of Neuroscience, Trinity College, Dublin 2, Ireland

Takeshi Saito Department of Hygiene and Preventive Medicine, Hokkaido University School of Medicine, Sapporo 060-8638, Japan

Johan Sandin Department of Neuroscience, Section of Behavioual Neuroscience, Karolinska Institute, S-171 77 Stockholm, Sweden

Lalania Schnexnayder Department of Pediatrics, Baylor College of Medicine, One Baylor Plaza, Houston, TX 77030, USA

Erin Schuman Caltech/Howard Hughes Medical Institute, Division of Biology, 114-96, Pasadena, CA 91125, USA

Alcino Silva Departments of Neurobiology, Psychiatry, Psychology and Brain Research Institute, University of California Los Angeles, Los Angeles, CA 90095, USA

Mark Thomas Departments of Neuroscience and Psychology, and Institute of Human Genetics, University of Minnesota, Minneapolis, MN 55455, USA

Susumu Tonegawa Picower Center for Learning and Memory, Howard Hughes Medical Institute, and RIKEN-MIT Neuroscience Research Center, Massachusetts Institute of Technology, Cambridge, MA 02139, USA

Richard Tsien Department of Molecular and Cellular Physiology, Beckman Center B105, Stanford University School of Medicine, Stanford, CA 94305-5345, USA

Shigeo Watanabe Department of Physiology, New York Medical College, Valhalla, NY 10595, USA

Matthew Wilson Picower Center for Learning and Memory and RIKEN-MIT Neuroscience Research Center, Massachusetts Institute of Technology, Cambridge, MA 02139, USA

Li-Lian Yuan Division of Neuroscience, Baylor College of Medicine, One Baylor Plaza, Houston, TX 77030, USA

Introduction

1. Long-term potentiation (LTP)

The issue of *Philosophical Transactions of the Royal Society* reprinted here celebrates the 30th anniversary of the first detailed description of long-term potentiation (LTP) in two papers published in 1973 in the *Journal of Physiology* (Bliss and Lømo 1973; Bliss and Gardner-Medwin 1973). These two papers brought to a wider audience a phenomenon that had been discovered by Lømo a few years earlier, and published as an abstract in 1966 (Lømo 1966). In LTP, the strength of synapses between neurons in the central nervous system is potentiated for prolonged periods following brief but intense synaptic activation. Thirty years of research have made this one of the most extensively studied topics in contemporary neuroscience. Yet LTP continues to puzzle and intrigue us today, with many of the fundamental questions relating to its cellular mechanisms and functional relevance remaining unanswered.

What is the basis of this continuing interest? Our answer to this question and the reason for holding a Discussion Meeting at The Royal Society is that LTP has, for neuroscientists, turned into something of a treasure chest. Its exploration has led to all manner of findings, issues and further questions. We can justly claim that LTP has been enhancing neuroscience for 30 years.

Two themes have dominated research in this area. The first key question is whether the neural mechanisms of LTP are the same as, or at least overlap with, those responsible for learning and memory. Is it a neural 'model' of memory formation, or is it the actual neural mechanism that is used by the brain to store at least some forms of acquired information? Second, and irrespective of the answer to the first question, can we find out more about how synapses work by studying the mechanisms by which they change in strength? Synapses communicate, and they can do this either weakly or strongly. Their ability to change in strength is therefore a critical property that we must understand if we are to comprehend the nervous system. These two themes, one functional and the other mechanistic, are fundamental to an understanding of how the nervous system works, and researchers have understandably been attracted to them as issues around which to exercise their scientific imagination.

The 30 years of research since 1973 have seen major developments in our conceptual understanding of activity-dependent synaptic plasticity, not least because of spectacular developments in experimental techniques. In the experiments leading up to the 1973 papers, LTP was elicited in the intact rabbit, initially in anaethetized animals at the University of Oslo (Bliss and Lømo 1973), and later in awake animals at University College London (Bliss and Gardner-Medwin 1973) using stimulation techniques that triggered activity in hundreds, or perhaps thousands of neurons. In Oslo, careful measurements of synaptic responses recorded on film by a camera placed in front of an oscilloscope screen provided a degree of quantitative rigour; in London, an early laboratory computer was pressed into service. Today, this approach (with film giving way to the desktop computer) is pursued alongside astonishing new technology, including multiphoton confocal microscopy that allows, for example, the imaging of synaptic transmission at single synapses, or the passage of receptor proteins to be monitored as they shuttle between the cytosol and the synaptic membrane. However sophisticated the technique that is used to study it, the phenomenon itself, robust and abrupt, continues to fascinate. To quote Bliss and Lynch (1988, p. 3): 'No matter how often one has witnessed the phenomenon, it is impossible not to retain a sense of amazement that such modest stimulation can produce so immediate, so profound, and so persistent an effect'.

For most, the defining property of LTP is its persistence. Would there be as much interest in LTP if the 'long' were replaced by 'short'—if it only lasted for a few minutes? The simple truth is that there would not. Inside our treasure chest is a neuronal 'magic wand' whereby extremely brief patterns of electrical stimulation (such as a short burst of high-frequency pulses) trigger biochemical and structural changes that long outlast the stimulation. This is a trick that the nervous system must perform if it is to make memories. And it is a trick that the nervous system does perform to express LTP. The correspondence teases the imagination.

However, persistence is only one of the treasures inside the chest. Other classical properties include input specificity and associativity, and more recently identified properties including metaplasticity, synaptic tagging and the converse phenomenon of long-term depression (LTD). Collectively, these are the kinds of properties that neural network engineers dream about when designing a biologically realistic system to emulate memory. The contributions in this issue describe and attempt to explain these and many other properties, and their functional implications.

2. Structure of the volume

The papers collected in this volume were delivered at a meeting to celebrate the 30th birthday of LTP held on 29 and 30 May 2003 at The Royal Society, London. Such is the effort going into research on activity-dependent synaptic plasticity that we could easily have held a much longer conference, but practicalities constrained us with respect to the aspects of synaptic plasticity that we could cover. The themes that we eventually chose are (a) *History*, (b) *Induction*, (c) *Expression*, (d) *Persistence*, (e) *Function* and (f) *Newdirections*. In extending invitations, we asked people who had made original contributions to one or more of these topics, but we did so in the uncomfortable knowledge that there are many others whom, with equal justification, we might have invited.

(a) History

How was LTP discovered? What happened? What happened next? And do the pioneers of the field agree about these first steps? For every history, there is a pre-history and in Chapter 1, this volume, Andersen takes readers back to one of the classical ages of neurophysiology—the extraordinary 20-year period from 1952 until around 1972. He emphasises the contribution of Sir John Eccles, who well understood that the primary issue was to demonstrate the existence of synapses in which activity-dependent changes in efficacy lasted for hours rather than minutes. In a separate chapter, Lømo (Chapter 2) describes the serendipitous circumstances that resulted in his discovery of LTP in 1966, and takes us through the experiments with Bliss in 1968–1969 that were eventually published in 1973. In Chapter 3, Bliss recalls how frustration with the complexity of the neocortex led him to the hippocampus, to Andersen's laboratory, and to the collaboration with Lømo. That the research they describe was largely completed four years before it was published is a reminder of a gentler age when matters were pursued at a more leisurely and arguably more reflective pace. Soon after the paper was published, Lømo left the field to pursue a distinguished career in another branch of neurophysiology. Bliss's interests also diverged for a few years, and it was Lynch's laboratory in California (see Chapter 4) and Andersen's in Oslo, both using the new *in vitro* hippocampal slice preparation, that were largely responsible for sustaining and promoting interest in LTP. By the late 1970s, LTP had begun to arouse interest worldwide. A Caledonian link also came early, with pioneering research on the properties and functions of LTP in the intact animal conducted in Graham Goddard's laboratory in Nova Scotia, as summarized by McNaughton in Chapter 5. Soon after, in 1983, came the discovery of the critical role of the N-methyl-D-aspartate (NMDA) receptor in the induction of LTP by Collingridge and colleagues at the University of British Columbia (see Chapter 6). Around the same time, Morris developed the watermaze in Scotland and conducted some of the early studies using this task that have revealed the importance of hippocampal LTP for spatial learning (see Chapter 7).

There is much more to be written about the history of LTP than we have space to cover here, but we hope that these articles, written in a more personal style than is usual in *Philosophical Transactions of the Royal Society*, where they were first published, will give a flavour of the intellectual climate in which the early advances were made.

(b) Induction

LTP is conventionally separated into two phases: induction and expression, with expression having several temporal components. Not all synapses are the same. Some show LTP, some do not; of those that do, many rely on the NMDA receptor, but others do not. The biophysical properties of the NMDA receptor, coupled with its regulation by GABA receptor-mediated inhibition, explains many of the defining characteristics of LTP where this receptor is the trigger for induction, including associativity and input-specificity. At other synapses, where induction is independent of NMDA receptors, there is growing evidence that another class of glutamate receptor— the kainate receptor—plays a pivotal part.

Synapses in which the induction of LTP is dependent on the NMDA receptor, as well as those in which it is not, can display activity-dependent LTD in synaptic efficacy. LTD in the hippocampus is more easily elicited in young animals and comes in two flavours. Once synapses are potentiated, the level of synaptic efficacy can be reversed by prolonged low-frequency stimulation in a process known as depotentiation, as first noted by Lynch and colleagues (Barrionuevo *et al.* 1980). In addition, it is also possible to induce LTD in 'naive' pathways (i.e. pathways in which LTP has not been experimentally induced). This type of LTD was first observed in the cerebellum by Ito and Kano (1982), but is now also widely studied in the hippocampus, and is sometimes referred to as *de novo* LTD to distinguish it from depotentiation. An important property of hippocampal plasticity is its bidirectionality; the same synapses can, according to circumstances, be potentiated, depotentiated or depressed.

Finally, recent research has validated Hebb's notion that the firing of the postsynaptic cell may be crucial for whether or not LTP occurs (Hebb 1949). In the simplest account of how neurons work, dendrites transduce incoming activity into synaptic currents, the cell-soma integrates these and generates an action potential once a threshold is exceeded. Axons then transmit action potentials away from the cell body, sometimes over long distances, to other neurons. Recent work has shattered the simplicity of this polarized world, in which activity proceeds in one direction, from dendrite to soma to axon. It is now known that action potentials can 'back-propagate' from the soma into the dendritic tree. The timing of these back-propagating action potentials relative to the synaptic input can play a critical part in determining the polarity of synaptic change.

These subjects are covered in this book by a set of three chapters. Bear (Chapter 8) discusses evidence supporting a theory of the induction of bidirectional plasticity as it applies to the visual cortex (Bienenstock *et al*. 1982). Bortolotto *et al*., in Chapter 9, describe the very different mechanisms of induction of potentiation at mossy fibre synapses in area CA3 of the hippocampus. And Johnston *et al*. transport us into the back-propagating world of spike timing-dependent plasticity in Chapter 10.

(c) Expression

The next step, LTP having been induced, is to reveal how the enhanced synaptic potentiation is expressed. Here, it is necessary to approach the treasure chest with care, for a veritable battleground is revealed within. In the left corner stand the marshalled forces of the presynaptic army. To make synapses stronger, they assert, it is only necessary for the synapse to release more transmitter or, at least, to release transmitter with a greater probability when an action potential invades the presynaptic terminal. That is what happens at axons of the neuromuscular junction, when one action potential rapidly follows another, and also at central synapses; so perhaps similar, longer-lasting mechanisms can also be pressed into service. In the right corner, across the narrow synaptic cleft, stand the battalions of the postsynaptic army. The NMDA receptor is on the postsynaptic side of hippocampal glutamatergic synapses, they proclaim. Since it is the 'locus of control' for the induction of the most prominent form of LTP, why should LTP expression be any more complex than a cascade of biochemical events inside postsynaptic dendritic spines whose net effect is to increase postsynaptic receptor efficacy? Whereas the presynaptic forces acknowledge the simplicity of an arrangement that assigns both induction and expression mechanisms to the postsynaptic side of the synapse, they claim that the necessary communication between the two sides could be accomplished by a retrograde messenger, signalling to the presynaptic side that the conditions for the induction of LTP have been met postsynaptically. The identity of the putative retrograde messenger remains elusive. (In another theatre of the campaign, a truce has been declared; most combatants agree that presynaptic mechanisms contribute to the expression of LTP at the mossy fibre pathway in the hippocampus, which, incidentally, was the first non-NMDA receptor-dependent form of LTP to be found; Harris and Cotman 1986.)

The opposing armies have fought a long and toughminded trench war and their struggles have led to major advances in our conceptual understanding of synaptic function, as well as new techniques and experimental protocols of great power and elegance. Work *in vivo* was quickly supplemented by the development of the *in vitro* brain slice, allowing greater precision and control. Discoveries about glutamate receptors came along, stimulated by the development of new agonists and antagonists that were deployed to reveal the relative contributions of NMDA receptor-mediated and AMPA receptor-mediated currents to LTP induction and expression. Creativity emerged in paradoxical ways in laboratories around the world, as in the analytical studies by which a postsynaptic channel-blocking drug (MK-801) was deployed to monitor changes in presynaptic transmitter release in short- and long-term forms of potentiation. For theoretically exacting studies, extracellular population recordings gave way to paired-recording techniques between identified neurons—hard work but necessary work—and more recently, several groups have enthusiastically embraced the potential of optical recording techniques to provide vivid and compelling pictures of synaptic function at the level of the single synapse. Conceptual developments are many and complex, as the papers in this section reveal, and they have also included a degree of lateral thinking about quantal analysis and synaptic biophysics. One example was the realization that a reduction in the number of transmission failures, conventionally regarded as a presynaptic change, might actually be postsynaptic in origin at central synapses. As a result of the inside-out thinking about this and related issues emerged the rediscovery of the concept of the 'silent synapse'. In contemporary guise, this is a synapse at which transmitter is released, but that lacks AMPA receptors on the postsynaptic membrane.

Bliss and his colleagues have long taken the view that LTP has a presynaptic component. Errington *et al.* (Chapter 11) summarize their earlier *in vivo* measurements of LTP-associated increases in extracellular glutamate, and then describe results obtained with a new weapon in the presynaptic armoury, the glutamate dialysis electrode, which allows real-time estimates of glutamate concentration to be made. In Chapter 12, Hosokawa *et al.* describe the use of optical recording techniques to examine changes in network behaviour following the induction of LTP in hippocampal slices, while Choi *et al.* (in Chapter 13) discuss the concept of fusion pore release in relation to glutamate transmitter release and how this idea might help us to think about silent synapses in a different way. Prominent among the postsynaptic army, Malinow, in Chapter 14, outlines the mechanisms by which AMPA receptors might be trafficked to and from the receptor membrane, a process that he teasingly describes as 'AMPAfication'. Duprat *et al.* (Chapter 15) follow up by discussing aspects of the relevant molecular mechanisms, notably the binding of specific proteins to the C-terminus of AMPA receptor subunits. Nicoll, in Chapter 16, summarizes a large body of data from his laboratory that supports a postsynaptic view of LTP expression at Schaffer commissural synapses on CA1 cells. Kullmann provides a cautionary note in Chapter 17. The first to introduce the concept of the silent synapse into the debate about the locus of the expression of LTP, he presents a cogent argument that some pieces of the jigsaw puzzle remain to be put in place.

(d) Persistence

So far, the papers have described the ways in which synaptic plasticity is induced and how it is expressed. However, the descriptions reveal that these processes are highly dynamic. Ion fluxes through ligand- and voltage-gated channels stimulate a rich and complex array of signal transduction pathways and protein–protein interactions, including classical processes such as protein phosphorylation. Given that proteins turn over relatively rapidly, the longevity of LTP presents us with an enormous puzzle. How does the change persist?

For the present, we do not know the answer to this question. Indeed, we do not even know how long LTP itself can last. If it is to be accepted as a valid model of memory, then the mechanisms responsible for the expression of LTP must be capable of sustaining enhanced synaptic strength for long periods, perhaps as long as a lifetime. Abraham (see Chapter 18) has long been interested in this enigma and by tweaking the induction parameters has found a set of conditions in which LTP can be shown to last for at least a year in the rat. This is a remarkable finding, although it does not establish that LTP-like changes normally last as long as this. There may also be important regional differences in the persistence of LTP.

The other authors in this section discuss possible mechanisms and approaches by which the puzzle of persistence could be tackled. In Chapter 19, Harris *et al.* describe anatomical studies at the level of the light and electron microscope that have revealed protein synthesis-dependent changes in dendritic spines. Schuman and Murase (Chapter 20) make the case for cadherins and local protein synthesis. Eric Kandel has, throughout his long career, juggled his interest in the hippocampus with his pioneering studies of an invertebrate neural system, the abdominal ganglion of *Aplysia*. His chapter with Pittenger (Chapter 21) puts forward the argument that a route to learning more about the genetic mechanisms by which long-lasting synaptic change are regulated might best be approached in the marine animal first. There are various reasons why the apparently simpler range of, for example, transcriptional controls, may make this preparation desirable for a first analysis.

(e) Function

Most discussion of the possible functions of LTP has, since its discovery, focused on the part that its underlying mechanisms might play in laying down memory traces in the brain. This is by no means its only possible function, nor indeed should it be thought that there may not be other mechanisms at the brain's disposal for ensuring lasting changes as a consequence of neuronal activity. However, the synaptic plasticity and memory hypothesis has been widely discussed.

One of the pioneers in the field was Barnes (Chapter 22) who was among the first to establish that the temporal persistence of LTP covaried with the persistence of memory. Was this correlation an accident, or might it reflect a causal relationship? To establish such a possibility, it was essential to find ways of blocking or enhancing LTP in behaving animals and then investigating whether they showed corresponding changes in their ability to learn certain tasks or to remember information once acquired. The problem with doing such experiments is that LTP may have different functional attributes when it occurs in different networks and circuits in the brain. That is, what LTP does in the amygdala may be functionally different from what it does in the hippocampus. In Chapter 23, Morris *et al.* discuss this subject in the particular context of their attempt to develop a neurobiological theory of the hippocampus in which LTP plays a part.

One of the exciting new developments of recent years in neuroscience has been the marriage of techniques across many different levels of analysis. This is particularly clear in the use of transgenic animals in behavioural studies. A molecular intervention is made—be it the overexpression or deletion of a gene—and the consequences of this intervention are examined at the highest level of analysis, namely that of behaviour. S. Tonegawa was a pioneer in this field and he and his colleagues describe his recent development of regional-specific alterations of the NMDA receptor and second-messenger transduction cascades and their impact on LTP, learning and the behaviour of neural ensembles (Chapter 24). In a similar vein, Hédou and Mansuy in Chapter 25, examine the consequences of inducible inactivation of protein phosphatases on LTP and behaviour, while Bozon *et al.* (Chapter 26) use transgenic and more traditional techniques to examine the relationship between gene expression, early and late LTP and short- and long-term memory.

(f) New directions

There may be a tendency for those outside the immediate field to suppose that research on LTP remains locked within the hippocampus, the brain area in which it was discovered. Not so. Part of what is exciting and invigorating about LTP is that the field is constantly expanding into new areas. The final four papers in the issue highlight examples of some new approaches. In Chapter 27, Thomas and Malenka discuss activity-dependent changes in the striatum, notably those induced by drugs of abuse that occlude the subsequent induction of striatal LTP. Demonstrating occlusion is a classic way of establishing commonality of underlying mechanisms—raising the intriguing and important possibility that the neurobiology of LTP could shed light on why drugs of abuse are so rewarding. Rowan *et al.* (Chapter 28) take us into the domain of animal models of Alzheimer's disease and discuss a range of different approaches—pharmacological and transgenic—that have revealed striking alterations in fast synaptic transmission and LTP in these models.

In the closing chapter, Lisman takes on the ambitious task of attempting to tie things together. In his comprehensive overview and synthesis of the molecular mechanisms underlying the expression of LTP he finds room for both presynaptic and postsynaptic components, bringing this anniversary volume to a consensual and harmonious conclusion.

Tim V. P. Bliss, London, UK
Graham L. Collingridge, Bristol, UK
Richard G. M. Morris, Edinburgh, UK

References

Barrionuevo, G., Shottler, F., and Lynch, G. (1980). The effects of repetitive low-frequency stimulation on control and 'potentiated' synaptic responses in the hippocampus. *Life Sci* **27**, 2385–91.

Bienenstock, E. L., Cooper, L. N., and Munro, P. W. (1982). Theory for the development of neuron selectivity: orientation specificity and binocular interaction in visual cortex. *J. Neurosci.* **2**, 32–48.

Bliss, T. V. P. and Gardner-Medwin, A. R. (1973). Long-lasting potentiation of synaptic transmission in the dentate area of the unanaesthetized rabbit following stimulation of the perforant path. *J. Physiol. (Lond.)* **232**, 357–74.

Bliss, T. V. P. and Lømo, T. (1973). Long-lasting potentiation of synaptic transmission in the dentate area of the anaesthetized rabbit following stimulation of the perforant path. *J. Physiol. (Lond.)* **232**, 331–56.

Bliss, T. V. P. and Lynch, M. A. (1988). Long-term potentiation of synaptic transmission in the hippocampus: properties and mechanisms. In *Long-term potentiation in the hippocampus: from biophysics to behavior* (ed. P. W. Landfield and S. A. Deadwyler), pp. 3–72. New York: Alan R. Liss.

Harris, E. W. and Cotman, C. W. (1986). Long-term potentiation of guinea pig mossy fiber responses is not blocked by *N*-methyl D-aspartate antagonists. *Neurosci. Lett.* **70**, 32–137.

Hebb, D. O. (1949). *The organization of behavior*. New York: Wiley.

Ito, M. and Kano, M. (1982). Long-lasting depression of parallel fiber–Purkinje cell transmission induced by conjunctive stimulation of parallel fibers and climbing fibers in the cerebellar cortex. *Neurosci. Lett.* **33**, 253–8.

Lømo, T. (1966). Frequency potentiation of excitatory synaptic activity in the dentate area of the hippocampal formation. *Acta. Physiol. Scand.* **68**, 128.

Lynch, G. (2003). Long-term potentiation in the Eocene. *Phil. Trans. R. Soc. Lond.* B **358**, 625–8. (DOI 10.1098/rstb. 2002.1253).

History

1

A prelude to long-term potentiation

Per Andersen

Searching for premonitory studies of hippocampal long-term potentiation (LTP), there is a paucity of data. While synaptic enhancement during repetitive activation was studied in several reports from many groups between 1955 and 1967, the reported after-effects were short, at the most lasting a few minutes. Responses lasting for more than 1 hour were not reported until 1973.

Keywords: long-term potentiation; synaptic plasticity; hippocampus; augmentation

1.1 A promising candidate

LTP is a highly popular topic in neuroscience research. The great interest is generated by its properties, making it a useful candidate for cellular processes supporting learning behaviour. From the outset of this research in the 1960s, the most interesting features were the enhanced synaptic efficiency and the long duration. Later discoveries were even more important, namely showing cooperativity between activated afferent fibres and associativity, meaning respectively that synaptic enhancement requires coactivation of a certain number of fibres, and that an efficient synaptic input leads to the improvement of a weaker input, provided it is activated in concert with the stronger one.

After two preliminary reports (Lømo 1966; Bliss and Lømo 1970), the LTP saga was initiated in earnest by two well-known reports in *The Journal of Physiology* in 1973 (Bliss and Gardner-Medwin 1973; Bliss and Lømo 1973). In many fields of science, a major advance is often preceded by a distinct period of ferment in which the ideas of several people gradually develop, often in a competitive interchange between several scientists. When a perceived advance is made, it is often triggered by a new approach or an improved technique. Were there such premonitions before the LTP discovery? In my view, there was surprisingly little such gradual build-up in the field of hippocampal synaptic plasticity. Nevertheless, it may be of interest to examine some of the efforts to provide examples of simple cellular models for learning that circulated among neurophysiologists and which, to some extent, may have influenced the LTP discovery.

1.2 Classes of models

For more than 100 years, neuroscientists have been interested in the relation between nerve cells and their connectivity on one hand and cognitive abilities on the other. In an influential review, Kandel and Spencer (1968) distinguished between neural concomitants of learning (where the experimenter uses near-physiological inputs and outputs) and neural analogues of learning (results acquired with greatly simplified preparations). Did such ideas influence the scientists who were working in this field before 1973? To me, the answer seems obvious.

With its peculiar histological arrangement and high amplitude sinusoidal electro-encephalographic signature (Jung and Kornmüller 1938), the hippocampus was seen as an interesting substrate for a search for basic cellular and synaptic analogues of learning. In particular, neuroscientists were looking for examples of long-lasting increases in synaptic transmission. Attempts to relate such activity to clinical memory studies came considerably later.

1.3 Facilitated synaptic transmission

Activity-dependent changes of synaptic responses come in several forms. These appear to be common to virtually all excitatory synapses, and have been particularly well studied by Magleby and Zengel (1975, 1976, 1982). After a single synaptic activation, excitatory synapses remain in a state that allows the synapse to release more trans-mitter for a period, peaking at around 10–20 ms and lasting for a few hundred milliseconds, a process called facilitation (Feng 1941). When the synapse is activated repeatedly, there is a marked enhancement of synaptic responses during, and for a few seconds after, the stimulating tetanus, a process Magleby called augmentation. Fol-lowing a period of sufficiently high-frequency synaptic stimulation, the system remains in a state with increased transmitter release for several minutes, called post-tetanic potentiation (PTP) (Feng 1941). Finally, at many excitatory synapses, perhaps mostly in the cortical tissue, a period of high-frequency synaptic activation is followed by an increased synaptic transmission efficiency, LTP. In the first analysis of this phenomenon, an event of 30 years ago, which is the reason for the present set of articles, Bliss and Lømo (1973) called the phenomenon long-lasting potentiation. A few years later, Douglas and Goddard (1975) proposed the name long-term potentiation, which has been generally accepted, perhaps because of its easily pronounced acronym. While both facilitation (Katz and Miledi 1968), augmentation and PTP (Magleby and Zengel 1982) are due to presynaptic increased calcium levels after the activation, LTP is probably more complex, employing a set of both pre- and postsynaptic processes each with a different time profile. First, during the first 20–40 min, there is a gradual decline of response amplitude, called short-term potentiation, followed by a seemingly steady state, the LTP proper. The latter is split into two parts, an early, around 3 h long form and a later process, many hours long, the latter requiring new protein synthesis.

1.4 Post-tetanic potentiation as a candidate for learning processes

Lloyd (1949) reported that PTP of monosynaptic spinal reflexes could last up to 7 min. Eccles (1953) proposed that spinal cord synapses could be 'capable of "learning" to operate more effectively' through PTP, in particular if they were in a disused state before the activation. Spencer and Wigdor (1965) and Beswick and Conroy (1965) both reported PTP durations in spinal reflex pathways lasting for several hours, but the tetanizing frequency and duration were far outside the range normally encountered. In a thalamo-cortical-bulbar pathway, Amassian and Weiner (1966) observed much larger

PTP mediated through cortical involvement than at spinal levels, but the duration was only 2.5 min. PTP is present in all hippocampal synapses tested, but it does not last for more than around 5 min after tetani of 100 Hz lasting for a few seconds.

In conclusion, in order to play a part in physiological mechanisms of learning, PTP is too short lasting to be a serious candidate.

1.5 Feeble premonitions of the LTP phenomenon

Were there any premonitions for the LTP discovery? The unusually large amplitude and synchronous appearance of the theta activity made several researchers feel that this transitory state might be correlated to a change in the state of the participating synapses. Several groups, therefore, studied the hippocampus, first with electroencephalographic techniques, later by recording signals evoked by stimulation of various afferent stations. Thus, Green and Arduini (1954) reported that the large theta waves were associated with phasic discharges of single hippocampal neurons. Green and Adey (1956) also recorded theta waves and felt they were changing in amplitude during learning. However, the relation between the large synchronous theta waves and the hippocampal function was difficult to analyse.

1.6 Augmentation responses

By contrast, the tremendously enhanced signals observed during periods of repetitive stimulation impressed researchers as a case of plasticity not easily matched by other nervous regions. In particular, many research groups were impressed by the augmentation process occurring during repetitive stimulation of afferent fibres to hippocampal neurons. The first to report this phenomenon were Cragg and Hamlyn (1955) who noted the strongly enhanced responses of CA1 neurons in anaesthetized rabbits to stimulation of stratum radiatum fibres at 5–30 Hz. They used the term facilitation for the phenomenon. They were also the first to distinguish between the presynaptic volley and the subsequent post-synaptic wave (fEPSP) and reported that the postsynaptic wave was the only wave to potentiate during the repetitive activation. Significantly, they did not report any activity to outlast the tetanic stimulation.

In a paper 2 years later Cragg and Hamlyn (1957) again reported on prominent augmentation effects and surmised that 'The facilitation at low repetition rates may well be a property peculiar to large interconnected assemblies of neurons'. However, they did not report any effects after the tetanic stimulation.

1.7 Effects following the augmentation

Several other groups subsequently noted remarkable augmentation in many dentate or hippocampal synapses. A number of these authors also found that the enhanced synaptic responses outlasted the tetanic period. Green and Adey (1956) noted that 'prolonged bursts would sometimes potentiate for several minutes', while Gloor et al. (1964) reported after-effects but only for a few seconds. Andersen (1960a,b) also

observed the augmentation, which he called frequency potentiation, during the tetanization. Following the tetani there were enhanced synaptic responses for 6 min in both
the Schaffer collateral/CA1 synapses and commissural/CA3 synapses. In the septo-
hippocampal system, the post-augmentation potentiation lasted up to 3 min (Andersen
et al. 1961). By contrast, following entorhinal activation of dentate granule cells, the
post-augmentation potentiated state only lasted 30 s, possibly because of the barbi-
turate anaesthesia used (Andersen et al. 1966). In their pioneering work on prepiriform
cortical slices, Yamamoto and McIlwain (1966) reported that stimulation of the
olfactory tract at 100 Hz for 10 s was followed by enhanced N-waves (fEPSPs) for
0.5–3 min, interpreted as PTP.

All of these groups were aware of the possible significance of the reported phase with
enhanced synaptic responses following a period with intense activation. However, we
all felt that the duration was not sufficiently long for these post-augmentation
changes by themselves to form a realistic mechanism for learning changes. However, in
cooperation with other processes they could be thought to play a part. For example,
Andersen and Lømo (1967; report from a symposium in 1965) characterized the progressively slower decay of post-augmentation potentiated CA1 responses to commissural stimulation: 'an example of a primitive synaptic learning'. Later, they proposed
'It appears, therefore, likely that the frequency potentiation (=augmentation) of cortical synaptic activity may be a factor involved in the establishment of neuronal circuits
of synaptic facilitated synaptic transfer as one might envisage happening during a
learning process'.

1.8 LTP was a new actor on the scene

The meagre data on durable changes of hippocampal synaptic responses reported
before 1966 are reflected in Bliss and Lømo (1973), which only refers to the early
preliminary abstract by Lømo (1966). There is no reference to other authors using
repetitive stimulation. There were two new aspects to their approach: first, the much
longer duration of the post-tetanus synaptic enhancement and, second, their use of two
divisions of the perforant path, a control pathway distributed to a virgin territory of
the dentate gyrus next to the tetanized pathway. Thus, they could link the synaptic
changes to the tetanized input and, later, show that the control synapses were, indeed,
also able to undergo LTP changes. Finally, Bliss and Lømo clearly set the LTP
phenomenon in relation to learning processes. Referring to Douglas (1967) and Olds
(1972) who both reviewed hippocampal involvement in memory, they state
'synapses... influenced by activity which may have occurred several hours previously
...a time scale long enough to be potentially useful for information storage'. The
prelude was over, the concert had started.

References

Amassian, V. E. and Weiner, H. (1966). Monosynaptic and polysynaptic activation of pyramidal
    tract neurons by thalamic stimulation. In The thalamus (ed. D. P. Purpura and M. D. Yahr),
    pp. 256–82. New York: Columbia University Press.

Andersen, P. (1960a). Interhippocampal impulses. II. Apical dendritic activation of CA1 neurons. *Acta Physiol. Scand.* **48**, 178–208.

Andersen, P. (1960b). Interhippocampal impulses. III. Basal dendritic activation of CA3 neurons. *Acta Physiol. Scand.* **48**, 209–30.

Andersen, P. and Lømo, T. (1967). Control of hippocampal output by afferent volley frequency. *Prog. Brain Res.* **27**, 400–12.

Andersen, P., Bruland, H., and Kaada, B. R. (1961). Activation of the dentate area by septal stimulation. *Acta Physiol. Scand.* **51**, 17–28.

Andersen, P., Holmqvist, B., and Voorhoeve, P. E. (1966). Entorhinal activation of dentate granule cells. *Acta Physiol. Scand.* **66**, 448–60.

Beswick, F. G. and Conroy, R. T. W. L. (1965). Optimal tetanic conditioning of heteronymous monosynaptic reflexes. *J. Physiol. (Lond.)* **180**, 134–46.

Bliss, T. V. P. and Gardner-Medwin, A. R. (1973). Long-lasting potentiation of synaptic transmission in the dentate area of the unanaesthetized hippocampus following stimulation of the perforant path. *J. Physiol. (Lond.)* **232**, 357–74.

Bliss, T. V. P. and Lømo, T. (1970). Plasticity in a monosynaptic cortical pathway. *J. Physiol. (Lond.)* **207**, 61.

Bliss, T. V. P. and Lømo, T. (1973). Long-lasting potentiation of synaptic transmission in the dentate area of the anaesthetized rabbit following stimulation of the perforant path. *J. Physiol. (Lond.)* **232**, 331–56.

Cragg, B. G. and Hamlyn, L. H. (1955). Action potentials of the pyramidal neurons in the hippocampus of the rabbit. *J. Physiol. (Lond.)* **129**, 608–27.

Cragg, B. G. and Hamlyn, L. H. (1957). Some commissural and septal connexions of the hippocampus in the rabbit. A combined histological and electrical study. *J. Physiol. (Lond.)* **135**, 460–85.

Douglas, R. J. (1967). The hippocampus and behavior. *Psychol. Bull.* **67**, 416–42.

Douglas, R. M. and Goddard, G. V. (1975). Long-term potentiation of the perforant path–granule cell synapse in the rat hippocampus. *Brain Res.* **86**, 205–15.

Eccles, J. C. (1953). *The neurophysiological basis of mind.* Oxford University Press.

Feng, T. P. (1941). Studies on the neuromuscular junction. XXVI. The changes of the end-plate potential during and after prolonged stimulation. *Chin. J. Physiol.* **16**, 341–72.

Gloor, P., Vera, C. L., and Sperti, L. (1964). Electrophysiological studies of hippocampal neurons. III. Responses of hippocampal neurons to repetitive perforant path volleys. *Electroenceph. Clin. Neurophysiol.* **17**, 353–70.

Green, J. D. and Adey, W. R. (1956). Electrophysiological studies of hippocampal connections and excitability. *Electroenceph. Clin. Neurophysiol.* **8**, 245–62.

Green, J. D. and Arduini, A. A. (1954). Hippocampal electrical activity in arousal. *J. Neurophysiol.* **17**, 533–57.

Jung, R. and Kornmüller, A. E. (1938). Eine Methodik der Ableitung lokalisierter Potentialschwankungen aus subcorticalen Hirngebieten. *Arch. Psychiat. Nervenkrank.* **109**, 1–30.

Kandel, E. R. and Spencer, W. A. (1968). Cellular neurophysiological approaches in the study of learning. *Physiol. Rev.* **48**, 65–134.

Katz, B. and Miledi, R. (1968). The role of calcium in neuromuscular facilitation. *J. Physiol. (Lond.)* **195**, 481–92.

Lloyd, D. P. C. (1949). Post-tetanic potentiation of response to in monosynaptic reflex pathways of the spinal cord. *J. Gen. Physiol.* **33**, 147–70.

Lømo, T. (1966). Frequency potentiation of excitatory synaptic activity in the dentate area of the hippocampal formation. *Acta Physiol. Scand.* **68**(Suppl. 277), 128.

Magleby, K. L. and Zengel, J. E. (1975). A dual effect of repetitive stimulation on post-tetanic potentiation of transmitter release at the frog neuromuscular junction. *J. Physiol. (Lond.)* **245**, 163–82.

Magleby, K. L. and Zengel, J. E. (1976). Augmentation: a process that acts to increase transmitter release at the frog neuromuscular junction. *J. Physiol. (Lond.)* **257**, 449–70.

Magleby, K. L. and Zengel, J. E. (1982). A quantitative description of stimulation-induced changes in transmitter release at the frog neuromuscular junction. *J. Gen. Physiol.* **80**, 613–38.

Olds, J. (1972). Learning and the hippocampus. *Rev. Can. Biol.* **31**(Suppl.), 215–38.

Spencer, W. A. and Wigdor, R. (1965). Ultra-late PTP of monosynaptic reflex responses in the cat. *Physiologist* **8**, 278.

Yamamoto, C. and McIlwain, H. (1966). Electrical activities in thin sections from the mammalian brain maintained in chemically-defined media *in vitro*. *J. Neurochem.* **13**, 1333–43.

Glossary

fEPSP   field excitatory postsynaptic potential
LTP   long-term potentiation
PTP   post-tetanic potentiation

2

The discovery of long-term potentiation

Terje Lømo

This paper describes circumstances around the discovery of long-term potentiation (LTP). In 1966, I had just begun independent work for the degree of *Dr medicinae* (PhD) in Per Andersen's laboratory in Oslo after an eighteen-month apprenticeship with him. Studying the effects of activating the perforant path to dentate granule cells in the hippocampus of anaesthetized rabbits, I observed that brief trains of stimuli resulted in increased efficiency of transmission at the perforant path-granule cell synapses that could last for hours. In 1968, Tim Bliss came to Per Andersen's laboratory to learn about the hippocampus and field potential recording for studies of possible memory mechanisms. The two of us then followed up my preliminary results from 1966 and did the experiments that resulted in a paper that is now properly considered to be the basic reference for the discovery of LTP.

Keywords: long-term potentiation; hippocampus; history of long-term potentiation; memory mechanisms

The discovery of LTP, as far as I am concerned, began in 1964. I was a doctor in the Norwegian Navy on leave to look for a job, when, by pure chance, I met Per Andersen in a street in Oslo. Per had recently returned from John Eccles' laboratory in Australia and was looking for people to work in his laboratory. Without that meeting, I would almost certainly not have ended up in neuroscience. As it was, I joined Per's laboratory in August 1964. Before then, I had spent a year at The Institute of Physiology in Pisa, Italy (1958–1959) and was therefore not completely naive in matters of research (Lømo and Mollica 1962).

I worked closely with Per for over a year, learning all that I needed to know to begin my own studies for a PhD (Dr medicinae) in his laboratory at the end of 1965. In those days, a PhD was expected to reflect essentially completely independent work and this suited me well. I needed to know that I could get along on my own. In 1969, I defended my thesis entitled 'Synaptic mechanisms and organization in the dentate area of the hippocampal formation', based on four single-author papers. The four papers were submitted to the journal *Experimental Brain Research* and two were published there (Lømo 1971*a,b*). The other two remain in my files unrevised and unrevisited. Because I believe that these papers still contain original and interesting observations, I want to modify them for eventual re-submission. They deal mainly with the longitudinal spread of excitation and inhibition on either side of a narrow transverse beam of excitation of dentate granule cells in the living animal. Subsequently, the *in vitro* transverse slice preparation conquered the field and, not many similar studies have been done.

Per and I agreed that my thesis should focus on 'frequency potentiation', a marked increase in neuronal firing that occurs during repetitive stimulation of axonal inputs. Frequency potentiation had already been described by Per in the perforant path input to the dentate area as a process 'requiring several seconds of tetanic stimulation to make itself manifest (and) conversely, after cessation of the tetanus, as a state of increased excitability of the granule cells lasting several seconds, sometimes for as long as half a minute' (Andersen *et al*. 1966, p. 457).

I began by recording field potentials in dendritic and cell body layers of the dentate area during repetitive stimulation of the perforant path and was impressed not only by the recruitment of cell discharges but also by the marked direct current shifts of different polarities that occurred in different layers. Soon, I also began looking for after-effects of repetitive stimulation, which were generally reported as short lasting (minutes) and akin to PTP (Green and Adey 1956; Gloor *et al*. 1964). PTP lasting hours was observed in the spinal cord but only after prolonged, high-frequency stimulation. Eccles (1964) and Kandel and Spencer (1968) discussed such after-effects as expressions of synaptic plasticity but not as possible mechanisms of learning (Eccles 1964; Kandel and Spencer 1968). Thus, Eccles writes: 'Perhaps the most unsatisfactory feature of the attempt to explain the phenomena of learning and conditioning by the demonstrated changes in synaptic efficacy is that long periods of excess use or disuse are required in order to produce detectable synaptic change', p. 260.

I presented my findings in Åbo (Turku, Finland) in August 1966 at a meeting of the Scandinavian Physiological Society (Lømo 1966). Figure 2.1 is a copy of the only slide that I still have and can remember that I presented at that meeting. Figure 2.1a shows recordings from the granule cell body layer during trains of stimuli at 12 Hz to the perforant path. The marked increase in amplitude and number of population spikes during each train is typical of frequency potentiation. In this experiment, trains of 120 pulses were delivered every 7 min except for the last two trains, which were separated by 22 min. For each new train, the second and third population spike in each discharge appeared earlier and earlier in the train (Fig. 2.1a,b). In addition, the amplitude of the monosynaptic first spike increased rapidly to a new maintained potentiated level, while its latency decreased progressively to a new and apparently stable low level (Fig. 2.1c).

Per and I were excited by these findings. In a paper prepared for a meeting in 1965 (but published in 1967) Per (with me as co-author) discussed a 'possible relationship between frequency potentiation and learning processes' in the following terms: '... the increase in EPSPs denoting an enhanced efficiency of synaptic transmission outlasts the stimulation by a certain period, from several seconds up to a few minutes. This duration is of the same order of magnitude as that of the post-tetanic potentiation. It is too short to account for the plastic changes in a neuronal circuit that might take place in learning processes of a higher kind. However, if frequency potentiation takes place in a set of neurons constituting a polysynaptic chain, the individual effects may be greatly enhanced...' (Andersen and Lømo 1967, p. 410).

By results such as those shown in Fig. 2.1, a possible relationship between frequency potentiation, its after-effects, and learning processes suddenly appeared much more likely. Further evidence that we thought so at the time is provided by Tim Bliss, who recollects that when he approached Per in the winter of 1967–1968 about coming to Oslo to learn about the hippocampus and field potential recording because of his continuing interest in the neural basis of learning and the conviction that he needed to work on a simpler brain structure, Per said something like 'well in that case you must come to Oslo and see what Terje Lømo has found' (T. Bliss, personal communication).

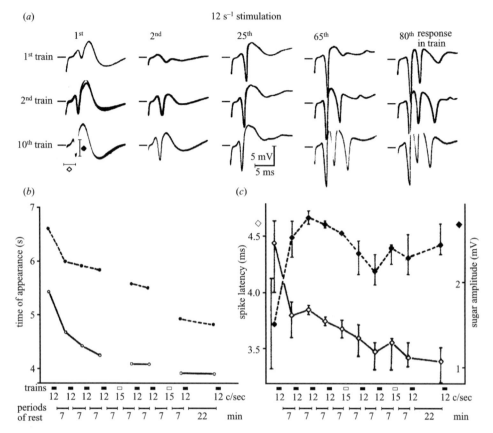

Fig. 2.1 Long-lasting increases in efficiency of transmission at synapses on dentate granule cells induced by repetitive trains of stimuli to the perforant path in anaesthetized rabbits. (*a*) Typical records of population spikes from the granule cell body layer during trains of stimuli at 12 Hz, each train lasting 10 s and repeated as indicated along the abscissa in (*b*) and (*c*). As the trains were repeated, a second and third population spike appeared earlier and earlier in each train ((*a*) and (*b*)). In addition, long-lasting decreases in latency and increases in amplitude appeared in the population spike evoked by single test stimuli before each train (*c*). In (*b*) dashed line, time of appearance of two spikes; solid line, time of appearance of three spikes. In (*c*) dashed line, spike amplitude (single volley); solid line, spike latency (single volley).

   Why did I not pursue and publish a fuller account of my findings in 1966? Because I was overcome by the complexity of the system and my lack of understanding of what was behind the findings. There was also no sense of urgency. Thus, when Tim and I published a full account in 1973 (Bliss and Lømo 1973), it still took years for the significance of the findings to be generally appreciated. To understand the system better, I therefore switched from studying frequency potentiation and its after-effects to studying single and paired pulse activation of orthodromic and antidromic inputs to the dentate area in combination with field potential and some intracellular recordings. This last work resulted in a relatively detailed description of the time-courses and spatial distributions of activity-induced excitability changes in the dentate area, which

I presented in the thesis that I defended in October 1969 just before I left to do postdoctoral work for one and half years at the Department of Biophysics, University College London. The study of frequency potentiation, which started me off, produced a fair amount of data, some of which I could probably recover but hardly publish today. With respect to the long-term after-effects of frequency potentiation, however, the arrival of Tim Bliss in Oslo in the autumn of 1968 made all the difference. Furthermore, by that time, I had acquired the experience and insight into the system that I felt was required.

When Tim arrived, we decided to carry out experiments together once a week on 'my' set-up to follow up on the findings presented in Åbo in 1966. The first experiment was immensely exciting. As shown in Fig. 2.2, each train of stimuli to the perforant path (tetanus at time of arrows) resulted in a progressive increase in the amplitude of the population spike of discharging granule cells on the tetanized side. By contrast, on the opposite control side, no potentiation occurred until that side was similarly tetanized at the end of the experiment late at night.

We then refined various technical aspects and did our last experiment in September 1969 before we both moved to London. The results, as mentioned, appeared in the *Journal of Physiology* in 1973. The reasons for the delay in publication are many. Again, the sense of urgency was nothing like what it would have been today. The time to think things over was longer then, which seemed to be confirmed by the relative lack

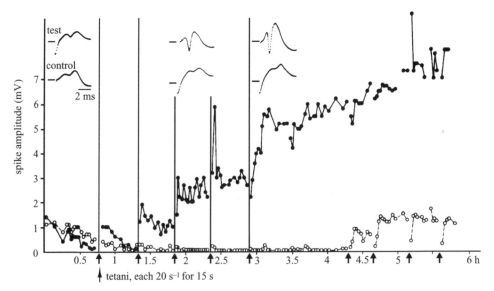

Fig. 2.2 Long-lasting increases in efficiency of transmission at synapses on dentate granule cells induced by repetitive trains of stimuli to the perforant path in anaesthetized rabbits. Insets show responses in the granule cell body layer to single test stimuli to the perforant path at times corresponding to their positions along the abscissa. Trains of stimuli at 20 Hz for 15 s were applied (arrows), first on one side (five trains) then on the opposite side (four trains). The trains caused an increase in the amplitude (and a decrease in the latency) of the population without affecting the contralateral control side. Furthermore, the changes persisted for the duration of the acute experiment.

of enthusiasm expressed by most people upon hearing the results. John Eccles was an exception. He became very interested when he saw the results during a visit to Oslo in 1968–1969 and presented variations of Fig. 2.2, which we never published, in several of his later books. There was also much analysis to be done, some of which had to await my return to Oslo in 1971, where the records were.

An intriguing but unanswerable question, of course, is if not me, then who would have discovered the long-lasting after-effects described above and when would that have happened? Certainly, Per Andersen set the scene for it all and appreciated its significance as a potential memory mechanism early. He has also been remarkably supportive in projecting me as the 'discoverer' of LTP from the beginning. Tim Bliss came to Oslo with the explicit aim of learning the hippocampus and studying potential memory mechanisms in a simpler cortical preparation than the one he had used in Montreal and London (Bliss *et al.* 1968). Thus, in the introduction to Bliss *et al.* (1968) it is made very clear that the intention of the work is to look for long-lasting facilitation of cortical synapses that might underlie learning. Without Tim's arrival in Oslo it is not clear when, if at all, I, or Per, would have followed up the findings reported in Åbo in 1966. As for me, it was certainly not prior interest in possible memory mechanisms that led me to a discovery that was in some ways accidental and in other ways the result of an intuition that has often, I feel, brought me to look for or see phenomena that turn out to be new and interesting.

I find it remarkable that the abstract from the Åbo meeting is sometimes cited for the discovery of LTP. This would hardly have happened, had not the introduction to Bliss and Lømo (1973) started 'These experiments arose from an observation made during a study of the phenomenon of frequency potentiation in the dentate area of the hippocampal formation' (Lømo 1966, p. 128). From the literature, it is clear that the phenomenon that I presented in 1966 represented something entirely new. It led directly to Bliss and Lømo (1973), of which Roger Nicoll has said: 'Why did this paper start this dramatic field? First of all, it describes all of the basic phenomena of the process of long-term potentiation. These include pathway specificity, saturation, and an increase in the coupling of the synaptic potential to the discharge of the granule cells. Second, there's not a single controversial result in that paper—a very remarkable thing in this field' (Bliss and Lømo 1995, p. 61).

Why did I not continue studying LTP? In fact, I did, first with Tim in London and then, after London, with Tony Gardner-Medwin in 1971–1972 in Oslo. However, we all failed in bringing the highly variable *in vivo* or *in vitro* preparations under such experimental control that we could fruitfully address underlying mechanisms. Tim left the LTP field for a time, while I returned to and then stayed with the nerve–muscle preparation that had given such wonderful and unexpected results in London.

Up until 1972 it was generally thought that motor neurons controlled the properties of skeletal muscle fibres outside the neuromuscular junctions by nerve-derived trophic factors that acted independently of impulse activity. According to Eccles (1964), the evidence for such factors was even conclusive. However, when we showed that direct muscle stimulation restored normal properties in denervated muscle with regard to acetylcholine sensitivity and resting membrane potential and mimicked the effects of cross-reinnervation on contractile speed, that view was turned upside down (Lømo and Rosenthal 1972; Lømo *et al.* 1974). Moreover, in the early 1970s, these results attracted much greater interest than LTP.

Do I regret that I left the LTP field? Not at all. For me, gaining new insights into how motor neurons set up neuromuscular junctions and control muscle cell phenotype has the same intrinsic value as similar work in other systems and excites me just as much. I like discovering new land, as occurred in the experiments on muscle referred to above or most recently when Gabriela Bezakova discovered that denervation caused wholesale changes in cytoskeletal organization that could be restored to normal by electrical muscle stimulation or external application of muscle agrin (Bezakova and Lømo 2001). These findings lead to new ideas about the function of muscle agrin, so far unknown, and how muscle activity controls the cytoskeleton to allow muscle fibres to handle the mechanical forces they generate or become exposed to.

The interest and activity created by the discovery of LTP has been amazing. I have been lucky to have played a small part and to live at a time where the opportunities for discovering new land in biology appear boundless.

References

Andersen, P. and Lømo, T. (1967). Control of hippocampal output by afferent volley frequency. *Prog. Brain Res.* **27**, 400–12.

Andersen, P., Holmqvist, B., and Voorhoeve, P. E. (1966). Entorhinal activation of dentate granule cells. *Acta Physiol. Scand.* **66**, 448–60.

Bezakova, G. and Lømo, T. (2001). Muscle activity and muscle agrin regulate the organization of cytoskeletal proteins and attached acetylcholine receptor (AChR) aggregates in skeletal muscle fibers. *J. Cell Biol.* **153**, 1453–63.

Bliss, T. and Lømo, T. (1973). Long-lasting potentiation of synaptic transmission in the dentate area of the anaesthetized rabbit following stimulation of the perforant path. *J. Physiol. (Lond.)* **232**, 331–56.

Bliss, T. V. P. and Lømo, T. (1995). Landmarks: long-lasting potentiation of synaptic transmission in the dentate area of the anaesthetized rabbit following stimulation of the perforant path. *J. NIH Res.* **7**, 59–67. Reprinted from *J. Physiol.* **232**, 991 (1979).

Bliss, T. V. P., Burns, B. D., and Uttley, A. M. (1968). Factors affecting the conductivity of pathways in the cerebral cortex. *J. Physiol. (Lond.)* **195**, 339–67.

Eccles, J. C. (1964). *The physiology of synapses.* Berlin: Springer.

Gloor, P., Vera, C. L., and Sperti, L. (1964). Electrophysiological studies of hippocampal neurons. III. Responses of hippocampal neurons to repetitive perforant path volleys. *Electrencephal. Clin. Neurophysiol.* **17**, 353–70.

Green, J. D. and Adey, W. R. (1956). Electrophysiological studies of hippocampal connections and excitability. *Electrencephal. Clin. Neurophysiol.* **8**, 245–62.

Kandel, E. R. and Spencer, W. A. (1968). Cellular neurophysiological approaches in the study of learning. *Physiol. Rev.* **48**, 65–34.

Lømo, T. (1966). Frequency potentiation of excitatory synaptic activity in the dentate area of the hippocampal formation. *Acta Physiol. Scand.* **68**(Suppl. 277), 128.

Lømo, T. (1971a). Patterns of activation in a monosynaptic cortical pathway: the perforant path input to the dentate area of the hippocampal formation. *Exp. Brain Res.* **12**, 18–45.

Lømo, T. (1971b). Potentiation of monosynaptic EPSPs in the perforant path–dentate granule cell synapse. *Exp. Brain Res.* **12**, 46–63.

Lømo, T. and Mollica, A. (1962). Activity of single units in primary optic cortex of the unanaesthetized rabbit during visual, auditory, olfactory and painful stimulation. *Arch. Ital. Biol.* **100**, 86–20.

Lømo, T. and Rosenthal, J. (1972). Control of ACh sensitivity by muscle activity in the rat. *J. Physiol. (Lond.)* **221**, 493–13.

Lømo, T., Westgaard, R. H., and Dahl, H. A. (1974). Contractile properties of muscle: control by pattern of muscle activity in the rat. *Proc. R. Soc. Lond.* B **187**, 99–103.

Glossary

LTP   long-term potentiation
PTP   post-tetanic potentiation

3

A journey from neocortex to hippocampus

T. V. P. Bliss

In the mid-1960s, it was generally agreed that the engram, the neural trace of previously experienced events, must be encoded by Hebb-like neurons in which synaptic efficacy could be modified by activity. Here, I describe my attempts as a PhD student at McGill University, Montreal, to find rules governing cortical plasticity in the neocortex, and having failed, why the hippocampus seemed to offer a far better prospect.

Keywords: neocortex to hippocampus; long-term potentiation; synaptic plasticity; Hebb; learning; memory

Sometime in the autumn of 1963 I went to see Ben Delisle Burns, then a professor in the Physiology Department at McGill University, Montreal, where I had taken my undergraduate degree, to talk about doing a PhD with him. 'There is one topic in which I am so passionately interested' said Burns, 'that if you come to my laboratory that is what I shall want you to work on'. His passionate interest—the neural basis of memory—was mine also. I signed up.

When I began my research in 1964, it was—then as now—widely, if not quite universally, assumed that the neural substrate of memory resided in the putative ability of cortical synapses to undergo long-term changes in efficacy as a result of particular patterns of activity. The synaptic theory of memory goes back at least as far as Cajal and Tanzi in the early part of the twentieth century, and is hinted at in the work of the nineteenth century psychologist William James. The first objective in the campaign to understand memory at the neural level was thus to identify synapses with the ability to sustain activity-dependent changes in efficacy for prolonged periods of time—in the limit, for the rest of the organism's life. David Lloyd in the 1940s (Lloyd 1949) and John Eccles in the early 1950s (Eccles and McIntyre 1953) had studied PTP in monosynaptic spinal pathways as a model for cortical plasticity, but by the early 1960s enthusiasm for PTP had waned; its time-course was simply too rapid to be useful. Burns expressed this disenchantment for existing models in his book on the properties of cortical ensembles published in 1958:

> Those mechanisms of synaptic facilitation which have been offered as candidates for an explanation of memory... have all proved disappointing.
>
> (Burns 1958, p. 96)

The mechanisms that Burns had in mind were PTP and reverberatory activity in self-re-exciting networks, a mechanism championed by Lorente de No in the 1930s and 1940s (Lorente de No 1939). The former was inherently too brief, and the latter was functionally too fragile to persist indefinitely.

The general frustration was echoed by Eccles a few years later at a meeting I shall return to below:

> Unfortunately, it has not been possible to demonstrate experimentally that excess use produces prolonged changes in synaptic efficacy.
>
> (Eccles 1966, p. 330)

Neurophysiologists have the option of turning to model neurons when the real things fail to please. Burns formulated a neural model of Pavlovian conditioning in which two cells A and B, A carrying the signal from the conditioned stimulus, and B the signal from the unconditioned stimulus, converged on a motor output cell M. Burns realized, like Konorski before him (Konorski 1948), that for conditioning to occur, the synaptic efficacy between B and M must be increased as a result of A and B being co-active. Sadly, he concluded, there was no evidence for 'such a peculiar property' (Burns 1958). Burns refers to his McGill colleague Hebb from time to time, but does not specifically mention his now famous 'neurophysiological hypothesis' (Hebb 1949):

> *When an axon of cell A is near enough to excite a cell B and repeatedly or persistently takes part in firing it, some growth process or metabolic change takes place in one or both cells such that A's efficiency, as one of the cells firing B, is increased.*[1], p. 62

It is strange now, writing at a time when Hebb's postulate must be the most quoted sentence in the literature of neuroscience, its only rival being Sherrington's magical metaphor of the brain as 'an enchanted loom where millions of flashing shuttles weave a dissolving pattern, always a meaningful pattern though never an abiding one',[2] to realise that neither Burns nor Eccles paid much attention to the neurophysiological postulate. Both, it is true, include Hebb with Ramon y Cajal, Tanzi and Konorski as among those who had identified activity-dependent changes at the synapse as the probable neural basis for memory. But for Burns and Eccles, the 'Hebb' synapse was little more than a self-evident conceptual embodiment of PTP, which Eccles and Lloyd had studied in spinal reflexes. The problem with PTP was that, except in pathological conditions involving a period of sensory deprivation by cutting the dorsal root, its duration was hopelessly inadequate for memory functions. In fact, Hebb's postulate is a good deal subtler than a simple restatement of homosynaptic potentiation. The artful phrase 'fires or takes part in firing' allows an input to share in the effect produced by another input, and thus endows his rule with the important property of associativity. It is nevertheless odd that Hebb did not draw this specific conclusion, extending his model to three neurons, as Burns was to do a few years later.

So it was obvious, by the time I started my PhD with Burns in 1964, that while spinal cord pathways may have been easy to isolate, they did not contain the stuff of which memories are made. There seemed no option but to look for electrophysiological evidence for synaptic plasticity in the brain itself, despite the then unfathomed neural tangle of cortical networks. Burns taught me how to record from single units in undercut slabs of cortical tissue in the intact cat, a preparation he had developed with the idea of reducing spontaneous activity, so that the firing of the recorded cell was more closely under the control of the experimenter. Test shocks were delivered to a stimulating electrode placed nearby in the isolated slab, and I took as a measure of the 'conductivity' of the pathway the probability of the test stimulus eliciting an action potential in the cell

I was recording from. My task was to see if I could produce long-lasting changes in conductivity by transient manipulations in the rate of stimulation. In some experiments, I had a second electrode, which allowed me to look for heterosynaptic effects. We were joined in the analysis of these experiments by the physicist Albert Uttley in whose division at the National Physical Laboratory in Teddington, near London, Burns and I had carried out the first experiments, and the results were published in 1968 (Bliss et al. 1968). I find the paper, with its heavy formalism, almost unreadable today. Moreover, the variability of the results and the generally polysynaptic nature of the responses conspired to make it impossible to draw any general conclusion about the rules governing activity-dependent changes at single synapses. Most experiments in which homosynaptic activity was briefly increased revealed an apparently anti-Hebbian reduction in 'conductivity' for a few tens of minutes (the duration of the effect limited by the length of time it was possible to hold the cell). Heterosynaptic stimulation led in most cases to facilitation of the homosynaptic pathway. However, the main conclusion I reached after devoting nearly 3 years to this approach was that it was misguided. The preparation was too complex; it was essential to simplify.

During this period, Eric Kandel had given a sparkling talk at McGill about his work with Tauc on synaptic plasticity in the sea slug *Aplysia* (Kandel and Tauc 1965). An animal with a nervous system consisting of a few nerve cells, each one identifiable from animal to animal, and a limited and reproducible behavioural repertoire, provided one clearly profitable way to simplify. But, perhaps as the result of my conventional English education, I preferred to stick to my own class, and so continued to work on mammals. It was while writing my thesis that I came across a book that would lead me in the direction of the hippocampus. In 1964 a conference on 'Brain and conscious experience' had been held, improbably, at the Vatican. The organizer was Sir John Eccles, who had won the Nobel Prize the year before, and who had long had an interest in the neural basis of memory. Among the speakers was Per Andersen, who had recently returned to Oslo after postdoctoral studies in Eccles' laboratory in Canberra, and who had steered Eccles towards the hippocampus, the detailed neural organization of which had been illuminated by the beautiful work of the Oslo school of neuroanatomists. In his chapter on memory in the proceedings of the Vatican conference—the book I had found in the library at McGill—Eccles speculated on what it was about cortical synapses (the presumptive neural seat of memory) that made them (again, presumably) more plastic than spinal cord synapses (Eccles 1966). He drew attention to the spine apparatus, found in or at the base of spines on neocortical and hippocampal pyramidal cells, and quoted a speculation of Hamlyn's (1963) that these structures, more prevalent in pyramidal cells of the hippocampus and neocortex than in spinal neurones, might contribute to the cellular machinery of memory. But it was Andersen's chapter (Andersen 1966) that made the greatest impact. He emphasized the relative simplicity of the hippocampal neural architecture, and the readily interpretable field potentials that stimulation of its stratified axonal projections elicited. Here was a way of recording synaptic efficacy in an identified monosynaptic pathway with extracellular electrodes. A superior preparation in every way—and in a structure that I knew to be important for memory. This is another McGill connection. In 1954, the patient known in the neurological literature as H.M. had undergone a bilateral resection of the temporal lobes, including the hippocampal formation, in an attempt to control his intractable epilepsy. The operation had resulted in a profound and permanent anterograde amnesia. H.M. was unable to form new episodic memories. His case established the importance of the hippocampus in the formation of new episodic or declarative memories in humans (Scoville and Milner 1957). Later work showed that other forms of learning and memory (for example, working memory, conditioning, priming, skill learning) were largely intact, demonstrating the existence of parallel and independent memory streams.

H.M.'s amnesia had first been studied by the McGill psychologist Brenda Milner, and his case was well known and much discussed in the seminar rooms of Montreal. In the autumn of 1967, when I came to Mill Hill, London, to continue working with Ben Burns who had become Head of the Division of Neurophysiology at the National Institute for Medical Research the year before, I had reached the inescapable conclusion that the hippocampus was the structure in which to continue the pursuit of the plastic synapse. I contacted Per Andersen shortly afterwards, to ask him if I could visit his laboratory to learn about the technique of field potential recording. With this indispensable technique, only possible in structures like the hippocampus that possess a rigorously laminated neural organization, synaptic responses could be monitored with extracellular recording electrodes. It was exactly what was needed to pursue changes in synaptic efficacy that, hopefully, might last for many hours.[3] The mnemonic engine of the brain was matched with the ideal technique for probing its mysteries. When Andersen heard of my reasons for wanting to work on the hippocampus, he told me that Terje Lømo, a PhD student in his laboratory, had discovered a phenomenon that would surely interest me. Lømo was writing his thesis, and had not had time to work on it further. If I came to Oslo, Andersen suggested, perhaps I might persuade him to take a break from writing? I made arrangements with an indulgent Medical Research Council to take a premature sabbatical, and a few months later, in the autumn of 1968, Terje Lømo and I did our first experiment together. We delivered a single tetanus to the perforant path, and the response to the test stimulus, reflecting the magnitude of the evoked synaptic response and therefore a measure of synaptic strength, was hugely potentiated. Over the following minutes the magnitude of the response dropped, as expected of PTP, but then levelled off well above the baseline. We watched with increasing excitement as the hours passed,[4] and the traces on our oscilloscope remained stubbornly elevated. We had confirmed what Lømo had found in 1966, and, unknown to me until I came to Oslo, had published in abstract form (Lømo 1966): tetanic stimulation of the perforant path leads to a persistent increase in synaptic efficacy. As I have said elsewhere, that experiment also engendered an equally persistent sense of amazement that 'such modest stimulation can produce so immediate, so profound, and so persistent an effect' (Bliss and Lynch 1988).

Lømo and I were aware of the significance of what we had seen, as was Per Andersen in whose laboratory the work was done and who did so much to encourage it. But we were careful not to claim too much for long-lasting potentiation, as we then called it. The last sentence of our paper attempts, in a flurry of clauses and subclauses, to emphasize that although we had found a cortical pathway in which changes in synaptic efficacy lasting for hours could be readily induced—clearly a good thing for a neural mnemonic device—our stimulus was wholly artificial, and we had no idea whether the effect that so delighted us did, in fact, play any part in the real life of the animal (Bliss and Lømo 1973). It is a salutary reminder of the difficulty of bridging the physiological and cognitive domains of enquiry that 30 years after writing that sentence we could rewrite it with almost equal validity today. We may suspect, but we do not know that LTP forms the neural basis of learning for any task in any animal. But perhaps a sub-Galilean murmur may be forgiven in this anniversary year: *surely, it must.*

Endnotes

1. A Google search on 28 November 2003 produced 276 hits for 'Hebb's postulate' and 153 hits for 'Sherrington enchanted loom'.
2. The italics are Hebb's. Switching to an italic font to notify the reader that the text so decorated constituted a significant statement was a technique introduced into popular literature by Stella Gibbons in Cold Comfort Farm (1932); its use by Hebb in his canonical postulate led to its adoption by at least one leading behavioural physiologist of the next generation.
3. Or for many days. The technique was equally adaptable to awake animals implanted with chronic recording and stimulating electrodes, as Tony Gardner-Medwin and I were to find after I returned to London (Bliss and Gardner-Medwin 1973).
4. Persistent excitement is something of a contradiction in terms. LTP and the last day of a closely fought 5-day cricket match provide two well-documented counter examples.

References

Andersen, P. O. (1966). Structure and function of archicortex. In *Brain and conscious experience* (ed. J. C. Eccles), pp. 59–84. New York: Springer.

Bliss, T. V. P. and Lømo, T. (1973). Long-lasting potentiation of synaptic transmission in the dentate gyrus of the anaesthetized rabbit. *J. Physiol. (Lond.)* **232**, 331–56.

Bliss, T. V. P. and Lynch, M. A. (1988). Long-term potentiation in the hippocampus: properties and mechanisms. In *Long-term potentiation: from biophysics to behavior* (ed. P. W. Landfield and S. A. Deadwyler), pp. 3–72. New York: Alan R. Liss.

Bliss, T. V. P., Burns, B. D., and Uttley, A. M. (1968). Factors affecting the conductivity of pathways in the cerebral cortex. *J. Physiol. (Lond.)* **195**, 339–67.

Bliss, T. V. P. and Gardner-Medwin, A. R. (1973). Long-lasting potentiation of synaptic transmission in the dentate area of the unanaestetized rabbit following stimulation of the perforant path. *J. Physiol. (Lond.)* **232**, 357–74.

Burns, B. D. (1958). *The mammalian cerebral cortex*. London: Edward Arnold.

Eccles, J. C. (1966). Conscious experience and memory. In *Brain and conscious experience* (ed. J. C. Eccles), pp. 314–44. New York: Springer.

Eccles, J. C. and McIntyre, A. K. (1953). The effects of disuse and of activity on mammalian spinal reflexes. *J. Physiol. (Lond.)* **121**, 492–516.

Hamlyn, L. H. (1963). An electron microscope study of pyramidal neurons in the Ammon's horn of the rabbit. *J. Anat. Lond.* **97**, 189–201.

Hebb, D. O. (1949). *Organization of behavior*. New York: Wiley.

Kandel, E. R. and Tauc, L. (1965). Heterosynaptic facilitation in neurones of the abdominal ganglion of *Aplysia depilans. J. Physiol. (Lond.)* **181**, 1–27.

Konorski, J. (1948). *Conditioned reflexes and neuron organization*. Cambridge University Press.

Lloyd, D. P. C. (1949). Post-tetanic potentiation of response in monosynaptic reflex pathways of the spinal cord. *J. Gen. Physiol.* **33**, 147–70.

Lømo, T. (1966). Frequency potentiation of excitatory synaptic activity in the dentate area of the hippocampal formation. *Acta Physiol. Scand.* **68** (Suppl. 277), 128.

Lorente de No, R. (1939). Transmission of impulses through cranial motor nuclei. *J. Neurophysiol.* **2**, 402–64.

Scoville, W. B. and Milner, B. (1957). Loss of recent memory after bilateral hippocampal lesion. *J. Neurol. Neurosurg. Psychiat.* **20**, 11–21.

Glossary

LTP   long-term potentiation
PTP   post-tetanic potentiation

4

Long-term potentiation in the Eocene

G. Lynch

The first ten years of long-term potentiation (LTP) research are reviewed. Surprisingly, given the intensity of current interest, the discovery paper did not trigger a wave of follow-on experiments. Despite this, the initial work laid out what ultimately became standard questions and paradigms. The application of the then still novel hippocampal slice technique oriented LTP towards basic neuroscience, perhaps somewhat at the cost of lesser attention to its functional significance. The use of slices led to the discovery of the events that trigger the formation of LTP and provided some first clues about its extraordinary persistence. Signs of the intense controversy over the nature of LTP expression (release vs receptors) emerged towards the end of the first decade of work. What appears to be lacking in the literature of that time is a widespread concern about LTP and memory. This may reflect a somewhat different attitude that neurobiologists then had towards memory research and a perceived need to integrate the new potentiation phenomenon into the web of established science before advancing extended arguments about its contributions to behaviour.

Keywords: long-term potentiation; early research; anatomical plasticity; induction; consolidation; memory

4.1 Motivations and diversions

My interest in LTP grew out of work on anatomical plasticity in adult hippocampus. Just before the appearance of the paper by Bliss and Lømo (1973), we had discovered that removal of the primary inputs to the dentate gyrus causes the remaining afferents to grow new synapses. How long this sprouting took was unclear; it started 5 days after lesions but then proceeded quickly, leaving open the possibility that contact formation might be fast enough to be involved in some stage of memory encoding. I remember reading the two LTP papers and wondering if this was physiologically induced anatomical plasticity. After all, the most startling feature of the new phenomenon was its longevity; something that I then (and now) had difficulty imagining could be achieved without structural changes. Given that we were already conducting electrophysiological studies of sprouting in hippocampus, it did not seem too great a step to search for those changes. However, a second paper derailed this plan even before the first electrode was lowered.

Within days of encountering LTP, I came across one of the papers by Yamamoto and McIlwain (1966) on hippocampal slices. Their results seemed astonishing because for whatever bizarre superstition (sanctity of the brain?), I simply couldn't picture slices of adult brain retaining their *in vivo* physiological properties. However, if this was the case, and the published results were certainly impressive, then it seemed that a revolution was at hand. Seen parochially, it meant that we would not have to search for a small population of synapses in a very large place but instead could stimulate multiple fibre populations converging on a defined dendritic location. (I belatedly realized that 'defined' means one thing at the light microscopic level and something altogether different in the electron microscope.) More generally, however, it was obvious that slices would vastly simplify electrophysiological studies and thereby allow for an unprecedented integration within neuroscience. Slices, in other words, seemed destined to complete the arrival of the hippocampus as the standard model for the cortical telencephalon and thereby allow for happy mingling of the tribes of brain scientists. Given all of this, our laboratory took a sharp turn towards this *in vitro* 'new dawn'.

Why a research group having no experience with culture methods would decide to launch slice experiments without first visiting McIlwain or Yamamoto is lost to memory. This is probably active repression because we had a truly horrible time with it. I remember at one point suggesting that we should move the physiology equipment into the animal colony where an oath would be taken that no one would leave until the slices lived or the rodent population was depleted. My colleagues (chiefly Sam Deadwyler and Tom Dunwiddie) took a second to be sure that this was in fact a joke. Eventually it became clear that we had seen complexity where there was only simplicity, after which slices became the routine business that they are today. Then it was on to LTP and physiologically induced sprouting.

Well, not quite. As the anatomical studies drew near, it seemed only prudent to pause and better define the new potentiation effect. I was surprised that there had not been a rush of papers doing exactly this. In fact, other than a fine replication from Graham Goddard (Douglas and Goddard 1975) and a report of potentiation in slices (and field CA1) (Schwartzkroin and Wester 1975), a strange sort of silence followed the discovery paper. Some possible reasons for this are noted later. Given this state of affairs, we thought it essential to at least confirm that the effect was present outside the dentate gyrus, because that structure, though the object of Bliss' attentions, is peculiar beyond all measure. If LTP was to be a substrate of memory, then we had to be sure that it would show up in more appropriate parts of brain. Then there was the question of whether we should be looking for changes in terminals or spines. Bliss *et al.* (1973) had provided good evidence that the potentiation effect is synapse specific but more could not be said on the basis of conventional physiological results alone. In addition, ahead of everything else, we had to know if it could be routinely obtained in our slice preparations. The first studies revealed LTP to be as robust in slices as in brain, and as prominent in field CA1 as in the dentate gyrus. Regarding location, one would assume that increases in transmitter receptors would amplify the response of the affected dendrites to applied transmitter. Testing this prediction produced a 'wrong' result—the only reliable change accompanying potentiation was a *depression* in the response to glutamate (Lynch *et al.* 1976, 1977). Some time later, Graham Collingridge carried out a much better version of this experiment and found that increased responses do appear, but only after considerable delays (Davies *et al.* 1989). With all that has been learned about glutamate receptors in the past few years, it might be a good idea to revisit this issue.

The depression effect led to systematic investigations of stimulation conditions and the idea of applying a fixed number of pulses at different frequencies. It transpired that high-frequency bursts induce potentiation whereas low-frequency trains cause depression (Dunwiddie and Lynch 1978). Thus, it was the in-between stimulation originally used to elicit LTP that reduced the responses to glutamate and heterosynaptic inputs. I suspect that the same low-frequency effect that was an annoyance in 1978 turned up years later as the much-discussed long-term depression. But the question *du jour* in the earlier period concerned the extent to which LTP was a laboratory artefact or, alternatively, part of the normal life of brain. Insight into this took years to arrive and then from an unlikely source. One day, while trying to make rats believe that electrical stimulation of the lateral olfactory tract was an odour, it suddenly became apparent to Ursula Staubli and myself that we were using completely arbitrary activation patterns. In this case it was a small matter to switch to more naturalistic stimulation (the sniffing pattern) and with this electric odours were born (Roman *et al.* 1987). As I walked away from this rather unlikely discovery, a collision with John Larson brought the realization that sniffing and hippocampal theta are just about the same thing. Within minutes the electric odour pattern, now recast as theta burst stimulation, was producing robust LTP in slices (Larson and Lynch 1986). Recognizing, as confirmed in subsequent experiments, that LTP has a special relationship with the most characteristic of hippocampal rhythms provided reassurance that it had correspondences in the real world.

Returning to 1977, with slices and appropriate stimulation parameters in hand, the search for the anatomical changes hypothesized to stabilize LTP was finally ready to begin. This project turned into a neuroscience equivalent of trench warfare, featuring on the one side an almost intractable problem and on the other a group of researchers driven mad by the idea that a result was just out of reach. Kevin Lee, the graduate student saddled with the project, assembled a team of undergraduate assistants, many of whom became casualties to the endless piles of electron micrographs. The project dragged on for so long that it became the subject of a scholarly book describing the horrors of frontline neurobiology (M. Lynch 1985 (no relation)).

Finally, evidence for anatomical modifications was obtained (Lee *et al.* 1980) and replicated by a separate group (Chang and Greenough 1984); since then there have been numerous studies demonstrating that changes in synaptic morphology accompany LTP. I still think of these as the most likely explanation for the stability of the potentiation effect, perhaps in the form developed a couple of years later in collaboration with Michel Baudry (Lynch and Baudry 1984). However, it has to be admitted that no one, at least to my knowledge, has yet shown that blocking the morphological adjustments causes LTP to lose its stability and simply decay away.

4.2 Early studies on the genesis of long-term potentiation

Even as we were beginning the structural studies, the group was being pulled ever more deeply into the puzzle of LTP's origins. It seemed best to break this large question into more digestible induction, expression and stabilization stages. Regarding the first of these, calcium was the only outside–in signalling device we knew of and indeed relatively small changes in its concentration proved to have large effects on the production of LTP (Dunwiddie and Lynch 1979). Shortly after this Phil Schwartzkroin reported on the use of intracellular applications of chelating agents to test if calcium is responsible for the afterhyperpolarization that follows bursts of discharges (Schwartzkroin and Stafstrom 1980). We eagerly adopted this technique and were delighted to find that buffering intracellular calcium did indeed completely block LTP induction (Lynch *et al.* 1983). At about the same time, Collingridge and McLennan discovered that antagonists of NMDA-type glutamate receptors suppress LTP (Collingridge *et al.* 1983);

when these receptors were found to admit calcium into the cell (Nowak *et al.* 1984), a neat story for the initial event in LTP production was complete. As a bonus, it turned out that the theta pattern, by a clever piece of cellular engineering, unblocks NMDA-receptors, a result that linked the induction step to rhythms occurring in real animals doing real learning. So within approximately 10 years the search for triggering events yielded both a standard model that has aged well and a satisfying amount of new biology.

The effort to identify events that follow the calcium influx got off to a fine start. Wilhelm Gispen visited the laboratory for a few weeks, ruled *ex cathedra* that LTP involves kinases, and together with Mike Browning quickly obtained evidence that high-frequency stimulation does indeed result in phosphorylation of synaptic proteins (Browning *et al.* 1979). Needless to say, I have since always envied that man's energy. Conversations with the newly arrived Michel Baudry led to a much more exotic candidate that seemed particularly appropriate for bridging the gap between calcium influx and long-lasting changes. This was calpain, a calcium-activated protease known from non-neural tissue to cleave cytoskeletal proteins. All of this seemed like genuine progress until the list of things that block LTP began to grow at an alarming rate. Soon, it became evident that LTP will not appear unless a great deal of normally present neuronal chemistry is, in fact, present. Despite all of that, calpain still holds a central spot in my ideas about LTP and recent work from various groups allows me to believe that this is more than simple nostalgia.

Finding the changes that express LTP also proved to be slow going, mainly because Baudry and I could not think of a way to distinguish increased release from more receptors. Bliss and colleagues had begun publishing papers showing that high-frequency afferent stimulation increases release but I could not go along with this because the trigger was clearly located postsynaptically. Why, other than sheer perversity, would induction be in one place and expression in another? Of course, what was really needed was an experimentally tractable prediction that distinguished the pre- and postsynaptic hypotheses. Somewhat later it occurred to me that the colocalization of two types of glutamate receptor in the hippocampal synapses provided for such a test: excluding special assumptions, increased release should result in almost equivalent changes in the currents mediated by the two groups of receptors, whereas postsynaptic changes *limited to one of the two groups of receptors* would not. Two versions of this experiment confirmed the postsynaptic prediction (Muller *et al.* 1988). Happily, Roger Nicoll had the same idea, did the same types of experiment and obtained the same result (Kauer *et al.* 1988). Thus, by the late 1980s, it seemed that expression had been narrowed down to a change in the number or operating properties of AMPA-type glutamate receptors. However, the release hypothesis soon came roaring back, this time in the form of studies using variants of quantal analysis. The resultant battle is certainly deserving of its own sociological analysis but takes us too close to the present for this review. Suffice it to say that today, judging from titles in the literature, most investigators agree with the minimal statement that changes in glutamate receptors are a major component of LTP expression, at least for the time-period measured in typical slice experiments.

Stabilization, the third and, to me, most fascinating of the questions from the late 1970s, proved to be even more resistant to analysis than expression. The structural hypothesis satisfied many of the constraints imposed by LTP phenomenology, most notably extreme duration, but called for spine chemistries that could rapidly reorganize and then restabilize synaptic anatomy. Calpain might satisfy the break-up requirement but we had no idea about how new synaptic architectures could be cemented in place. Indeed, it took almost 10 years for a suitable candidate to come along. Thinking back to those times I realize, with some irritation, that I overlooked an important clue from my own laboratory about stabilization. This was a result showing that LTP can be fully reversed by low-frequency stimulation if the stimulation is delivered immediately after induction (Barrionuevo *et al.* 1980). This apparently fell right into an intellectual blind spot. I simply did not realize what was obvious: LTP must have a consolidation period during which it becomes resistant to disruption and is converted into a persistent form. Had that point been developed in 1980, we would have realized much sooner that at least one aspect of stabilization occurs over a time-course that excludes a vast array of candidate mechanisms.

4.3 Long-term potentiation and memory

One of the more curious features of the early literature is the relative lack of discussion about LTP's potential significance for ideas about memory. An early paper of mine sidestepped the subject by using the expression 'behavioural plasticity' in place of 'learning'. All of this seems strange now but only, I think, because we cannot help but impose on the neuroscience of the 1970s the prominence that memory enjoys today. This anachronism distorts the picture. True, the years leading up to Bliss and Lømo's work established a behavioural context that elevated their results from the status of an interesting observation to a major discovery. Most relevant was the intensifying search during the 1960s for the synaptic correlates of learning in various model systems. The idea going back to the nineteenth century, and aggressively argued by J. C. Eccles, that repetitive afferent activity would produce neurophysiological changes lasting for very long periods had been confirmed, probably most clearly in the seminal work of Eric Kandel on simple forms of learning in *Aplysia*. Thompson and Spencer's extremely influential analysis of habituation/sensitization, followed by Thompson's studies of these effects in spinal neurons, led to the general expectation that use-dependent synaptic plasticity would soon be isolated, even in mammals. But those years also saw claims about the neurobiology of memory—for example, the successful transfer of specific memories via injections into naive animals of RNA from trained counterparts—that were, to say the least, controversial. I suspect that mainstream neuroscientists without the behavioural sophistication of Kandel, Thompson *et al.* were affected by all of this, and consequently much more conservative than is the case now, when proposing new substrates for memory. This socio-historical hypothesis might be tested with a survey of how often the word 'memory' was used in neurobiological papers with no behavioural components during the 1970s relative to later decades.

The above argument might also help explain the initially slow expansion of LTP research. Other factors would be the time needed for adoption of the hippocampus as a model system and for converting slices into a routine technique. By the mid 1980s, these steps had been taken, the memory controversies had begun to fade, and the explosive growth in LTP research was underway. Adding fuel to this were the above-noted successes in attaching at least some parts of potentiation to recognizable cellular substrates. In the sense of the philosopher Willard Quine, LTP was becoming enmeshed in that network of associations that stretches across all of science (the 'web of science') and thereby was itself becoming a scientific datum. LTP, rather than an isolated physiological effect, was now simply another element of neurobiology, albeit one with several properties suggestive of an encoding device. Finally, the identification of cellular substrates brought with it, and indeed was partly based upon, tools for blocking the induction step. Using these in behavioural studies provided what seemed to be a direct way of testing for a contribution of LTP to memory formation. Richard Morris was the first to see these possibilities and the first to generate experimental evidence linking potentiation to particular instances of memory (Morris *et al.* 1986). With this, LTP crossed its Rubicon and set in motion yet another round of debate.

References

Barrionuevo, G., Schottler, F., and Lynch, G. (1980). The effects of repetitive low frequency stimulation on control and 'potentiated' synaptic responses in the hippocampus. *Life Sci.* **27**, 2385–91.

Bliss, T. V. P. and Lømo, T. (1973). Long-lasting potentiation of synaptic transmission in the dentate area of the anaesthetized rabbit following stimulation of the perforant path. *J. Physiol. (Lond.)* **232**, 331–56.

Bliss, T. V. P., Lømo, T., and Gardner-Medwin, A. R. (1973). Synaptic plasticity in the hippocampal formation. In *Macromolecules and behaviour* (ed. G. Ansell and P. B. Bradley), pp. 193–203. London: MacMillan.

Browning, M., Dunwiddie, T., Bennett, W., Gispen, W., and Lynch, G. (1979). Synaptic phosphoproteins: specific changes after repetitive stimulation of the hippocampal slice. *Science* **203**, 60–2.

Chang, F. L. and Greenough, W. T. (1984). Transient and enduring morphological correlates of synaptic activity and efficacy change in the rat hippocampal slice. *Brain Res.* **309**, 35–46.

Collingridge, G. L., Kehl, S. J., and McLennan, H. (1983). Excitatory amino acids in synaptic transmission in the Schaffer collateral–commissural pathway of the rat hippocampus. *J. Physiol.* **334**, 33–46.

Davies, S. N., Lester, R. A., Reymann, K. G., and Collingridge, G. L. (1989). Temporally distinct pre- and post-synaptic mechanisms maintain long-term potentiation. *Nature* **338**, 500–3.

Douglas, R. M. and Goddard, G. V. (1975). Long-term potentiation of the perforant path-granule cell synapse in the rat hippocampus. *Brain Res.* **86**, 205–15.

Dunwiddie, T., and Lynch, G. (1978). Long-term potentiation and depression of synaptic responses in the rat hippocampus: localization and frequency dependency. *J. Physiol.* **276**, 353–67.

Dunwiddie, T. V. and Lynch, G. (1979). The relationship between extracellular calcium concentrations and the induction of hippocampal long-term potentiation. *Brain Res.* **169**, 103–10.

Kauer, J. A., Malenka, R. C., and Nicoll, R. A. (1988). A persistent postsynaptic modification mediates long-term potentiation in the hippocampus. *Neuron* **1**, 911–17.

Larson, J. and Lynch, G. (1986). Induction of synaptic potentiation in hippocampus by patterned stimulation involves two events. *Science* **232**, 985–8.

Lee, K. S., Schottler, F., Oliver, M., and Lynch, G. (1980). Brief bursts of high-frequency stimulation produce two types of structural change in rat hippocampus. *J. Neurophysiol.* **44**, 247–58.

Lynch, G. and Baudry, M. (1984). The biochemistry of memory: a new and specific hypothesis. *Science* **224**, 1057–63.

Lynch, G., Larson, J., Kelso, S., Barrionuevo, G., and Schottler, F. (1983). Intracellular injections of EGTA block induction of hippocampal long-term potentiation. *Nature* **305**, 719–21.

Lynch, G. S., Dunwiddie, T., and Gribkoff, V. (1977). Heterosynaptic depression: a postsynaptic correlate of long-term potentiation. *Nature* **266**, 737–9.

Lynch, G. S., Gribkoff, V. K., and Deadwyler, S. A. (1976). Long term potentiation is accompanied by a reduction in dendritic responsiveness to glutamic acid. *Nature* **263**, 151–3.

Lynch, M. (1985). *Art and artifact in laboratory science: a study of shop work and shop talk in a research laboratory*. London: Routledge and Kegan Paul.

Morris, R. G. M., Anderson, E., Lynch, G. S., and Baudry, M. (1986). Selective impairment of learning and blockade of longterm potentiation by an N-methyl-D-aspartate receptor antagonist, AP5. *Nature* **319**, 774–6.

Muller, D., Joly, M., and Lynch, G. (1988). Contributions of quisqualate and NMDA receptors to the induction and expression of LTP. *Science* **242**, 1694–7.

Nowak, L., Bregestovski, P., Ascher, P., Herbet, A., and Prochiantz, A. (1984). Magnesium gates glutamate-activated channels in mouse central neurones. *Nature* **307**, 462–5.

Roman, F., Staubli, U., and Lynch, G. (1987). Evidence for synaptic potentiation in a cortical network during learning. *Brain Res.* **418**, 221–6.

Schwartzkroin, P. A. and Stafstrom, C. E. (1980). Effects of EGTA on the calcium-activated afterhyperpolarization in hippocampal CA3 pyramidal cells. *Science* **210**, 1125–6.

Schwartzkroin, P. A. and Wester, K. (1975). Long-lasting facilitation of a synaptic potential following tetanization in the *in vitro* hippocampal slice. *Brain Res.* **89**, 107–19.

Yamamoto, C. and McIlwain, H. (1966). Potentials evoked *in vitro* in preparations from the mammalian brain. *Nature* **210**, 1055–6.

Glossary

LTP   long-term potentiation
NMDA   *N*-methyl-D-aspartate

5

Long-term potentiation, cooperativity and Hebb's cell assemblies: a personal history

Bruce L. McNaughton

The early history of the experimental work leading to the discovery that long-term potentiation (LTP) embodies Hebb's principle of association is described. In addition, the fallacy underlying the sometimes presumed distinction between 'cooperativity' and 'associativity' in the induction of LTP is pointed out.

Keywords: Hebb; cooperativity; associative; kindling; long-term enhancement; cell assembly

Few people, perhaps scientists least of all, are able to agree on present reality. The likelihood of there being much agreement about history, especially among those who participated in it, is thus vanishingly small. And so it was with considerable reservation that I accepted the invitation to write a historical perspective on the early days of LTP research in the laboratory of Graham Goddard in Halifax, Nova Scotia, Canada. Indeed, I would not have accepted, were it not for the fact that much of the excitement about the LTP phenomenon derives from the astonishing prescience of a Canadian psychologist, Donald Hebb, who, some 20 years before the discovery of LTP, had postulated such a phenomenon and had outlined its implications concerning the mechanism of associative memory (Hebb 1949). Few would disagree that Hebb's ideas form the fundamental basis of our increasingly sophisticated understanding of the properties of neural networks, both in the abstract and as implemented in real nervous systems. Hebb also founded a tradition in Canadian universities and elsewhere of attempting to explain the observations and concepts of psychology in terms of physiological observables. Graham Goddard was a 'grand-student' of Hebb, having worked at McGill under Hebb's student Peter Milner, who both introduced inhibitory control into the cell assembly theory (Milner 1957) and later formulated the first hypotheses on the use of oscillations to solve the binding problem. As an undergraduate, several of my teachers similarly traced their intellectual lineage directly back to Hebb. Thus, out of my deep respect for Hebb and his contribution, I feel some obligation to attempt to write this brief, personal history of his influence on the early developments in LTP research in Canada, and on the direction of my own research career then and now.

When I was 16 years old, my father gave me two books to read. One was Penfield's and Roberts' (1959) *Speech and brain mechanisms*, wherein he described his observations of the mnemonic retrieval effects of electrical stimulation on the temporal lobe. Penfield had concluded that 'the hippocampus of the two sides is, in fact, the repository of the ganglionic patterns that preserve the record of the stream of consciousness. If not the repository, then each hippocampus plays an important role in the mechanism of reactivation of that record'. The other book was Hebb's *The organization of behavior*. So I was, in some sense, 'primed' for a research career involving the hippocampus, synaptic plasticity and memory. Later, as a beginning graduate student in Ottawa, I attended a seminar course on memory, conducted by Dan MacIntyre, a former student of Goddard's and a major contributor to the kindling field (Goddard and McIntyre 1969). I confess that my real reason for taking this course was not primarily my interest in memory, but involved a certain other graduate student in the course by the name of Carol Barnes. Carol was then a student of Peter Fried, also a former Goddard student. In any case, for my term project, I undertook to present to the class the recent ideas of David Marr (1969, 1970, 1971), who was perhaps the first to take Hebb's concepts and formalize them mathematically in the context of the known anatomical organization of synaptic circuits in the brain. Little did I anticipate the difficulty of this undertaking. Marr's 'pre-Hopfield' mathematical framework has proven almost impossibly difficult to follow, even by today's specialists in computational theory. Indeed, some have suggested that the mathematics were just plain wrong (Willshaw and Buckingham 1990); but the strength of Marr's early papers was not in the mathematics, but in his fundamental ideas on the properties of associative networks, such as pattern completion and error correction; on the roles of the various cellular elements of real networks, such as modifiable recurrent collateral synapses and inhibitory synapses with 'shunting' effects; and on the basic activity parameters necessary for a network to store associations, such as sparse, orthogonal patterns. All of these concepts are now fundamental components of our understanding of how networks store experiences. Marr's writings on associative memory in the cerebellum, neocortex and hippocampus preceded the formal publication of the discovery of LTP, but he may have caught wind of it, as there is a 'note in proof' on Lømo's early brief report on synaptic facilitation in the dentate gyrus and also, according to Tim Bliss (personal communication), Marr was a friend of Tony Gardner-Medwin.

A few months later, in the summer of 1973, I had the opportunity to attend a three-week summer school on synaptic transmission, held in Erice, Sicily. The meeting was directed by Sir Bernard Katz, and the field was small enough at the time that most of the major players were in attendance as lecturers. One of the informal lectures was given by Terje Lømo, who had just published his work with Tim Bliss on 'long-lasting potentiation' in the dentate gyrus of the hippocampus. Clearly, I was primed to receive this information as the verification of the ideas of both Hebb and Marr. Upon my return to Canada, I had to wait impatiently for photocopies of the Bliss, Lømo and Gardner-Medwin papers from inter-library loan. I read them eagerly when they arrived but was astonished to find that neither Hebb nor Marr was even mentioned. It was clear to me that there was an opportunity for a dissertation project here and I decided I would have to move to London or Oslo to pursue it.

By this time, my relationship with Carol Barnes had become rather more than academic, and we both decided that LTP was the right course for us. Carol's interest was in memory and ageing and it was obvious to her that a loss of LTP functionality might well be an important factor in age-related memory impairment, a conjecture that she has systematically and elegantly verified (see Chapter 22, this volume). At this point, Peter Fried informed us that there was no need to go abroad to pursue these interests. As it happened, a graduate student in Goddard's laboratory in Halifax, Rob M. Douglas (not to be confused with R. J. Douglas who earlier contributed much to the experimental psychology literature on hippocampus and behaviour) had already replicated the Bliss and Gardner-Medwin experiments, with chronically implanted electrodes in rats (Douglas and Goddard 1975). Graham had spent a sabbatical visit with Tim Bliss at University College London in 1974, where they had attempted, unsuccessfully according to Tim, to induce LTP in rats. Graham had exported the evoked hippocampal field potential method to Halifax where he apparently had had more success, and Douglas was in the process of refining the stimulus parameters and stimulus locations that eventually led to considerably more reliability in producing the phenomenon than had been evident in the 1973 *Journal of Physiology* paper. Douglas had shown that short, high-frequency (200–400 Hz) bursts, mimicking, it was thought, the normal activity of central neurons, was a much more reliable protocol than the extended, relatively low-frequency, long-duration stimuli used by Bliss *et al.*, which had been derived from the earlier 'frequency potentiation' studies of the Oslo group. Douglas had also made very effective use of one of the first laboratory minicomputers, a 12-bit Linc-8, the size of a large refrigerator, with around 4 kb of memory and an approximately 100 kb tape drive. This was programmed in binary assembly code to enable the routine collection and analysis of the large amounts (for the time) of physiological data that would be necessary for a really systematic study of the LTP phenomenon. Later, Graham's laboratory acquired a 16-bit PDP-11 with 32 kilobytes of memory and 1.6-megabyte removable hard disk storage packs, which seemed to us a miracle. In addition to his early direct contributions to improving LTP reliability and to understanding the postsynaptic nature of the locus of LTP induction (Douglas and Goddard 1982), Rob contributed indirectly but enormously to the early LTP research by the selfless sharing of his computer programs with many researchers in the field (myself and Tim Bliss to mention two) at a time when it was simply not possible to buy an effective data acquisition package for such experiments.

Peter Fried arranged an interview for Carol and me with Graham Goddard, who agreed to accept us into his laboratory. Graham, who, in Hebb's tradition, always encouraged innovative research efforts in his students, agreed, in anticipation of our arrival, to purchase a large cohort of adult and ageing rats for Carol's planned ageing research on LTP. That summer, Carol and I were married and departed the same day for the 1000-mile drive to Halifax.

Dalhousie Psychology in the mid 1970s was an extremely exciting place for a young student of the neurosciences because, within a framework of quantitative experimental psychology provided by people like Vern ('working memory') Honig, it had a focus of interest in synaptic plasticity, from early development to associative learning. To highlight a few individuals: Robert Sutherland, who subsequently became a major contributor to hippocampal learning theory and experimental neuropsychology, was a member of the graduate student cohort, and was trying to condition single neurons to fire using brain stimulation reward. Max Cynader and Donald Mitchell were studying the role of experience and correlated activity in the early development of the visual system. M. Yoon was developing increasingly sophisticated experimental models to elucidate retino-tectal innervation. Ian Meinertzhagen was doing exquisitely detailed anatomical studies on the development of the insect visual system. Some early work in computer modelling of neural networks was also in progress. And Lynn Nadel was there as a visiting lecturer, putting the finishing touches on a long-promised volume with John O'Keefe on the 'Hippocampus as a cognitive map' (O'Keefe and Nadel 1978) that, whatever the final analysis reveals, would revolutionize research into the way the hippocampus processes information. Lynn had been a graduate student in

Hebb's department at McGill, and frequently contributed to deep and lofty discussions about cell assemblies and associative memory at the local watering hole.

Part of Goddard's reason for accepting me as a graduate student was that I had had considerable experience in electron microscopy. Goddard had earlier discovered the 'kindling phenomenon', through which repeated daily electrical stimulation of certain brain structures eventually led to electrical after-discharge and behavioural seizures (Goddard 1967). Kindling was, and is, a powerful experimental model for epilepsy research; but Goddard's main interest was in memory, not epilepsy. He saw in the kindling effect, and in epilepsy in general, 'the brain's mechanism for memory gone awry'. During the 5-year period prior to my arrival in Halifax, Graham had been using electron microscopy in the attempt to find evidence for the 'growth process', possibly the increase in the area of synaptic contact synapse, that Hebb had postulated would underlie the associative mechanism. Goddard's 5-year study attempting to find kind-ling-related synaptic structural changes in the amygdala had come to nothing. Even if structural changes had been the basis of LTP, the amygdala is simply too complex and diverse a structure, and the EM methods of the day were simply too imprecise and time consuming to yield statistically reliable results in any reasonable period of time. Graham set me the task of using the LTP phenomenon in the dense, homogeneous and monosynaptic connections of the perforant path in the dentate gyrus, to look for Hebb's growth process following LTP.

I was naive enough to the pitfalls and arduousness of such an EM analysis that I agreed to undertake Graham's assignment. I was not so naive, however, as to believe that it was likely, even in the nearly ideal experimental system provided by the per-forant path–dentate gyrus, that the LTP derived from stimulation at a single site would alter enough of the relevant synapses to make the needle emerge from the haystack. I knew from the anatomical studies of Hjorth-Simonsen (1972) and Steward (1976) that the perforant-path projection to the dorsal hippocampus arose from a large area of entorhinal cortex, encompassing both its medial and lateral subdivisions, and that only a rather small proportion of the total synaptic population was likely to be activated from one stimulus location. I thought that I might increase my odds of success if I could sequentially induce LTP from many sites across the axis of this projection pathway. Because LTP was, by definition, long lasting, the effects from one site would persist as I systematically moved the stimulating electrode in order to include most of the inputs. Only then would I perfuse the animal and prepare the tissue for electron microscopy. But was the entire entorhinal projection capable of exhibiting LTP? This was not yet known, and had to be investigated first. However, with the high current strengths (300–500 μA) then in standard use to evoke large field EPSP and population spike responses in the dentate gyrus, it would be hard to know how far the stimulus field extended, and therefore hard to know which fibres were responsible for any observed LTP. I decided to do an exploratory study using relatively weak stimulation (around 50 μA), set well below the threshold for evoking a population spike, and systematically to map the mediolateral axis of the perforant path for LTP expression. My first preparation was a complete failure. The brief bursts that previously had induced LTP hardly left any trace at all, certainly nothing lasting. In order to preserve the improved spatial resolution of using low-intensity stimuli, I decided to try trains of longer duration: 100–200 pulses at 200 Hz. Such stimulation was often known to induce seizures when delivered at high intensity, but I thought that since there would be less postsynaptic discharge, there might be less risk of seizures. I was rather astounded to find that this stimulation indeed induced rather large increments in synaptic efficacy, particularly in the lateral parts of the entorhinal system, but it was transient, decaying smoothly back to baseline in a few minutes. Perhaps LTP was not always long-term. Something about the shape of the decay function reminded me of a recent series of papers by Magleby and Zengel (1975, 1976) on synaptic plasticity in the neuromuscular junction. There was an initial fast decay, followed by a slower one, which, when plotted semilogarithmically, yielded two components that looked very much like what the latter authors had termed 'Augmentation' (3–5 s) and 'Potentiation' which lasted a few minutes and had been described in the early literature as 'post-tetanic' (PTP). Perhaps LTP was merely long-lasting PTP? This was rather disheartening to me, as I knew that these phenomena were entirely presynaptic in their origin, and hence could not embody Hebb's rule. This caused me to begin to think critically of what was the essence of Hebb's idea. It was that a weak synapse could only potentiate if it was activated while the postsynaptic cell was firing. To get the postsynaptic cell to fire in the first place there must be either a coactive strong synapse, or the equivalent, a lot of coactive weaker synapses (which was what Hebb had assumed was typically the case). In my experimental setup at the time, I only had room to get one stimulating electrode in the perforant path. How could I test the effects on a weak input of coactivating it with a strong (i.e. more numerous) input? Clearly, the way to do this was to use low-intensity test pulses, increase the intensity during the high frequency so as to recruit a much larger number of fibres in addition to the test set, and then revert to the low-intensity stimulation for subsequent testing (see Figs 5.1 and 5.2). I would still be activating the test fibres,

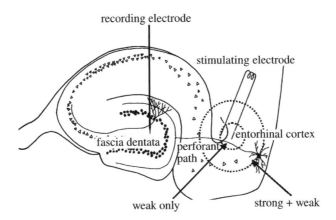

Fig. 5.1 Illustration of the recording and stimulation set-up for the original experiments on cooperativity of coactive inputs in LTP induction. These experiments compared the effects of high-frequency stimulation of a 'weak pathway', that is, a small number of afferent fibres, with the effects on the same pathway when it was stimulated in association with a 'strong pathway', that is, a large number of afferents. This comparison was made using a single electrode. The weak input was activated using a weak stimulus. The combination of strong and weak inputs was achieved by increasing the stimulus intensity during the high-frequency train, and then returning to the weak stimulus for further testing. The same experiment can be carried out with two electrodes, but the principle is the same.

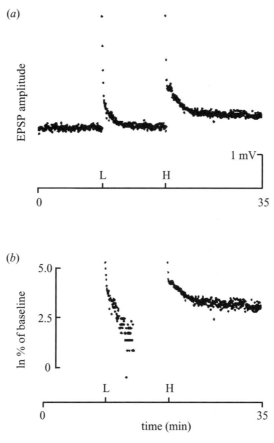

Fig. 5.2 Results of the experiment described in Fig. 5.1 are shown in linear and semilogarithmic coordinates in (*a*) and (*b*), respectively. Activating the weak pathway at high frequency (L) produced a large but transient increase in the perforant-path EPSP. The dual exponential decay is characteristic of the processes of 'augmentation' and 'potentiation' which involve an increase in transmitter release probability. Activating the weak pathway in association with a strong one (H) produced the same two fast components and also a third, very slow component, now identified as LTP. This 'cooperativity' was the first indication that LTP embodied Hebb's principle of association.

and would therefore accomplish the goal of activating a weak and a strong input together at high frequency. Sure enough, the first time I tried it, I observed robust LTP, riding on top of which was apparently the short-lasting 'Augmentation and Potentiation', which was the only effect of stimulating the weak pathway alone.

Hebb had also emphasized that his proposal implied the 'association of two afferent fibres of the same order—in principle a sensori-sensory association', and not just a linear association. By this time, we had realized that the medial and lateral components of the perforant path were separate fibre systems with different sources of input, different biochemistry and different synaptic physiology (McNaughton and Barnes 1977). Could the two pathways, which were both presynaptic to the dentate gyrus granule cells and hence, from that perspective, of the same 'order', cooperate with one another to induce LTP? The answer was clearly yes. Not only could both pathways exhibit LTP on their own, if enough fibres were coactivated, but at low stimulus strength which induced no LTP in either pathway activated by itself, robust LTP occurred when they were coactive. Clearly, the factors underlying the induction of LTP in some way embodied Hebb's associative principle: exactly how would not become clear until several years later, when the properties of the N-methyl-D-aspartate receptor and its role in LTP induction were discovered (Collingridge and Kehl 1983; Harris and Ganong 1984).

In preparing these results for publication (McNaughton and Douglas 1978), I made two tactical errors in my choice of vocabulary. The first error was in my choice of the word 'cooperativity'. In subsequent years, several groups repeated almost the identical experiments I described, but used two separate stimulating electrodes to induce their 'strong' and 'weak' synaptic inputs rather than varying the stimulus intensity at a single electrode. They called the resulting LTP 'associative' as though there were some logical distinction pertaining to how the weak and strong inputs had been activated. The misconception that 'cooperativity' and 'associativity' somehow relate to different phenomena has, unfortunately, persisted in the minds of some, and has been a source of considerable confusion to newcomers to the field. The second tactical error was to attempt to change the name 'long-term potentiation' to 'long-term enhancement'. There was, I thought, a very good reason to do so. The cooperativity/associativity effect clearly suggested that 'LTE' was not 'LTP', if by potentiation one was referring to the phenomenon defined as 'potentiation' by the neuromuscular and spinal cord physiologists. Moreover, I had also provided indirect, but reasonably compelling, evidence (see McNaughton 1982) that hippocampal 'potentiation' as well as 'augmentation' involved an increased transmitter release probability, as had been shown at the neuromuscular junction, whereas 'enhancement' did not (see Fig. 5.3). Thus 'enhancement' and 'potentiation' were clearly separate mechanisms and I felt it would be useful to the field to keep the distinction clear. As it turned out, the ease with which an acronym 'trips off the tongue' was considered more important. Perhaps so.

There is a final anecdote that is of some historical interest. Donald Hebb was born in a small Nova Scotia town not far from Dalhousie University. He retired there about the time that the cooperativity studies were nearing completion. He was awarded an emeritus professorship in our department and given a small office adjacent to the front door, with a large, black leather, easy-chair. He was there frequently, and his door was always open. After I was convinced that our experiments adequately corroborated his 'neurophysiological postulate' I took the data to his office and explained them to him. He listened carefully and politely, and made a few helpful suggestions, but finally asked why there was so much excitement about this particular part of his theory. The basic idea was, he said, an old one, dating at least to Lorente de No, and the principle was obvious to anyone who had considered the principles of associative learning. Something like cooperativity *had* to be present in the nervous system, there was no other plausible means of association. His suggestion to me was that I would have a much more interesting career if I focused on his cell assembly and phase sequence concepts. I think that he was definitely correct on that score, and his advice was also partly responsible for the fact that the over-ambitious electron microscopy project that was indirectly responsible for the initial confirmation of his neurophysiological postulate was quietly dropped.

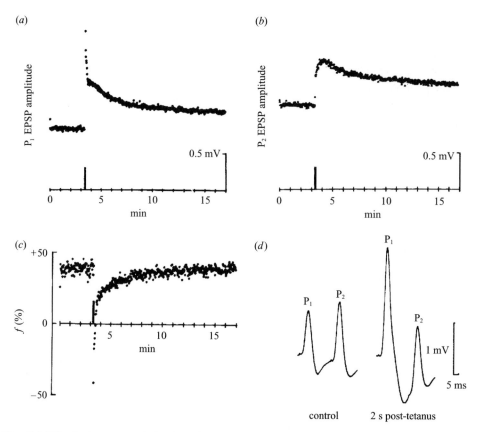

Fig. 5.3 What's in a name? Early evidence that LTP is fundamentally different from the 'potentiation' of neurotransmitter release that had been studied in many types of synapses prior to the discovery of LTP. (Reproduced, with permission, from *J. Physiol.* (*Lond.*) 1982, pp. 249–262, Fig. 5.) This study demonstrated the presence in hippocampal synapses of two short-term processes with kinetics identical to the 'augmentation' and 'potentiation' effects (Magleby and Zengel 1975, 1976), which were known to involve increased transmitter release probability. Both processes are elicited in the absence of LTP by weak, high-frequency stimulation, and are especially evident in the lateral perforant path where the resting release probability is inherently low. Augmentation and potentiation decay with exponential time constants of around 5 and 90 s, respectively. When probed using pairs of stimuli at intervals (25 ms) much shorter than their decay time-constants, an increase in synaptic depression is observed during both processes, in proportion to the elevation in absolute EPSP magnitude. The same effect is observed when transmitter release probability is increased by other means such as elevated calcium ion in the bath. When the same stimulus train is delivered at a higher intensity that produces a lasting enhancement of the EPSP (i.e. LTP), and the result is again probed using paired stimuli, there is an increase in relative depression of the second response of each pair; however, this depression disappears with the same time-course as when there is no long-term change, even though there may be a substantial persistent enhancement of the EPSP. These results showed that LTP is not long-term 'potentiation', but some other process.

References

Collingridge, G. and Kehl, S. (1983). Excitatory amino acids in synaptic transmission in the Schaffer collateral-commissural pathway of the rat hippocampus. *J. Physiol.* (*Lond.*) **334**, 3–46.

Douglas, R. M. and Goddard, G. V. (1975). Long-term potentiation of the perforant path-granule cell synapse in the rat hippocampus. *Brain Res.* **86**, 205–15.

Douglas, R. M. and Goddard, G. V. (1982). Inhibitory modulation of long-term potentiation: evidence for a postsynaptic locus of control. *Brain Res.* **240**, 259–72.

Goddard, G. V. (1967). The development of epileptic seizures through brain stimulation at low intensity. *Nature* **214**, 1020–1.

Goddard, G. V. and McIntyre, D. C. (1969). A permanent change in brain function resulting from daily electrical stimulation. *Exp. Neurol.* **25**, 295–30.

Harris, E. W. and Ganong, A. H. (1984). Long-term potentiation in the hippocampus involves activation of N-methyl-D-aspartate receptors. *Brain Res.* **323**, 132–7.

Hebb, D. O. (1949). *The organization of behavior.* New York: Wiley.

Hjorth-Simonsen, A. (1972). Projection of the lateral part of the entorhinal area to the hippocampus and fascia dentata. *J. Comp. Neurol.* **146**, 219–32.

Milner, P. M. (1957). The cell assembly: mark II. *Psychol. Rev.* **64**, 242–52.

McNaughton, B. L. (1982). Long-term synaptic enhancement and short-term potentiation in rat fascia dentata act through different mechanisms. *J. Physiol.* (*Lond.*) **324**, 249–62.

McNaughton, B. L. and Barnes, C. A. (1977). Physiological identification and analysis of dentate granule cell responses to stimulation of the medial and lateral perforant pathways in the rat. *J. Comp. Neurol.* **175**, 439–54.

McNaughton, B. L. and Douglas, R. M. (1978). Synaptic enhancement in fascia dentata: cooperativity among coactive afferents. *Brain Res.* **157**, 277–93.

Magleby, K. L. and Zengel, J. E. (1975). A quantitative description of tetanic and post-tetanic potentiation of transmitter release at the frog neuromuscular junction. *J. Physiol.* (*Lond.*) **245**, 183–208.

Magleby, K. L. and Zengel, J. E. (1976). Augmentation: a process that acts to increase transmitter release at the frog neuromuscular junction. *J. Physiol.* (*Lond.*) **257**, 449–70.

Marr, D. (1969). A theory of cerebellar cortex. *J. Physiol.* (*Lond.*) **202**, 437–70.

Marr, D. (1970). A theory of cerebral neocortex. *Proc. R. Soc. Lond.* B **176**, 161–234.

Marr, D. (1971). Simple memory: a theory for archicortex. *Phil. Trans. R. Soc. Lond.* B **262**, 23–81.

O'Keefe, J. and Nadel, L. (1978). *The hippocampus as a cognitive map.* Oxford: Clarendon Press.

Penfield, W. and Roberts, L. (1959). *Speech and brain-mechanisms.* Princeton University Press.

Steward, O. (1976). Topographic organization of the projections from the entorhinal area to the hippocampal formation of the rat. *J. Comp. Neurol.* **167**, 285–314.

Willshaw, D. J. and Buckingham, J. T. (1990). An assessment of Marr's theory of the hippocampus as a temporary memory store. *Phil. Trans. R. Soc. Lond.* B **329**, 205–15.

Glossary

EM	electron microscopic
EPSP	excitatory postsynaptic potential
LTE	long-term enhancement
LTP	long-term potentiation
PTP	post-tetanic potentiation

6

The induction of *N*-methyl-D-aspartate receptor-dependent long-term potentiation[†]

Graham L. Collingridge

The role of *N*-methyl-D-aspartate (NMDA) receptors in the induction of long-term potentiation (LTP) was established during the 1980s. In this article I present a personal reflection upon the role that my colleagues and I played in the discovery of the mechanism of induction of NMDA receptor-dependent LTP.

Keywords: long-term potentiation; *N*-methyl-D-aspartate; hippocampus; synaptic plasticity; magnesium; glutamate

6.1 1980–1982: Potential excitement

I hope my NMDA receptors were working well in the 1980s as I try to recall the events leading up to the establishment of the mechanism of induction of LTP. My story begins in 1980 as I start my first postdoctoral position in the laboratory of Hugh McLennan, in Vancouver. Hugh was interested in L-glutamate as a neurotransmitter in the brain and was one of the pioneers in the identification of multiple classes of glutamate receptor. His PhD student, Stephen Kehl, was studying the actions of L-glutamate on CA1 neurons in the hippocampal slice preparation, when I arrived looking for a project. At that time also, a visitor to Hugh's laboratory, David West, was working on LTP in this slice preparation. When I first saw LTP demonstrated by David, I was hooked and decided to spend the next two years working on this fascinating process. I was already well aware of the existence of multiple types of glutamate receptor, having spent a PhD in London studying with another major player in the glutamate field—John Davies. I asked myself the question whether different subtypes of glutamate receptor may be involved in the mediation of synaptic transmission and the induction of LTP; and this, with Hugh's approval, is what I set out to investigate.

There was no *a priori* reason to suspect one type of glutamate receptor over another with respect to a specific role in synaptic plasticity. I therefore decided to investigate the subtypes in a random order. The first agonist I found in the freezer was kainate. In my first experiment I found that a brief focal application of kainate induced a pronounced, long-lasting facilitation of the population spike recorded from the CA1 cell body region (Collingridge and McLennan 1981). Although this effect superficially resembled LTP it was immediately evident that kainate was not inducing LTP since the potentiation was associated with a sustained depression of the dendritically recorded fEPSP. Furthermore, there was no occlusion between kainate and tetanus-induced facilitation. Indeed, subsequent experiments also revealed a depression of synaptic

[†]Dedicated to Jeff C. Watkins for his discovery of the NMDA receptor.

inhibition that accounted for the increased excitability (Kehl *et al.* 1984). (I was to return to these effects many years later when improved pharmacological tools enabled the identification of presynaptic kainate receptors regulating both L-glutamate (Chittajallu *et al.* 1996) and GABA release (Clarke *et al.* 1997) in the CA1 region of the hippocampus.) However, as far as LTP was concerned there was no obvious role for kainate receptors at Schaffer collateral/commissural–CA1 synapses. (Ironically, the situation proved to be very different at another synapse in the hippocampus where LTP is independent of the activation of NMDA receptors, the mossy fibre–CA3 synapse (see Chapter 9, this volume).)

The next agonist I tested was what I thought was *N*-methyl-DL-aspartate, which had little effect in the CA1 region of the hippocampus. I felt unhappy with this result since my previous experiments in the substantia nigra had shown that NMDA was an extremely potent excitant of these neurons (Collingridge and Davies 1979). Although this could obviously be due to a regional difference in sensitivity, I was sufficiently concerned to want to test *bona fide* NMDA, which at the time was not commercially available. On a visit to Bristol I raised my concern with Jeff Watkins who let me have samples, not only of NMDA but also two of his latest glutamate antagonists, (D,L)-2-amino-5-phosphonopentanoate (AP5; note that Jeff originally called his antagonist 2-amino-5-phosphonovalerate according to the earlier chemical nomenclature and the compound is often hence abbreviated as APV—we have switched to Jeff's preferred name of AP5) and DGG. On my return to Vancouver in the spring of 1981 I applied NMDA by ionophoresis to CA1 dendrites and observed dramatic effects. First was a depression of synaptic transmission, which we attributed to depolarization of CA1 neurons, but this was followed by a potentiation of the fEPSP (Collingridge *et al.* 1983*a*). In my heart I knew at that point that NMDA receptors were a trigger for the induction of LTP. The obvious experiment was to test Jeff's specific NMDA receptor antagonist, AP5. This had no effect on basal synaptic transmission or pre-established LTP but blocked the induction of LTP in a reversible manner (Collingridge *et al.* 1983*a*). My head now agreed with my heart. In these same experiments I tested DGG, which is a weak antagonist of AMPA and kainate receptors, and this depressed synaptic transmission. Thus the original hypothesis, that different classes of glutamate receptor mediate synaptic transmission and the induction of LTP, turned out to be correct. The NMDA receptor was identified as the trigger for the induction of LTP and some type of non-NMDA glutamate receptor as the mediator of synaptic transmission. (Beautiful autoradiographic images, produced by Dan Monaghan and Carl Cotman, of AMPA and NMDA receptors showed very high concentrations of both types of receptor in the dendritic layers of area CA1 (Monaghan *et al.* 1983) suggesting that AMPA receptors are the mediators of the synaptic response. Indeed the development of more selective pharmacological tools has confirmed that it is the AMPA receptor, rather than the kainate receptor, which serves this role.)

The amount of AP5 that was available in these first two sets of experiments was so little that we applied the antagonist by ionophoresis, directly into the synaptic region of the slice. However, by the time of my next visit to Bristol, Jeff had synthesized more batches of AP5 and its resolved isomers. We therefore applied these via the perfusate and found that the activity resided in the D isomer and that a concentration of 50 μM was required to fully block the induction of LTP. We also tested the effects of D-AP5 on synaptic responses at a further five excitatory pathways in the hippocampus and found no effect on basal synaptic transmission in any of these (Collingridge *et al.* 1983*b*). It seemed plausible that the concept that NMDA receptors mediate the induction of LTP but not basal synaptic transmission was a general principle. However, before I could test this directly my two-year postdoctorate was over and my application for a Canadian MRC scholarship to continue this work in Vancouver had been turned down. Next port of call—Sydney—and a change of scene to GABA. During this six-month sojourn with Peter Gage I developed an interest in synaptic channel kinetics (Collingridge *et al.* 1984), a subject that I was to return to when Tim Benke suggested using non-stationary fluctuation analysis to investigate the expression mechanism of NMDA receptor-dependent LTP (Benke *et al.* 1998)—but that is another story.

6.2 1984–1985: Gathering excitation

I returned to Bristol, for a faculty position, and was joined in 1984 by two graduate students, Elizabeth Coan and Robin Lester, and a postdoctoral student, Caroline Herron. Although the role of NMDA receptors as a trigger for the induction of LTP was established, and other groups had started to work in this area, the mechanism of their involvement was not known. We therefore set out to try to establish this process. Our first experiment was to omit Mg^{2+} from the perfusate. Evans, Francis and Watkins had already shown that Mg^{2+} was a potent non-competitive NMDA receptor antagonist (Evans *et al.* 1977) and so it seemed reasonable to assume that this ion was somehow involved in the induction process. (Indeed, Stephen Kehl and I had briefly explored the effects of Mg^{2+}-free medium on synaptic transmission in the hippocampus but we saw such an extreme increase in excitability that we assumed that the slice had turned epileptic beyond salvation.) In Bristol, we again noted a dramatic increase in synaptic transmission and the appearance of evoked epileptiform activity. However, significantly most of the increase in excitability was reversed by application of D-AP5 (Coan and Collingridge 1985; see also Herron *et al.* 1985*a*). This told us that NMDA receptors could be activated during basal synaptic transmission but that the presence of Mg^{2+} in the perfusate, in concentrations present in the extracellular fluid, was preventing their activation. What we did not know was what was special about high-frequency stimulation, used to induce LTP.

The paper by Ascher and colleagues was an instant revelation. Nowak *et al.* (1984) showed that the Mg^{2+} block of NMDA receptors was a direct interaction with the ion channel and that this channel block was strongly voltage-dependent, decreasing with depolarization. Thus based on the knowledge that (i) NMDA receptors are the trigger for LTP induction (Collingridge *et al.* 1983*a*), (ii) Mg^{2+} prevents the synaptic activation of NMDA receptors during basal synaptic transmission (Coan and Collingridge 1985), and (iii) the Mg^{2+} block of NMDA receptors is strongly voltage-dependent (Mayer *et al.* 1984; Nowak *et al.* 1984), the first part of the scheme for the induction of LTP fell into place (Collingridge 1985; Fig. 6.1; see also Wigström and Gustafsson 1985). The idea that AMPA receptors provide the depolarization to enable the unblocking of the NMDA receptors during high-frequency synaptic transmission quickly gained widespread acceptance and the scheme has since appeared in many guises. More generally, the concept that NMDA receptors are a coincidence detector of conjoint pre- and postsynaptic activity was established by these experiments.

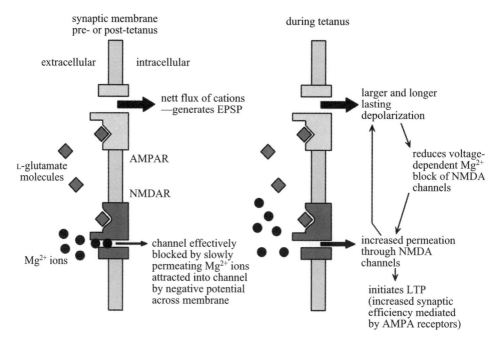

Fig. 6.1 A scheme for the induction of NMDA receptor-dependent LTP. (Redrawn from Collingridge (1985).)

I recall the conversation Caroline Herron and I had in the Highbury Vaults, a watering hole well known to most visitors to Bristol University's Medical School. We wondered why NMDA receptors were not appreciably activated at resting membrane potentials, since the Mg^{2+} block was not complete at -70 mV but intensified as neurons were hyperpolarized. It seemed to us that GABA inhibition provided the reason. The experiment was simple and involved the application of a $GABA_A$ receptor antagonist, which as we expected enabled a single stimulus to elicit an NMDA receptor-mediated response in the presence of Mg^{2+} (Herron et al. 1985b). There was, fortunately, only a short-lived resistance to our proposal that the hyperpolarizing influence of $GABA_A$ receptor-mediated inhibition was more important than the conductance shunt in limiting the synaptic activation of NMDA receptors (which contradicted the textbook view of the role of inhibition at the time). The ability of GABAergic inhibition to limit the synaptic activation of NMDA receptors also explained the earlier finding that GABA antagonists could greatly facilitate the induction of LTP. A logical prediction from these experiments was that artificial depolarization of the neuron should enable the synaptic activation of NMDA receptors despite the presence of synaptic inhibition. We found that this was indeed the case (see below). We were acutely aware that such depolarization would probably enable single shock stimulation to induce LTP and were careful to avoid this complicating factor, which could hinder our analysis of synaptic responses. Others took the view that such a pairing of depolarization and low-frequency synaptic activation provided insights into the 'Hebbian' functioning of these synapses and produced elegant studies demonstrating this (e.g. Kelso *et al.* 1986; Wigström *et al.* 1986).

6.3 1986–1988: Kinetics and competition

At the time that we started working on the induction mechanisms of LTP the prevailing view was that NMDA receptors mediated a slow component of synaptic transmission because they provided excitation via polysynaptic circuits; an idea formed from studies in the spinal cord. In all our schemes we assumed to the contrary that the synaptic activation of NMDA receptors was monosynaptic. The motivation for this was a combination of Occam's razor and the elegant studies of Dale and Roberts (1985) who showed that NMDA receptors mediated a slow monosynaptic EPSP in *Xenopus* motor neurons. Robin Lester, Caroline Herron and I tested this idea directly by blocking $GABA_A$ receptor-mediated inhibition, depolarizing CA1 neurons to remove the Mg^{2+} block and thereby increase the size of the NMDA receptor-mediated component further, voltage-clamping the neuron and applying D-AP5 to block this synaptic component. What was left was a fast, AMPA receptor-mediated EPSC. Subtraction of this synaptic current from the total EPSC revealed, for the first time, a slow rising and decaying NMDA receptor-mediated EPSC (Collingridge *et al.* 1987, 1988*a*). Note that the converse experiment of blocking the AMPA receptor component was not possible at the time as available antagonists were not sufficiently potent.

The kinetics of the NMDA receptor-mediated EPSC spoke volumes. The slow rise explained why there was essentially no synaptic activation during low-frequency stimulation; by the time that the conductance is significantly activated, coactivated GABAergic inhibition hyperpolarizes the neuron into a region of substantial Mg^{2+} block. The slow decay, however, enables effective temporal summation at times when the neuron is not hyper-polarized, in particular, by synaptically released GABA. At about the same time an NMDA receptor-mediated EPSC with slow kinetics was also reported in cultured hippocampal neurons by Forsythe and Westbrook (1988). These authors did not discuss the slow rise of the NMDA receptor-mediated current as they attributed this at the time to a voltage-clamp artefact. We knew the slow rise was not an artefact; the simple experiment showing that blockade of $GABA_A$ inhibition enabled single shock activation of NMDA receptors told us that the regulation had physiological significance. We assumed, but were not in a position to test, that the slow rise and decay of the NMDA receptor-mediated EPSC was an intrinsic property of NMDA receptors. Robin Lester, after leaving my laboratory for a postdoctoral position in the laboratory of Craig Jahr, performed the definitive experiment, which elegantly described the kinetic basis of the slow NMDA receptor-mediated EPSC (Lester *et al.* 1990). I was happy to see our ideas given a sound biophysical basis.

The view that high-frequency stimulation enabled the synaptic activation of NMDA receptors was demonstrated by determining the sensitivity of low- and high-frequency stimulation to AP5. As would be predicted, from the above properties of NMDA receptors, the NMDA receptor-mediated component was visible in the presence of Mg^{2+} and intact synaptic inhibition during high-frequency stimulation (Herron *et al.* 1986). This frequency-dependent synaptic component had the appropriate slow time-course and voltage dependence, and was clearly visible when evoked from resting membrane potentials (Collingridge *et al.* 1988*b*). What was readily apparent, however, was that it was not the algebraic sum of the equivalent number of appropriately spaced low-frequency synaptic responses—the level of depolarization was far too great during high-frequency stimulation given the dominance of synaptic inhibition during low-frequency stimulation.

At around this time, we heard rumours that Tage Honoré had discovered a family of potent and selective AMPA receptor antagonists and was talking about these for the first time at the European Winter Conference on Brain Research (Tignes, France). We therefore booked a ski holiday in Tignes and gate-crashed the session. The quinox-alinedione antagonists were fantastically effective, and Tage kindly let us have a sample of the most selective compound CNQX. This enabled Jo Blake in my laboratory to demonstrate the slow kinetics and monosynaptic nature of the NMDA receptor-mediated synaptic response directly (Blake *et al.* 1988); any lingering doubts of remaining sceptics were fully and finally dispelled.

6.4 1989–1991: Losing one's inhibition

New people joined the laboratory; notably a postdoctoral student, Stephen Davies, and a PhD student, Ceri Davies. Our minds once again turned to synaptic inhibition. It was already known at the time that GABAergic synaptic inhibition was transiently inhibited during periods of repetitive stimulation and the mechanism of this effect was being investigated with respect to epileptiform activity. We wondered if the activity-dependent depression of synaptic inhibition had a physiological function—namely to temporarily suppress the synaptic activation of $GABA_A$ receptor-mediated synaptic inhibition just sufficiently for the appropriate synaptic activation of NMDA receptors (as required to induce LTP). Until that time, synaptic inhibition in the hippocampus had been difficult to study directly, because of the concomitant activation of glutamatergic synapses that both affected synaptic inhibition via polysynaptic activation and produced overlapping synaptic potentials. We needed to be able to study synaptic inhibition without these complications resulting from synaptic excitation. The discovery of CNQX provided us with this opportunity. We blocked both AMPA and NMDA receptor-mediated synaptic transmission, using CNQX and D-AP5, and directly stimulated GABAergic inhibition using an appropriately positioned stimulating electrode (Davies and Collingridge 1989). This led to the characterization of monosynaptic GABAergic inhibition.

To study acute plasticity of the GABAergic system we initially investigated paired-pulse depression of IPSCs. In these studies (Davies *et al.* 1990) we found a pronounced depression of the second IPSC with a maximally effective interval of between 100 and 200 ms (5–10 Hz). Importantly, there was no depression of a second pulse delivered 10 ms after the first, showing that these inhibitory synapses could follow high frequencies (at least 100 Hz) and, therefore, that the depression was due to some active process. The depression induced by a single stimulus had a powerful influence because, at its peak, it could depress inhibition, typically, by 75% and the effect lasted for a few seconds. In addition, it depressed both $GABA_A$ and $GABA_B$ receptor-mediated synaptic inhibition to the same extent. This profile suggested to us that a receptor-mediated presynaptic inhibition was operating. At the time there was no evidence for functional autoreceptors in the central nervous system but the principle was well established in the peripheral nervous system. Also the pharmacological inhibition of neurotransmitter release by various neurotransmitter agonists was well known; indeed, in this context it had been recently shown that activation of $GABA_B$ receptors, using baclofen, resulted in a depression of synaptic inhibition in the hippocampus (Harrison *et al.* 1988). This all pointed to the existence of $GABA_B$ autoreceptors that provided a powerful regulation of the synaptic release of GABA in the hippocampus. Consistent with this hypothesis, paired-pulse inhibition of IPSCs was largely blocked by the best available $GABA_B$ antagonist, 2-hydroxy-saclofen (Davies *et al.* 1990).

The next step was to determine whether this autoreceptor mechanism is responsible for the activity-dependent depression of synaptic inhibition that enables the induction of LTP. For this we required a more potent and selective $GABA_B$ antagonist. As luck would have it, I happened to be sitting next to Mario Pozza, a scientist from Ciba-Geigy, at a conference dinner and mentioned this to him. His company had a long-standing interest in $GABA_B$ receptors and Mario immediately informed me about their latest $GABA_B$ antagonist, CGP35348. Together we set out to test the theory. We reasoned that a 'priming' protocol described by Diamond *et al.* (1988), whereby a single stimulus is delivered approximately 200 ms before a short burst (typically four stimuli at 100 Hz), had temporal characteristics that pointed to a role of $GABA_B$ autoreceptors. Consistent with the hypothesis, CGP35348 prevented the depression of $GABA_A$ receptor-mediated inhibition during the high-frequency burst and fully blocked the induction of priming-induced LTP (Davies *et al.* 1991). As would be predicted from an understanding of the mechanism, $GABA_B$ antagonists do not invariably block the induction of LTP—for example, in the presence of a $GABA_A$ receptor antagonist or during longer high-frequency trains (see Davies and Collingridge (1993, 1996) for a detailed explanation). The role of $GABA_B$ autoreceptors is critically dependent upon the induction parameters employed. They are important when patterns of activation that mimic natural firing activity are used. In this context it is probably no coincidence that the optimal frequency for the $GABA_B$ autoreceptor-mediated depression of synaptic inhibition corresponds to the theta frequency. Therefore, while in many studies (such as those designed to study the expression mechanisms of LTP) $GABA_A$ receptor-mediated inhibition is blocked pharmacologically (with, for example, picrotoxin), from a physiological perspective $GABA_B$ receptors have a crucial role in the induction process—one that has yet to be rigorously explored in the context of learning and memory. From this point onwards we have emphasized the role of activity-dependent changes in synaptic inhibition in the induction of NMDA receptor-dependent LTP (e.g. Collingridge and Singer 1990; Fig. 6.2).

6.5 Afterthoughts: significance of NMDA receptor-dependent LTP

The mechanism of induction of NMDA receptor-dependent LTP seems to have captured the imagination of many neuroscientists. There are probably several reasons for this. Not least, the *Hebbian* properties of synapses can now be given a molecular basis; namely that synaptically released L-glutamate signals presynaptic activity and post-synaptic depolarization indicates the level of postsynaptic activity—with the NMDA

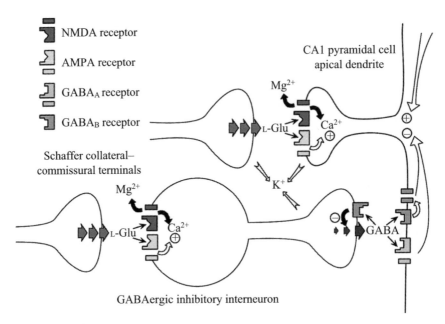

Fig. 6.2 A refinement of the scheme for the induction of NMDA receptor-dependent LTP, incorporating activity-dependent changes in synaptic inhibition. (Redrawn from Collingridge and Singer (1990).)

receptor acting as the coincidence detector. The requirement for L-glutamate to activate the NMDA receptor can explain *input specificity* as depolarization alone will not activate the NMDA receptor; the precision of specificity will be determined by the extent that L-glutamate can 'spill-over' onto neighbouring synapses in sufficient amounts. *Cooperativity* and *associativity* can be explained on the basis that a single input, or small number of inputs, will not be able to provide enough depolarization to sufficiently relieve the Mg^{2+} block of NMDA receptors. However, the coordinated activation of sets of fibres (cooperativity) or the arrival of appropriately timed activity from other pathways (associativity) will provide, or enable, the sufficient depolarization. The coordinated activity is required for the depolarization but not to provide sufficient L-glutamate; the activity of a single synapse provides enough L-glutamate to induce LTP at that synapse—this is clearly demonstrated in a single fibre, pairing experiment where the recording electrode can provide the necessary depolarization to negate the cooperativity requirement of LTP.

The NMDA receptor is clearly important for normal physiological function. Equally clear is how potentially dangerous it can be. If activated inappropriately it may lead to aberrant synaptic plasticity, and such mechanisms may occur during epilepsy—as modelled by kindling. In greater excess, it may lead to death of neurons via the excitotoxic flood of Ca^{2+} into neurons (e.g. Meldrum and Garthwaite 1990). It is widely assumed that this occurs during stroke and trauma, when excessive amounts of L-glutamate act on depolarized neurons. More speculatively, similar mechanisms have been considered to contribute to neurodegenerative disorders. Conversely, it has been considered that hypoactivity of NMDA receptors may contribute to psychiatric and cognitive dysfunction. The finding that phencyclidine is a potent NMDA receptor antagonist (Anis *et al.* 1983) has, given the prominent use of PCP as a model for schizophrenia, led people to wonder whether aberrant NMDA receptor-dependent LTP is at the heart of this disease. Similarly, the idea of boosting NMDA receptor function underpins certain strategies for developing cognitive enhancing drugs. Indeed, the scientific rationale behind 'AMPAkines' is that by facilitating the activity of AMPA receptors this will enhance the synaptic activation of NMDA receptors and hence LTP, as outlined in figure 6.1.

Paradoxically, NMDA receptor antagonists may actually prove beneficial in cognitive disorders, such as Alzheimer's disease. Indeed, the weak NMDA receptor channel blocking agent memantine is used in the clinic for this purpose. Again there is a scientific rationale for this effect. Inappropriate activation of the NMDA receptors, as first modelled by bathing slices in Mg^{2+}-free medium (Coan *et al.* 1989), results in a loss of LTP that can be restored by applying an appropriate dose of an NMDA receptor antagonist (i.e. that is sufficient to dampen down the inappropriate activation but not the coordinated activation of NMDA receptors). This model was used to provide the scientific rationale for the beneficial effects of memantine (Parsons *et al.* 1999).

6.6 Concluding remarks

That, in summary, is how I remember the events of the 1980s. In each case the experiments were carried out to test predictions arising from the hypothesis (rather than the hypothesis being retrospectively created to fit the data). Fortunately, the hypothesis was correct (in the sense that it has gained widespread acceptance). My recollections along the way have been helped by writing the occasional review which, in addition to those listed above, include Collingridge (1987) and Collingridge and Bliss (1987) (which to my amazement was the most cited *Trends in Neurosciences* article in their historical survey of 1995), Collingridge (1992) and Bliss and Collingridge (1993) (which to my even greater amazement was the most cited article in neuroscience during the decade of the brain) and Collingridge and Bliss (1995). The level of citations says a lot about the importance the world's scientific community places on the phenomenal phenomenon of LTP!

I especially thank all my friends who contributed to the work reviewed here—without them none of this would have happened. I also thank the MRC and The Wellcome Trust for their financial support.

References

Anis, N. A., Berry, S. C., Burton, N. R., and Lodge, D. (1983). The dissociative anaesthetics, ketamine and phencyclidine, selectively reduce excitation of central mammalian neurons by N-methyl-aspartate. *Br. J. Pharmacol.* **79**, 565–75.

Benke, T. A., Lüthi, A., Isaac, J. T. R., and Collingridge, G. L. (1998). Modulation of AMPA receptor unitary conductance by synaptic activity. *Nature* **393**, 793–7.

Blake, J. F., Brown, M. W., and Collingridge, G. L. (1988). CNQX blocks acidic amino acid induced depolarizations and synaptic components mediated by non-NMDA receptors in rat hippocampal slices. *Neurosci. Lett.* **89**, 182–6.

Bliss, T. V. P. and Collingridge, G. L. (1993). A synaptic model of memory: long-term potentiation in the hippocampus. *Nature* **361**, 31–9.

Bortolotto, Z. A., Lauri, S., Isaac, J. T. R., and Collingridge, G. L. (2003). Kainate receptors and the induction of mossy fibre long-term potentiation. *Phil. Trans. R. Soc. Lond.* B **358**, 657–66.

Chittajallu, R., Vignes, M., Dev, K. K., Barnes, J. M., Collingridge, G. L., and Henley, J. M. (1996). Regulation of glutamate release by presynaptic kainate receptors in the hippocampus. *Nature* **379**, 78–81.

Clarke, V. R. J. Ballyk, B. A., Hoo, K. H., Mandelzys, A., Pellizzari, A., Bath, C. P., *et al.* (1997). A hippocampal GluR5 kainate receptor regulating inhibitory synaptic transmission. *Nature* **389**, 599–603.

Coan, E. J. and Collingridge, G. L. (1985). Magnesium ions block an N-methyl-D-aspartate receptor-mediated component of synaptic transmission in rat hippocampus. *Neurosci. Lett.* **53**, 21–6.

Coan, E. J., Irving, A. J., and Collingridge, G. L. (1989). Low-frequency activation of the NMDA receptor system can prevent the induction of LTP. *Neurosci. Lett.* **105**, 205–10.

Collingridge, G. L. (1985). Long term potentiation in the hippocampus: mechanisms of initiation and modulation by neurotransmitters. *Trends Pharmacol. Sci.* **6**, 407–11.

Collingridge, G. L. (1987). The role of NMDA receptors in learning and memory. *Nature* **330**, 604–5.

Collingridge, G. L. (1992). The mechanism of induction of NMDA receptor-dependent long-term potentiation in the hippocampus. *Exp. Physiol.* **77**, 771–97.

Collingridge, G. L. and Bliss, T. V. P. (1987). NMDA receptors—their role in long-term potentiation. *Trends Neurosci.* **7**, 288–93.

Collingridge, G. L. and Bliss, T. V. P. (1995). Memories of NMDA receptors and LTP. *Trends Neurosci.* **18**, 54–6.

Collingridge, G. L. and Davies, J. (1979). An evaluation of D-α-aminoadipate and D-(and DL-) α-aminosuberate as selective antagonists of excitatory amino acids in the substantia nigra and mesencephalic reticular formation of the rat. *Neuropharmacology* **18**, 193–9.

Collingridge, G. L. and McLennan, H. (1981). The effect of kainic acid on excitatory synaptic activity in the rat hippocampal slice preparation. *Neurosci. Lett.* **27**, 31–6.

Collingridge, G. L. and Singer, W. (1990). Excitatory amino acid receptors and synaptic plasticity. *Trends Pharmacol. Sci.* **11**, 290–6.

Collingridge, G. L., Kehl, S. J., and McLennan, H. (1983*a*). Excitatory amino acids in synaptic transmission in the Schaffer collateral-commissural pathway of the rat hippocampus. *J. Physiol.* **334**, 33–46.

Collingridge, G. L., Kehl, S. J., and McLennan, H. (1983*b*). The action of an N-methylaspartate antagonist on synaptic processes in the rat hippocampus. *J. Physiol.* (*Lond.*) **338**, 27P.

Collingridge, G. L., Gage, P. W., and Robertson, B. (1984). Inhibitory post-synaptic currents in rat hippocampal CA1 neurones. *J. Physiol.* **356**, 551–64.

Collingridge, G. L., Herron, C. E., and Lester, R. A. J. (1987). NMDA receptor involvement in synaptic potentials evoked by low-frequency stimulation in rat hippocampus *in vitro*. *J. Physiol.* (*Lond.*) **394**, 151P.

Collingridge, G. L., Herron, C. E., and Lester, R. A. J. (1988*a*). Frequency-dependent N-methyl-D-aspartate receptor-mediated synaptic transmission in rat hippocampus. *J. Physiol.* (*Lond.*) **399**, 301–12.

Collingridge, G. L., Herron, C. E., and Lester, R. A. J. (1988*b*). Synaptic activation of N-methyl-D-aspartate receptors in the Schaffer collateral-commissural pathway of rat hippocampus. *J. Physiol.* (*Lond.*) **399**, 283–300.

Dale, N. and Roberts, A. (1985). Dual-component amino acid-mediated synaptic potentials: excitatory drive for swimming in *Xenopus* embryos. *J. Physiol.* (*Lond.*) **363**, 35–59.

Davies, C. H. and Collingridge, G. L. (1993). The physiological regulation of synaptic inhibition by GABA$_B$ autoreceptors in rat hippocampus. *J. Physiol. (Lond.)* **472**, 245–65.

Davies, C. H. and Collingridge, G. L. (1996). Regulation of EPSPs by the synaptic activation of GABA$_B$ autoreceptors in rat hippocampus. *J. Physiol. (Lond.)* **496**, 451–70.

Davies, S. N. and Collingridge, G. L. (1989). Role of excitatory amino acid receptors in synaptic transmission in area CA1 of rat hippocampus. *Proc. R. Soc. Lond.* B **236**, 373–84.

Davies, C. H., Davies, S. N., and Collingridge, G. L. (1990). Paired-pulse depression of monosynaptic GABA-mediated inhibitory postsynaptic responses in rat hippocampus. *J. Physiol.* **424**, 513–31.

Davies, C. H., Starkey, S. J., Pozza, M. F., and Collingridge, G. L. (1991). GABA$_B$ autoreceptors regulate the induction of LTP. *Nature* **349**, 609–11.

Diamond, D. M., Dunwiddie, T. V., and Rose, G. M. J. (1988). Characteristics of hippocampal primed burst potentiation *in vitro* and in the awake rat. *J. Neurosci.* **8**, 4079–88.

Evans, R. H., Francis, A. A., and Watkins, J. C. (1977). Selective antagonism by Mg^{2+} of amino acid-induced depolarizations of spinal neurons. *Experientia* **33**, 489–91.

Forsythe, I. A. and Westbrook, G. L. (1988). Slow excitatory postsynaptic currents mediated by N-methyl-D-aspartate receptors on cultured mouse central neurones. *J. Physiol. (Lond.)* **396**, 515–33.

Harrison, N. L., Lange, G. D., and Barker, J. L. (1988). (−)-Baclofen activates presynaptic GABA$_B$ receptors on GABAergic inhibitory neurons from embryonic rat hippocampus. *Neurosci. Lett.* **85**, 105–9.

Herron, C. E., Lester, R. A. J., Coan, E. J., and Collingridge, G. L. (1985a). Intracellular demonstration of an N-methyl-D-aspartate receptor medicated component of synaptic transmission in the rat hippocampus. *Neurosci. Lett.* **60**, 19–23.

Herron, C. E., Williamson, R., and Collingridge, G. L. (1985b). A selective N-methyl-D-aspartate antagonist depresses epileptiform activity in rat hippocampal slices. *Neurosci. Lett.* **61**, 255–60.

Herron, C. E., Lester, R. A. J., Coan, E. J., and Collingridge, G. L. (1986). Frequency-dependent involvement of NMDA receptors in the hippocampus: a novel synaptic mechanism. *Nature* **322**, 265–8.

Kehl, S. J., McLennan, H., and Collingridge, G. L. (1984). Effects of folic and kainic acids on synaptic responses of hippocampal neurones. *Neuroscience* **11**, 111–24.

Kelso, S. R., Ganong, A. H., and Brown, T. H. (1986). Hebbian synapses in hippocampus. *Proc. Natl Acad. Sci. USA* **83**, 5326–30.

Lester, R. A. J., Clements, J. D., Westbrook, G. L., and Jahr, C. E. (1990). Channel kinetics determine the time course of NMDA receptor-mediated synaptic currents. *Nature* **346**, 565–7.

Mayer, M. L., Westbrook, G. L., and Guthrie, P. B. (1984). Voltage-dependent block by Mg^{2+} of NMDA responses in spinal cord neurones. *Nature* **309**, 261–3.

Meldrum, B. and Garthwaite, J. (1990). Excitatory amino-acid neurotoxicity and neurodegenerative disease. *Trends Pharmacol. Sci.* **11**, 379–7.

Monaghan, D. T., Holets, V. R., Toy, D. W., and Cotman, C. W. (1983). Anatomical distribution of four pharmacologically distinct ^{3}H-L-glutamate binding sites. *Nature* **306**, 176–9.

Nowak, L., Bregestovski, P., Ascher, P., Herbert, A., and Prochiantz, A. (1984). Magnesium gates glutamate-activated channels in mouse central neurones. *Nature* **307**, 462–5.

Parsons, C. G., Danysz, W., and Quack, G. (1999). Memantine is a clinically well tolerated N-methyl-D-aspartate (NMDA) receptor antagonist—a review of preclinical data. *Neuropharmacology* **38**, 735–67.

Wigström, H. and Gustafsson, B. (1985). On long lasting potentiation in the hippocampus: a proposed mechanism for its dependence on coincident pre- and postsynaptic activity. *Acta Physiol. Scand.* **123**, 519–22.

Wigström, H., Gustafsson, B., Huang, Y. Y., and Abraham, W. C. (1986). Hippocampal long-term potentiation is induced by pairing single afferent volleys with intracellularly injected depolarizing current pulses. *Acta Physiol. Scand.* **126**, 317–9.

Glossary

AMPA	α-amino-3-hydroxy-5-methyl-4-isoxazolepropionic acid
AP5	(D,L)-2-amino-5-phosphonopentanoate
DGG	γ-D-glutamylglycine
EPSC	excitatory postsynaptic current
EPSP	excitatory presynaptic potential
fEPSP	field excitatory presynaptic potential
IPSC	inhibitory postsynaptic current
LTP	long-term potentiation
NMDA	N-methyl-D-aspartate

7

Long-term potentiation and memory

Richard G. M. Morris

The discovery of long-term potentiation (LTP) transformed research on the neurobiology of learning and memory. This did not happen overnight, but the discovery of an experimentally demonstrable phenomenon reflecting activity-driven neuronal and synaptic plasticity changed discussions about what might underlie learning from speculation into something much more concrete. Equally, however, the relationship between the discovery of LTP and research on the neurobiology of learning and memory has been reciprocal; for it is also true that studies of the psychological, anatomical and neurochemical basis of memory provided a developing and critical intellectual context for the physiological discovery. The emerging concept of multiple memory systems, from 1970 onwards, paved the way for the development of new behavioural and cognitive tasks, including the watermaze described in this paper. The use of this task in turn provided key evidence that pharmacological interference with an LTP induction mechanism would also interfere with learning, a finding that was by no means a foregone conclusion. This reciprocal relationship between studies of LTP and the neurobiology of memory helped the physiological phenomenon to be recognized as a major discovery.

Keywords: long-term potentiation; learning; memory; spatial memory; watermaze

7.1 Perspectives on memory of 1973 and 2003

The perspective that we have of memory systems in 2003 is radically different from that prevailing in 1973. We now know of several interdependent brain systems that mediate different types of memory and, within these, the distinctive processes of memory encoding, storage, consolidation and retrieval (Schachter and Tulving 1994, pp. 269–310). These include explicit (declarative) and implicit (nondeclarative) systems, and various sub-systems such as those responsible for spatial, episodic and semantic memory on the one hand, and for skill learning and priming on the other. These distinct brain systems have different operating characteristics, distinct patterns of cerebral localization and network architecture, and subserve discrete aspects of cognitive function. In 1973, by contrast, we had little more than a suspicion that learning involved both associative and non-associative mechanisms, and that short- and long-term memory were likely to be mediated by different neuronal mechanisms. The range of behavioural tasks at our disposal to study learning was equally limited, ranging from the word-list learning tasks of the 'verbal learning' era of human psychology through to operant schedules, alleyways and simple mazes for animals.

Observations about human global amnesia were emerging, starting with the seminal observations on patient H.M. (Scoville and Milner 1957). Following a medial temporal lobectomy for the relief of epilepsy, this now extensively studied patient was found to have intact short-term memory, reasonable memory for information acquired earlier in his life, but an apparent inability to form new long-term memories after the operation.

Brenda Milner later advanced what she referred to as a 'consolidation' account in which the hippocampus, this being the brain area most clearly damaged, was held to be critical for transferring information from short- to long-term memory (Milner 1966).

This proposal was not without its problems. First, it was already apparent to Milner by 1970 that H.M. could learn and retain motor skills. Thus, some information was getting through to long-term memory. Second, it was apparent that other amnesic patients, notably those with damage to the mamillary bodies and dorso-medial thalamus, presented with a very severe retrograde amnesia. This led Warrington and Weizkrantz (1968) to advance the then controversial idea that at least some of the memory problems of amnesic patients were due to a failure of retrieval rather than of consolidation. Their argument was that their patients were failing to remember events that, before the onset of their amnesia, they could clearly recall—events such as marriage and the birth of their children. This profile cannot be due to a failure to assimilate information into the long-term memory, but could perhaps be due to dysfunctional retrieval processes.

Neuropsychological studies on animals were proceeding with a range of tasks that, surprisingly, revealed little or no deficits in learning when experimental lesions were made to the hippocampus. This led some researchers to wonder if rodents, and even primates, were different from people in their neuroanatomical organization of mechanisms of learning. At the same time, a revolution was happening in animal learning theory with old behaviourist concepts about the determinants of classical and instrumental conditioning, dating back to Pavlov and Thorndike, in the process of being swept away. New ideas were emerging out of some ingenious experiments, such as Kamin's discovery of 'blocking' (Kamin 1968) and Rescorla's studies of 'contingency effects' in conditioning. These led to a radical new *zeitgeist* beginning with the Rescorla–Wagner theory, in which conditioning was held only to occur when the US that followed the CS was unexpected (Rescorla and Wagner 1972). Although immensely influential in psychological circles, then and to this day, this departure from the notion that the mere coincidence of CSs and USs was all that mattered for associative learning did not impact substantially on physiologists. Later, mathematical modelling of Hebbian and other learning rules contributed to the developing sense that there must be multiple types of learning and memory with different functions.

7.2 The changing perspective around 1973

Several developments led to major changes in the way that the neurobiology of learning and memory was studied in mammals. Numerous papers had an impact, but that impact differed across the various scientific sub-cultures examining the neurobiology of memory. Examples include McGaugh's advocacy of post-training drug administration protocols to explore the neuropharmacology of memory consolidation (McGaugh 1966), Marr's theory of archicortex (Marr 1971), the development of new one-trial recognition memory paradigms for primates (Gaffan 1974; Mishkin and Delacour 1975) and the introduction of the radial maze as a way of looking at short- and long-term spatial memory simultaneously (Olton and Samuelson 1976).

However, I believe that it was physiological findings that really changed the scene: O'Keefe and Dostrovsky's discovery of place cells in the hippocampus (O'Keefe and

Dostrovsky 1971) and Bliss and Lømo's detailed description of long-lasting potentiation (Bliss and Lømo 1973). Over the next decade, as these findings were reproduced by others and the properties of LTP began to be documented, attention in the learning and memory community began to turn from merely asking where learning happened in the brain to identifying the physiological events that might trigger the 'growth process' at neuronal connections that Hebb (1949) had predicted, and the nature of the representations once formed.

7.3 The watermaze

I first met Lynn Nadel and John O'Keefe in 1973. They told me about place cells and emphasized the need for new ways to study spatial learning. I was intrigued by the assertion that was later to become the first two sentences of their 1978 book: 'Space plays a role in all our behaviour. We live in it, move through it, explore it, defend it' (O'Keefe and Nadel 1978). I carried out my last behavioural experiment in an operant chamber in 1972 and have never been tempted back into the world of response rates and schedules of reward and punishment. Instead, I tried to re-invent tasks reminiscent of an earlier era of animal learning in which navigation through extended space was critical, but in a manner that better fitted the new physiological findings. A key issue for me was that place cells fired where they did irrespective of local cues—they could not be strictly sensory cells, whether unimodal or polymodal, they had to depend on some kind of memory processing. However, I also wanted to study the possible relationship between learning and plasticity, rather than just spatial perception and representation. To achieve this, I reasoned, I had to get rid of local cues completely but in a true learning task.

Upon joining the University of St Andrews in Scotland in 1977, I was assigned laboratory space outside the Department in the remarkable but somewhat antiquated Gatty Marine Laboratory located on the West Sands of St Andrews' north facing, and often bleak, shoreline. It was a slightly strange place to work, quite apart from not infrequently having to battle my way down the path along the shore through the winds of a northerly winter gale that had blown in from Russia. Once indoors, I got to my laboratory past tank after tank of sea creatures of various shapes and forms, some of whom might have been the subject of Adrian Horridge's recently completed studies of invertebrate interneurons (Horridge 1968). One day, it occurred to me that rats might be able to learn while swimming and that this might help solve the local cue problem. I wondered if they could escape from water onto a platform that was hidden beneath the water surface and so was neither visible, audible, offered no olfactory cues and could not be identified using somatosensory cues until after the animal had already successfully navigated to it. This might be the solution to the local cue problem.

The first 'watermaze' was built from hardboard and yacht resin by myself with the help of Chris Barman, an animal technician. We completed it in the workshop over the weekend, these being the days when staff still had access to workshops at weekends and Health and Safety Officers were still over the horizon. To my amazement and delight, the rats learned the task very quickly (Fig. 7.1). I ran some essential control conditions and a paper on 'place navigation' followed soon (Morris 1981). The observation that this type of learning is severely impaired by hippocampal lesions was made a year later

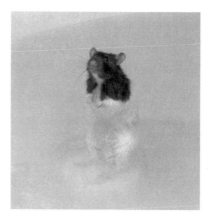

Fig. 7.1 The watermaze. A rat stands on the hidden escape platform inspecting distal cues. After very limited amounts of training, the animal learns to navigate relatively directly to this location in space from any starting point.

(Morris *et al.* 1982). We tracked the animals by tracing a path with a felt-tip pen onto clear film that we had taped over a video monitor. A year or so later, the British Broadcasting Corporation (BBC) introduced the BBC Computer with 128 K of memory and an easily learned software language called BBC Basic. Some colleagues and I wrote a little program and, using a commercially available tracking device that John O'Keefe had used to track place cell firing, we were soon able to track the paths of the swimming rats directly. This was a revelation for, to my knowledge, studies of spatial learning had hitherto relied on observer reports. It was a small step towards better objectivity.

7.4 Using the watermaze to study long-term potentiation and memory

I presented these findings at what came to be known as the 'Schloss Hippocampus' meeting of 1982. This was a meeting at a castle in southern Bavaria owned by the Max-Planck Society at which, in the views of many, the hippocampal field was to change direction irrevocably (Siefert 1983). Until then, work had been very much on the 'septo-hippocampus' with particular emphasis on the cholinergic and other inputs from the midbrain. It was at this meeting that many in the field first heard Carol Barnes describe her tantalizing observations that the persistence of LTP correlated with the persistence of memory in her circular arena task (Barnes 1983), although a journal paper had appeared earlier (Barnes 1979). While there, I met Gary Lynch who mesmerized us all with his remarkable observations on LTP. These included his work confirming the homosynaptic nature of the synaptic change when studied in hippocampal slices *in vitro*, the role of calcium in LTP induction, and the structural changes in spines viewed at the electron microscopic level (Lynch *et al.* 1983*a,b*). It was immediately apparent that LTP was much more than a persistent change in synaptic efficacy induced by tetanic stimulation, as Bliss and Lømo (1973) had described 10 years earlier. It was also a change that was associated, at the point of induction, with an ionic current different from that used to mediate normal synaptic transmission and a change expressed in a manner that could have the very storage capacity required of the network model of Marr (1971) incorporating the Hebb synapse. The following year, Lynch and Baudry (1984) produced their remarkable *Science* paper in which glutamate receptors (*sic.*) were inserted into membranes to express the enhanced synaptic efficacy. If this concept has a contemporary ring to it, bear in mind that the paper is now nearly 20 years old. It is not always cited as often as it should be, perhaps because a cardinal plank of their evidence turned out to be changes in glutamate transport rather than in the expression of the synaptic receptor. However, the concept of a simple postsynaptic mechanism to express the change in synaptic weights had already emerged. Current debates on AMPA receptor trafficking have not moved on conceptually so very far from these early ideas, even if the techniques available now are spectacular by comparison to what was around then.

I resolved to go and work with Lynch and was fortunate to be able to do so in 1984, courtesy of a Medical Research Council Fellowship scheme that released University teaching staff to focus on research for a while. In this, and many other ways, I owe a great deal to the MRC. Lynch's laboratory was then working on a range of projects, including a serine protease inhibitor called leupeptin that was thought to inhibit the proteolytic mechanism that he and Michel Baudry had implicated in the glutamate receptor insertion process. In laboratory experiments on olfactory learning conducted in the Irvine laboratory, I had mixed success, possibly because we were using the very discrimination learning tasks that were proving insensitive to hippocampal lesions in rats and primates. Ursula Staubli was later to have success in using this drug to block LTP (Staubli *et al.* 1988), but its effects on learning were generally quite modest, even in the watermaze (Morris *et al.* 1987). However, while in Irvine, and contrary to the 'house rules' that reflected the friendly rivalry between the Lynch and Cotman laboratories, I discussed these experiments with Eric Harris, then a postdoc with Carl Cotman. He drew my attention to the recently published paper by Collingridge *et al.* (1983) on the role of the NMDA-receptor in LTP and the drug AP5. Sadly, it was time to go home, but Gary and I discussed some experimental options for when I got back to my laboratory.

Upon returning to St Andrews, Jeff Watkins at Bristol University kindly made available a small supply of the racemic mixture of an NMDA-antagonist (D,L-AP5) and I began work. At that point, no one knew whether AP5 would work *in vivo* or, indeed, be very effective in crossing the blood–brain barrier. Its structure did not augur well in this regard. Accordingly, using the same ICV minipump procedure that had been tried in Irvine with leupeptin, I did some acute *in vivo* experiments on dentate LTP. These experiments were exactly as Bliss and Lømo (1973) had carried out long before, but now in the rat rather than the rabbit and after chronically infusing D,L-AP5 or saline for several days. The blockade of LTP *in vivo* was complete, across a range of test pulse intensities, and without any apparent effect on baseline synaptic transmission. I was amazed and excited.

The obvious next step was to try this in swimming rats and, to my delight, Elizabeth Anderson and I found that rats treated with the drug were unable to learn the reference memory spatial version of the watermaze. Those given saline or the inactive isomer, L-AP5, were unimpaired. Strangely, we did not work with D-AP5 at that stage. I cannot remember why. Concerned that the deficit with D,L-AP5 might be sensory in

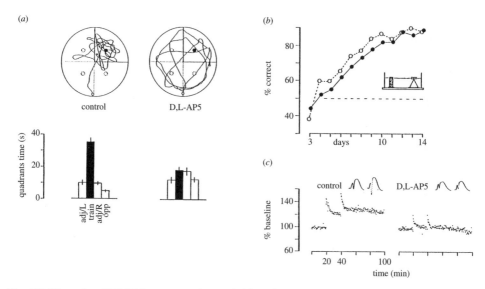

Fig. 7.2 The role of NMDA-receptors in spatial learning. (*a*) An original drawing of the first set of probe test data obtained in the watermaze after chronic infusion of D,L-AP5. (*b*) Normal visual discrimination learning, a task unimpaired by hippocampal lesions. Control represented by open circles; D,L-AP5 infusion results represented by filled circles. (*c*) LTP of f-excitatory post-synaptic potential. Chronic intraventricular infusion of D,L-AP5 blocks dentate gyrus LTP *in vivo*.

nature, I deliberately tried the very discrimination tasks that animals with hippocampal lesions can learn and I observed, now with a mounting sense of disbelief, that they could. Both behavioural experiments were replicated 'blind'. Thus, chronic intraventricular infusions of D,L-AP5 at a dose sufficient to block LTP *in vivo*, without affecting fast synaptic transmission in the hippocampus, caused an apparently selective impairment of hippocampal-dependent place navigation (Fig. 7.2). The animals could see, could move around properly and could learn another equally difficult task, but they could not find their way in a task that needed place cells and apparently required NMDA-receptor-dependent LTP. Gary Lynch came to St Andrews to help write the paper that was published in 1986 (Morris *et al.* 1986). In the same year, McNaughton *et al.* (1986) took a complementary step forward by establishing the causal role of activity-dependent synaptic enhancement in learning in a different way. They observed that prior physiological saturation of LTP impaired subsequent spatial learning. This was to prove a controversial finding, but one for which Bruce McNaughton and his colleagues were later vindicated (Moser *et al.* 1998).

7.5 Reflections

LTP might have turned out to be a physiological curiosity. It might have been a physiological phenomenon that displayed persistence of a duration commensurate with it being a basis for learning, but unrelated to the actual mechanisms used by the brain.

However, there are now two primary reasons for thinking that synaptic plasticity and memory are intimately intertwined (Martin *et al.* 2000; Martin and Morris 2002). First, a generation of work on the physiological properties and cell-biological mechanisms reveals it to possess many other important characteristics of a memory mechanism. The discovery of Bliss and Lømo (1973) did indeed unleash a scientific party as Andersen notes (Andersen 2003). Second, LTP and long-term depression have now been shown to meet at least three of the four criteria that need to be met to establish it as a mechanism that is both 'necessary and sufficient for the information storage underlying the type of memory mediated by the brain area in which that plasticity is observed' (Martin and Morris 2002, p. 609).

(i) Changes in synaptic weights are detectable after learning.
(ii) Interfering with (or altering) the mechanisms responsible for the induction and expression of synaptic plasticity does indeed interfere (or alter) the rate of learning in a variety of relevant learning paradigms.
(iii) Altering the pattern of synaptic weights after learning also affects the ability of animals to remember a previous learning experience.

The fourth criterion, surely not yet met, is mimicry: were it feasible to alter the pattern of synaptic weights in a network in an appropriate manner, the animal should behave as if it remembered something that, in practice, had not happened. Tim Bliss calls this the 'Marilyn Monroe' criterion. This one weakness of the available data apart, a rich array of physiological, pharmacological, molecular engineering and other techniques, allied to behavioural studies, have now tightened up the link between activity-dependent synaptic plasticity and memory to a point where it is reasonable to set aside a scientist's natural scepticism about the central principle.

I was lucky in several ways. I entered the field at a time of great change, and was in a position to profit from the important foundations laid by others. I met several key individuals who advised and very generously helped me, particularly in giving me the opportunity to travel abroad and work in a very exciting laboratory at a critical time. Finally, I also had the good fortune to hold my first university lectureship in a Department with no laboratory space. I love walking along the beach in St Andrews and I look up wistfully at the dark and somewhat forbidding grey, stonewalls of the Gatty Marine Laboratory with secret affection.

The author is grateful to Christopher Barman and Elizabeth Anderson who both helped so much in the early watermaze and AP5 experiments. The author's research group has long been fortunate to have core support from the Medical Research Council, latterly as a Programme Grant. The author is indebted to them.

References

Andersen, P. (2003). A prelude to long-term potentiation. *Phil. Trans. R. Soc. Lond.* B **358**, 613–15. (DOI 10.1098/rstb. 2002.1232.)

Barnes, C. A. (1979). Memory deficits associated with senescence: a neurophysiological and behavioral study in the rat. *J. Comp. Physiol. Psychol.* **93**, 74–104.

Barnes, C. A. (1983). The physiology of the senescent hippocampus. In *Neurobiology of the hippocampus* (ed. W. Siefert), pp. 87–108. London: Academic Press.

Bliss, T. V. P. and Lømo, T. (1973). Long-lasting potentiation of synaptic transmission in the dentate area of the anaesthetized rabbit following stimulation of the perforant path. *J. Physiol. (Lond.)* **232**, 331–56.

Collingridge, G. L., Kehl, S. J., and McLennan, H. (1983). Excitatory amino acids in synaptic transmission in the Schaffer collateral-commissural pathway of the rat hippocampus. *J. Physiol.* **334**, 33–46.

Gaffan, D. (1974). Recognition impaired and association intact in the memory of monkeys after transection of the fornix. *J. Comp. Physiol. Psychol.* **86**, 1100–9.

Hebb, D. O. (1949). *The organization of behavior*. New York: Wiley.

Horridge, A. (1968). *Interneurons*. San Francisco: W. H. Freeman.

Kamin, L. J. (1968). Attention-like processes in classical conditioning. In *Miami Symp. on the prediction of behavior: aversive stimulation* (ed. M. R. Jones), pp. 9–33. University of Miami Press.

Lynch, G. and Baudry, M. (1984). The biochemistry of memory: a new and specific hypothesis. *Science* **224**, 1057–63.

Lynch, G., Halpain, S., and Baudry, M. (1983a). Structural and biochemical effects of high-frequency stimulation in the hippocampus. In *Neurobiology of the hippocampus* (ed. W. Siefert), pp. 253–64. London: Academic Press.

Lynch, G., Larson, J., Kelso, S., Barrionuevo, G., and Schottler, F. (1983b). Intacellular injections of EGTA block induction of hippocampal long-term potentiation. *Nature* **305**, 719–21.

McGaugh, J. L. (1966). Time-dependent processes in memory storage. *Science* **153**, 1351–8.

McNaughton, B. L., Barnes, C. A., Rao, G., Baldwin, J., and Rasmussen, M. (1986). Long-term enhancement of hippocampal synaptic transmission and the acquisition of spatial information. *J. Neurosci.* **6**, 563–71.

Marr, D. (1971). Simple memory: a theory for archicortex. *Phil. Trans. R. Soc. Lond.* B **262**, 23–81.

Martin, S. J. and Morris, R. G. M. (2002). New life in an old idea: the synaptic plasticity and memory hypothesis revisited. *Hippocampus* **12**, 609–36.

Martin, S. J., Grimwood, P. D., and Morris, R. G. (2000). Synaptic plasticity and memory: an evaluation of the hypothesis. *A. Rev. Neurosci.* **23**, 649–711.

Milner, B. (1966). Amnesia following operations on the temporal lobes. In *Amnesia* (ed. O. L. Zangwill and C. W. M. Wa), pp. 109–133. London: Butterworth.

Mishkin, M. and Delacour, J. (1975). An analysis of short-term visual memory in the monkey. *J. Exp. Psychol.* **1**, 326–34.

Morris, R. G. M., Hagan, J. J., Nadel, L., Jensen, J., Baudry, M., and Lynch, G. S. (1987). Spatial learning in the rat: impairment induced by the thiol-proteinase inhibitor, leupeptin, and an analysis of [3H]glutamate receptor binding in relation to learning. *Behav. Neur. Biol.* **47**, 333–45.

Morris, R. G. M. (1981). Spatial localisation does not depend on the presence of local cues. *Learn. Motiv.* **12**, 239–60.

Morris, R. G. M., Garrud, P., Rawlins, J. N. P., and O'Keefe, J. (1982). Place navigation impaired in rats with hippocampal lesions. *Nature* **297**, 681–3.

Morris, R. G. M., Anderson, E., Lynch, G. S., and Baudry, M. (1986). Selective impairment of learning and blockade of longterm potentiation by an N-methyl-D-aspartate receptor antagonist, AP5. *Nature* **319**, 774–6.

Moser, E. I., Krobert, K. A., Moser, M. B., and Morris, R. G. (1998). Impaired spatial learning after saturation of long-term potentiation. *Science* **281**, 2038–42.

O'Keefe, J. and Dostrovsky, J. (1971). The hippocampus as a spatial map. Preliminary evidence from unit activity in the freely-moving rat. *Brain Res.* **34**, 171–5.

O'Keefe, J. and Nadel, L. (1978). *The hippocampus as a cognitive map*. Oxford, UK: Clarendon Press.

Olton, D. S. and Samuelson, R. J. (1976). Remembrance of places passed: spatial memory in rats. *J. Exp. Psychol.* **2**, 97–116.

Rescorla, R. A. and Wagner, A. R. (1972). A theory of Pavlovian conditioning: the effectiveness of reinforcement and nonreinforcement. In *Classical conditioning II: current research and theory* (ed. A. H. Black and W. F. Prokasy), pp. 64–99. New York: Appleton-Century-Crofts.

Schachter, D. and Tulving, E. (1994). *Memory systems*. Cambridge, MA: MIT Press.

Scoville, W. B. and Milner, B. (1957). Loss of recent memory after bilateral hippocampal lesions. *J. Neurol. Neurosurg. Psychiat.* **20**, 11–21.

Siefert, W. (1983). *Neurobiology of the hippocampus*. London: Academic Press.

Staubli, U., Larson, J., Thibault, O., Baudry, M., and Lynch, G. (1988). Chronic administration of a thiol-proteinase inhibitor blocks long-term potentiation of synaptic responses. *Brain Res.* **444**, 153–8.

Warrington, E. K. and Weizkrantz, L. (1968). New method of testing long-term retention with special reference to amnesic patients. *Nature* **217**, 972–4.

Glossary

AMPA α-amino-3-hydroxy-5-methylisoxazole-4-propionic acid
CS   conditioned stimulus
ICV   intracerebroventriculae
LTP   long-term potentiation
NMDA   *N*-methyl-D-aspartate
US   unconditioned stimulus

Induction

8

Bidirectional synaptic plasticity: from theory to reality

Mark F. Bear

Theories of receptive field plasticity and information storage make specific assumptions for how synapses are modified. I give a personal account of how testing the validity of these assumptions eventually led to a detailed understanding of long-term depression and metaplasticity in hippocampal area CA1 and the visual cortex. The knowledge of these molecular mechanisms now promises to reveal when and how sensory experience modifies synapses in the cerebral cortex.

Keywords: long-term depression; metaplasticity; visual cortex; ocular dominance plasticity; Hebb; Bienenstock–Cooper–Munro (BCM) theory

8.1 Hebb synapses as a basis for receptive field plasticity in visual cortex

How are synapses in the cerebral cortex modified by experience to store information? Important clues have come from studies of how neuronal activity changes in response to a changing environment. A consistent finding is that as the environment changes and new information is stored, cells gain responsiveness to some stimuli and lose responsiveness to others. In other words, neuronal receptive fields are modified by experience. These changes in receptive fields reflect synaptic modifications that, distributed over many neurons, store information. Thus, we can reframe the question: what is the synaptic basis of receptive field plasticity in the cerebral cortex?

A good example of receptive field plasticity can be found in the visual cortex during early postnatal life. When a visual cortical neuron receives information from the two eyes that is *correlated*, as is often the case during normal binocular vision, the cell becomes responsive to both eyes. When the correlation breaks down, as occurs during a period of monocular deprivation or strabismus, then the cell becomes monocularly responsive in a 'winner-takes-all' fashion. Thus, input patterns can *associate* or *compete* depending on how well they are correlated (Wiesel 1982). The correlation detector must be the postsynaptic neuron, because it has available information from both eyes, and a reasonable assumption is that the degree of correlation among converging inputs is reflected in the firing rate of the neuron.

In 1949, Donald Hebb postulated that associative memories are formed in the brain by a process of synaptic modification that strengthens connections when presynaptic activity correlates with postsynaptic firing (Hebb 1949). Thus, 'Hebb synapses' were enthusiastically embraced as a likely basis for receptive field plasticity in the visual cortex (and receptive field plasticity in the visual cortex was enthusiastically embraced as a model for associative memory). However, it was also immediately apparent that 'Hebbian' modification alone would not be sufficient to account for receptive field plasticity—there must also exist a synaptic basis for weakening connections when presynaptic activity is poorly correlated with postsynaptic firing. Thus, in 1973 Gunther Stent made the influential proposal that connections weaken when they are inactive at the same time that the postysnaptic neuron is active (owing to the influence of competing inputs). According to this way of thinking, postsynaptic activity, driven by a set of well-correlated inputs, initiates the physiological processes that potentiate the active synapses *and* depress the inactive ones (which, interestingly, Stent envisaged to be the stabilization or elimination of postsynaptic receptors). To account for the effects of the behavioural state on visual cortical plasticity, Wolf Singer (1979) added the provision that postsynaptic activity has to cross a threshold to be permissive for synaptic modifications. Singer, also ahead of his time, made the further suggestion that the permissive postsynaptic factor for receptive field plasticity is dendritic calcium entry.

8.2 Hippocampus and visual cortex collide

I joined Wolf Singer as a post-doctoral fellow in 1984 to investigate the modulation of visual cortical plasticity by cholinergic and noradrenergic inputs. Modulation seemed like a ripe target for establishing a molecular mechanism for visual cortical plasticity. Although I accepted the necessity of assuming that Hebb synapses account for receptive field plasticity, such theories seemed very abstract in the absence of a clue as to how the active postsynaptic neuron could distinguish active from inactive inputs and reward and punish them, respectively. Suddenly, this situation changed, because of three key discoveries made in hippocampal area CA1 between 1983 and 1986. First, induction of LTP became NMDAR and Ca^{2+} dependent; second, NMDARs became detectors of coincident presynaptic and postsynaptic activity; third, and most importantly, LTP became Hebbian (reviewed by Bliss and Collingridge 1993; see also Collingridge 2003). These studies showed that an active (strongly depolarized) neuron could recognize a simultaneously active presynaptic input by the local Ca^{2+} flux through the postsynaptic NMDARs, and reward it by making this synapse stronger.

These discoveries had a huge impact on how we subsequently approached the problem of visual cortical plasticity. LTP became a molecular metaphor for Hebbian plasticity. We started to pay close attention to what was happening in the hippocampus to gain insights into the molecular basis for receptive field plasticity. Additionally, of course, we now had a potential mechanism for Hebbian modifications based on the properties of NMDARs. People started infusing the NMDAR antagonist APV everywhere Hebbian modifications were suspected to occur—into rat hippocampus during learning; into frog optic tectum during development; and, in our case, into kitten visual cortex during a period of monocular deprivation—and there was universal agreement: blocking NMDARs disrupts experience-dependent synaptic plasticity (Morris *et al.* 1986; Cline *et al.* 1987; Kleinschmidt *et al.* 1987).

As Stent had recognized many years before, however, Hebbian modifications are, at most, only half the story. There must also be mechanisms for synaptic depression, certainly to account for the dramatic effects of monocular deprivation in the visual cortex. Students of visual cortical plasticity, unlike many of our hippocampal colleagues, shared a deep conviction that there must also be a mechanism of LTD. However,

I began to have doubts about Stent's specific proposal. According to Stent, synaptic weakening occurs by *heterosynaptic depression*—activity in one set of synpases leads to depression of a second, inactive set. Yet, many studies of LTP in CA1 (my focus, for reasons stated above) had failed to reveal this phenomenon (although it had been reported to occur in the dentate gyrus by Abraham and Goddard (1983)). Closer to home, studies in Singer's laboratory, using a manipulation of visual experience called reverse-suture, showed that monocular deprivation could rapidly depress synaptic responses even when postsynaptic neurons were relatively silent. This finding seemed to violate the principle that postsynaptic activation beyond a threshold is required for receptive field plasticity. I also began to question the precise role of dendritic Ca^{2+} in visual cortical plasticity, which now seemed more likely to be instructive than permissive.

8.3 A physiological basis for the Bienenstock–Cooper–Munro theory

I started to consider alternative ideas, and became interested in a different theory for visual cortical receptive field plasticity, developed by theoretical physicist Leon Cooper and his colleagues. Therefore, when Leon and Ford Ebner offered me a faculty position in their Centre for Neural Science at Brown University, I gladly accepted. We spent much of 1986 discussing the theory, the new understanding of the biology of synaptic transmission in the cortex, and how these might be related. Because we spoke different languages (those of mathematics and biology), these conversations could be painful (eased occasionally by Leon's stash of fine single malt). However, as we came to understand each other, a very interesting picture started to emerge.

As in previous Hebbian models, Cooper *et al.* (1979) had suggested that active synapses grow stronger when postsynaptic activity exceeds a 'modification threshold', θ_m. However, instead of assuming that quiet synapses simultaneously depress, they proposed that depression occurs at presynaptically *active* synapses when postsynaptic activity falls below θ_m (but remains above a lower threshold, defined as zero). Thus, the proposal was that presynaptic activity triggers synaptic depression or potentiation depending on the concurrent level of postsynaptic activity (i.e. the degree of correlation). To explain competition and provide stability, Bienenstock *et al.* (1982), in what is now called the BCM theory, made the additional proposal that the value of θ_m varies as a function of the history of integrated postsynaptic activity. As average activity falls or rises, so does the value of θ_m. I was particularly attracted to this 'sliding threshold' idea, as it seemed to account for the effects of reverse-suture in visual cortex.

How might such a form of modification be implemented by glutamatergic synapses? I considered the possibility that θ_m corresponds to the threshold level of postsynaptic response at which NMDAR-dependent Ca^{2+} flux is sufficient to induce LTP. Two interesting predictions followed. First, input activity that consistently fails to activate postsynaptic neurons (elevate postsynaptic Ca^{2+}) sufficiently to induce LTP should induce LTD instead. Second, the threshold level of stimulation required to achieve LTP should vary depending on the history of cellular activity, which I reasoned could be accomplished by alterations in the voltage- or glutamate-sensitivity of NMDARs. These proposals were published (Bear *et al.* 1987), and testing them was the first priority of my newly established laboratory.

8.4 Homosynaptic long-term depression in hippocampus

My goal was to establish models of synaptic plasticity in slices of visual cortex, copying the approach that had been so successful in area CA1 of the hippocampus. At the time, few data were available on LTP in the neocortex, and I quickly discovered why—they were very difficult to elicit (a problem later solved in my laboratory by Alfredo Kirkwood). Fortunately, in the meantime, Serena Dudek joined me as a graduate student. Serena had spent some time in Gary Lynch's laboratory, so she arrived with considerable hippocampal slice experience. Therefore, we decided to search for LTD in area CA1, where the Hebbian properties of LTP had already been established. Our approach was to emulate the conditions that, in theory, should produce LTD—lots of presynaptic activity under conditions that yield postsynaptic responses too weak to induce LTP. Of course, this was electrophysiology for the resource challenged; we were recording extracellular synaptic field potentials, and had no way of directly manipulating postsynaptic voltage. However, it had been established that LTP is reliably induced by high-frequency stimulation of a bundle of Schaffer collateral axons because the temporal summation of synaptic responses strongly depolarizes postsynaptic neurons in CA1. Therefore, our approach was to vary the frequency, intensity and duration of the synaptic stimulation, searching for the sweet spot that might yield LTD. This is obviously a large parameter space, and despite the additional help of Joel Gold, a Brown undergraduate, many months of failure ensued. However, we were determined. This was one of those cases where to see it, one had to believe in it. We were believers.

The breakthrough came in 1991. We discovered that at an intensity just below threshold for producing population spikes, prolonged stimulation (900 pulses) at 0.5–3 Hz reliably induced LTD in CA1. However, there were some immediate reasons for concern. Previous reports in the literature suggested that similar types of stimulation do not alter baseline synaptic transmission (which we ascribed to significant differences in experimental conditions). More worryingly, however, these same studies reported that a 1 Hz stimulation could be quite effective in reversing LTP if it was delivered shortly after induction (Barrionuevo *et al.* 1980; Staubli and Lynch 1990; Fujii *et al.* 1991). This retrograde disruption of LTP, a phenomenon called depotentiation, could also be produced by such non-specific manipulations as temporary anoxia (Arai *et al.* 1990*b*), bath application of adenosine (Arai *et al.* 1990*a*) or inducing seizure activity (Hesse and Teyler 1976).

Therefore, the challenge became to convince ourselves, and what we anticipated would be a very critical audience of hippocampal physiologists, that LTD indeed was a form of synaptic modification. After all, there are several manipulations that can make synaptic transmission depress that are not synaptic plasticity (frying the fibres with too much stimulation current or bumping the air table, for example). Global changes in slice health were eliminated by demonstrating that the LTD was input specific, and therefore *homosynaptic*. To address the concern of using so many stimulus pulses, Serena varied the frequency while holding the number of pulses constant. Remarkably, she derived a plasticity function that was virtually identical to that proposed in the BCM theory, if we assumed that variations in frequency were translated into variations in postsynaptic response during conditioning stimulation.

The missing piece was mechanism. Our initial hunch was that LTD is triggered by activation of the recently discovered mGluR (Bear 1988; Dudek and Bear 1989). Unfortunately, no good mGluR antagonists were available to test this hypothesis. However, we already had the NMDAR antagonist APV. We made an attempt, reasoning that it should at least shift the frequency–response function. We were utterly amazed to discover that APV blocked induction of LTD. Homosynaptic LTD, like LTP, was NMDAR-dependent! NMDARs were not 'switches', engaged only during Hebbian plasticity, as was commonly believed. Rather, they could function as analogue detectors of the degree of presynaptic and postsynaptic correlation.

We also had an early indication that there might be more to the LTD story in CA1. We consistently found that LTD magnitude increased substantially in slices that were maintained *in vitro* for more than 5–6 h. This LTD caused concern, however, because it could only be partly blocked by APV. In the laboratory, this became known as the 'late-in-the-day effect', and for years we were very mindful to avoid it in our experiments. We now know that the late-in-the-day effect reflects the added contribution of a second form of LTD that is mGluR- and protein-synthesis-dependent (Huber *et al.* 2000). The delayed expression of this LTD *in vitro* remains a mystery, but we believe it reflects the time it takes for protein synthesis to recover from the trauma of slice preparation.

Our findings on NMDAR-dependent LTD were debuted at the Society for Neuroscience Meeting in 1991. I was anxious about how they might be received, as I was a newcomer to the field of hippocampal synaptic plasticity. I gave a preview of the poster to Rob Malenka—a close friend, my roommate for the meeting, and one of the outstanding young hippocampal slice physiologists. His enthusiastic reaction convinced me that we were ready for prime time. We came home and submitted our paper for publication.

8.5 Common forms of synaptic plasticity in hippocampus and neocortex

Serena and I advanced as far as we could with field potential experiments, subsequently showing that CA1 LTD was saturable, reversible, the functional inverse of LTP and age-dependent (Dudek and Bear 1992, 1993). I considered that the next crucial issue was to determine if synapses in our model of receptive field plasticity, the visual cortex, behave like those in CA1. Fortunately, by this time Alfredo Kirkwood had discovered how to reliably elicit LTP in layer III of the visual cortex. We went on to demonstrate that visual cortical LTP is Hebbian, that LTP and LTD could be reliably elicited with high- and low-frequency stimulation, respectively, and that both forms of synaptic plasticity are NMDAR-dependent (Kirkwood *et al.* 1993; Kirkwood and Bear 1994*a,b*). Thus, it appeared that insights gained by the study of CA1 could indeed be applied to the visual cortex and the problem of receptive field plasticity.

Subsequent work from several laboratories, in species ranging from mice to humans, revealed that very similar principles guide synaptic plasticity in widely different regions of the cerebral cortex. As Leon Cooper had originally proposed, active synapses can be bidirectionally modified as a function of postsynaptic voltage. This plasticity occurs because voltage provides graded control of the NMDAR-dependent changes in

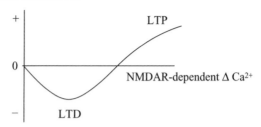

Fig 8.1 Function that governs the bidirectional modification of synaptic transmission mediated by AMPARs at glutamatergic synapses in area CA1 of the hippocampus and the superficial layers of the neocortex.

postsynaptic Ca^{2+} that trigger LTD or LTP (Fig. 8.1). In a colloquium paper I suggested we refer to bidirectionally modifiable synapses with these properties as 'Cooper synapses' for obvious reasons (Bear 1996). I remember Eric Kandel remarking at the time that he did not think the name would catch on. He was right.

8.6 Metaplasticity and the sliding modification threshold

Our characterization of bidirectional synaptic plasticity in layer III of the visual cortex had finally put us in a position to test the next key assumption of the BCM theory: the sliding modification threshold. If this idea is correct, reducing average visual cortical activity by a period of binocular deprivation should alter the properties of synaptic plasticity, favouring LTP over LTD. We confirmed this prediction, showing that binocular deprivation shifts the LTP threshold to lower stimulation frequencies, and that this can be reversed by restoring normal vision (Kirkwood *et al.* 1996). Thus, all the key assumptions of the BCM theory had now been validated: (i) active synapses are bidirectionally modifiable; (ii) the sign or polarity of the modification (LTD or LTP) depends on the level of postsynaptic response relative to a modification threshold; and (iii) the value of the modification threshold varies with the history of cortical activity.

The sliding threshold of the BCM theory is an example of what Cliff Abraham and I called *metaplasticity*, the plasticity of synaptic plasticity (Abraham and Bear 1996). There is now abundant evidence from several systems that the properties of synaptic plasticity depend importantly on the recent history of synaptic or cellular activity. In the visual cortex, we have identified an attractive mechanism for the sliding threshold, based on experience-dependent alterations in NMDARs. Ben Philpot has recently shown that unitary NMDAR-mediated EPSCs are slowed after a period of binocular deprivation, and that restoring normal vision rapidly reverses this change. These relatively small changes in kinetics have a large impact on EPSC summation (and therefore Ca^{2+} entry) at different stimulation frequencies (Philpot *et al.* 2001). Ben and Betsy Quinlan further found that the changes in NMDAR properties are probably explained by alterations in the subunit composition of synaptically expressed receptors. Receptors containing the NR2A subunit are delivered to synapses by visual experience, and are replaced by NR2B-containing receptors after a period of binocular deprivation (Quinlan *et al.* 1999*a,b*; Fig. 8.2). These changes in subunit composition alter the affinity of the receptor for glutamate (we made a good guess in 1987); however, it remains to be determined if the modifications of EPSC duration are alone responsible for the observed metaplasticity in the visual cortex. This question is now being examined using mice in which NMDARs have been genetically modified.

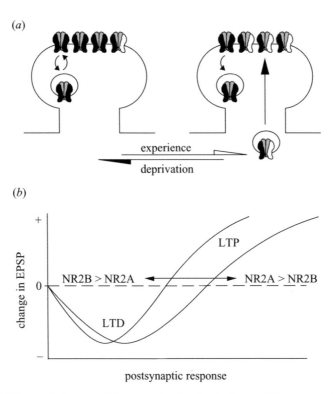

Fig. 8.2 NMDAR regulation provides a molecular basis for a sliding synaptic modification threshold in visual cortex. (*a*) In the absence of visual experience, high constituitive expression of NR2B (black subunits) and reduced expression of NR2A (white subunits) leads to an increase in NR1/NR2B diheteromeric NMDARs at the synapse, and slower NMDAR-mediated EPSCs. Visual experience triggers increased NR2A expression and the rapid delivery of NR1/NR2A/ NR2B triheteromeric receptors to the synapse, compensated by a net loss of surface NR1/NR2B diheteromers. (*b*) Model relating NMDAR subunit regulation to the properties of synaptic modification. The *y*-axis represents the lasting change in synaptic strength following conditioning stimulation at different levels of integrated postsynaptic response (*x*-axis). The curves are schematized from the data of Kirkwood *et al.* (1996). An increase in the NR2A/B ratio, as seen with light exposure after a period of dark-rearing, is proposed to be responsible for sliding the LTD–LTP crossover point (θ_m) to the right, thus decreasing the likelihood that synaptic strengthening will occur. Conversely, a fall in the NR2A/B ratio, as seen with binocular deprivation, slides θ_m to the left, favouring LTP over LTD. According to this model, the properties of synaptic modification depend upon the history of cortical activity, as originally proposed in the BCM theory, because of the activity-dependent expression of NR2A-containing NMDARs at cortical synapses. (Figure adapted from Philpot *et al.* (2001).)

8.7 Altered AMPAR function during LTD

One of the things that made the discovery of LTD in the hippocampus exciting is that it appeared to be the mirror image of LTP, at least for AMPAR-mediated transmission. Thus, the study of LTD potentially offered a new way to address some of the sticky issues of the day, such as the site of LTP expression. At the time that LTD was discovered, it was believed that postsynaptic calcium/calmodulin-dependent protein kinase II (CaMKII) activity was essential for LTP induction. Inspired by a proposal from John Lisman (1989), Rob Malenka went on to show that LTD induction requires activation of a postsynaptic phosphatase cascade (Mulkey et al. 1994). These findings suggested that synaptic strength is bidirectionally regulated by the phosphorylation state of a set of postsynaptic proteins. The phosphoprotein of greatest interest was the postsynaptic AMPAR (Bear and Malenka 1994).

This set the stage for a memorable meeting I had with Rick Huganir during a visit to Johns Hopkins University in 1993. His laboratory had characterized multiple phosphorylation sites on the GluR1 subunit of AMPARs, and they were developing phosphorylation site-specific antibodies. He ushered me into his office, closed the door and started pressing me for information on how he might pharmacologically induce LTP in hippocampal slices. His idea was to induce LTP at a large population of synapses, and then use the phosphorylation site-specific antibodies to detect changes in receptor phosphorylation. I offered my opinion that this approach would be difficult, because LTP seems to require brief increases in postsynaptic Ca^{2+} that are difficult to achieve with bath applied drugs. A few days later, however, it suddenly occurred to me that LTD, which was induced by prolonged stimulation of NMDARs, might be more amenable to this approach. Hey-Kyoung Lee accepted the challenge, and was able to demonstrate that brief bath application of NMDA can induce LTD at a large population of CA1 synapses.

We went on to show that GluR1 was indeed dephosphorylated after induction of LTD. To our surprise, however, it was not the CaMKII site (ser-831) on GluR1 that was altered, but the PKA site (ser-845) instead (Lee et al. 1998). In subsequent experiments, we demonstrated that synaptically induced LTD and LTD reversal (dedepression) are induced by dephosphorylation and phosphorylation, respectively, of postsynaptic PKA substrates (Kameyama et al. 1998; Lee et al. 2000). These findings contrast with LTP and depotentiation, which are associated with bidirectional regulation of the CaMKII site on GluR1 (Barria et al. 1997; Lee et al. 2000). LTD and LTP are not, therefore, mirror symmetric (Fig. 8.3).

More recently, studies performed on hippocampal neurons in culture have revealed that AMPARs dephosphorylated at GluR1 ser-845 are rapidly internalized in response to NMDAR activation (Ehlers 2000). As in LTD, this change can be mimicked by inhibiting, and reversed by activating, PKA. Current opinion is that a reduction in the number of postsynaptic AMPARs is likely to be the major expression mechanism for LTD (Malinow and Malenka 2002). Consistent with this notion, Arnie Heynen and Betsy Quinlan showed that a redistribution of synaptic AMPAR protein occurs after induction of LTD in CA1 of adult rats in vivo (Heynen et al. 2000). These findings are important because they demonstrate that LTD has a molecular fingerprint that can be detected in vivo. As will be discussed, this information can be used to determine if naturally occurring synaptic modifications use the same mechanism.

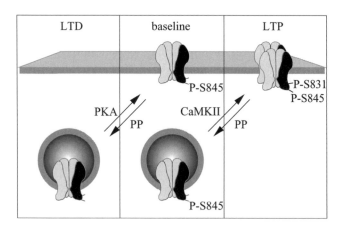

Fig. 8.3 Model of bidirectional modifications of AMPAR phosphorylation and surface expression during LTD and LTP. In the basal state, ser-845 of the GluR1 subunit (shaded black) is phosphorylated. Induction of LTD leads to dephosphorylation of ser-845 by protein phosphastases (PP) and the internalization of AMPARs. These changes can be reversed by activating PKA. By contrast, induction of LTP from the basal state alters phosphorylation of the CaMKII site on GluR1, ser-831. CaMKII activation also leads to the delivery of AMPARs to the surface.

8.8 Is long-term depression a substrate for receptive field plasticity in visual cortex?

The BCM theory, devised to account for receptive field plasticity in the visual cortex, has obviously been very influential by pointing us in directions we might not have explored otherwise. In addition to being a guiding light, a theory can serve as a bridge to connect the molecular mechanisms of synaptic plasticity with their functional consequences. Implementing the BCM theory in neural network models shows that the mechanisms of LTP, LTD and metaplasticity *can* account for receptive field plasticity. However, the difficult experimental question remains, *do they*?

In 1997, a group of experts gathered at a Dahlem conference in Berlin to debate what formal criteria must be met to conclude that LTP is a substrate for learning. Simply stated, it was decided that: (i) learning must induce LTP; and (ii) induction of LTP must produce learning. Obviously this group was not concerned with the practicalities of achieving these standards. Satisfying them requires that we be able to measure and induce LTP in the selected population (which could be large and widely dispersed) of synapses that are modified during learning. A third criterion, that *the mechanism of LTP must be necessary for learning*, is more easily achieved. However, it is based on the assumption that LTP might be the *only* mechanism for a particular type of learning. Finding that learning survives the deletion of LTP would not be grounds for rejecting the hypothesis that LTP is a substrate for learning (Carew *et al.* 1998).

We are tackling a conceptually similar problem in the visual cortex. Is LTD a substrate for receptive field plasticity? One of the interesting predictions of the BCM theory is that the synaptic depression induced by monocular deprivation is not a consequence of retinal inactivity, as Stent assumed, but rather is caused by the residual 'noise' in the deprived eye. Cindi Rittenhouse confirmed this prediction by showing that inactivation of the retina with tetrodotoxin produces much less synaptic depression in the cortex than does simply closing the eyelid. Thus, deprivation-induced synaptic depression, like LTD, is homosynaptic (Rittenhouse *et al.* 1999). These findings then led us to wonder whether visual deprivation also triggers the same molecular changes as LTD. Remarkably, Arnie Heynen and Bongjune Yoon were able to show that 24 h of monocular deprivation during a sensitive period of postnatal life precisely mimics NMDAR-dependent LTD for altered phosphorylation and decreased neuronal surface expression of AMPARs. Cheng-Hang Liu went on to find that the changes induced by monocular deprivation occlude the subsequent expression of homosynaptic LTD at synapses *ex vivo* (Heynen *et al.* 2003). These findings demonstrate that *monocular deprivation induces LTD*.

The primary functional consequence of brief monocular deprivation is a reduction in visually evoked responses through the deprived eye. What are the functional consequences of inducing LTD? Arnie and Bongjune have recently found that prolonged low-frequency stimulation of the dorsal LGN, the thalamic relay of visual information, will induce NMDAR-dependent LTD of LGN-evoked field potentials and dephosphorylation of GluR1 ser-845 in primary visual cortex (Heynen *et al.* 2003). We also found that *induction of LTD produces a reduction in visually evoked responses*, comparable to that caused by monocular deprivation.

Work is in progress to establish if the third Dahlem criterion will also be met, with the caveats already mentioned above. In the meantime, we can reconstruct, at least in part, the molecular chain of events that is set in motion by monocular deprivation in the visual cortex. The data support a model in which the activity in the deprived retina, relayed to the visual cortex by the LGN, weakly activates postsynaptic NMDARs. The activation is weak because it rarely correlates with responses evoked by visual stimulation of the open eye. Activated NMDARs admit Ca^{2+} ions into the postsynaptic neuron that, in turn, regulate a network of protein phosphatases and kinases. Among the consequences of the modest rise in intracellular calcium is dephosphorylation of postsynaptic PKA substrates, including ser-845 of the AMPAR GluR1 subunit, and the net loss of synaptic glutamate receptors. Consequently, the deprived eye no longer effectively drives synaptic excitation in the visual cortex.

8.9 Concluding remark

None of the theories discussed here—those of Hebb, Stent and Cooper—provide a complete description of receptive field plasticity and information storage in the cerebral cortex (see Shouval *et al.* 2002). However, they all provided a framework that helped guide us towards the questions that are most relevant. Hebb's theory for a synaptic basis for memory in the cerebral cortex motivated the characterization of LTP by Bliss and Lømo (1973). The BCM theory motivated our characterization of LTD and the sliding modification threshold. These theories have been extraordinarily useful because they are simple enough for the consequences to be traced to assumptions, and concrete enough to be tested experimentally.

The author acknowledges his mentors, Ford Ebner, Wolf Singer, and Leon Cooper, current faculty colleagues Barry Connors, Michael Paradiso, Arnold Heynen, Ben Philpot, and

Harel Shouval, assistants Suzanne Meagher and Erik Sklar, and all the students and post-doctoral students in his laboratory who carried out the work. The research described in this article was supported by the National Institutes of Health, the US Office of Naval Research and the Howard Hughes Medical Institute.

References

Abraham, W. and Bear, M. (1996). Metaplasticity: the plasticity of synaptic plasticity. *Trends Neurosci.* **19**, 126–30.

Abraham, W. C. and Goddard, G. V. (1983). Asymmetric relationships between homosynaptic long-term potentiation and heterosynaptic long-term depression. *Nature* **305**, 717–9.

Arai, A., Kessler, M., and Lynch, G. (1990*a*). The effects of adenosine on the development of long-term potentiation. *Neurosci. Lett.* **119**, 41–4.

Arai, A., Larson, J., and Lynch, G. (1990*b*). Anoxia reveals a vulnerable period in the development of long-term potentiation. *Brain Res.* **511**, 353–357.

Barria, A., Muller, D., Derkach, V., Griffith, L. C., and Soderling, T. R. (1997). Regulatory phosphorylation of AMPA-type glutamate receptors by CaM-KII during long-term potentiation. *Science* **276**, 2042–5.

Barrionuevo, G., Schottler, F., and Lynch, G. (1980). The effects of low frequency stimulation on control and 'potentiated' synaptic responses in the hippocampus. *Life Sci.* **27**, 2385–91.

Bear, M. F. (1988). Involvement of excitatory amino acid receptor mechanisms in the experience-dependent development of visual cortex. In *Frontiers in excitatory amino acid research* (ed. E. A. Cavalheiro, J. Lehmann and L. Turski), pp. 393–401. New York: Alan R. Liss.

Bear, M. F. (1996). A synaptic basis for memory storage in the cerebral cortex. *Proc. Natl Acad. Sci. USA* **93**, 13 453–9.

Bear, M. F. and Malenka, R. C. (1994). Synaptic plasticity: LTP and LTD. *Curr. Opin. Neurobiol.* **4**, 389–99.

Bear, M. F., Cooper, L. N., and Ebner, F. F. (1987). A physiological basis for a theory of synaptic modification. *Science* **237**, 42–8.

Bienenstock, E. L., Cooper, L. N., and Munro, P. W. (1982). Theory for the development of neuron selectivity: orientation specificity and binocular interaction in visual cortex. *J. Neurosci.* **2**, 32–48.

Bliss, T. V. P. and Collingridge, G. L. (1993). A synaptic model of memory: long-term potentiation in the hippocampus. *Nature* **361**, 31–9.

Bliss, T. V. P. and Lømo, T. (1973). Long-lasting potentiation of synaptic transmission in the dentate area of the anaethetized rabbit following stimulation of the perforant path. *J. Physiol.* **232**, 331–56.

Carew, T. J., Menzel, R., and Shatz, C. J. (ed.) (1998). *Mechanistic relationships between development and learning.* New York: Wiley.

Cline, H. T., Debski, E., and Constantine-Paton, M. (1987). NMDA receptor antagonist desegregates eye-specific stripes. *Proc. Natl Acad. Sci. USA* **84**, 4342–5.

Collingridge, G. L. (2003). The induction of *N*-methyl-D-aspartate receptor-dependent long-term potentiation. *Phil. Trans. R. Soc. Lond.* B **358**, 635–41. (DOI 10.1098/rstb.2002. 1241.)

Cooper, L. N., Liberman, F., and Oja, E. (1979). A theory for the acquisition and loss of neuron specificity in visual cortex. *Biol. Cybern.* **33**, 9–28.

Dudek, S. M. and Bear, M. F. (1989). A biochemical correlate of the critical period for synaptic modification in the visual cortex. *Science* **246**, 673–5.

Dudek, S. M. and Bear, M. F. (1992). Homosynaptic long-term depression in area CA1 of hippocampus and effects of N-methyl-D-aspartate receptor blockade. *Proc. Natl Acad. Sci. USA* **89**, 4363–7.

Dudek, S. M. and Bear, M. F. (1993). Bidirectional long-term modification of synaptic effectiveness in the adult and immature hippocampus. *J. Neurosci.* **13**, 2910–8.

Ehlers, M. D. (2000). Reinsertion or degradation of AMPA receptors determined by activity-dependent endocytic sorting. *Neuron* **28**, 511–25.

Fujii, S., Saito, K., Miyakawa, H., Ito, K.-I., and Kato, H. (1991). Reversal of long-term potentiation (depotentiation) induced by tetanus stimulation of the input to CA1 neurons of guinea pig hippocampal slices. *Brain Res.* **555**, 112–22.

Hebb, D. O. (1949). *Organization of behavior.* New York: Wiley.

Hesse, G. W. and Teyler, T. J. (1976). Reversible loss of hippocampal long term potentiation following electroconvulsive seizures. *Nature* **264**, 562–4.

Heynen, A. J., Quinlan, E. M., Bae, D. C., and Bear, M. F. (2000). Bidirectional, activity-dependent regulation of glutamate receptors in the adult hippocampus *in vivo. Neuron* **28**, 527–6.

Heynen, A. J., Yoon, B.-J., Liu, C.-H., Chung, H. J., Huganir, R. L., and Bear, M. F. (2003). Molecular mechanism for loss of visual cortical responsiveness following brief monocular deprivation. *Nature Neurosci* **6**, 854–62.

Huber, K. M., Kayser, M. S., and Bear, M. F. (2000). Role for rapid dendritic protein synthesis in hippocampal mGluR-dependent long-term depression. *Science* **288**, 1254–7.

Kameyama, K., Lee, H. K., Bear, M. F., and Huganir, R. L. (1998). Involvement of a post-synaptic protein kinase A substrate in the expression of homosynaptic long-term depression. *Neuron* **21**, 1163–75.

Kirkwood, A. and Bear, M. F. (1994*a*). Hebbian synapses in visual cortex. *J. Neurosci.* **14**, 1634–45.

Kirkwood, A. and Bear, M. F. (1994*b*). Homosynaptic long-term depression in the visual cortex. *J. Neurosci.* **14**, 3404–12.

Kirkwood, A., Dudek, S. M., Gold, J. T., Aizenman, C. D., and Bear, M. F. (1993). Common forms of synaptic plasticity in the hippocampus and neocortex *in vitro. Science* **260**, 1518–21.

Kirkwood, A., Rioult, M. G., and Bear, M. F. (1996). Experience-dependent modification of synaptic plasticity in visual cortex. *Nature* **381**, 526–8.

Kleinschmidt, A., Bear, M. F., and Singer, W. (1987). Blockade of 'NMDA' receptors disrupts experience-dependent modifications of kitten striate cortex. *Science* **238**, 355–8.

Lee, H. K., Kameyama, K., Huganir, R. L., and Bear, M. F. (1998). NMDA induces long-term synaptic depression and dephosphorylation of the GluR1 subunit of AMPA receptors in hippocampus. *Neuron* **21**, 1151–62.

Lee, H. K., Barbarosie, M., Kameyama, K., Bear, M. F., and Huganir, R. L. (2000). Regulation of distinct AMPA receptor phosphorylation sites during bidirectional synaptic plasticity. *Nature* **405**, 955–9.

Lisman, J. (1989). A mechanism for the Hebb and the anti-Hebb processes underlying learning and memory. *Proc. Natl Acad. Sci. USA* **86**, 9574–8.

Malinow, R. and Malenka, R. C. (2002). AMPA receptor trafficking and synaptic plasticity. *A. Rev. Neurosci.* **25**, 103–26.

Morris, R. G. M., Anderson, E., Lynch, G. S., and Baudry, M. (1986). Selective impairment of learning and blockade of long-term potentiation by an N-methyl-D-aspartate receptor antagonist, APV. *Nature* **319**, 774–6.

Mulkey, R. M., Endo, S., Shenolikar, S., and Malenka, R. C. (1994). Calcineurin and inhibitor-1 are components of a protein-phosphatase cascade mediating hippocampal LTD. *Nature* **369**, 486–8.

Philpot, B. D., Sekhar, A. K., Shouval, H. Z., and Bear, M. F. (2001). Visual experience and deprivation bidirectionally modify the composition and function of NMDA receptors in visual cortex. *Neuron* **29**, 157–69.

Quinlan, E. M., Olstein, D. H., and Bear, M. F. (1999*a*). Bidirectional, experience-dependent regulation of N-methyl-D-aspartate receptor subunit composition in the rat visual cortex during postnatal development. *Proc. Natl Acad. Sci. USA* **96**, 12 876–80.

Quinlan, E. M., Philpot, B. D., Huganir, R. L., and Bear, M. F. (1999*b*). Rapid, experience-dependent expression of synaptic NMDA receptors in visual cortex *in vivo. Nature Neurosci.* **2**, 352–7.

Rittenhouse, C. D., Shouval, H. Z., Paradiso, M. A., and Bear, M. F. (1999). Monocular deprivation induces homosynaptic long-term depression in visual cortex. *Nature* **397**, 347–50.

Shouval, H. Z., Bear, M. F., and Cooper, L. N. (2002). A unified model of NMDA receptor-dependent bidirectional synaptic plasticity. *Proc. Natl Acad. Sci. USA* **99**, 10 831–6.

Singer, W. (1979). Central-core control of visual cortex functions. In *The neurosciences fourth study program* (ed. F. O. Schmitt and F. G. Worden), pp. 1093–109. Cambridge, MA: MIT Press.

Staubli, U. and Lynch, G. (1990). Stable depression of potentiated synaptic responses in the hippocampus with 1–5 Hz stimulation. *Brain Res.* **513**, 113–8.

Stent, G. S. (1973). A physiological mechanism for Hebb's postulate of learning. *Proc. Natl Acad. Sci. USA* **70**, 997–1001.

Wiesel, T. N. (1982). Postnatal development of the visual cortex and the influence of the environment. *Nature* **299**, 583–92.

Glossary

AMPAR	α-amino-3-hydroxy-5-methylisoxazole-propionic acid receptor
APV	2-amino-5-phosphonovaleric acid
BCM	Bienenstock–Cooper–Munro
EPSC	excitatory postsynaptic current
LGN	lateral geniculate nucleus
LTD	long-term depression
LTP	long-term potentiation
mGluR	metabotropic glutamate receptor
NMDA	*N*-methyl-D-aspartate
NMDAR	*N*-methyl-D-aspartate receptor
PKA	protein kinase A

9

Kainate receptors and the induction of mossy fibre long-term potentiation

Zuner A. Bortolotto, Sari Lauri, John T. R. Isaac, and Graham L. Collingridge

There is intense interest in understanding the molecular mechanisms involved in long-term potentiation (LTP) in the hippocampus. Significant progress in our understanding of LTP has followed from studies of glutamate receptors, of which there are four main subtypes (α-amino-3-hydroxy-5-methyl-4-isoxazolepropionic acid (AMPA), N-methyl-D-aspartate (NMDA), mGlu and kainate). This article summarizes the evidence that the kainate sub-type of glutamate receptor is an important trigger for the induction of LTP at mossy fibre synapses in the CA3 region of the hippocampus. The pharmacology of the first selective kainate receptor antagonists, in particular the GLU_{K5} subunit selective antagonist LY382884, is described. LY382884 selectively blocks the induction of mossy fibre LTP, in response to a variety of different high-frequency stimulation protocols. This antagonist also inhibits the pronounced synaptic facilitation of mossy fibre transmission that occurs during high-frequency stimulation. These effects are attributed to the presence of presynaptic GLU_{K5}-subunit-containing kainate receptors at mossy fibre synapses. Differences in kainate receptor-dependent synaptic facilitation of AMPA and NMDA receptor-mediated synaptic transmission are described. These data are discussed in the context of earlier reports that glutamate receptors are not involved in mossy fibre LTP and more recent experiments using kainate receptor knockout mice, that argue for the involvement of GLU_{K6} but not GLU_{K5} kainate receptor subunits. We conclude that activation of pre-synaptic GLU_{K5}-containing kainate receptors is an important trigger for the induction of mossy fibre LTP in the hippocampus.

Keywords: synaptic plasticity; long-term potentiation; hippocampus; glutamate

9.1 Introduction

Since its discovery, first documented in full 30 years ago (Bliss and Lømo 1973; Bliss and Gardner-Medwin 1973), LTP has become the most popular experimental model for understanding the synaptic processes that are involved in learning and memory and many other functions of the nervous system (Bliss and Collingridge 1993). Two distinct forms have since been identified in the mammalian CNS, which are distinguished by their induction mechanisms. The most widely expressed form of LTP is induced by the synaptic activation of NMDA receptors (Collingridge *et al.* 1983). The mechanism of induction of NMDA receptor-dependent LTP is established, and has been described elsewhere (Collingridge 1985; Bliss and Collingridge 1993; see also Chapter 6, this volume). The other form of LTP is distinguished by its independence from the synaptic activation of NMDA receptors. The best characterized form of NMDA receptor-independent LTP is at mossy fibre synapses in the hippocampus (Harris and Cotman 1986). Recent experiments have begun to shed light on the induction mechanisms of

LTP at this synapse, and in particular the role of kainate receptors. We summarize our experiments that led to the discovery of the role of kainate receptors in the induction of LTP, and in the related synaptic facilitation, at mossy fibre synapses, and present previously unpublished information obtained during the course of these experiments.

Early work suggested that mossy fibre LTP was independent of the activation of glutamate receptors since it could be induced during application of glutamate receptor antagonists such as kynurenic acid and CNQX (Ito and Sugiyama 1991; Castillo *et al.* 1994; Weisskopf and Nicoll 1995; Yeckel *et al.* 1999). Indeed, one simple model proposed that mossy fibre LTP was triggered by Ca^{2+} entry into the presynaptic terminal via entry through voltage-gated Ca^{2+} channels. However, we were always intrigued by the observation that the mossy fibre pathway was strikingly different from other hippocampal pathways in that it was associated with a relatively low density of NMDA receptor binding sites and an extremely high density of kainate receptor binding sites (Monaghan and Cotman 1982). We therefore wondered whether kainate receptors might serve an analogous function to NMDA receptors at other hippocampal pathways; namely, act as a trigger for the induction of mossy fibre LTP. However, to explore this possibility required the development of selective kainate receptor antagonists.

9.2 Kainate receptor pharmacology

Pharmacological experiments clearly identified kainate receptors as a distinct class of glutamate receptor (Davies *et al.* 1979; McLennan and Lodge 1979), which together with AMPA and NMDA receptors constitute the three classes of ionotropic glutamate receptors present in the CNS (Watkins and Evans 1981). Molecular cloning revealed five kainate receptor subunits (Bettler and Mulle 1995), which are named, according to IUPHAR nomenclature (Lodge and Dingledine 2000), GLU_{K5}, GLU_{K6}, GLU_{K7}, GLU_{K1} and GLU_{K2} (also known as GluR5 or iGlu5, GluR6 or iGlu6, GluR7 or iGlu7, KA-1 and KA-2, respectively). These subunits may exist as certain homomeric assemblies, although native receptors are most likely to be heteromeric assemblies. Kainate is a potent agonist at both AMPA and kainate receptors. However, its actions on kainate receptors can be studied by blocking AMPA receptors with selective antagonists such as GYKI53655. In addition, potent selective kainate receptor agonists have been described. The most widely used selective agonist is 2-amino-3-(3- hydroxy-5-*tert*-butylisoxazol-4-yl)propanoic acid (Clarke *et al.* 1997), which is very potent at GLU_{K5} receptors and only affects AMPA receptors and other kainate receptors in considerably higher concentrations.

Early, so-called, non-NMDA receptor antagonists such as kynurenic acid and the quinoxalinediones (e.g. CNQX and NBQX) antagonize both AMPA and kainate receptors to varying degrees. The first selectivity towards kainate receptors was obtained when a series of decahydroisoquinolines, synthesized by Paul Ornstein at Eli Lilly, was screened against AMPA and kainate receptor subunits expressed in HEK293 cells. These compounds had the expected AMPA receptor antagonist activity but surprisingly also antagonized homomeric GLU_{K5} receptors. The first compound, LY293558, was roughly equipotent at GLU_{K5} and AMPA-receptor subunits (Bleakman *et al.* 1996) but subsequent compounds, such as LY294486 (Clarke *et al.* 1997) and its active isomer LY377770 (O'Neill *et al.* 2000; Smolders *et al.* 2002) showed improved selectivity for GLU_{K5} receptors. The most selective GLU_{K5} receptor antagonist that is currently available is LY382884 (O'Neill *et al.* 1998; Bortolotto *et al.* 1999). This compound antagonizes GLU_{K5} receptors with a K_i value of 4.0 µM and is much less active on AMPA receptors. Like other decahydroisoquinolines, it is essentially inactive on other kainate receptor subunits. Importantly, but not surprisingly, it is roughly equipotent on homomeric GLU_{K5} receptors and heteromers containing the GLU_{K5} subunit (Bortolotto *et al.* 1999). In native tissue, LY382884 blocks a variety of effects of kainate receptor activation at a concentration (10 µM) that does not affect AMPA receptor-mediated synaptic transmission in the mossy fibre pathway (Bortolotto *et al.* 1999). It has been tested on a variety of other receptor systems and found to be inactive at this concentration (Lauri *et al.* 2001*b*). It is therefore a very useful compound with which to explore the functions of kainate receptors.

Recent studies in the spinal cord of mice have shown that LY382884 strongly inhibits kainate currents in wild-type and $GLU_{K6-/-}$ mice but is inactive in $GLU_{K5-/-}$ mice (Kerchner *et al.* 2002). This further confirms the selectivity of LY382884 for GLU_{K5} receptors. Interestingly, the current density in $GLU_{K5-/-}$ mice and wild-types was similar. This shows that GLU_{K5}-dependent functions in wild-type mice can be compensated for in $GLU_{K5-/-}$ mice. This result has important implications for the interpretation of experiments using kainate receptor knockout mice.

9.3 Kainate receptor antagonists block the induction of LTP at mossy fibre synapses

The selective kainate receptor antagonist LY382884, applied at a concentration (10 µM) that did not affect mossy fibre synaptic transmission, completely blocked the induction of mossy fibre LTP in a fully reversible manner (Bortolotto *et al.* 1999). LY382884 had no effect on basal synaptic transmission, on pre-established LTP or on LTP induced by direct stimulation of adenylyl cyclase with forskolin. This shows that its action is specific for LTP induction. Furthermore, LY382884 had no effect on NMDA receptor-dependent LTP evoked in the same neurons by activation of assoc./comm. fibres. This provided the first, and to our minds compelling, evidence that kainate receptors are involved in the induction of mossy fibre LTP.

It has been suggested that different forms of mossy fibre LTP can coexist, and may have different expression mechanisms (Urban and Barrionuevo 1996). We have therefore investigated the sensitivity to LY382884 of additional induction protocols; B-HFS, which comprised 10 pulses at 100 Hz repeated eight times at 5 s intervals, and L-HFS, which comprised 100 pulses at 100 Hz repeated three times at 10 s intervals (Urban and Barrionuevo 1996). As illustrated in Fig. 9.1, 10 µM LY382884 fully blocked the induction of mossy fibre LTP in a reversible manner when either protocol was used.

Since our conclusion that kainate receptors were triggers for the induction of LTP disagreed with the reports that kynurenate and CNQX do not block the induction of mossy fibre LTP (Ito and Sugiyama 1991; Castillo *et al.* 1994; Weisskopf and Nicoll 1995; Yeckel *et al.* 1999; but see Urban and Barrionuevo 1996) it became necessary to repeat these experiments using these non-selective AMPA/kainate receptor antagonists. These experiments were complicated by the depression of AMPA receptor-mediated synaptic transmission; however, in all experiments a second non-tetanized input was

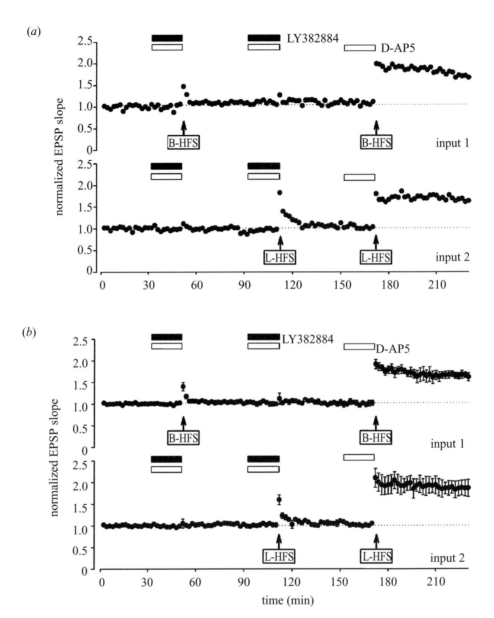

Fig. 9.1 GLU$_{K5}$-containing kainate receptors are triggers for the induction of mossy fibre LTP. (*a*) A single experiment, plotting field EPSP slope (averages of four successive responses) versus time. Tetani were delivered at the times indicated by arrows, in the presence of D-AP5 (50 μM; duration of application indicated by bar) to ensure that only mossy fibre LTP was being investigated. Two independent mossy fibre inputs were studied simultaneously. In input 1, B-HFS, and in input 2, L-HFS were delivered. Note that LY382884 (10 μM) fully blocked the induction of LTP in a reversible manner in both inputs. (*b*) Pooled data (mean ± s.e. mean) from four similar experiments.

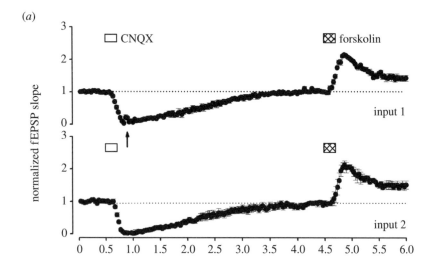

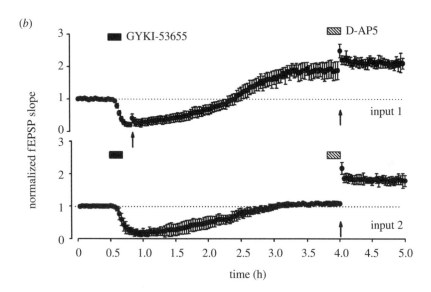

Fig. 9.2 CNQX but not NBQX blocks the induction of mossy fibre LTP. (*a*) Pooled data from five two-input fEPSP experiments showing that CNQX (10 μM) blocked the induction of mossy fibre LTP, as assessed following recovery of AMPA receptor-mediated synaptic transmission. A single tetanus (100 Hz, 1 s, test intensity) was delivered to input 1 (at the time indicated by the arrow). Subsequent application of forskolin (50 μM) resulted in LTP in both inputs. (*b*) Pooled data for five equivalent experiments using GYKI53655 (30 μM). Note that the tetanus delivered to input 1 induced LTP, as assessed following recovery of AMPA receptor-mediated synaptic transmission. A second tetanus delivered to this input elicited very little additional LTP (due to saturation), whereas a tetanus delivered for the first time to input 2 elicited normal LTP.

used as a control to ensure stability of the recordings. Both kynurenate (10 mM) and CNQX (10 μM) reversibly blocked the induction of mossy fibre LTP, as determined after AMPA receptor-mediated synaptic transmission had recovered following wash-out of the antagonist (Bortolotto *et al.* 1999). Experiments reported in Bortolotto *et al.* (1999), but not previously illustrated, showing the block of mossy fibre LTP by 10 μM CNQX are presented in Fig. 9.2*a*. Significantly, the potency of these three structurally distinct compounds (LY382884, kynurenic acid and CNQX) as GLU$_{K5}$ antagonists correlated with their potency at blocking the induction of mossy fibre LTP (Bortolotto *et al.* 1999). Conversely, selective inhibition of AMPA receptors, using GYKI53655, did not impair the induction of mossy fibre LTP, once again determined after AMPA receptor-mediated synaptic transmission had been restored. These experiments, noted in Bortolotto *et al.* (1999), are illustrated for the first time in Fig. 9.2*b*.

Our conclusion that kainate receptors are involved in the induction of mossy fibre LTP was challenged (Nicoll *et al.* 2000) because of the earlier failures to observe antagonism using kynurenic acid or CNQX. However, the group that disputed our findings subsequently confirmed that CNQX can block the induction of mossy fibre LTP (Schmitz *et al.*, 2003). Also, it has been shown that mossy fibre LTP is absent in certain kainate receptor knockout mice (Contractor *et al.* 2001). Therefore, an involvement of kainate receptors in mossy fibre LTP seems now to be generally accepted. What has yet to be fully resolved is the relative importance of the various kainate receptor subunits. In the study of Contractor *et al.* (2001) it was reported that LTP was reduced in GLU$_{K6-/-}$ mice but not affected in GLU$_{K5-/-}$ mice. Given the high degree of selectivity of LY382884 for GLU$_{K5}$ versus other kainate-receptor subunits, we propose that the normal role of GLU$_{K5}$ is compensated for in GLU$_{K5-/-}$ mice. This conclusion is supported by the compensation reported for kainate actions on spinal neurons (Kerchner *et al.* 2002) and for synaptic facilitation (see below). Whether the reduction in the magnitude of LTP observed in the GLU$_{K6-/-}$ mouse is due to the acute loss of this subunit or a developmental consequence of the absence of this receptor throughout development is not currently known. GLU$_{K6}$-subtype-selective antagonists would be useful to address this issue.

9.4 The synaptic activation of kainate receptors at mossy fibre synapses

High-frequency stimulation of the mossy fibre pathway elicits a postsynaptic kainate receptor-mediated EPSC (Castillo *et al.* 1997; Vignes and Collingridge 1997). This EPSC was identified by blocking AMPA receptor-mediated synaptic transmission using GYKI53655. The residual synaptic current is sensitive to CNQX (Castillo *et al.* 1997; Vignes and Collingridge 1997) and the more selective GLU$_{K5}$ kainate receptor antagonists LY293558 and LY294486 (Vignes *et al.* 1998). This kainate receptor-mediated EPSC is not readily observed with single shock stimulation at mossy fibres but is rapidly recruited during the stimulus train, such that it is evident by the second stimulus. This enhancement during the train is due to the slow kinetics of the kainate receptor-mediated response, which promotes temporal summation, and the facilitation of glutamate release that occurs during repetitive stimulation (Salin *et al.* 1996). Unlike NMDA receptors, which also summate effectively during high-frequency stimulation (Herron *et al.* 1986), there is no voltage dependence to the synaptic kainate receptor-mediated response. The reason for the slow kinetics of synaptic kainate receptor-mediated currents is not known, but probably relates to intrinsic channel properties.

The recruitment of a kainate receptor-mediated EPSC is not the only occurrence during high-frequency stimulation of mossy fibres. Recordings made during the tetanus, used to induce mossy fibre LTP, showed that AMPA receptor-mediated synaptic transmission was rapidly enhanced and this enhancement was sustained throughout the high-frequency train (Bortolotto *et al.* 1999; Lauri *et al.* 2001*a*). This enhancement of the synaptic response was therefore very distinct from that seen during tetanic stimulation at CA1 synapses where AMPA receptor-mediated synaptic transmission was depressed but NMDA receptor-mediated synaptic transmission was greatly facilitated (Herron *et al.* 1986). The nature of the synaptic response during the tetanus at mossy fibres was most simply explained by a rapid, facilitatory autoreceptor mechanism resulting in enhanced glutamate release, and hence more AMPA receptor activation in response to every stimulus (following the initial one). Its sensitivity to LY382884 suggested that this putative autoreceptor was a kainate receptor. However, a synaptically elicited facilitatory autoreceptor had not been observed in the mammalian CNS before and, like any positive feedback process, could represent a highly unstable mechanism—particularly given that L-glutamate is potentially excitotoxic. We therefore set out to establish the existence (or otherwise) of such a mechanism.

9.5 The synaptic activation of a facilitatory kainate autoreceptor

Whole-cell patch-clamp recordings confirmed the existence of a facilitatory kainate autoreceptor at mossy fibre synapses and enabled many of its properties to be established (Lauri *et al.* 2001*a*). These findings entered the public domain at the meeting of the Federation of European Neuroscience (Brighton, June 2000) and Fig. 9.3 shows data as presented at this meeting, some of which were subsequently published in Lauri *et al.* (2001*a*). Note the rapid facilitation of synaptic transmission at mossy fibre synapses but not assoc./comm. synapses and the selective effect of 10 μM LY382884 on mossy fibre responses (Fig. 9.3*a*). Note also that LY382884 had no effect on the first EPSC in the high-frequency train, consistent with its lack of effect on low-frequency AMPA receptor-mediated synaptic transmission, but antagonized the subsequent four EPSCs by around 50%. Figure 9.3*b* presents data from a train of five stimuli delivered at 100 Hz. Note again the lack of effect on the first EPSC but substantial antagonism of subsequent EPSCs in the train. Thus, the onset latency was less than 10 ms, suggesting an ionotropic receptor mechanism. In this example, exponentials were fitted to the decay of the synaptic response—the decay comprises an early component mediated by AMPA receptors and a late component that is due to the synaptic activation of postsynaptic kainate receptors. The finding that both components are depressed equally is suggestive of a presynaptic locus of action of LY382884; namely inhibition of a facilitatory autoreceptor mechanism. Further evidence for a presynaptic action of LY382884 is the finding that the facilitation of mossy fibre transmission by low concentrations of kainate (Kehl *et al.* 1984; Lauri *et al.* 2001*a*; Schmitz *et al.* 2001) that presumably results from direct depolarization of presynaptic elements, is blocked by this antagonist (Fig. 9.3*c*).

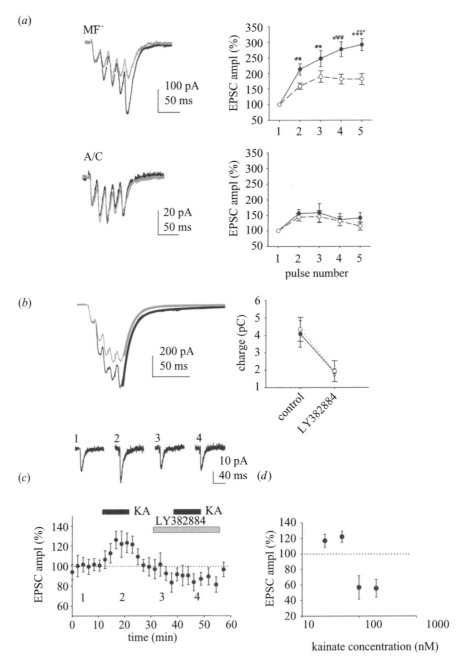

Fig. 9.3 GLU$_{K5}$-containing kainate receptors mediate synaptic facilitation of AMPA receptor-mediated mossy fibre synaptic transmission. (*a*) AMPA receptor-mediated EPSCs in response to five shocks at 50 Hz under control conditions (black) and in the presence of LY382884 (grey) for mossy fibre (MF) and assoc./comm. (A/C) inputs. The graphs plot pooled data of EPSC amplitude, normalized with respect to the first EPSC in the train, for six neurons. (Data replotted from Lauri *et al.* (2001*a*).) (*b*) AMPA receptor-mediated mossy fibre EPSCs in response to five

Based on the extensive pharmacological characterization of LY382884 it seems extremely likely that its effect on synaptic facilitation is due to antagonism of GLU_{K5}-containing kainate receptors. This conclusion is supported by experiments using knockout mice (S. E. Lauri, J. T. R. Isaac, and G. L. Collingridge, unpublished observations). We have found very pronounced synaptic facilitation, induced by 50 Hz stimulation, in both the $GLU_{K5-/-}$ and wild-type littermates that is not significantly different in magnitude. However, while LY382884 antagonizes synaptic facilitation in wild-type mice, in a similar manner to that in rats, it is inactive in $GLU_{K5-/-}$ mice. Thus, the $GLU_{K5-/-}$ mouse must compensate for the lack of GLU_{K5} receptors. What the consequences of this compensation are for synaptic function at mossy fibres remains to be fully explored.

Synaptic facilitation can also be observed by using the NMDA receptor-mediated component of synaptic transmission at mossy fibres as a monitor of synaptic glutamate release (Lauri et al. 2001b; Schmitz et al. 2001). This enables the non-selective AMPA/ kainate receptor antagonists, such as CNQX and NBQX, to be used. As expected, these agents mimicked the effects of LY382884 on synaptic facilitation (Fig. 9.4). However, the use of the NMDA receptor-mediated synaptic component is limited in two respects. First, the level of facilitation is much less when compared with that observed using AMPA receptor-mediated synaptic transmission. Second, the effect of kainate receptor antagonists is less evident until later in the train (Fig. 9.4). Therefore, NMDA receptor-mediated EPSCs, compared with AMPA receptor-mediated EPSCs, are a poor reporter of synaptically released L-glutamate. These two differences can be explained by the higher affinity of NMDA receptors, compared with AMPA receptors, for L-glutamate resulting in greater occupancy of NMDA receptors during mossy fibre transmission.

In contrast to a facilitatory function for kainate receptor on mossy fibres, other work conducted in parallel to our own work concluded that L-glutamate released synaptically from either mossy fibre synapses or assoc./comm. synapses resulted in depression of mossy fibre transmission—i.e. an inhibitory auto and heteroreceptor function (Schmitz et al. 2000). In a reappraisal of their work, these authors subsequently reported bi-directional modifications of mossy fibre synaptic transmission depending on the number of pulses delivered at 200 Hz to assoc./comm. fibres (Schmitz et al. 2001). Thus, 3 pulses resulted in facilitation of an NMDA receptor-mediated EPSC while 10 pulses resulted in depression. This unusual sensitivity to stimulus number is specific to assoc./comm. influences since facilitation within mossy fibres persists throughout a long high-frequency train (e.g. 100 stimuli delivered at 100 Hz) when measured using AMPA receptor-mediated synaptic responses (Lauri et al. 2001a).

---

shocks at 100 Hz under control conditions (black) and in the presence of LY382884 (grey). Double exponential fits (thick black and grey traces) are superimposed upon the EPSC decays. The graph plots the charge associated with the fast (black circles) (AMPA receptor-mediated EPSC) and slow (open circles) (kainate receptor-mediated EPSC) components. Note the parallel inhibition by LY382884. (c) Pooled data from four experiments to illustrate facilitation of AMPA receptor-mediated mossy fibre transmission by 50 nM kainate (KA) and its inhibition by 10 μM LY382884. The mossy fibre EPSCs were obtained at the times indicated (1–4). (Data replotted from Lauri et al. (2001a).) (d) Concentration-dependent effects of kainate on mossy fibre synaptic transmission. Each point is the mean of at least four experiments. $*p < 0.05$; $**p < 0.01$; $***p < 0.005$.

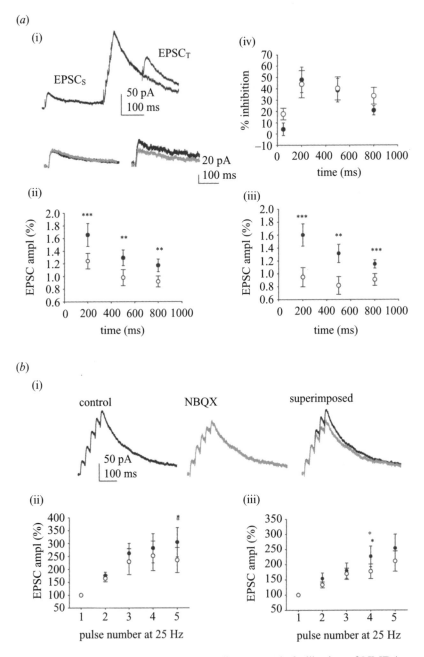

Fig. 9.4 GLU_{K5}-containing kainate receptors mediate synaptic facilitation of NMDA receptor-mediated mossy fibre synaptic transmission. (a) (i) Upper recording shows NMDA receptor-mediated EPSCs (recorded at +40 mV) evoked by a single stimulus ($EPSC_S$) and five stimuli delivered at 100 Hz followed by a test pulse ($EPSC_T$) delivered 200 ms later. The traces are superimposed upon responses to the same stimulus protocol but without the test pulse. The lower recordings show single stimuli and test pulses under control conditions (black traces) and in the presence of NBQX (20 µM; grey trace). Note the inhibition of synaptic facilitation by NBQX.

During the course of our experiments we asked whether L-glutamate released from one population of mossy fibres can regulate the release from another via activation of presynaptic kainate receptors in a heterosynaptic manner. To explore this possibility we stimulated two sets of mossy fibres and determined the influence of delivering 5 or 10 shocks to one input on NMDA receptor-mediated EPSCs at the other input. Heterosynaptic facilitation, antagonized by NBQX, was observed in each experiment (Fig. 9.5).

9.6 Presynaptic kainate receptors mediate the induction of mossy fibre LTP

The finding that both pre- and postsynaptic kainate receptors are readily activated by synaptically released L-glutamate at mossy fibre synapses means that either or both could be involved in the induction of mossy fibre LTP. However, we found that a concentration of LY382884 (10 μM) that fully blocked the induction of mossy fibre LTP was able to completely inhibit kainate-mediated facilitation of mossy fibre synaptic transmission and inhibit synaptic facilitation without affecting postsynaptic kainate currents in CA3 neurons (Lauri et al. 2001a). Thus, LY382884 is a selective inhibitor of presynaptic kainate receptors at mossy fibre synapses. This therefore strongly suggests that presynaptic kainate receptors are involved in the induction of mossy fibre LTP. One piece of evidence that was cited against a role of GLU_{K5}-containing kainate receptors in the induction of LTP is the low levels of expression of GLU_{K5} message in the hippocampus (Nicoll et al. 2000). However, dentate granule cells, like CA3 pyramidal neurons, express detectable levels of GLU_{K5} message (Bahn et al. 1994) and presynaptic kainate receptors would, most probably, need only one GLU_{K5} subunit to confer sensitivity to GLU_{K5} antagonists.

The finding that kainate receptor-dependent mossy fibre LTP can be induced following selective blockade of AMPA receptors with GYKI53655 (Bortolotto et al. 1999) shows that activation of these receptors is not required. Although NMDA receptors can be readily activated synaptically by mossy fibre stimulation, NMDA receptors are not required for mossy fibre LTP (Harris and Cotman 1986). Indeed, mossy fibre LTP is often studied in the presence of an NMDA receptor antagonist to prevent the induction of LTP at assoc./comm. fibres that could be activated inadvertently. However, mGlu receptors may act as a parallel induction trigger since certain mGlu receptor

---

(ii) The level of facilitation ($EPSC_T/EPSC_S$) plotted versus inter-pulse interval (time between first stimulus in 100 Hz train and test pulse) for 12 experiments. Control conditions, black; NBQX: open. (iii) Equivalent experiments using LY382884 (10 μM; $n = 10$). Control conditions, black; LY382884, open. (iv) Plot of percentage inhibition of synaptic facilitation versus inter-pulse interval. The first points plot the peak response during the tetanus. Note the similarity between NBQX (open) and LY382884 (black). (Data analysis expanded from Lauri et al. (2001b).) (b) Analysis during a high-frequency train. (i) NMDA receptor-mediated EPSCs (recorded at +40 mV) evoked by five shocks delivered at 25 Hz before (black) and in the presence of NBQX (20 μM; grey) and their superimposition. Note the lack of effect of NBQX until later in the response. (ii) The graph plots the amplitude of each EPSC in the train, normalized to the first, for 12 NBQX experiments. Control conditions, black; NBQX, open. (iii) Equivalent data for eight LY382884 experiments. Control conditions, black; NBQX, open. $*p < 0.05$; $**p < 0.01$; $***p < 0.005$.

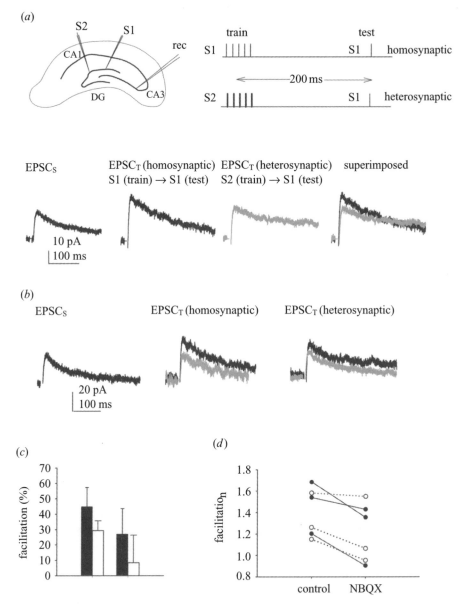

Fig. 9.5 Kainate receptor-dependent heterosynaptic facilitation of mossy fibre synaptic transmission. (*a*) NMDA receptor-mediated EPSCs were evoked by stimulation of two inputs and a train (five shocks at 100 Hz) delivered 200 ms before a test pulse. The traces show, from left to right, EPSC$_S$ and EPSC$_T$ (homosynaptic), EPSC$_T$ (heterosynaptic) and the superimposition of the two EPSC$_T$s. (*b*) The traces show EPSC$_S$, EPSC$_T$ (homosynaptic) and EPSC$_T$ (heterosynaptic) and the effects of NBQX (grey; 20 µM); control conditions are shown in black. (*c*) The histograms plot the level of homosynaptic (black bars) and heterosynaptic (open bars) facilitation for three experiments, in response to five shocks delivered at 100 Hz or 10 shocks delivered at 200 Hz. (*d*) The graphs plot the level of homosynaptic (black) and heterosynaptic (open) facilitation for three experiments, in response to five shocks delivered at 100 Hz, under control conditions and in the presence of NBQX (20 µM).

antagonists, such as (S)-α-methyl-4-carboxyphenylglycine, can block the induction of mossy fibre LTP (Bashir et al. 1993; Yeckel et al. 1999; Contractor et al. 2001).

Although we have found that LY382884, kynurenic acid and CNQX readily block the induction of mossy fibre LTP, one needs to take account of previous reports that the latter two compounds do not affect mossy fibre LTP (Ito and Sugiyama 1991; Castillo et al. 1994; Weisskopf and Nicoll 1995; Yeckel et al. 1999; but see Urban and Barrionuevo 1996). One possibility is that in these earlier studies, mossy fibre LTP was not investigated due to contamination by inadvertent activation of other fibres. Another explanation is that it may be possible, under certain circumstances, to induce mossy fibre LTP without the need for the synaptic activation of kainate receptors.

9.7 Bypassing the need for kainate receptor activation to induce mossy fibre LTP

In an attempt to understand how in several previous studies mossy fibre LTP could be induced in the presence of kainate receptor antagonists, we explored differences in the experimental protocols adopted by the various laboratories. To our surprise we found that the ability of LY382884 to block mossy fibre LTP, induced by a single tetanus comprising 100 stimuli delivered at 100 Hz, was highly dependent on the Ca^{2+} concentration in the bathing medium (Lauri et al. 2003). Thus, in our standard medium (Ca 2 : Mg 1) LY382884 fully blocked the induction of mossy fibre LTP whilst in elevated divalents (e.g., Ca 4 : Mg 4) LY382884 failed to inhibit the induction of mossy fibre LTP. This might explain the failure of earlier reports to inhibit mossy fibre LTP with other kainate receptor antagonists (i.e., CNQX and kynurenic acid) since elevated divalent cation concentrations were often used in these studies (to suppress excitability).

A second parameter that can affect the sensitivity of mossy fibre LTP to kainate receptor antagonists is the number of stimuli delivered during the tetanus (Schmitz et al. 2003). Even, in elevated divalents (Ca 4 : Mg 4) CNQX was able to fully inhibit the induction of mossy fibre LTP, monitored as the amplitude of NMDAR-EPSCs recorded in the presence of GYKI53655, when 12 or 24 stimuli were delivered at 25 Hz. However, when 48 pulses were delivered it was less effective and when 125 pulses were used normal levels of LTP were induced.

So what are the mechanisms that account for the compensation? In the case of elevated Ca^{2+} we have found that Ca^{2+} entry via presynaptic L-type Ca^{2+} channels can compensate for the need for kainate receptors (Lauri et al. 2003). Thus, in Ca 2 : Mg 1, the trigger for mossy fibre LTP appears to be Ca^{2+} permeation via kainate receptors which then triggers Ca^{2+} release from intracellular stores. In Ca 4 : Mg 4, there is also sufficient Ca^{2+} entry via L-type Ca^{2+} channels to provide an alternative source of the required Ca^{2+}.

A key question that remains to be addressed is the importance of kainate receptors for the induction of mossy fibre LTP in the living animal. Given that the lower Ca^{2+} concentration is the more physiological and that granule cells are more likely to discharge at high frequencies for brief, rather than prolonged, periods of time we suspect that kainate receptors will be shown to be important triggers for this process.

9.8 The relationship between synaptic facilitation and mossy fibre LTP

The observation that LY382884 inhibits synaptic facilitation and the induction of mossy fibre LTP could mean that the two functions are causally linked; or they could be two independent consequences of presynaptic kainate receptor activation. This is another area requiring further investigation. A surprising observation is that LY382884-sensitive synaptic facilitation is selectively occluded following the induction of mossy fibre LTP (Lauri *et al.* 2001*a*). Thus, following LTP induction, the level of synaptic facilitation is markedly reduced and the residual facilitation is insensitive to the actions of LY382884. This suggests that the kainate receptor-dependent component of synaptic facilitation shares mechanisms in common with the expression of mossy fibre LTP—in which case, studying the former may give clues to the latter.

9.9 Concluding remarks

For the last 20 years of its 30-year lifetime, most interest has focused on the NMDA receptor-dependent form of LTP, such as that exhibited at Schaffer collateral-commissural fibres in the CA1 region, perforant path synapses in the dentate gyrus and at assoc./comm. synapses in the CA3 region of the hippocampus. Now that tools equivalent to NMDA receptor antagonists are available for studying mossy fibre LTP, in particular kainate receptor antagonists, it is likely that research in this form of LTP will intensify. Several immediate questions come to mind. These include the following. (i) What are the roles of the various kainate receptor subtypes in mossy fibre LTP? (ii) Under what conditions can the involvement of kainate receptors be bypassed? (iii) What is the physiological role of kainate receptor-dependent mossy fibre LTP? (iv) Do other forms of NMDA receptor-independent LTP in the brain involve kainate receptor dependency? Perhaps the most interesting question is whether the biophysical properties of kainate receptors confer important functional properties on kainate receptor-dependent LTP analogous to the role of NMDA receptors in NMDA receptor-dependent LTP.

This work was supported by the MRC and The Wellcome Trust.

References

Bahn, S., Volk, B., and Wisden, W. (1994). Kainate receptor gene expression in the developing rat brain. *J. Neurosci.* **14**, 5525–47.

Bashir, Z. I., Bortolotto, Z. A., Davies, C. H., Berretta, N., Irving, A. J., Seal, A. J., *et al.* (1993). The synaptic activation of glutamate metabotropic receptors is necessary for the induction of LTP in the hippocampus. *Nature* **363**, 347–50.

Bettler, B. and Mulle, C. (1995). AMPA and kainate receptors. *Neuropharmacology* **34**, 123–39.

Bleakman, D., Schoepp, D. D., Ballyk B., Bufton, H., Sharpe, E. F., Thomas, K., *et al.* (1996). Pharmacological discrimination of GluR5 and GluR6 kainate receptor subtypes by (3S,4aR,6R,8aR)-6-[2-(1(2)*H*-tetrazole-5-yl)ethyl]decahydroisoquinoline-3 carboxylic acid. *Mol. Pharmacol.* **49**, 581–5.

Bliss, T. V. P. and Collingridge, G. L. (1993). A synaptic model of memory—long-term potentiation in the hippocampus. *Nature* **361**, 31–9.

Bliss, T. V. P. and Gardner-Medwin, A. R. (1973). Long-lasting potentiation of synaptic transmission in the dentate area of the unanaestetized rabbit following stimulation of the perforant path. *J. Physiol. (Lond.)* **232**, 357–74.

Bliss, T. V. P. and Lømo, T. (1973). Long-lasting potentiation of synaptic transmission in the dentate area of the anaesthetized rabbit following stimulation of the perforant path. *J. Physiol. (Lond.)* **232**, 331–56.

Bortolotto, Z. A., Clarke, V. R., Delany, C. M., Parry, M. C., Smolders, I., Vignes, M., *et al.* (1999). Kainate receptors are involved in synaptic plasticity. *Nature* **402**, 297–301.

Castillo, P. E., Weisskopf, M. G., and Nicoll, R. A. (1994). The role of Ca^{2+} channels in hippocampal mossy fiber synaptic transmission and long-term potentiation. *Neuron* **12**, 261–9.

Castillo, P. E., Malenka, R. C., and Nicoll, R. A. (1997). Kainate receptors mediate a slow postsynaptic current in hippocampal CA3 neurons. *Nature* **388**, 182–6.

Clarke, V. R. J., Ballyk, B. A., Hoo, K. H., Mandelzys, A., Pellizzari, A., Bath, C. P., *et al.* (1997). A hippocampal GluR5 kainate receptor regulating inhibitory synaptic transmission. *Nature* **389**, 599–603.

Contractor, A., Swanson, G., and Heinemann, S. F. (2001). Kainate receptors are involved in short- and long-term plasticity at mossy fiber synapses in the hippocampus. *Neuron* **29**, 209–16.

Collingridge, G. L. (1985). Long-term potentiation in the hippocampus: mechanisms of initiation and modulation by neurotransmitters. *Trends Pharmacol. Sci.* **6**, 407–11.

Collingridge, G. L. (2003). The induction of N-methyl-D-aspartate receptor-dependent long-term potentiation. *Phil. Trans. R. Soc. Lond.* B **358**, 635–41.

Collingridge, G. L., Kehl, S. J., and McLennan, H. (1983). Excitatory amino acids in synaptic transmission in the Schaffer collateral–commissural pathway of the rat hippocampus. *J. Physiol.* **334**, 33–46.

Davies, J., Evans, R. H., Francis, A. A., and Watkins, J. C. (1979). Excitatory amino acid receptors and synaptic excitation in the mammalian central nervous system. *J. Physiol. (Paris)* **75**, 641–54.

Harris, E. W. and Cotman, C. W. (1986). Long-term potentiation of guinea pig mossy fibre responses is not blocked by N-methyl-D-aspartate antagonists. *Neurosci. Lett.* **70**, 132–7.

Herron, C. E., Lester, R. A. J., Coan, E. J., and Collingridge, G. L. (1986). Frequency-dependent involvement of NMDA receptors in the hippocampus: a novel synaptic mechanism. *Nature* **322**, 265–8.

Ito, I. and Sugiyama, H. (1991). Roles of glutamate receptors in long-term potentiation at hippocampal mossy fiber synapses. *NeuroReport* **2**, 333–6.

Kehl, S. J. Mclennan, H., and Collingridge, G. L. (1984). Effects of folic and kainic acids on synaptic responses of hippocampal neurones. *Neuroscience* **11**, 111–24.

Kerchner, G. A., Wilding, T. J., Huettner, J. E., and Zhuo, M. (2002). Kainate receptor subunits underlying presynaptic regulation of transmitter release in the dorsal horn. *J. Neurosci.* **22**, 8010–17.

Lauri, S. E., Bortolotto, Z. A., Bleakman, D., Ornstein, P. L., Lodge, D., Isaac, J. T. R., *et al* (2001*a*). A critical role of a facilitatory kainate autoreceptor in mossy fibre LTP. *Neuron* **32**, 697–709.

Lauri, S. E., Delany, C., Clarke, V. R. J., Bortolotto, Z. A., Ornstein, P. L., Isaac, J. T. R., *et al.* (2001*b*) Synaptic activation of a presynaptic kainate receptor facilitates AMPA receptor-mediated synaptic transmission at hippocampal mossy fibre synapses. *Neuropharmacology* **41**, 907–15.

Lauri, S. E., Bortolotto, Z. A., Nistico, R., Bleakman, D., Ornstein, P. L., Lodge, D., *et al.* (2003). A role for Ca^{2+} stores in kainate receptor-dependent synaptic facilitator and LTP at mossy fiber synapses in the hippocampus. *Neuron* **39**, 327–41.

Lodge, D. and Dingledine, R. (2000). Ionotropic glutamate receptors. In *The IUPHAR compendium of receptor characterization and classification*, 2nd edn. London: IUPHAR Media Ltd.

McLennan, H. and Lodge, D. (1979). The antagonism of amino acid-induced excitation of spinal neurones in the cat. *Brain Res.* **169**, 83–90.

Monaghan, D. T. and Cotman, C. W. (1982). The distribution of [H^3] kainic acid binding-sites in rat brain CNS as determined by autoradiography. *Brain Res.* **252**, 91–100.

Nicoll, R. A., Mellor, J., Frerking, M., and Schmitz, D. (2000). Kainate receptors and synaptic plasticity. *Nature* **406**, 957.

O'Neill, M. J., Bond, A., Ornstein, P. L., Ward, M. A., Hicks, C. A., Hoo, K., *et al.* (1998). Decahydroisoquinolines: novel competitive AMPA/kainate antagonists with neuroprotective effects in global cerebral ischaemia. *Neuropharmacology* **37**, 1211–22.

O'Neill, M. J., Bogaert, L., Hicks, C. A., Bond, A., Ward, M. A., Ebinger, G., *et al.* (2000). LY377770, a novel iGluR5 kainate receptor antagonist with neuroprotective effects in global and focal cerebral ischaemia. *Neuropharmacology* **39**, 1575–88.

Salin, P. A., Scanziani, M., Malenka, R. C., and Nicoll, R. A. (1996). Distinct short-term plasticity at two excitatory synapses in the hippocampus. *Proc. Natl Acad. Sci. USA* **93**, 13 304–9.

Schmitz, D., Frerking, M., and Nicoll, R. A. (2000). Synaptic activation of presynaptic kainate receptors on hippocampal mossy fiber synapses. *Neuron* **27**, 327–38.

Schmitz, D., Mellor, J., and Nicoll, R. A. (2001). Presynaptic kainate receptor mediation of frequency facilitation at hippocampal mossy fibre synapses. *Science* **291**, 1972–6.

Schmitz, D., Mellor, J., Breustedt, J., and Nicoll, R. A. (2003). Presynaptic kainate receptors impart an associative property to hippocampal mossy fiber long-term potentiation. *Nat Neurosci.* **6**, 1058–63.

Smolders, I., Bortolotto, Z. A., Clarke, V. R., Warre, R., Khan, G. M., O'Neill, M. J., *et al.* (2002). Antagonists of GLU_{K5}-containing kainate receptors prevent pilocarpine-induced limbic seizures. *Nature Neurosci.* **5**, 796–804.

Urban, N. N. and Barrionuevo, G. (1996). Induction of Hebbian and non-Hebbian mossy fiber long-term potentiation by distinct patterns of high-frequency stimulation. *J. Neurosci.* **16**, 4293–9.

Vignes, M. and Collingridge, G. L. (1997). The synaptic activation of kainate receptors. *Nature* **388**, 179–82.

Vignes, M., Bleakman, D., Lodge, D., and Collingridge, G. L. (1998). The synaptic activation of the GluR5 subtype of kainate receptor in area CA3 of the rat hippocampus. *Neuropharmacology* **36**, 1477–81.

Watkins, J. and Evans, R. H. (1981). Excitatory amino acid transmitters. *A. Rev. Pharmacol. Toxicol.* **21**, 165–204.

Weisskopf, M. G. and Nicoll, R. A. (1995). Presynaptic changes during mossy fibre LTP revealed by NMDA receptor-mediated synaptic responses. *Nature* **376**, 256–9.

Yeckel, M. F., Kapur, A., and Johnston, D. (1999). Multiple forms of LTP in hippocampal CA3 neurons use a common postsynaptic mechanism. *Nature Neurosci.* **2**, 625–33.

Glossary

B-HFS   brief high-frequency stimulation
CNS   central nervous system
EPSC   excitatory postsynaptic current
EPSP   excitatory post-synaptic potential
L-HFS   long high-frequency stimulation
LTP   long-term potentiation
NBQX   2,3-dihydroxy-6-nitro-7-sulphamoyl-benz(F) quinoxaline
NMDA   *N*-methyl-D-aspartate

10

Active dendrites, potassium channels and synaptic plasticity

*Daniel Johnston, Brian R. Christie, Andreas Frick, Richard Gray,
Dax A. Hoffman, Lalania K. Schexnayder, Shigeo Watanabe,
and Li-Lian Yuan*

The dendrites of CA1 pyramidal neurons in the hippocampus express numerous types of voltage-gated ion channels, but the distributions or densities of many of these channels are very non-uniform. Sodium channels in the dendrites are responsible for action potential (AP) propagation from the axon into the dendrites (back-propagation); calcium channels are responsible for local changes in dendritic calcium concentrations following back-propagating APs and synaptic potentials; and potassium channels help regulate overall dendritic excitability. Several lines of evidence are presented here to suggest that back-propagating APs, when coincident with excitatory synaptic input, can lead to the induction of either long-term depression (LTD) or long-term potentiation (LTP). The induction of LTD or LTP is correlated with the magnitude of the rise in intracellular calcium. When brief bursts of synaptic potentials are paired with postsynaptic APs in a theta-burst pairing paradigm, the induction of LTP is dependent on the invasion of the AP into the dendritic tree. The amplitude of the AP in the dendrites is dependent, in part, on the activity of a transient, A-type potassium channel that is expressed at high density in the dendrites and correlates with the induction of the LTP. Furthermore, during the expression phase of the LTP, there are local changes in dendritic excitability that may result from modulation of the functioning of this transient potassium channel. The results support the view that the active properties of dendrites play important roles in synaptic integration and synaptic plasticity of these neurons.

Keywords: hippocampus; CA1 neurons; long-term potentiation; long-term depression; Ca^{2+}

10.1 Introduction

The dendrites of neurons in the central nervous system have been studied for many years because of their presumed role in coordinating synaptic input and in regulating the strengths of those inputs. Historically, there have been great debates about whether dendrites were active or passive, and whether synaptic inputs on the distal portions of dendritic trees were too far away from the cell body to have much effect on neuronal excitability (for reviews, see Shepherd 1991; Johnston *et al.* 1996). In the hippocampus, CA1 pyramidal neurons have received the most attention in this regard. The dendrites of these neurons, as well as many other neurons in the hippocampus, neocortex, olfactory bulb and cerebellum, are now known to express a wide array of voltage-gated ion channels (reviewed in Magee 1999). For example, in CA1 pyramidal neurons Na^+ channels, which support the active back-propagation of APs, are expressed at a relatively uniform density from the initial segment of the axon to at least three quarters of the length of the main apical dendrite (Magee and Johnston 1995; Colbert and Johnston

1996; Mickus *et al.* 1999; Colbert and Pan 2002; Gasparini and Magee 2002). Ca^{2+} channels, which are opened by both synaptic potentials and dendritic APs, are also at a relatively uniform total density from the soma into the distal dendrites, but the distribution of the various subtypes of Ca^{2+} channel is quite heterogeneous—L- and N-type channels are more numerous in the soma and proximal dendrites, whereas R- and T-type channels are more numerous in the distal dendrites (Magee *et al.* 1995; Sabatini and Svoboda 2000). Hyperpolarization-activated h-channels, which affect temporal summation of synaptic inputs and overall neuronal excitability (Poolos *et al.* 2002), are expressed non-uniformly with a very high density in the distal dendrites (Magee 1998). Finally, there are two broad classes of K^+ channels in the dendrites of these neurons inactivating and non-inactivating, both of which have profound effects on dendritic signalling. The non-inactivating class is expressed with a uniform density, while the inactivating class is non-uniformly distributed with the highest density in the distal dendrites (Hoffman *et al.* 1997). Clearly, CA1 pyramidal neuron dendrites cannot be considered passive.

Based on these and other findings, the issues about dendritic function have moved significantly past the active versus passive debate and have become much more complicated and specific. For example, some of the more recent questions about how dendrites work relate to:

  (i) which molecular subunits are responsible for the dendritic channels;
 (ii) how are they targeted to dendrites;
(iii) what is the smallest synaptic integration zone (for example, spines, side branches or main trunk);
 (iv) what is the function of dendritic APs;
  (v) how do dendritic channels affect the spatial and temporal summation of synaptic inputs;
 (vi) do dendritic channels undergo activity-dependent modification; and
(vii) do dendritic channels regulate the induction of various forms of synaptic plasticity?

It is now well known that the AP of these neurons is actively propagated into the apical dendrites as well as being locally generated under certain conditions (Jaffe *et al.* 1992; Spruston *et al.* 1995; Golding and Spruston 1998; Golding *et al.* 2001, 2002). The so-called b-AP is an attractive candidate mechanism for regulating certain forms of Hebbian-type synaptic plasticity (Magee and Johnston 1997), but many questions remain concerning precise mechanisms.

We have addressed some of these questions in recent years, and although the picture is far from clear, some answers are beginning to emerge. We have focused much of our attention on a particular type (or class) of K^+ channel, the A-type K^+ channel. This channel shows rapid activation and inactivation and, as mentioned above, is expressed at a high density in apical dendrites of CA1 pyramidal neurons. We will review some of the recent work related to active dendrites and their role in synaptic plasticity in CA1 neurons, paying particular attention to this transient, A-type K^+ channel.

10.2 Long-term depression

Work on LTD was the first to show that b-APs could play an integral role in the induction of long-term synaptic plasticity. This work stemmed from studies showing that low-frequency stimulation (LFS: 1–3 Hz) provides a reliable means to induce LTD in the CA1 region of the hippocampus (Dudek and Bear 1992; Mulkey and Malenka 1992). When small, sub-threshold EPSPs are evoked with LFS and recorded at the resting membrane potential, LTD is not usually induced in CA1 neurons (Christie *et al.* 1996*b*; Fig. 10.1*a*). When these same synaptic stimuli are paired with APs triggered with somatic current injection, however, LTD is reliably elicited (Fig. 10.1*c*). Administration of b-APs at 1–3 Hz alone does not produce LTD, indicating that there is some need for coincident pre- and postsynaptic activity. This requirement may also be met by giving an intensity of synaptic stimulation sufficient to elicit APs (suprathreshold EPSPs). This procedure also elicits a robust LTD that is indistinguishable from that observed with the pairing protocol (Fig. 10.1*d*).

The role of $[Ca^{2+}]_i$ in LTD comes from a variety of observations. First, LTD can be blocked by the intracellular injection of postsynaptic Ca^{2+} chelators (Mulkey and Malenka 1992). Second, the LTD from pairing sub-threshold EPSPs and APs is correlated with rises in $[Ca^{2+}]_i$ in the dendritic regions produced by the b-APs during the induction protocol (Christie *et al.* 1996*b*). Finally, LFS-induced LTD is also blocked by Ca^{2+} channel blockers and NMDA antagonists (Camodeca *et al.* 1998; Christie *et al.* 1996*a,b*, 1997; Dudek and Bear 1992; Mulkey and Malenka 1992; Mockett *et al.* 2002).

When similar pairings of sub-threshold EPSPs and b-APs were given over a wide range of frequencies (1–200 Hz), a transition from LTD to LTP was observed in the 10–30 Hz range (Schexnayder 1999; Fig. 10.2). The transition from LTD to LTP was also correlated with the rise in dendritic $[Ca^{2+}]$ (Fig. 10.3). Although higher concentrations of D,L-APV (50 µM) blocked the plasticity at all frequencies (Fig. 10.2), lower concentrations (10 µM), or the addition of the L-type Ca^{2+} channel blocker nimodipine to the bath, shifted the transition in the plasticity–stimulus frequency curve to higher frequencies so that in the range of 10–100 Hz, LTD was induced instead of LTP (Schexnayder 1999). These data again suggested a role for dendritic Ca^{2+} influx via b-APs in the induction of both LTD and LTP in CA1 neurons.

10.3 Long-term potentiation

Strong support for the importance of back-propagating APs and LTP induction was provided by a technically challenging set of experiments carried out by Jeff Magee (Magee and Johnston 1997). Dendritic recordings were made during synaptic stimulation alone, and when EPSPs were paired with b-APs. When the EPSPs and b-APs were paired, the amplitudes of the b-APs in the distal dendrites were boosted in a supralinear fashion, and LTP was induced. The key experiment in that study was the local and reversible application of TTX to the proximal apical dendrites during the LTP induction protocol. Such local application of TTX blocked the propagation of the b-APs from the soma to the site of the stimulated synapses. Although APs still occurred in the cell body and synaptic input was still elicited in the dendrites, the TTX prevented (disconnected?) the b-APs from reaching the synapses during the pairing paradigm. When the propagation of the APs into the dendrites was interrupted in this fashion, LTP induction was prevented. After a few minutes the local TTX washed away and an identical pairing of EPSPs and b-APs was given. The b-APs now fully propagated into the dendritic regions of the stimulated synaptic input (demonstrated

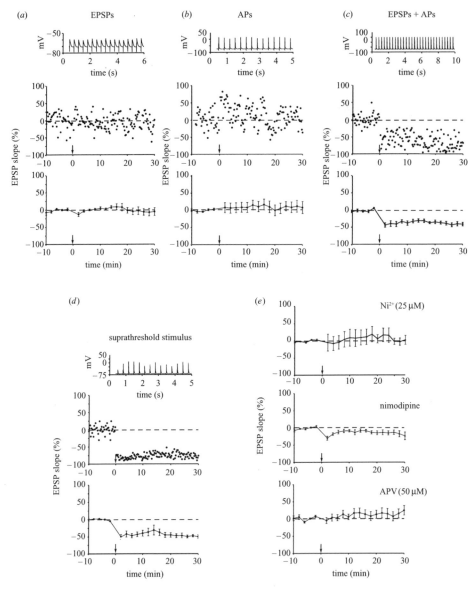

Fig. 10.1 LTP by pairing Schaffer collateral EPSPs and APs in CA1 pyramidal neurons. (*a*) EPSPs, sub-threshold for AP generation, fail to induce LTD (3 Hz for 900 stimuli). The top trace in this and panels (*a–d*) is a portion of the stimulus train (EPSPs in this panel) recorded with a whole-cell pipette in the soma. The EPSP slope as a function of time for one experiment is shown in the middle trace, while the average for four experiments is given in the bottom trace. The arrow in this and all panels represents the time of the 3 Hz train. (*b*) Similar to (*a*) except that a 3 Hz (900 stimuli) train of postsynaptic APs was substituted for the EPSP train. The APs were triggered by 1–2 ms current pulses to the soma and back-propagated into the dendrites. (*c*) Similar to (*a*) and (*b*) except that the APs triggered by brief somatic current injections were paired with the EPSPs. LTD was induced in all experiments using this pairing protocol. (*d*) The intensity of Schaffer collateral stimulation was increased so that now the EPSPs triggered APs on their own

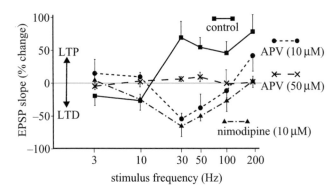

Fig. 10.2 Changes in synaptic strength as a function of stimulus frequency. Sub-threshold EPSPs from Schaffer collateral stimulation were paired with APs triggered by brief somatic current injections (900 stimuli at each frequency, $n = 3–7$ for each point, similar protocol to that shown in figure 10.1c). Plasticity versus frequency curves were also obtained in low (filled circles; 10 μm) and high (crosses; 50 μm) APV (D,L) and in nimodipine (filled triangles; 10 μm). Although high APV blocked all plasticity, lower concentrations of APV and nimodipine shifted the transition frequency from LTD to LTP to higher frequencies. Control represented by filled squares. (Taken from Schexnayder (1999), with permission.)

by Ca^{2+} imaging), and LTP was induced. This experiment led to the conclusion that, at least for this type of LTP protocol in which small EPSPs are paired with postsynaptic APs, the back-propagation of the APs is required for the induction of LTP. Furthermore, the strict notion of Hebbian plasticity, in which APs in the postsynaptic neuron are critically important, received strong support from these results.

These experiments, however, also raised many other important questions about the nature of the mechanisms boosting the b-APs during the pairing protocol and whether the boosting was somehow necessary for the LTP induction. At approximately the same time as the Magee experiments, Dax Hoffman discovered a very high density of transient, A-type K^+ channels in the distal dendrites of CA1 pyramidal neurons (Hoffman et al. 1997). These channels prevented the b-AP from reaching full amplitude, and suggested the hypothesis that EPSPs in dendrites could inactivate the K^+ channels, allowing b-APs occurring within around 10–15 ms following the peak of the EPSP to be boosted or increased in amplitude. The boosted b-APs could then be an effective depolarization to unblock NMDA receptors, increase the Ca^{2+} influx through voltage-gated Ca^{2+} channels, and induce LTP at the activated synapses. The theoretical basis for this hypothesis was explored in several modelling studies (Migliore et al. 1999; Johnston et al. 2000).

without depolarizing current to the soma. The suprathreshold stimulus train also induced LTD in all experiments. (e) The protocol of sub-threshold EPSPs paired with postsynaptic APs shown in (c) was given with different pharmacological agents in the bath during the pairing protocol. For Ni^{2+}, $n = 5$; nimodipine, $n = 5$; and D,L-APV, $n = 6$. (From Christie et al. (1996b) and reprinted with permission from *Learning and Memory*. Copyright © 1996 Cold Spring Harbor Laboratory Press.)

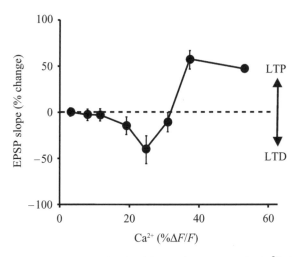

Fig. 10.3 Relationship between synaptic plasticity and postsynaptic Ca^{2+} (measured in apical dendrites) for the experiments performed in control saline shown in Fig. 10.2. Ca^{2+} was measured with a high-speed, cooled CCD camera by using similar methods to those described in Christie *et al.* (1996*b*). (Taken from Schexnayder (1999), with permission.)

10.4 Regulation of dendritic K^+ channels

Because the high density of A-type K^+ channels in CA1 dendrites appeared to have such a strong influence on the amplitude of b-APs, synaptic potentials, and dendritic electrical signals in general, it was of some interest to explore the regulation of these channels by neuromodulatory neurotransmitters and second messenger systems. Activation of PKA and PKC was found to shift the activation curve of the K^+ channels to more positive potentials, thereby reducing their probability of opening (Hoffman and Johnston 1998). The result of this modulation was to decrease the activity of the channels and thus to increase the amplitude of b-APs (Hoffman and Johnston 1999; Johnston *et al.* 1999). Although the molecular subunit comprising the dendritic, A-type K^+ channels is not known with certainty, there is good evidence for the involvement of Kv4.2 (Sheng *et al.* 1992; Maletic-Savatic *et al.* 1995; Serodio and Rudy 1998; Ramakers and Storm 2002). Phosphorylation sites on Kv4.2 have been identified for PKA, PKC, Ca^{2+}-calmodulin-dependent protein kinase II and MAPK (Adams *et al.* 2000; Anderson *et al.* 2000), and the phosphorylation of Kv4.2 by MAPK is regulated by both PKA and PKC (Yuan *et al.* 2002). We recently tested whether the downregulation of the dendritic, A-type K^+ channels by PKA and PKC was acting through MAPK and found that the increase in b-AP amplitude by either PKA or PKC was blocked by MAPK inhibitors in a similar manner to that shown for Kv4.2 (Yuan *et al.* 2002). These results provide further support for the role of Kv4.2 in the native K^+ current, but also highlight the complex manner in which signal transduction pathways interact to regulate dendritic channels (Schrader *et al.* 2002).

10.5 Changes in dendritic signalling during the expression of long-term potentiation

It is well known that several protein kinases are activated either transiently or persistently with the induction of LTP (Roberson *et al.* 1996). Because A-type K^+ channels in the dendrites are modulated by many of these same protein kinases, we tested whether a change in K^+ channel function could be detected locally in the dendrites after LTP induction. One consequence of a decrease in K^+ channel activity would be an increase in b-AP amplitude. In previous experiments we have shown that Ca^{2+} signals from b-APs in the dendrites are very good indicators of AP amplitude (Jaffe *et al.* 1992; Miyakawa *et al.* 1992; Magee and Johnston 1997; Magee *et al.* 1998). We therefore measured the amplitude of Ca^{2+} signals from b-APs before and after inducing LTP (using a similar protocol of pairing sub-threshold EPSPs with somatically triggered APs, at 100 Hz, as described in Figs. 10.1–10.3). The results were consistent with the hypothesis of a decrease in K^+ channel activity during the early expression phase of LTP. We found that the Ca^{2+} signals from b-APs were increased within the region of the dendrites (±25 μm) where the synapses were stimulated (Fig. 10.4) (Schexnayder 1999).

10.6 K^+ channels and induction of long-term potentiation

We investigated the role of A-type K^+ channels in LTP induction at Schaffer collateral synapses by using a thetaburst pairing (TBP) protocol (see also Hoffman *et al.* 2002). The protocol was similar to that used by Magee and Johnston (1997) and described

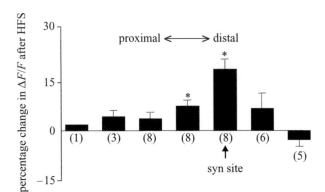

Fig. 10.4 Changes in dendritic Ca^{2+} signals after LTP induction. The histograms represent percentage change in $\Delta F/F \pm$ s.e.m. for adjacent 25 μm segments of the dendrite before, and 5 min after, inducing LTP with a 100 Hz pairing regime (see text). The segment of the dendrite corresponding to the location of the synapse (as determined from measurements of sub-threshold Ca^{2+} signals; see Magee *et al.* 1995) is marked with an arrow (syn site). The Ca^{2+} signals resulted from a train of 5 b-APs at 20 Hz triggered by brief current injections via a whole-cell patch pipette on the soma. The distances were normalized with respect to the location of the activated synapses, and the percentage change was averaged over all experiments for each region. Significant changes are marked with an asterisk, and the number of observations is shown in parentheses. (Taken from Schexnayder (1999), with permission.)

above, except that we chose the minimum number of b-APs that would elicit reliable LTP (Fig. 10.5; Watanabe *et al.* 2002). With two b-APs timed to coincide with the last two EPSPs in the train, LTP was induced. When the EPSPs and the b-APs were unpaired, however, no plasticity was observed. Furthermore, when the pairing protocol

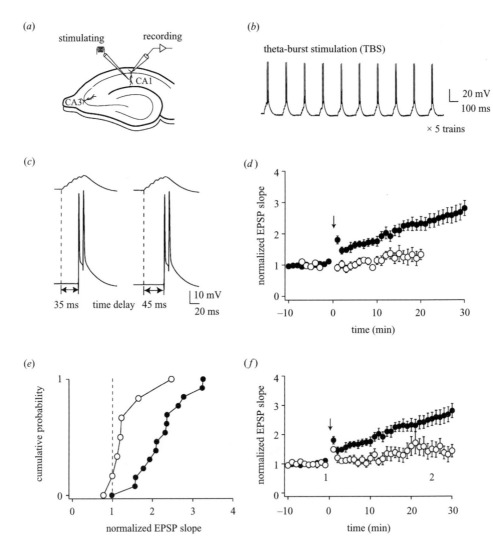

Fig. 10.5 LTP induction by pairing sub-threshold EPSPs and postsynaptic APs in a theta-burst pattern. (*a*) Schematic of a hippocampal slice showing stimulating and recording sites. (*b*) A sample of the TBP protocol. (*c*) Representative traces of subthreshold EPSPs and b-APs at two different time delays. (*d*) Time-course and magnitude of the test EPSP before and after the TBP (filled circles) procedure (arrow) for the 35 ms delay and for similar but unpaired (open circles) stimulation. (*e*) Cumulative probability plots (rank ordering of magnitude changes) for all experiments for TBP at 35 ms (filled circles) and 45 ms (open circles) delays. (*f*) Summary for all the experiments (35 ms, filled circles; 45 ms, open circles). (Taken from Watanabe *et al.* (2002), with permission.)

was changed so that the b-APs were delayed by 10 ms and only one b-AP was paired with an EPSP, LTP was significantly reduced. Recordings of these b-APs in the dendrites indicated that when the two b-APs were paired with the EPSPs, they were both boosted in amplitude, as seen previously by Magee and Johnston (1997), but when shifted by 10 ms, only one b-AP was increased in amplitude.

The results of this experiment, that is, that b-APs are boosted in amplitude when they are paired with EPSPs, were in keeping with the hypothesis previously mentioned, that inactivation of dendritic K^+ channels by the EPSPs would allow b-APs to propagate at increased amplitude. The results, however, also suggested that the boosting of b-AP amplitudes was essential for LTP induction. We further tested the proposed role of the K^+ channels by taking advantage of the finding that MAPK inhibitors shift the activation curve for A-type K^+ channels in the hyperpolarized direction and thereby increase their probability of opening (Watanabe *et al.* 2002). We found that the MAPK inhibitor U0126 decreased the amplitude of b-APs, decreased the boosting of b-APs during the TBP protocol, and decreased LTP induction. Although the MAPK inhibitor could be having multiple effects on channels and other signal transduction pathways, we did find that we could overcome the block of LTP by increasing the number of APs given during the TBP paradigm. The results are consistent with the hypothesis that the A-type K^+ channels in dendrites regulate the induction of LTP under certain conditions.

10.7 Discussion

Given the numerous types of voltage-gated channel in dendrites, important questions exist concerning the function of these channels in regulating synaptic integration and synaptic plasticity. The b-AP is an attractive candidate for providing a feedback signal from the cell body to the synaptic regions of the dendrites to show that an output of the neuron has occurred. Such a feedback signal may be an important enabler for LTP and LTD induction at active synapses and in certain dendritic branches, although b-APs are certainly not required for LTP/LTD induction under all conditions (e.g. Brown *et al.* 1990). The Ca^{2+} influx that accompanies the b-APs, and which occurs during the LTP induction protocols, may also regulate the expression and/or modulation of dendritic ion channels. Such mechanisms (e.g. Fig. 10.4) may play a role in so-called E-S potentiation where changes in the excitability of postsynaptic neurons have been shown to accompany LTP of the synaptic response (Chavez-Noriega *et al.* 1990).

In this report we have presented some of the experiments involving b-APs and LTD and LTP induction in CA1 pyramidal neurons. These experiments have demonstrated:

(i) a strong correlation between b-APs and the induction of several forms of synaptic plasticity;
(ii) that the amplitude of b-APs in the dendrites is an important variable for LTP induction;
(iii) that A-type K^+ channels in dendrites are highly regulated by several types of protein kinases and membrane potential;
(iv) that the induction of LTP using a TBP protocol depends on the activation/inactivation state of these K^+ channels;

(v) that the timing of pre- and postsynaptic events is critical for the induction of LTP and that this timing is determined in part by dendritic K^+ channels; and

(vi) that after the induction of LTP there are changes in the excitability of the dendrites in the vicinity of the activated synapses.

Several previous studies have shown that the induction of LTD/LTP depends on the relative timing of pre- and postsynaptic APs (Bi and Poo 1998, 2001; Markram *et al.* 1997; Debanne *et al.* 1998; Feldman 2000). The b-AP, and the boosting of the b-AP, may be an important mechanism in those studies as well, although there are clearly mechanisms other than dendritic K^+ channels that may be involved. For example, Stuart and Hausser (2001) have shown that the pairing of EPSPs and b-APs in neocortical pyramidal neurons boosts b-AP amplitude through an increased activation of Na^+ channels rather than the decreased activity of K^+ channels, as proposed here. Furthermore, in the most distal dendritic regions of CA1 neurons, in stratum lacunosum-moleculare, the local initiation of a dendritic AP by synaptic input rather than a b-AP propagated from the cell soma appears to be critical for LTP induction (Golding *et al.* 2002). Nevertheless, for Schaffer collateral synapses in the middle region of CA1 pyramidal neuron dendrites (stratum radiatum) from adult animals, a role for A-type K^+ channels in the induction and expression of LTP is well supported by several different types of experiment (see Ramakers and Storm 2002). Clearly, however, much more work is needed before the role of active dendrites in the induction and expression of synaptic plasticity is fully understood.

This work was supported by NIH grants MH44754, MH48432, and NS37444.

References

Adams, J. P., Anderson, A. E., Varga, A. W., Dineley, K. T., Cook, R. G., Pfaffinger, P. J., *et al.* (2000). The A-type potassium channel Kv4.2 is a substrate for the mitogen-activated protein kinase ERK. *J. Neurochem.* **75**, 2277–87.

Anderson, A. E., Adams, J. P., Qian, Y., Cook, R. G., Pfaffinger, P. J., and Sweatt, J. D. (2000). Kv4.2 phosphorylation by cyclic AMP-dependent protein kinase. *J. Biol. Chem.* **275**, 5337–46.

Bi, G.-Q. and Poo, M.-M. (1998). Synaptic modifications in cultured hippocampal neurons: dependence on spike timing, synaptic strength, and postsynaptic cell type. *J. Neurosci.* **18**, 10464–72.

Bi, G. and Poo, M. (2001). Synaptic modification by correlated activity: Hebb's postulate revisited. *A. Rev. Neurosci.* **24**, 139–66.

Brown, T. H., Kairiss, E. W., and Keenan, C. L. (1990). Hebbian synapses: biophysical mechanisms and algorithms. *A. Rev. Neurosci.* **13**, 475–511.

Camodeca, N., Rowan, M. J., and Anwyl, R. (1998). Induction of LTD by increasing extracellular Ca^{2+} from a low level in the dentate gyrus *in vitro. Neurosci. Lett.* **255**, 53–6.

Chavez-Noriega, L. E., Halliwell, J. V., and Bliss, T. V. P. (1990). A decrease in firing threshold observed after induction of the EPSP-spike (E-S) component of long-term potentiation in rat hippocampal slices. *Exp. Brain Res.* **79**, 633–41.

Christie, B. R., Magee, J. C., and Johnston, D. (1996*a*). Dendritic calcium channels and hippocampal long-term depression. *Hippocampus* **6**, 17–23.

Christie, B. R., Magee, J. C., and Johnston, D. (1996*b*). The role of dendritic action potentials and Ca^{2+} influx in the induction of homosynaptic long-term depression in hippocampal CA1 pyramidal neurons. *Learn. Memory* **3**, 160–9.

Christie, B. R., Schexnayder, L. K., and Johnston, D. (1997). Contribution of voltage-gated Ca^{2+} channels to homosynaptic long-term depression in the CA1 region *in vitro. J. Neurophysiol.* **77**, 1651–5.

Colbert, C. M. and Johnston, D. (1996). Axonal action-potential initiation and Na^+ channel densities in the soma and axon initial segment of subicular pyramidal neurons. *J. Neurosci.* **16**, 6676–86.

Colbert, C. M. and Pan, E. (2002). Ion channel properties underlying axonal action potential initiation in pyramidal neurons. *Nature Neurosci.* **5**, 533–8.

Debanne, D., Gähwiler, B. H., and Thompson, S. M. (1998). Long-term synaptic plasticity between pairs of individual CA3 pyramidal cells in rat hippocampal slice cultures. *J. Physiol. (Lond.)* **507**, 237–47.

Dudek, S. M. and Bear, M. F. (1992). Homosynaptic long-term depression in area CA1 of hippocampus and effects of N-methyl-D-aspartate receptor blockade. *Proc. Natl Acad. Sci. USA* **89**, 4363–7.

Feldman, D. E. (2000). Timing-based LTP and LTD at vertical inputs to layer II/III pyramidal cells in rat barrel cortex. *Neuron* **27**, 45–56.

Gasparini, S. and Magee, J. C. (2002). Phosphorylation-dependent differences in the activation properties of distal and proximal dendritic Na^+ channels in rat CA1 hippocampal neurons. *J. Physiol.* **541**, 665–72.

Golding, N. L. and Spruston, N. (1998). Dendritic sodium spikes are variable triggers of axonal action potentials in hippocampal CA1 pyramidal neurons. *Neuron* **21**, 1189–200.

Golding, N. L., Kath, W. L., and Spruston, N. (2001). Dichotomy of action-potential backpropagation in CA1 pyramidal neuron dendrites. *J. Neurophysiol.* **86**, 2998–3010.

Golding, N. L., Staff, N. P., and Spruston, N. (2002). Dendritic spikes as a mechanism for cooperative long-term potentiation. *Nature* **418**, 326–31.

Hoffman, D. A. and Johnston, D. (1998). Downregulation of transient K^+ channels in dendrites of hippocampal CA1 pyramidal neurons by activation of PKA and PKC. *J. Neurosci.* **18**, 3521–8.

Hoffman, D. A. and Johnston, D. (1999). Neuromodulation of dendritic action potentials. *J. Neurophysiol.* **81**, 408–11.

Hoffman, D. A., Magee, J. C., Colbert, C. M., and Johnston, D. (1997). K^+ channel regulation of signal propagation in dendrites of hippocampal pyramidal neurons. *Nature* **387**, 869–75.

Hoffman, D. A., Sprengel, R., and Sakmann, B. (2002). Molecular dissection of hippocampal theta-burst pairing potentiation. *Proc. Natl Acad. Sci. USA* **99**, 7740–5.

Jaffe, D. B., Johnston, D., Lasser-Ross, N., Lisman, J. E., Miyakawa, H., and Ross, W. N. (1992). The spread of Na^+ spikes determines the pattern of dendritic Ca^{2+} entry into hippocampal neurons. *Nature* **357**, 244–6.

Johnston, D., Magee, J. C., Colbert, C. M., and Christie, B. R. (1996). Active properties of neuronal dendrites. *A. Rev. Neurosci.* **19**, 165–86.

Johnston, D., Hoffman, D. A., Colbert, C. M., and Magee, J. C. (1999). Regulation of backpropagating action potentials in hippocampal neurons. *Curr. Opin. Neurobiol.* **9**, 288–92.

Johnston, D., Hoffman, D. A., Magee, J. C., Poolos, N. P., Watanabe, S., Colbert, C. M., *et al.* (2000). Dendritic potassium channels in hippocampal pyramidal neurons. *J. Physiol. (Lond.)* **525**, 75–81.

Magee, J. C. (1998). Dendritic hyperpolarization-activated currents modify the integrative properties of hippocampal CA1 pyramidal neurons. *J. Neurosci.* **18**, 7613–24.

Magee, J. C. (1999). Voltage-gated ion channels in dendrites. In *Dendrites* (ed. G. Stuart, N. Spruston and M. Hausser), pp. 139–60. Oxford University Press.

Magee, J. C. and Johnston, D. (1995). Characterization of single voltage-gated Na^+ and Ca^{2+} channels in apical dendrites of rat CA1 pyramidal neurons. *J. Physiol. (Lond.)* **487**, 67–90.

Magee, J. C. and Johnston, D. (1997). A synaptically controlled, associative signal for Hebbian plasticity in hippocampal neurons. *Science* **275**, 209–13.

Magee, J. C., Christofi, G., Miyakawa, H., Christie, B., Lasser-Ross, N., and Johnston, D. (1995). Subthreshold synaptic activation of voltage-gated Ca^{2+} channels mediates a localized Ca^{2+} influx into the dendrites of hippocampal pyramidal neurons. *J. Neurophysiol.* **74**, 1335–42.

Magee, J. C., Hoffman, D., Colbert, C., and Johnston, D. (1998). Electrical and calcium signaling in dendrites of hippocampal pyramidal neurons. *A. Rev. Physiol.* **60**, 327–46.

Maletic-Savatic, M., Lenn, N. J., and Trimmer, J. S. (1995). Differential spatiotemporal expression of K^+ channel polypeptides in rat hippocampal neurons developing *in situ* and *in vitro. J. Neurosci.* **15**, 3840–51.

Markram, H., Lübke, J., Frotscher, M., and Sakmann, B. (1997). Regulation of synaptic efficacy by coincidence of postsynaptic APs and EPSPs. *Science* **275**, 213–15.

Mickus, T., Jung, H. Y., and Spruston, N. (1999). Properties of slow, cumulative sodium channel inactivation in rat hippocampal CA1 pyramidal neurons. *Biophys. J.* **76**, 846–60.

Migliore, M., Hoffman, D. A., Magee, J. C., and Johnston, D. (1999). Role of an A-type K^+ conductance in the back-propagation of action potentials in the dendrites of hippocampal pyramidal neurons. *J. Comput. Neurosci.* **7**, 5–15.

Miyakawa, H., Ross, W. N., Jaffe, D., Callaway, J. C., Lasser-Ross, N., Lisman, J. E., *et al.* (1992). Synaptically activated increases in Ca^{2+} concentration in hippocampal CA1 pyramidal cells are primarily due to voltage-gated Ca^{2+} channels. *Neuron* **9**, 1163–73.

Mockett, B., Coussens, C., and Abraham, W. C. (2002). NMDA receptor-mediated metaplasticity during the induction of long-term depression by low-frequency stimulation. *Eur. J. mNeurosci.* **15**, 1819–26.

Mulkey, R. M. and Malenka, R. C. (1992). Mechanisms underlying induction of homosynaptic long-term depression in area CA1 of the hippocampus. *Neuron* **9**, 967–75.

Poolos, N. P., Migliore, M., and Johnston, D. (2002). Pharmacological upregulation of h-channels reduces the excitability of pyramidal neuron dendrites. *Nature Neurosci.* **5**, 767–74.

Ramakers, G. M. and Storm, J. F. (2002). A postsynaptic transient K^+ current modulated by arachidonic acid regulates synaptic integration and threshold for LTP induction in hippocampal pyramidal cells. *Proc. Natl Acad. Sci. USA* **99**, 10 144–9.

Roberson, E. D., English, J. D., and Sweatt, J. D. (1996). A biochemist's view of long-term potentiation. *Learn. Memory* **3**, 1–24.

Sabatini, B. L. and Svoboda, K. (2000). Analysis of calcium channels in single spines using optical fluctuation analysis. *Nature* **408**, 589–3.

Schexnayder, L. K. (1999). Postsynaptic mechanisms for the induction of long-term potentiation and long-term depression of synaptic transmission in CA1 pyramidal neurons. PhD dissertation, Division of Neuroscience, Baylor College of Medicine.

Schrader, L. A., Anderson, A. E., Mayne, A., Pfaffinger, P. J., and Sweatt, J. D. (2002). PKA modulation of Kv4.2-encoded A-type potassium channels requires formation of a supramolecular complex. *J. Neurosci.* **22**, 10 123–33.

Serodio, P. and Rudy, B. (1998). Differential expression of Kv4 K^+ channel subunits mediating subthreshold transient K^+ (A-type) currents in rat brain. *J. Neurophysiol.* **79**, 1081–91.

Sheng, M. Tsaur, M., Jan, Y. N., and Jan, L. Y. (1992). Subcellular segregation of two A-type K^+ channel proteins in rat central neurons. *Neuron* **9**, 271–4.

Shepherd, G. M. (1991). *Foundations of the neuron doctrine.* Oxford University Press.

Spruston, N., Schiller, Y., Stuart, G., and Sakmann, B. (1995). Activity-dependent action potential invasion and calcium influx into hippocampal CA1 dendrites. *Science* **268**, 297–300.

Stuart, G. J. and Hausser, M. (2001). Dendritic coincidence detection of EPSPs and action potentials. *Nature Neurosci.* **4**, 63–71.

Watanabe, S., Hoffman, D. A., Migliore, M., and Johnston, D. (2002). Dendritic K^+ channels contribute to spike-timing dependent long-term potentiation in hippocampal pyramidal neurons. *Proc. Natl Acad. Sci. USA* **99**, 8366–71.

Yuan, L. L., Adams, J. P., Swank, M., Sweatt, J. D., and Johnston, D. (2002). Protein kinase modulation of dendritic K^+ channels in hippocampus involves a mitogen-activated protein kinase pathway. *J. Neurosci.* **22**, 4860–8.

Glossary

AP	action potential
b-AP	back-propagating action potential
EPSP	excitatory postsynaptic potential
LFS	low-frequency stimulation
LTD	long-term depression
LTP	long-term potentiation
MAPK	mitogen-activated protein kinase
NMDA	N-methyl-D-aspartate
PKA	cAMP-dependent protein kinase
PKC	protein kinase C
TTX	tetrodotoxin

Expression

11

Long-term potentiation in the dentate gyrus of the anaesthetized rat is accompanied by an increase in extracellular glutamate: real-time measurements using a novel dialysis electrode

M. L. Errington, P. T. Galley, and T. V. P. Bliss

We have used a glutamate-specific dialysis electrode to obtain real-time measurements of changes in the concentration of glutamate in the extracellular space of the hippocampus during low-frequency stimulation and following the induction of long-term potentiation (LTP). In the dentate gyrus, stimulation of the perforant path at 2 Hz for 2 min produced a transient increase in glutamate current relative to the basal value at control rates of stimulation (0.033 Hz). This activity-dependent glutamate current was significantly enhanced 35 and 90 min after the induction of LTP. The maximal 2 Hz signal was obtained during post-tetanic potentiation (PTP). There was also a more gradual increase in the basal level of extracellular glutamate following the induction of LTP. Both the basal and activity-dependent increases in glutamate current induced by tetanic stimulation were blocked by local infusion of the N-methyl-D-aspartate receptor antagonist D-APV. In areas CA1 and CA3 we were unable to detect a 2 Hz glutamate signal either before or after the induction of LTP, possibly owing to a more avid uptake of glutamate in the pyramidal cell fields. These results demonstrate that LTP in the dentate gyrus is associated with a greater concentration of extracellular glutamate following activation of potentiated synapses, either because potentiated synapses release more transmitter per impulse, or because of reduced uptake by glutamate transporters. We present arguments favouring increased release rather than decreased uptake.

Keywords: long-term potentiation; hippocampus; synaptic plasticity; glutamate

11.1 Introduction

An uneasy peace occupied most of the first decade of the 30 years' war between the pre- and post-expressionists—that is, between those who maintain that the expression of NMDA receptor-dependent LTP has a presynaptic component, and those who claim it is entirely postsynaptic.[1] The first salvo was fired in 1981 by the presynaptic forces. Skrede and Malthe-Sørenssen measured the efflux of radiolabelled aspartate from hippocampal slices and noted an increase in both basal and stimulated efflux after tetanization in area CA1 (Skrede and Malthe-Sørenssen 1981). Using a push–pull cannula with attached recording electrodes, we observed a similar increase in the efflux of radiolabelled glutamate following the induction of LTP in the dentate gyrus of the anaesthetized rat (Dolphin *et al.* 1982), and accordingly declared ourselves for the presynaptic cause.[2] In the latter study, we first established that the technique was sensitive enough to detect an increase in the concentration of glutamate in the extracellular space under conditions in which, assuredly, there was an increase in glutamate release—that is, when the rate of stimulation and the number of fibres stimulated were simultaneously increased. We then showed that following the induction of LTP there was a sustained increase (lasting more than 1 h) in the concentration of extracellular glutamate, and that when the induction protocol failed to induce LTP there was no such increase. These experiments were carried out 1–2 years before publication of the first method for blocking the induction of LTP in the dentate gyrus (by pairing the tetanus to the perforant path with activation of the inhibitory commissural input; Douglas *et al.* 1983) and the seminal discovery of the block of LTP by D-APV, a specific antagonist of the NMDA receptor (Collingridge *et al.* 1983). In later push–pull experiments we measured endogenous glutamate and confirmed that LTP was associated with an increase in glutamate efflux. Moreover, both LTP and the associated increase in glutamate efflux were blocked by commissural stimulation (Bliss *et al.* 1986) and by perfusion with D-APV (Errington *et al.* 1987). We interpreted these results as indicating that LTP was associated with an increase in transmitter release, and hence that there was a presynaptic component to the expression of LTP (reviewed in Bliss *et al.* 1990). We were, however, unable to exclude the possibility that a persistent reduction in glutamate uptake contributed to the observed increase. Moreover, our results gave us information only on basal and not on stimulus-dependent glutamate efflux, which might be expected to be a more sensitive measure of increased release from terminals of potentiated synapses. Another disadvantage of HPLC-based glutamate measurements using the push–pull technique is the poor time resolution; samples have to be collected for 10–15 min to collect sufficient perfusate for reliable assays. We have re-approached the question using a glutamate-sensitive electrode developed by Albery, Galley and colleagues (Albery *et al.* 1987; Galley 1991) that has allowed us to make real-time measurements of changes in glutamate concentration in the hippocampus of the anaesthetized rat.

Using this real-time device, we have confirmed our previous observation that LTP in the dentate gyrus is associated with an increase in the basal concentration of extracellular glutamate. We also report a sustained increase in a stimulus-dependent component of extracellular glutamate that most probably reflects an increase in glutamate release from potentiated fibres. In areas CA1 and CA3, in striking contrast to our findings in the dentate gyrus, we were unable to detect a stimulus-dependent increase in glutamate efflux unless we used stimulus parameters that led to seizure activity. The most likely reason for this failure is a greater density of glutamate transporters in this region than in the dentate gyrus.

11.2 Methods

(a) Surgery

Adult male Sprague–Dawley rats (250–400 g), bred in the NIMR animal facility, were anaesthetized with urethane (1.5 g kg^{-1}, injected intraperitoneally, a dose sufficient to maintain anaesthesia for the duration of the experiment) and placed in a head-holder with the skull horizontal. Temperature was monitored with a rectal thermometer and maintained by means of an overhead lamp to within $\pm 0.5\,°C$ of initial body temperature. The skull was exposed, and two holes drilled, one exposing the cortex overlying the dorsal hippocampus, and the other over the angular bundle. The dura was deflected to allow insertion of the dialysis and recording electrode assembly through the first hole, and a stimulating electrode through the second.

All experiments described in this report were carried out in accordance with the UK Animals (Scientific Procedures) Act, 1986.

(b) Stimulating and recording

To activate fibres of the perforant path, a bipolar stimulating electrode (Rhodes Electromedical) was placed in the angular bundle (coordinates with respect to bregma: 8 mm posterior, 4.4 mm lateral, depth adjusted to maximize the synaptic potential evoked in the dentate gyrus). Test stimuli were delivered at a frequency of 0.033 Hz, and consisted of monophasic rectangular pulses, pulse width 50 µs. Intensity was chosen to produce a population spike of around 1 mV at the start of the experiment. LTP was induced in the dentate gyrus by a sequence of three trains (250 Hz for 200 ms) delivered at intervals of 60 s, with a single test shock interpolated 30 s after each train. In areas CA1 and CA3 the tetanus consisted of a sequence of two trains (100 Hz for 500 ms) at an interval of 60 s, with a test shock delivered 30 s after the first train. Field potentials were monitored with two Teflon-coated stainless steel wires (125 µm o.d., Clark Electromedical, UK) attached with epoxy resin to the sides of the microdialysis electrode. The separation between the cut ends of the two electrodes was around 750 µm, so that when the upper electrode was in the molecular layer the lower end was in the hilus.

The dialysis and recording electrode assembly (coordinates: 3.9 mm posterior to bregma and 2.5 mm lateral to midline, on the same side as the stimulating electrode) was advanced slowly into the dorsal hippocampus through the overlying cortex, while test stimuli were delivered at 0.033 Hz. The electrode was advanced until the field EPSP at the upper of the two recording electrodes was maximally negative. At this point, the upper recording electrode was in the terminal region of the medial perforant path in the middle of the molecular layer, the exposed dialysis membrane straddled the molecular layer, and the epoxy plug and the lower recording electrode were in the hilus, below the granule cell layer.

For stimulating and recording in the CA1 and CA3 pyramidal cell fields the following electrode positions were used: CA1, dialysis electrode 4.1 mm posterior to bregma, 2.5 mm lateral to midline; stimulating electrode in contralateral ventral hippocampal commissure, 4.0 mm posterior to bregma, 0.5 mm lateral. CA3, dialysis electrode 3.0 mm posterior to bregma, 2.2 mm lateral to midline; stimulating electrode in contralateral ventral hippocampal commissure, 3.0 mm posterior to bregma, 0.5 mm lateral to midline. The depth of the recording electrode was adjusted to maximize negative-going synaptic potentials in stratum oriens or in stratum radiatum. In some experiments a second stimulating electrode was placed in the hilus of the ipsilateral dentate gyrus to activate mossy fibres. The depth of this electrode was adjusted to maximize the antidromic population spike recorded in the dentate gyrus.

The collection of evoked potentials, and the timing and intensity of stimulation, were under computer control (software written by Dr R. M. Douglas, University of British Columbia). The output from the potentiostat was sampled at 100 Hz, and means of 500 responses were computed at 5 s intervals, using a second computer.

(c) The dialysis electrode

The underlying principles of the dialysis electrode and details of its fabrication have been given in detail elsewhere (Albery *et al.* 1987; Galley 1991; Walker *et al.* 1995), and will only be briefly considered here. The glutamate electrode, as indicated in Fig. 11.1*a*, depends on the oxidation of glutamate by glutamate oxidase that, in the presence of molecular oxygen, produces hydrogen peroxide by means of the linked reactions depicted in Fig. 11.1*b*. The coenzyme flavin adenine dinucleotide, essential for electron transfer, is irreversibly bound to glutamate oxidase during manufacture. The reaction is contained within the interior of the dialysis tubing, which is freely permeable to glutamate, but impermeable to the enzyme. Hydrogen peroxide is reoxidized at the surface of the platinum electrode, which is held at a potential of 650 mV, producing two electrons for each molecule of H_2O_2. Glutamate oxidase was a gift from Dr H. Kusakobe, Yamasa Corporation, Chosi, Japan.

(d) Construction of the dialysis electrode

The working electrode consists of platinum wire inserted into a 9 mm length of microdialysis tubing (o.d. 230 µm; Gambro, UK). The wire is coated with Teflon (Goodfellow, UK) except for a 1.5 mm length at its distal end, where it is bent double, exposing two around 600 µm lengths of uninsulated platinum (see Fig. 11.1*a*). The exposed platinum was coated with Nafion or, in later experiments, with polyphenylene diamine to reduce the signal from other electroactive interferents (see next section). The assembly is strengthened and supported at the top by an inner layer of polythene tubing, and an outer layer of glass tubing, and is sealed at the top and bottom with epoxy cement which leaves only the lower 0.5 mm length of dialysis tubing exposed. Two Teflon-insulated 75 µm silver wires, with 2 mm of exposed silver, one chlorided except at the cut tip, and the other unchlorided, were inserted into the chamber to act as reference and counter electrodes, respectively, for the potentiostat (see below). Inflow and outflow pipes, made from vitreous silica tubing (o.d. 140 µm; SGE Scientific, Milton Keynes, UK) were provided to enable the chamber to be filled with appropriate media. (Similar dialysis electrodes can be obtained pre-assembled from Sycopel International, Jarrow, UK.) Electrodes were connected to 1 mm gold pins (AWP, Redhill, UK). The preparation of the electrode for *in vitro* and *in vivo* use is described below.

(e) Specificity

Potential sources of artefact are of two principal kinds: electroactive metabolites other than H_2O_2 that generate a signal at 650 mV, and impurities in the enzyme which could allow a signal to be generated by amino acids other than glutamate. In respect of the first type, the major interferent is ascorbate, which is present at a concentration of 100–500 µM in cerebrospinal fluid, and at 650 mV is oxidized to dehydroascorbate. Interference from ascorbate, as well as other possible anionic interferents such as dopamine and its metabolite DOPAC, homovanillic acid and uric acid, was minimized initially by coating the electrode with Nafion, a negatively charged sulphonated polymer, or, subsequently and more effectively, by electropolymerizing a

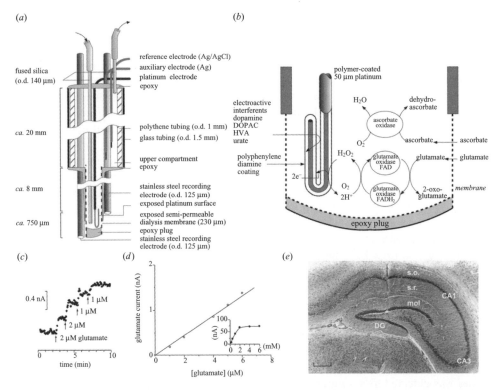

Fig. 11.1 The glutamate dialysis electrode. (*a*) Construction details. The working part of the electrode is at the bottom, immediately above the epoxy plug. Here, the semi-permeable dialysis membrane is exposed, and small extracellular molecules are free to diffuse into the dialysis chamber. The platinum electrode within the chamber is uninsulated at this level, and is hooked to increase surface area. a.c.s.f., glutamate oxidase and ascorbate oxidase can be infused into the chamber via the polythene tubing inlet and outlet. The three electrodes are connected to a high-impedance potentiostat that monitors the current generated at the platinum electrode. To monitor synaptically evoked field potentials two wire electrodes with exposed ends staggered by 750 μm are attached to the electrode assembly with epoxy cement. (*b*) Summary of redox reactions. Electro-active molecules, including glutamate and ascorbate, diffuse into the dialysis chamber from extracellular space. The oxidation of glutamate by glutamate oxidase leads to the production of H_2O_2, which is electroactive in the presence of oxygen, producing two electrons for each molecule of H_2O_2 (see text). Ascorbate, the major electroactive interferent, is oxidized to the inactive dehydroascorbate by ascorbate oxidase. Other interferents include dopamine, 3,4-dihydroxy-phenylacetic acid (DOPAC), homovanillic acid (HVA) and urate. (*c,d*) *In vitro* calibration of the electrode. Data from two electrodes. The electrode was immersed in a.c.s.f. in a small beaker, and aliquots of glutamate added to produce step-changes of 1 or 2 μM in the concentration of glutamate. The electrode shows a linear response curve up to 1 mM; at higher concentrations the response saturates (*d*, inset). (*e*) Coronal section through the hippocampal formation, stained with cresyl violet, showing the track of the glutamate electrode as it was advanced through area CA1 into the molecular layer of the dentate gyrus; scale bar, 500 μm. Abbreviations: s.o., stratum oriens; s.r., stratum radiatum; mol, molecular layer; DG, dentate gyrus; CA1, CA3, pyramidal cell fields of areas CA1 and CA3.

polyphenylene diamine coat onto the platinum electrode immediately before use. The polymer coating excludes interferents on the basis of size. Further reduction in the ascorbate signal with either coating was obtained by adding ascorbate oxidase ($1 \, \text{U} \, \mu\text{l}^{-1}$) to the solution in the dialysis chamber, to oxidize ascorbate before it reached the platinum electrode; the oxidation product, dehydroascorbate, is not itself electro-active. Utilizing these precautions, no stimulus-dependent increase in electrode current attributable to ascorbate could be detected (Fig. 11.2b). The enzyme showed negligible sensitivity to other physiological L-amino acids tested (Dr H. Kusakobe, personal communication), with the exception, in early batches, of glutamine, presumably as the result of contamination with glutamine oxidase. The glutamine signal saturated at 20 μM, a concentration which is less than that reported for extracellular fluid in hippocampus (Lerma et al. 1986); it is thus unlikely that any increases in signal observed in these experiments can be explained by an increase in the concentration of glutamine. Later batches of the enzyme showed no glutaminase activity. Similar results were obtained with glutamine-sensitive and glutamine-insensitive enzyme, and data from the two sources have been pooled.

(f) Potentiostat

The current generated by the oxidation of H_2O_2 was measured with a potentiostat operating in a three-electrode configuration (Energy Microsystems, Newbury, UK). A potential of 650 mV was applied between the working platinum electrode and the reference electrode, while the current flowing between the working and counter electrodes was detected as a voltage at the output of the current-to-voltage circuitry of the potentiostat.

(g) Calibration and use of the electrode

To prepare the electrode, the dialysis chamber was filled with a.c.s.f. (composition in mM: NaCl 120, KCl 3, KH_2PO_4 1.2, Mg_2SO_4 1.18, $NaHCO_3$ 23, $CaCl_2$ 2, glucose 10, pre-gassed with 95% O_2, 5% CO_2) using a perfusion pump (CMA/100, Carnegie). Electrodes were sometimes prepared on the day they were to be used, and sometimes on the previous day and stored overnight at 4 °C. Immediately before first use, platinum electrodes that had not already been coated with Nafion were protected by electropolymerization; a positive potential (650 mV) was applied for 20 min while the electrode was immersed in a solution containing 5 mM polyethylene diamine. a.c.s.f. in the chamber was then replaced with a.c.s.f. containing glutamate oxidase ($0.05 \, \text{U} \, \mu\text{l}^{-1}$), and ascorbate oxidase ($1 \, \text{U} \, \text{l}^{-1}$) in a.c.s.f. The electrode was calibrated *in vitro* by immersion in a small pot containing a.c.s.f., to which aliquots of glutamate were added. A linear relationship between glutamate concentration and current was routinely observed in the range 0–1 mM (Fig. 11.1c,d). Following *in vitro* calibration, which was carried out before each experiment, the electrode was lowered into the hippocampus, as described above. In some cases, the electrode fluid was replaced with a.c.s.f. containing ascorbate oxidase but with glutamate oxidase omitted, to obtain a glutamate-independent baseline (Fig. 11.2b). We found that it was necessary to leave the electrode in place for 4–5 h before a stable baseline and reliable activity-dependent responses could be obtained, presumably because of high background levels of glutamate released by

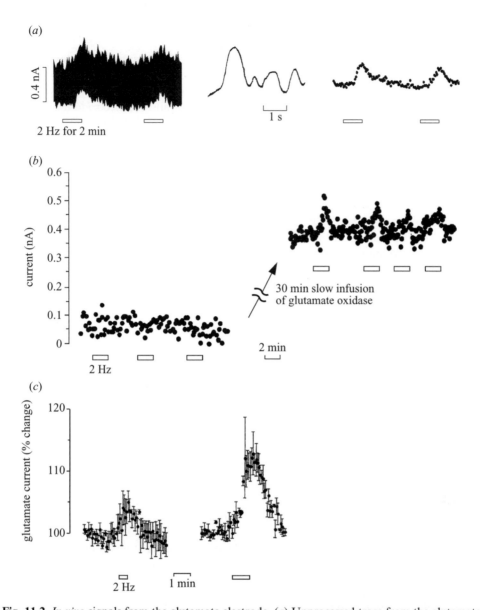

Fig. 11.2 *In vivo* signals from the glutamate electrode. (*a*) Unprocessed trace from the glutamate electrode (left), showing the increase in signal generated by increasing the rate of stimulation from 0.033 to 2 Hz (open bars here and in subsequent figures). The middle trace displays the unprocessed signal at an expanded time-scale. Note the strong 1 Hz component. The relatively noise-free trace on the right was computed by sampling the unprocessed signal at 100 Hz, and averaging successive sets of 500 consecutive values, to obtain a mean value every 5 s. All glutamate signals in this and subsequent figures were obtained in this way. (*b*) The glutamate electrode generates a small non-specific current *in vivo* in the absence of glutamate oxidase owing to the presence of electroactive contaminants. Slow infusion of glutamate oxidase resulted in an increase in basal current from approximately 0.05 to 0.38 nA. An interval of 4 h elapsed between the 30 min infusion of glutamate oxidase and the record of glutamate current shown on the right. A 2 Hz glutamate signal (open bars) was only obtained when glutamate oxidase was present. (*c*) The amplitude and duration of the 2 Hz signal depends on the duration of stimulation. The traces are averages from a single animal in which episodes of 2 Hz stimulation were given for 30 and 60 s ($n = 3$ in both cases).

damaged tissue. The electrode was usually recalibrated at the end of the experiment. Where this was done, we invariably noted a reduction in sensitivity, probably through coating of the membrane with extracellular proteins. Previously used electrodes could be cleaned by sonication, electrolyte and enzyme replaced, and the electrode recalibrated.

(h) Kinetics of the response to glutamate and consideration of rate-limiting factors

Although there is an absolute requirement for oxygen, the oxygen tension in a.c.s.f. and in the extracellular fluid of the brain is sufficiently high that the availability of oxygen is not a factor that limits the glutamate current either *in vitro* or *in vivo*. The rate-limiting step in the reaction is the diffusion of glutamate through the dialysis membrane. The kinetics of the electrode *in vitro* can be estimated from Fig. 11.1*c*. The time-constant to step increases of glutamate concentration in the external medium is approximately 15 s.

11.3 Results

(a) Response of the glutamate electrode in vivo

The glutamate signal from the dialysis electrode was contaminated by a much larger endogenous rhythmic electrical activity at a frequency in the range 1–2 Hz, arising from a combination of respiratory, electrocardiogram and electroencephalogram activity. We did not find a satisfactory way of eliminating or filtering the signal, and instead extracted the glutamate signal from the uncorrelated noise by averaging. The computer was programmed to sample the potentiostat output at 10 ms intervals, and the mean value was computed and plotted on-line at 5 s intervals (representing 500 samples). Figure 11.2*a* shows examples of the non-averaged output from the potentiostat plotted on a chart recorder at slow and fast paper speeds, and of the corresponding computer-derived mean signal obtained over successive 5 s sampling episodes, when the rate of stimulation was increased from 0.033 to 2 Hz for 2 min. Note the delay, typically 30–60 s, between the onset of 2 Hz stimulation and the onset of the response.

(b) Estimation of resting glutamate concentration

Our attempts to obtain estimates of the absolute concentration of glutamate were frustrated by two factors. The first was the fact, mentioned above, that insertion into the brain reduced the sensitivity of the probe, as indicated by subsequent *in vitro* recalibration. Thus, for any given experiment we had, at best, only an upper and lower limit of sensitivity. The second factor can be clarified by reference to the experiment illustrated in Fig. 11.2*b*. In order to estimate the component of the total signal due to electroactive interferents, in some experiments the electrode assembly was initially advanced into the hippocampus with the microdialysis chamber filled with a.c.s.f. containing ascorbate oxidase but without glutamate oxidase. Five hours were allowed for the basal signal to stabilize. The original solution was then replaced, using an infusion pump (0.05 μl min^{-1}), with a.c.s.f. containing both ascorbate oxidase and glutamate oxidase. In the experiment shown, this procedure resulted in a gradual rise in current to a new, stable level. The percentage of the total resting current due to glutamate can be expressed as the ratio of the increase in current with glutamate oxidase in the electrode to the total current: in this case the glutamate current was 87.5% of the total current. In other cases, however, when this protocol was followed, addition of glutamate oxidase to the electrode solution resulted in a prolonged period of instability in the current signal, sometimes lasting for 1–2 h, before the signal stabilized at a new level, which was sometimes, for unknown reasons, lower than that previously measured in the absence of glutamate oxidase. We also attempted to develop an *in vivo* calibration protocol. A cannula (23 gauge needle) was attached to the glutamate electrode with its tip adjacent to the region of exposed membrane. Glutamate was injected over a range of concentrations and injection rates. In favourable cases this allowed an estimate to be made of the increase, in μM, of the concentration of glutamate following a 2 Hz simulation or the induction of LTP. We would only have been able to make an estimate of absolute values of glutamate concentration if we had been able to combine both of the above techniques in the same experiment. In the event, neither method was sufficiently reliable for routine use. Our results are therefore all expressed as percentage changes with respect to baseline glutamate current.

(c) Activity-dependent release in the dentate gyrus

We did not detect any difference in glutamate current when switching from stimulation of the perforant path at the test frequency of 0.033 Hz to no stimulation at all (data not shown). However, we consistently observed an increase in current when the rate of stimulation of the perforant path was increased from 0.033 to 2 Hz, provided the electrode contained glutamate oxidase (Fig. 11.2a,b). The amplitude of the 2 Hz signal was a function of the duration of stimulation (Fig. 11.2c). It was essential that the exposed platinum surface of the glutamate electrode was positioned in the molecular layer as no 2 Hz signal could be obtained in the cell body layer or the hilus.

(d) LTP in the dentate gyrus is associated with an increase in both basal and activity-dependent glutamate efflux

The experiments illustrated in Figs 11.3 and 11.4 illustrate the principal result obtained. They demonstrate that LTP in the dentate gyrus is accompanied by a sustained increase in both basal and activity-dependent glutamate signals. The experimental protocol required a pre-tetanus period of at least 1 h during which stimulation at the test frequency of 0.033 Hz was interrupted by one or more episodes of 2 Hz stimulation for 2 min. LTP was then induced and monitored for 2–5 h, test stimuli again being interspersed with episodes of 2 Hz stimulation. An individual experiment of this sort is shown in Fig. 11.3, with the slope of the population EPSP plotted in Fig. 11.3a, and the glutamate-dependent current in Fig. 11.3b. Note that the signal corresponding to zero glutamate is known in this case (the same experiment as illustrated in Fig. 11.2b), so that changes in the current can be expressed as a percentage change in extracellular glutamate concentration relative to the pre-tetanus level. The mean peak value (± s.e.m.) of the change in glutamate current induced by 2 Hz stimulation before the tetanus was 19.3 ± 0.9%, compared with the post-tetanus mean of 32.6 ± 3.9% 90 min

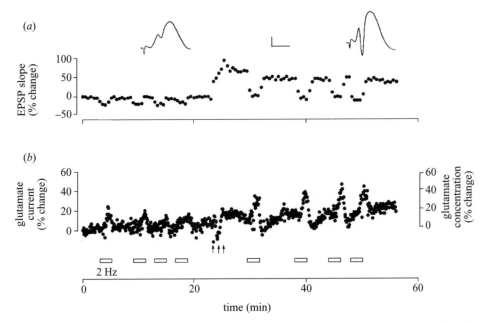

Fig. 11.3 Increase in basal and stimulus-dependent extracellular glutamate concentration following the induction of LTP. Records obtained from a single animal (same experiment as in Fig. 11.2*b*). (*a*) The slope of the EPSP was sampled at 30 s intervals. Episodes of 2 Hz stimulation for 2 min were given at the times indicated by the open bars in (*b*). Note the reduction in slope of the EPSP during 2 Hz stimulation. LTP was induced by a protocol consisting of three sets of trains (50 stimuli at 250 Hz, arrows), with an inter-train interval of 1 min, and a test stimulus between each train. Sample field potentials obtained 1 min before (left) and 30 min after (right) the induction of LTP are shown above. Calibration 2 mV, 5 ms. (*b*) Percentage change in glutamate current aligned with the slope of the EPSP. Following the induction of LTP, there were statistically significant increases both in the 2 Hz signal and in basal glutamate concentration (see text).

post-tetanus ($n = 4$ before and after tetanus; $p < 0.02$, unpaired, two-tailed *t*-test). Peaks were measured from basal values immediately before the onset of the 2 Hz stimulation in each case. The basal level was $8.7 \pm 0.6\%$ for the 20 values immediately preceding the tetanus; this increased to $22.8 \pm 0.6\%$ for the 20 values immediately preceding the final 2 Hz episode ($p < 0.0001$, *t*-test).

The normalized and averaged results of a series of experiments in which test stimulation was interrupted by periods of 2 Hz stimulation for 2 min, starting 15 min before, 30 min after and again 90 min after the tetanus, are shown in Fig. 11.4. It is noticeable that the increase in the basal glutamate signal following tetanization (Fig. 11.4*a,b*) has an onset that is considerably slower than the almost immediate increase in the evoked response. The averaged values of the glutamate signal elicited by the 2 Hz stimulation are displayed in Fig. 11.4*c* for all 11 animals with glutamate oxidase-filled electrodes in which LTP was induced. There was a marked increase in magnitude and duration, and a decrease in onset of the activity-dependent glutamate current at both 35 and 90 min after induction of LTP (Fig. 11.4*c*). To estimate the statistical significance of these increases the area under the current–time curve generated by the electrode in the 3 min following the onset of the 2 Hz stimulation was computed. This procedure gives a

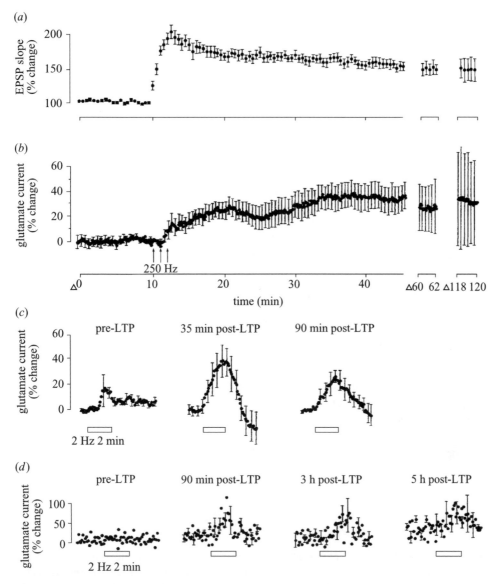

Fig. 11.4 LTP is associated with an increase in both basal and activity-dependent extracellular glutamate concentration. (*a–c*) Group data from a series of 11 experiments. (*a*) The slope of the EPSP plotted as a function of time. (*b*) Corresponding timecourse of percentage change in glutamate current. The open triangles beneath the abscissa indicate the times at which episodes of 2 Hz stimulation for 2 min were given. Note the slow rise in the basal glutamate current after the tetanus (arrows), compared to the immediate increase in the slope of the EPSP. (*c*) The 2 Hz signal is significantly increased 35 and 90 min after the induction of LTP. (*d*) A single experiment in which the 2 Hz signal was monitored for 5 h after the induction of LTP. Note that in this experiment, there was no 2 Hz signal before induction. The three post-induction time points are approximate, since at each interval two or three episodes of 2 Hz, 2 min stimulation were given over a period of around 10 min. The means ± s.e.m. of the percentage change in glutamate current are displayed at each interval.

measure of the percentage increase in charge generated at the electrode by the 2 Hz induced rise in glutamate concentration during each of the three periods. The means ($\pm$ s.e.m., $n = 11$) of the values, expressed in arbitrary units were: pre-tetanus, 107.7 ± 3.9; 30 min post-tetanus, 1070.6 ± 346.8 ($p < 0.01$) and 600.2 ± 155.5 ($p < 0.05$). (The p values indicating the statistical significance of the increase in signal at 35 and 90 min compared with the pre-tetanus value were computed using the non-parametric Wilcoxon paired test because of the wide spread of variances). No increase in background or activity-dependent release was seen in three experiments with electrodes not containing glutamate oxidase (data not shown). In one animal, in which no 2 Hz activity was detected before induction, activity-dependent glutamate changes were monitored 90 min, 3 and 5 h after the induction of LTP; the response was maximal at 90 min but was still detectable at 5 h (Fig. 11.4d).

(e) Basal and stimulus-dependent increases in glutamate concentration induced by tetanic stimulation are NMDA receptor-dependent

If the increase in glutamate concentration detected by the glutamate-sensitive electrode is related to the induction of LTP rather than to some other unsuspected consequence of tetanic stimulation, the effect should be blocked by drugs or procedures that block induction. In the experiments illustrated in Fig. 11.5 the NMDA-receptor antagonist D-APV (200 μM, 8 μl at 0.25 μl min^{-1}) was infused into the dentate gyrus through a thin-bore vitreous silica tube attached to the glutamate electrode, with its tip adjacent to the exposed membrane. Tetanic stimulation applied 1 h later induced PTP but not LTP (Fig. 11.5a) and there was no post-tetanus increase in basal glutamate concentration, or in the 2 Hz signal obtained 35 min after the tetanus (Fig. 11.5b,c). After a further 3 h, to allow time for a reduction in the concentration of D-APV by diffusion, the tetanus was reapplied and LTP was successfully induced (Fig. 11.5d). Accompanying LTP was the usual slowly developing increase in basal glutamate current and an enhancement in the 2 Hz current (Fig. 11.5e,f).

(f) Granule cells are not the source of the tetanus-induced increase in glutamate concentration

The most straightforward explanation of the increased glutamate current observed after tetanization is that it reflects an increase in the quantal content of the activated terminals of the perforant path. This interpretation would be turned on its head if the increased current at the glutamate electrode were the result of increased release from axon collaterals of the target granule cells and not from perforant path fibres. The increased signal would then have a postsynaptic rather than a presynaptic origin. We thought this unlikely, given the spatial selectivity of the glutamate electrode already mentioned. Nevertheless, we tested explicitly whether the electrode could detect glutamate released from terminals of granule cell axons (mossy fibres) by placing a second stimulating electrode in the hilus where the axons run en route to their target cells in the CA3 pyramidal cell field. In three animals we were unable to pick up a 2 Hz signal when stimulating the mossy fibres (confirmed by the presence of a characteristic antidromic population spike in the granule cell layer), either before or after the

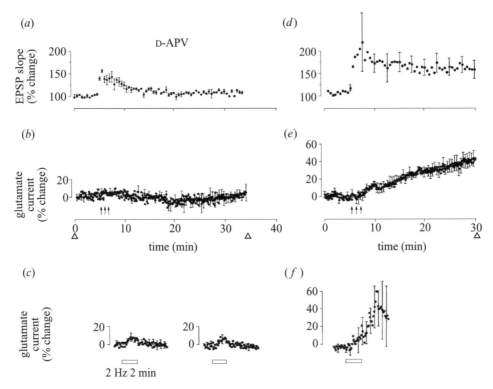

Fig. 11.5 The NMDA antagonist D-APV blocks the tetanus-induced increase in basal and activity-dependent extracellular glutamate concentration. Mean data from three experiments. (*a*) Tetanic stimulation (arrows in *b*) in the presence of locally infused D-APV induced PTP but not LTP. There was no change in either (*b*) basal glutamate current or (*c*) the activity-dependent glutamate signal, measured before (left) and 30 min after (right) the induction of LTP. (*c*,*d*) After an interval of 3 h, to allow time for diffusion of D-APV from the infusion site, the tetanus was repeated, now producing (*d*) robust LTP, (*e*) a delayed increase in basal current, and (*f*) a substantial increase in glutamate current generated by 2 Hz, 2 min stimulation. Open triangles indicate the times at which the 2 Hz samples were taken.

induction of LTP in the perforant path. Interleaved 2 Hz trains to the perforant path elicited the typical glutamate response, which was enhanced following induction of LTP (Fig. 11.6*a*). This result rules out a significant contribution from granule cell firing to the enhanced glutamate signal; it also renders unlikely the possibility that depolarization-induced reversal of a dendritic glutamate transporter makes a significant contribution, since back-propagating action potentials in dendrites should have triggered any such release.

(g) The activity-dependent increase in glutamate efflux is greatest during PTP

There is indirect evidence that PTP, which is the immediate consequence of high-frequency stimulation and which, in the hippocampus, lasts for a few minutes, reflects an increase in transmitter release from activated synapses (Wu and Saggau

(a)

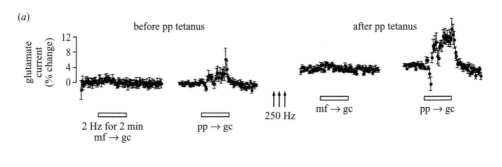

(b)

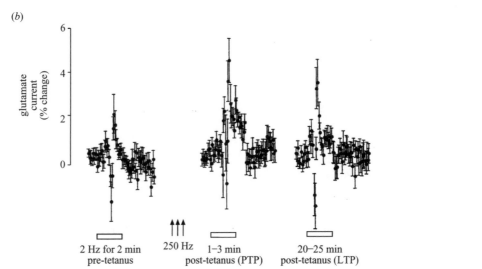

Fig. 11.6 (*a*) Antidromic activation of granule cells does not lead to an increase in extracellular glutamate concentration in the molecular layer. In this series of three experiments, stimulating electrodes were placed both in the perforant path (PP) and in the hilus to activate the axons (mossy fibres, mf) of granule cells (gc). In each animal, episodes of 2 Hz stimulation for 2 min were repeated two or three times for each pathway before and after the induction of LTP. The group data shown are, in each case, means of a total of eight sets of 2 Hz data collected from the three animals. No 2 Hz signal could be detected with mossy fibre stimulation, either before or after the induction of LTP in the perforant path. By contrast, a 2 Hz signal could be detected with perforant path activation, and this was markedly increased after the induction of LTP. Abbreviations: mf, mossy fibre; gc, granule cell; pp, perforant path. (*b*) Activity-dependent increases in glutamate concentration are greater during PTP than during LTP. In a group of three animals PTP was induced multiple times by repeated tetanization. Although LTP rapidly saturates with this procedure, each tetanus still elicits PTP. In addition, repeated episodes of 2 Hz stimulation were given in each animal before the induction of LTP, during PTP, and 20–25 min after each tetanus. Means ± s.e.m. are plotted for responses obtained before the induction of LTP ($n = 15$), and beginning 1–3 min after a tetanus ($n = 16$) or 20–25 min after a tetanus ($n = 15$).

1994). It is thus surprising that the signal from the glutamate electrode did not achieve maximal values during PTP, but grew slowly to a plateau over the following 20–30 min (Fig. 11.4*b*). However, the basal glutamate signal at test rates of stimulation probably reflects non-activity-dependent glutamate release (see Section 11.4). To establish whether activity-dependent release was higher during PTP than during LTP, we compared the peak glutamate current elicited by 2 Hz stimulation for 2 min, starting 1–3 min after the induction of LTP, with the values obtained 20–25 min after induction. In agreement with prediction, in three animals in which multiple episodes of tetanic stimulation were given at intervals of around 30 min to induce PTP several times, the 2 Hz glutamate current during PTP (1–3 min post-tetanus) was of greater magnitude and duration than that obtained during LTP (20–25 min post-tetanus; Fig. 11.6b). (Note the initial decrease in the 2 Hz glutamate signal; we saw this pattern of response in some animals, but it was not a consistent finding and we have not investigated it further.)

(h) In areas CA1 and CA3, activation of afferent fibres at 2 Hz does not lead to an increase in signal from the glutamate electrode, and LTP in these areas is not associated with an increase in basal glutamate concentration

In contrast to the dentate gyrus, where 2 Hz stimulation almost always resulted in a transiently enhanced glutamate signal, we were consistently unable to detect any such increase in areas CA1 or CA3 during 2 Hz stimulation of commissural–associational axons. In our first experiments, the electrode assembly was positioned in the apical dendritic field of the stratum radiatum in area CA1, and Schaffer-commissural afferents were activated through a stimulating electrode placed in the contralateral ventral hippocampal commissure. In six experiments we failed to elicit a 2 Hz response in the stratum radiatum, either before or after the tetanus, despite large and characteristic synaptic responses and robust LTP (Fig. 11.7a,c). In another three experiments, we positioned the glutamate electrode in the basal dendritic field (stratum oriens) of area CA1. In this position, the electrode lay above the pyramidal cell layer, avoiding damage to the cell bodies. However, we had no more success in the stratum oriens than in the stratum radiatum. A similar failure attended experiments in which the electrode was positioned in the stratum oriens of area CA3, where again the pyramidal cell layer escaped penetration by the electrode. Moreover, in none of the three locations was LTP associated with a change in the basal concentration of glutamate (see Fig. 11.7b for experiments in the stratum radiatum; results from the stratum oriens in CA1 and CA3 are not shown).

(i) Seizure activity is accompanied by massive changes in extracellular glutamate concentration in the dentate gyrus and in area CA1

Seizure activity is readily induced in the dentate gyrus and in area CA1 by 10 Hz stimulation of the perforant path or the Schaffer-commissural projection, respectively. In both areas, this procedure led to a prolonged increase in basal glutamate concentration. The onset of the increase is characteristically biphasic in both regions (Fig. 11.7d,e), reflecting initial synchronous exocytosis followed by efflux owing to depolarization-driven reversal of uptake carriers (Nicolls and Attwell 1991; Obrenovitch and Urenjak 1997). Although the initial rate of rise is slower and the magnitude of the increase is somewhat less in area CA1 than in the dentate gyrus, the peak increase in glutamate current is 2–3-fold in both cases. Thus, in all hippocampal regions the glutamate electrode can readily detect the large and pathological changes in

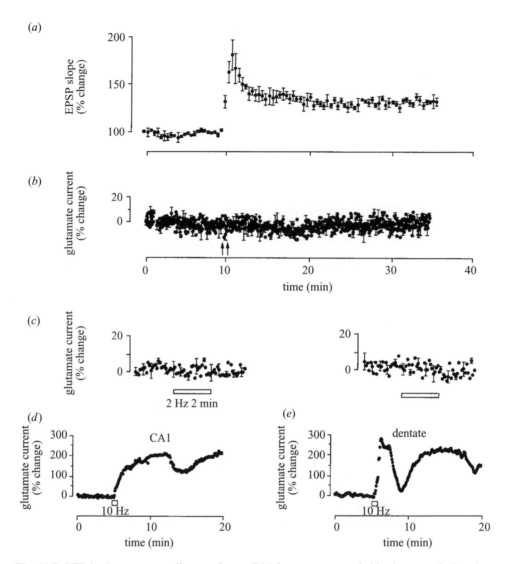

Fig. 11.7 LTP in the stratum radiatum of area CA1 is not accompanied by increases in basal or activity-dependent extracellular glutamate concentration. (*a*) LTP induced in area CA1 by a two-train tetanus (arrows in *b*) delivered to the contralateral ventral hippocampal commissure. Group data from six animals. (*b*) Basal glutamate current was not affected by the tetanus. (*c*) Activity-dependent 2 Hz signals were not seen either before or 30 min after the induction of LTP. Similar results were obtained when the glutamate electrode was placed in the stratum oriens of area CA1 or CA3. (*d*) Seizures induced in area CA1 by stimulating the commissural pathway at 10 Hz for 1 min are associated with large biphasic changes in current. The record shows a typical response from a single animal with a glutamate electrode positioned in stratum radiatum. (*e*) Seizures induced in the dentate gyrus also led to large biphasic changes in glutamate current. Data from another animal.

extracellular glutamate that occur in circumstances of synchronous release from large numbers of excitatory terminals.

11.4 Discussion

(a) Basal glutamate concentration and activity-dependent increases in concentration

The basal level of glutamate current detected here may reflect the spontaneous release of glutamate by vesicular exocytosis or reverse uptake, rather than activity-driven release, since abolition of activity with tetrodoxin had no effect on basal glutamate levels measured with conventional microdialysis in the striatum (Shiraishi *et al.* 1997). Our basal stimulation rate was low, and we saw no difference in glutamate current when we stopped stimulating. However, when we increased the stimulus rate to 2 Hz for 2 min, we consistently observed an increase in signal from the glutamate electrode (Figs 11.2 and 11.3). The increase was delayed, with an onset of 15–30 s. Some of this delay is imposed by the design of the glutamate electrode, since there was a delay of around 10–15 s before any change was signalled by the electrode following step changes in glutamate concentration *in vitro* (Fig. 11.1*c*). Coating of the dialysis membrane with cellular debris during implantation of the electrode may explain the slightly longer delay *in vivo*. It is also possible that in the initial post-tetanus phase of low-frequency stimulation the uptake mechanisms are able to cope with the extra efflux of glutamate, before eventually becoming saturated; only at that point does glutamate concentration in the extrasynaptic space sensed by the glutamate electrode begin to rise.

(b) Increase in basal and activity-dependent glutamate concentration following the induction of LTP

An increase in basal concentration of extracellular glutamate was also seen in our earlier studies which combined perfusion of the hippocampus using a push–pull cannula with off-line measurements of radiolabelled or endogenous glutamate (Dolphin *et al.* 1982; Bliss *et al.* 1986). The temporal resolution of this technique (perfusates were collected in 10–15 min fractions) is two orders of magnitude less than that offered by the glutamate electrode. However, even taking that factor into account, there was little if any evidence of a delay in the onset of the rise in glutamate concentration after the induction of LTP. The slow increase reported here (Figs 11.2 and 11.3) implies either that there is a parallel rise in spontaneous glutamate release, or that the uptake mechanisms themselves become less effective with a time-course that is the inverse of the increase in glutamate current. We are not able to differentiate between these two non-exclusive possibilities. If the latter were the case, then the latency of the 2 Hz signal should be greater 10–15 min after the tetanus than at later times. Our data do not allow us to come to any firm conclusion on that point, though it is notable that the onset latency is considerably less at 35 and 90 min post-induction than it is before the induction of LTP (Fig. 11.4*c*).

The results presented here conflict with an earlier report, also using a dialysis electrode but with external detection, in which no changes in glutamate concentration were observed following the induction of LTP in the dentate gyrus of anaesthetized rats

(Jay *et al.* 1999). In the approach adopted by Jay *et al.*, a.c.s.f. was perfused through a dialysis chamber inserted into the brain, and the dialysate was then pumped to an external amperometric apparatus, where glutamate concentration was estimated by the same reaction, based on glutamate oxidase, as used here (Fig. 11.1*b*). An advantage of external detection is that it allows an absolute estimate of glutamate concentration to be made, as the electrode remains outside the brain and is not exposed to the *in vivo* contamination that occurs with the integrated electrode we have used. However, the study suffered from the problem that the system could not reliably detect a glutamate signal when the perforant path was stimulated at 2 Hz for 10 min. Activity-dependent changes in extracellular glutamate could therefore not be usefully studied. More puzzlingly, Jay *et al.* (1999) did not see an increase in basal glutamate concentration following the induction of LTP, but again there was an absence of a positive control. (In both our studies and those by Jay *et al.*, large biphasic increases in glutamate concentration could be detected in pathological condition—either during seizure activity (Fig. 11.7*d,e*) or in terminal ischaemia (Jay *et al.* 1999; Fig. 11.2).) Negative results were also reported by Aniksztejn *et al.* (1989) using a push–pull system, but again this study did not include positive controls to show that the method was capable of detecting an increase in glutamate concentration if it occurred. A similar stricture applies to our negative results in CA1 and CA3.

(c) Enhanced release or reduced uptake?

The interpretation of our data depends critically on the source of the increase in extracellular glutamate. We have ruled out the axon terminals of granule cells as a source (Fig. 11.6*a*), but contributions to the basal signal could originate from terminals of the perforant path fibres, from glial cells or from the dendrites of granule cells. Depolarization of any of these elements could, in principle, cause an increase in extracellular glutamate by a decrease in uptake through the reversal of voltage-dependent glutamate transporters (reviewed by Danbolt 2001). The issue is not easy to address directly, since our attempts at local infusion of uptake inhibitors into the hippocampus invariably led to seizures. However, it is unlikely that all our data can be explained in this way. Changes in uptake would be expected to affect basal and activity-induced glutamate in a similar way. This was not always the case, as is most clearly seen in the data on PTP; the 2 Hz signal is greater at 3 min than at 25 min (Fig. 11.6*b*), while for basal release the opposite is the case. Moreover, there were individual animals in which there was an increase in the 2 Hz signal after the induction of LTP without an increase in basal release.

In conditions of physiological homeostasis, increased release of glutamate is accompanied by increased levels of uptake (Danbolt 2001). In the hippocampus, recording of glial transporter currents in area CA1 has revealed an increase in current during PTP (Diamond *et al.* 1998; Lüscher *et al.* 1998), consistent with other evidence suggesting that PTP is presynaptic in origin (McNaughton 1982; Kauer *et al.* 1988; Muller and Lynch 1988). However, there was no increase in transporter currents during LTP itself, suggesting that LTP is not associated with an increase in transmitter release. Our results throw no further light on the situation in area CA1 as we were unable to measure activity-dependent glutamate currents in the pyramidal cell fields. Conversely, there are no reported measurements of glial transporter currents in the dentate gyrus in the context of LTP. A decrease in uptake could lead to an increase in excitability and a potentiation of synaptic transmission, and could thus provide a mechanism for LTP. However, this possibility is not supported by the observation that LTP in area CA1 is associated with an increase in glutamate uptake (Levenson *et al.* 2002). Thus, the most straightforward interpretation of our results is that LTP in the dentate gyrus is accompanied by an increase in both spontaneous and stimulated glutamate release from potentiated terminals.

(d) In areas CA1 and CA3 LTP is not linked to changes in glutamate concentration

Having found a consistent increase in extracellular glutamate concentration when we stimulated at 2 Hz in the dentate gyrus, we had every expectation that we would see a similar effect in areas CA1 and CA3. We were, therefore, somewhat taken aback to find that we were completely unable to reproduce the observation in the pyramidal cell fields. The evidence that glutamate is the endogenous transmitter at excitatory synapses in areas CA1 and CA3 is perhaps less overwhelming than the evidence that glutamate receptors are the target for the endogenous transmitter. But if not glutamate, what? There is no other credible candidate. Although aspartate is co-packaged with glutamate in synaptic vesicles at excitatory synapses in stratum radiatum of area CA1, and with glutamate is released and taken up into glial cells following depolarization (Gundersen *et al.* 1998), it has a negligible affinity for AMPA (α-amino-3-hydroxy-5-methyl-4-isoxazolepropionic acid) receptors (Curras and Dingledine 1992). An alternative explanation for our results is that glutamate is more enthusiastically removed from extracellular space in the pyramidal cell fields than in the dentate gyrus. There is some evidence to support this possibility since uptake of glutamate into synaptosomes prepared from hippocampal subfields is higher in area CA1 than in the terminal fields of the perforant path (Taxt and Storm-Mathisen 1984).

11.5 Conclusions

We have demonstrated that changes in extracellular glutamate concentration can be detected in the dentate gyrus of the anaesthetized rat in real time with a glutamate-sensitive dialysis electrode. Low-frequency (2 Hz) stimulation of the perforant path leads to an increase in glutamate concentration, and the size of this increase is enhanced in an NMDA-receptor-dependent manner following the induction of LTP. This observation is consistent with an LTP-associated decrease in glutamate uptake or an activity-dependent increase in glutamate release from potentiated terminals. We were unable to detect changes in glutamate release following 2 Hz stimulation either before or after the induction of LTP in areas CA1 and CA3, possibly because of more efficient glutamate uptake in the pyramidal cell fields.

Endnotes

1. The terms pre- and post-expressionist derive from the sci-art movement that developed towards the end of this period.

2. The 'presynapticists' have on the whole fought a more limited campaign than their adversaries on the other side of the synaptic divide; unlike the latter, they have lacked the experimental ammunition to lay claim to the entire territory of expression mechanisms and their battle hymn has resounded to the more modest refrain 'the expression of LTP is at least in part presynaptic'.

References

Albery, W. J., Bartlett, P. N., and Cass, E. G. (1987). Amperometric enzyme electrodes. *Phil. Trans. R. Soc. Lond.* B **316**, 107–19.

Aniksztejn, L., Roisin, M. P., Amsellem, R., and Ben-Ari, Y. (1989). Long-term potentiation is not associated with a sustained enhanced release of endogenous excitatory amino acids. *Neuroscience* **28**, 387–92.

Bliss, T. V. P., Douglas, R. M., Errington, M. L., and Lynch, M. A. (1986). Correlation between long-term potentiation and release of endogenous amino acids from dentate gyrus of anaesthetized rats. *J. Physiol.* (*Lond.*) **377**, 391–408.

Bliss, T. V. P., Errington, M. L., Lynch, M. A., and Williams, J. H. (1990). Presynaptic mechanisms in hippocampal long-term potentiation. In *The brain* (ed. E. R. Kandel, T. Sejnowski and C. F. Stevens). Cold Spring Harbor Symp. Quantitative Biology, vol. 55, pp. 119–30. Cold Spring Harbor Laboratory Press.

Collingridge, G. L., Kehl, S. J., and McLennan, H. (1983). Excitatory amino acids in synaptic transmission in the Schaffer collateral-commissural pathway of the rat hippocampus. *J. Physiol.* (*Lond.*) **334**, 33–46.

Curras, M. C. and Dingledine, R. (1992). Selectivity of amino acid transmitters acting at N-methyl-D-aspartate and amino-3-hydroxy-5-methyl-4-isoxazolepropionate receptors. *Mol. Pharmacol.* **41**, 520–6.

Danbolt, N. C. (2001). Glutamate uptake. *Prog. Neurobiol.* **65**, 1–105.

Diamond, J. S., Bergles, D. E., and Jahr, C. E. (1998). Glutamate release monitored with astrocyte transporter currents during LTP. *Neuron* **21**, 425–33.

Dolphin, A. C., Errington, M. L., and Bliss, T. V. P. (1982). Long-term potentiation of the perforant path *in vivo* is associated with increased glutamate release. *Nature* **297**, 496–8.

Douglas, R. M., McNaughton, B. L., and Goddard, G. V. (1983). Commissural inhibition and facilitation of granule cell discharge in fascia dentata. *J. Comp. Neurol.* **219**, 285–94.

Errington, M. L., Lynch, M. A., and Bliss, T. V. P. (1987). Long-term potentiation in the dentate gyrus: induction and increased glutamate release are blocked by D(−)aminophosphonovalerate. *Neuroscience* **20**, 279–84.

Galley, P. T. (1991). The development of enzyme electrodes for neurophysiology. PhD thesis. Imperial College, University of London.

Gundersen, V., Chaudhry, F. A., Bjaalie, J. G., Fonnum, F., Ottersen, O. P., and Storm-Mathisen, J. (1998). Synaptic vesicular localization and exocytosis of L-aspartate in excitatory nerve terminals: a quantitative immunogold analysis in rat hippocampus. *J. Neurosci.* **18**, 6059–70.

Jay, T. M., Zilkha, E., and Obrenovitch, T. P. (1999). Long-term potentiation in the dentate gyrus is not linked to increased extracellular glutamate concentration. *J. Neurophysiol.* **81**, 1741–8.

Kauer, J. A., Malenka, R. C., and Nicoll, R. A. (1988). A persistent postsynaptic modification mediates long-term potentiation in the hippocampus. *Neuron* **1**, 911–17.

Lerma, J., Herranz, A. S., Herreras, O., Abraira, V., and Martin del Rio, R. (1986). *In vivo* determination of extracellular concentrations of amino acids in the rat hippocampus. A method based on brain dialysis and computerized analysis. *Brain Res.* **384**, 145–55.

Levenson, J., Weeber, E., Selcher, J. C., Kategaya, L. S., and Sweatt, J. D. (2002). Long-term potentiation and contextual fear conditioning increase neuronal glutamate uptake. *Nature Neurosci.* **5**, 155–61.

Lüscher, C., Malenka, R. C., and Nicoll, R. A. (1998). Monitoring glutamate release during LTP with glial transporter currents. *Neuron* **21**, 435–41.

McNaughton, B. L. (1982). Long-term synaptic enhancement and short-term potentiation in rat fascia dentata act through different mechanisms. *J. Physiol. (Lond.)* **324**, 249–62.

Muller, D. and Lynch, G. (1988). Long-term potentiation differentially affects two components of synaptic responses in hippocampus. *Proc. Natl Acad. Sci. USA* **85**, 9346–50.

Nicolls, D. and Attwell, D. (1991). The release and uptake of excitatory amino acids. *Trends Pharmacol.* **11**, 462–8.

Obrenovitch, T. P. and Urenjak, J. (1997). Altered glutamatergic transmission in neurological disorders: from high extracellular glutamate to excessive synaptic efficacy. *Prog. Neurobiol.* **51**, 39–87.

Shiraishi, M., Kamiyama, Y., Huttemeier, P. C., and Benveniste, H. (1997). Extracellular glutamate and dopamine measured by microdialysis in the rat striatum during blockade of synaptic transmission in anesthetized and awake rats. *Brain Res.* **759**, 221–7.

Skrede, K. K. and Malthe-Sørenssen, D. (1981). Increased resting and evoked release of transmitter following repetitive electrical tetanization in hippocampus: a biochemical correlate to long-lasting synaptic potentiation. *Brain Res.* **208**, 436–41.

Taxt, T. and Storm-Mathisen, J. (1984). Uptake of D-aspartate and L-glutamate in excitatory axon terminals in hippocampus: autoradiographic and biochemical comparison with gamma-aminobutyrate and other amino acids in normal rats and in rats with lesions. *Neuroscience* **11**, 79–100.

Walker, M. C., Galley, P. T., Errington, M. L., Shorvon, S. D., and Jefferys, J. G. R. (1995). Ascorbate and glutamate release in the rat hippocampus after perforant path stimulation: a 'dialysis electrode' study. *J. Neurochem.* **65**, 725–31.

Wu, L. G. and Saggau, P. (1994). Presynaptic calcium is increased during normal synaptic transmission and paired-pulse facilitation, but not in long-term potentiation in area CA1 of hippocampus. *J. Neurosci.* **14**, 645–54.

Glossary

a.c.s.f. artificial cerebrospinal fluid
AMPA   α-amino-3-hydroxy-5-methylisoxazole-4-propionic acid
D-APV   D-2-amino-5-phosphonovaleric acid
EPSP   excitatory postsynaptic potential
LTP   long-term potentiation
NMDA   *N*-methyl-D-aspartate
PTP   post-tetanic potentiation

12

Imaging spatio-temporal patterns of long-term potentiation in mouse hippocampus

Toshiyuki Hosokawa, Masaki Ohta, Takeshi Saito, and Alan Fine

Spatio-temporal patterns of neuronal activity before and after the induction of long-term potentiation in mouse hippocampal slices were studied using a real-time high-resolution optical recording system. After staining the slices with voltage-sensitive dye, transmitted light images and extracellular field potentials were recorded in response to stimuli applied to CA1 stratum radiatum. Optical and electrical signals in response to single test pulses were enhanced for at least 30 minutes after brief high-frequency stimulation at the same site. In two-pathway experiments, potentiation was restricted to the tetanized pathway. The optical signals demonstrated that both the amplitude and area of the synaptic response were increased, in patterns not predictable from the initial, pretetanus, pattern of activation. Optical signals will be useful for investigating spatio-temporal patterns of synaptic enhancement underlying information storage in the brain.

Keywords: long-term potentiation; voltage-sensitive dye; optical recording; synaptic plasticity

12.1 Introduction

It is commonly supposed that memories are laid down in the brain as distributed patterns of altered synaptic strength. Testing this hypothesis, however, has been extremely difficult, largely because of the lack of experimental methods for visualizing spatial and temporal patterns of synaptic plasticity. LTP of synaptic transmission, wherein high-frequency stimulation of excitatory pathways results in a persistent increase in synaptic strength (Bliss and Lømo 1973), is the most widely studied model of memory formation in the mammalian brain (Bliss and Collingridge 1993). Typically LTP is monitored at one or a few sites by means of intracellular or extracellular electrodes, with excellent temporal resolution but little ability to resolve spatial patterns of activation. Multisite optical recording, using voltage-sensitive dyes, provides an alternative approach with greatly increased spatial resolution (Orbach *et al.* 1985). Here, we use a fast digital imaging system in conjunction with a voltage-sensitive absorbance dye to monitor evoked synaptic responses in acutely prepared hippocampal slices. By comparing responses to identical stimuli before and after induction of LTP we are able to extract the spatio-temporal pattern by which synaptic enhancement is expressed in this network.

12.2 Material and methods

(a) Hippocampal slice preparation

Male *ddy* mice ($n = 11$; Hokudo, Sapporo, Japan), 4–5 weeks of age, were decapitated under ether anaesthesia. The brain was rapidly removed into ice-cold physiological saline, then mounted onto the stage of a vibroslicer, and 300–320 µm thick horizontal slices were cut through the hippocampus. The slices were stored for at least 1 h in a holding chamber filled with ACSF containing (in mM): NaCl, 120; KCl, 3; $NaHCO_3$, 23; NaH_2PO_4, 1.2; glucose, 11; $CaCl_2$, 2.4; $MgSO_4$, 1.2; bubbled with a 95% O_2/5% CO_2 gas mixture yielding pH 7.3.

(b) Electrophysiological recording

After staining (see Section 2c), the slice was transferred to a recording chamber on the stage of an inverted microscope (TMD-300; Nikon) and was continuously superfused with oxygenated ACSF at 33 °C at a rate of 2–3 ml min^{-1}. Electrical test pulses (up to 40 V, constant voltage, 50 µs duration; Master-8 stimulator with Iso-flex isolator; A.M.P.I., Israel) were applied at a rate of 0.033 Hz via a bipolar tungsten electrode (5 µm tip, 5 MΩ; A-M systems, Inc., WA, USA). One electrode was placed in CA1 stratum radiatum to stimulate Schaffer collateral inputs; a second was placed some distance from the first to stimulate a different set of afferent fibres, either in stratum radiatum or stratum oriens. A test stimulus was applied via this second electrode 100 ms after each test stimulus through the first electrode. The evoked PS or fEPSP in response to the test stimuli was recorded through a glass extracellular electrode (filled with 2 M NaCl and 5% brilliant blue) placed in CA1 stratum pyramidale or stratum radiatum. Responses were amplified (MEG-1251, Nihon Koden, Tokyo, Japan), digitized (ITC-16; Instru-Tech, NY, USA) and input to a Macintosh computer. Experimental control and analysis were carried out via A/DVANCE software (McKellar Designs, Vancouver, Canada). Stimulus intensity was adjusted to evoke a half-maximal fEPSP. LTP was induced in either pathway ('potentiated pathway') by the application of a tetanus consisting of four 1 s bursts of 100 Hz stimulation (50 µs duration and same strength as the test stimuli) with 3 s intervals between bursts, to one stimulating electrode ('S2, potentiated pathway'). No stimulus was applied to the other stimulating electrode ('S1, reference pathway') during the tetanus. After the tetanus, test stimuli were applied at rate of 0.033 Hz to both pathways as before. PS amplitude or fEPSP slope was measured and plotted with A/DVANCE, with LTP expressed as per cent change from the pretetanus baseline.

(c) Optical recording

Immediately before transfer to the recording chamber, slices were stained for 10 min with voltage-sensitive oxonol dye, NK-3630 (Nihon Kanko Shikiso Kenkyusho, Okayama, Japan) (Momose-Sato et al. 1999) diluted in ACSF at a final concentration of 0.25–0.5 mg ml^{-1}. A Deltaron (Fujifilm, Tokyo, Japan) imager with a 128 × 128 MOS photodetector array and 0.6 ms frame interval was attached to the camera port of the microscope for optical recording. Details of the Deltaron system have been described elsewhere (Kita et al. 1995). The image of the hippocampal slice was focused on the photodetector array by means of a magnification × 4, 0.20 N.A. objective (Nikon). With this arrangement, the array detected an area of 1.7 mm × 1.7 mm in the plane of the hippocampal slice (i.e. each pixel covered approximately 13 µm × 13 µm in the specimen plane). The slice was transilluminated for 1 s in each trial by a stabilized high-intensity tungsten filament lamp via a 700/30 nm interference filter, corresponding to the major absorption peak of the dye NK-3630.

At the beginning of each optical recording trial, a reference image was taken 600 ms before application of the test stimuli and stored in the Deltaron's memory. Each of the subsequent frames was subtracted from this reference, amplified 400 times, and stored in the memory as a difference image. The frame rate of the system was 0.6 ms, and 512 frames (i.e. total sequence *ca.* 300 ms) were recorded for each trial. The timing of stimulus test pulses with respect to the start of the optical recording was constant from trial to trial.

(d) Image processing and data analysis

From the reference and difference images, absorbance changes at each pixel at each time point were calculated as fractional change in light intensity, $\%\Delta I/I = 100((d/400)I)$, where d is the value of the pixel in the difference image, and I is the pixel's intensity in the reference image. Calculated $\%\Delta I/I$ image series were viewed using IMAGEJ (W. Rasband, NIH). For each experiment, the optical recordings were carried out twice, once just prior to the application of tetanus and a second time 20 min after the tetanus. For optical analysis of synaptic plasticity, after 3×3 median filtering of each image, the percentage of potentiation (%LTP) was calculated as 100(post-tetanus image − pretetanus image)/(pretetanus image) for each corresponding image pair in the two series. Pixels from each frame with %LTP greater than twice the standard deviation were projected to a single plane with IMAGEJ, and superimposed on the reference image using Adobe Photoshop to visualize the total spatial extent of plasticity.

12.3 Results

The voltage-sensitive dye used here had no overt pharmacological effects, with no conspicuous differences noted between the electrical responses in stained and unstained preparations. This is in agreement with previous results using the same dye (Momose-Sato *et al.* 1999). Bleaching was relatively slow under the conditions of these experiments, and was not corrected.

Montages of every third difference image in optical recordings of a representative preparation just before and 30 min after tetanic stimulation are shown in Fig. 12.1*a,b*, respectively. (The reference image of the slice can be seen in the last tile in the montage of Fig. 12.1*a*, and at larger magnification as the grey-scale component of Fig. 12.1*e*.) These $\%\Delta I/I$ images were calculated as described in Section 12.2d, and false coloured according to the indicated scale. In the pretetanus trial (Fig. 12.1*a*), strong optical responses were elicited close to each stimulating electrode immediately after stimulation through each, with the expected 100 ms interval. In both cases the optical signals propagated orthodromically towards the subiculum, generally passing across stratum pyramidale to involve both stratum radiatum and stratum oriens. Qualitatively similar patterns of signal propagation were obtained in 10 out of 10 other preparations; in some of these, antidromic activation could also be detected with shorter latencies than the orthodromic signals. Orthodromic propagating signals, but not antidromic signals, were completely abolished in each of two separate experiments following the application of 20 μM CNQX (data not shown), confirming that the propagating optical signals reflected excitatory glutamate mediated postsynaptic responses.

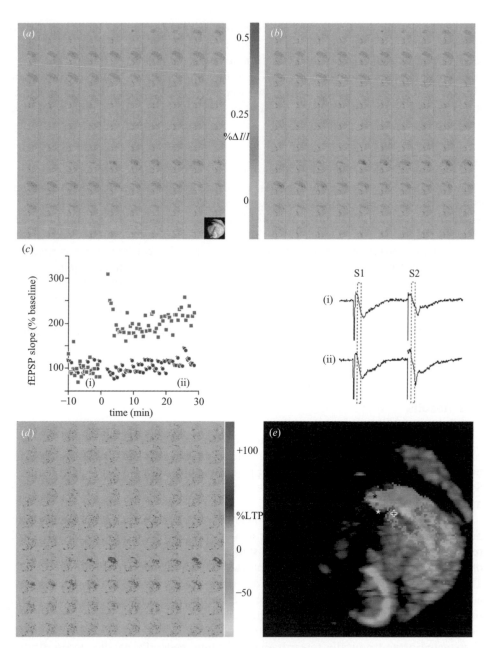

Fig. 12.1 Optical imaging of synaptic responses and potentiation in a hippocampal slice. (a) Optical signals in response to two stimuli at 100 ms intervals, just prior to high-frequency stimulation. Images were obtained at 0.6 ms intervals; every third image is shown in this montage, i.e. at intervals of 1.8 ms, reading left to right and top to bottom. (An ordinary image of the slice is visible in the last element of the montage, and at higher magnification in part (e), where the positions of the stimulating and recording electrodes are indicated.) The false-colour scale indicates the fractional change in intensity in per cent, $\%\Delta I/I$. (b) Optical signals recorded as in (a), 20 min after high-frequency stimulation applied via the second stimulating electrode. The

In the post-tetanus optical recording (Fig. 12.1b), both stimuli evoked signals that propagated toward the subiculum as in Fig. 12.1a. However, the optical response to the second stimulus reached higher amplitudes and was more spatially extensive than before the tetanus.

Representative extracellularly recorded electrical responses are shown on the right-hand side of Fig. 12.1c; both stimuli evoked compound fEPSPs. The fEPSP slopes are plotted over time on the left-hand side of Fig. 12.1c. The tetanus resulted in a clear and stable potentiation of the EPSP in the potentiated pathway (S2), with no change in the response of the reference pathway (S1).

In the computed %LTP images (Fig. 12.1d), there is little difference between responses to the first stimulus (the small apparent reduction in this response may be an artefact of dye bleaching), but a robust potentiation of the response to the second stimulus is evident. Similar results were obtained in all other preparations following the induction of LTP. In several experiments, the magnitudes of the optically detected synaptic responses and/or LTP magnitude were larger at locations distant from, as compared to close to, the recording electrode.

A projection of all pixels in which the post-tetanus optical signal was more than two standard deviations beyond the pretetanus signal at any point during the recording is shown in Fig. 12.1e. Although this usefully summarizes the spatial extent and magnitude of potentiation, it masks the temporal component. Figure 12.2 shows all frames (at 0.6 ms intervals) beginning just prior to the second stimulus, during the pretetanus trial (Fig. 12.2a) and in the corresponding frames of the computed %LTP series (Fig. 12.2b). Whereas the synaptic activation (Fig. 12.2a) propagates as a coherent volume moving towards the subiculum, the potentiation signal moves as a roughly circular expanding wavefront (Fig. 12.2b).

12.4 Discussion

Optical recordings of voltage-sensitive dye signals have been used previously to monitor spatio-temporal patterns of synaptic activation in the hippocampus (Grinvald et al. 1982; Bonhoeffer and Staiger 1988; Plenz and Aertsen 1993; Barish et al. 1996; Iijima et al. 1996; Jackson and Scharfman 1996; Nakagami et al. 1996; Sekino et al. 1997;

---

response to the second stimulus is increased. (c) Electrical responses to two-pathway stimulation, recorded prior to, and after, potentiation of the second stimulated pathway. On the left is plotted the fEPSP slope in response to 0.033 Hz stimuli applied to electrode 1 (blue circles) and electrode 2 (red squares). At time 0, a brief high-frequency stimulus was applied via electrode 2, resulting in potentiation of the synaptic response. The traces on the right were obtained at the times labelled (i) and (ii) on the left; the dashed regions correspond to the intervals over which the EPSP slopes were measured. (d) Optical image of synaptic potentiation, obtained by frame-by-frame digital subtraction of the series shown in (a) from the series in (b). The false-colour scale shows the percentage change in the optical signal, %LTP. (e) The spatial extent of significant LTP (post-tetanus optical signal more than two standard deviations different from the pretetanus level) is indicated by coloured areas, superimposed on the grey-scale reference image of the slice. False colours correspond to the scale in (d). Black and white stars indicate positions of S1 and S2 stimulating electrodes, respectively; the white cross indicates the position of the recording electrode. The filamentous shadows are cast by lens paper on which the slice is mounted in the perfusion chamber. The field of view is 1.7 mm on each side. (See Plate 1 of the Plate Section, at the centre of this book.)

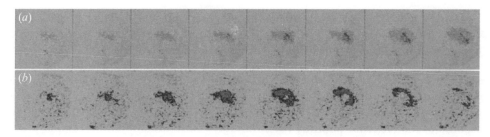

Fig. 12.2 The spatio-temporal pattern of potentiation is not predictable from the pattern of the baseline synaptic response. (*a*) All frames, at 0.6 ms intervals, are now shown of the portion of the optical recording (%Δ*I/I*) in Fig. 12.1*a* covering the onset of the response to S2. The colour scale is as in Fig. 12.1*a*. (*b*) The equivalent frames at 0.6 ms intervals from the %LTP series of Fig. 12.1(*d*). The potentiation appears as an expanding wavefront. The colour scale is as in Fig. 12.1(*d*). (See Plate 2 of the Plate Section, at the centre of this book.)

Chesi *et al.* 1998; Antic *et al.* 1999; Otsu *et al.* 2000; Sato *et al.* 2000; Inoue *et al.* 2001). Such recordings have also detected the induction of LTP as an increase in the amplitude (Saggau *et al.* 1986; Bonhoeffer *et al.* 1989; Tominaga *et al.* 2000) and a reduction in latency (Nakagami *et al.* 1997) of the synaptically evoked voltage-sensitive dye signal. However, voltage-sensitive dyes have not previously been used to visualize the spatio-temporal pattern of potentiation.

The data presented here demonstrated that such patterns of potentiation can be monitored with high spatial and temporal resolution. Their shapes and trajectories are complex, reflecting the underlying connectivity of the network and possibly the history of activation. The ability to monitor these patterns in this relatively non-invasive manner may be of use in deciphering the encoding of natural memory in the brain.

The authors thank B. Hoyt for assistance with data analysis, and Dr T. V. P. Bliss and Dr L. B. Cohen for helpful comments. This work was supported by the Japan Society for the Promotion of Science, the Human Frontier Science Program and the Natural Science and Engineering Research Council of Canada.

References

Antic, S., Major, G., and Zecevic, D. (1999). Fast optical recordings of membrane potential changes from dendrites of pyramidal neurons. *J. Neurophysiol.* **82**, 1615–21.

Barish, M. E., Ichikawa, M., Tominaga, T., Matsumoto, G., and Iijima, T. (1996). Enhanced fast synaptic transmission and a delayed depolarization induced by transient potassium current blockade in rat hippocampal slice as studied by optical recording. *J. Neurosci.* **16**, 5672–87.

Bliss, T. V. P. and Collingridge, G. L. (1993). A synaptic model of memory: long-term potentiation in the hippocampus. *Nature* **361**, 31–9.

Bliss, T. V. P. and Lømo, T. (1973). Long-lasting potentiation of synaptic transmission in the dentate area of the anaesthetized rabbit following stimulation of the perforant path. *J. Physiol. (Lond.)* **232**, 331–56.

Bonhoeffer, T. and Staiger, V. (1988). Optical recording with single cell resolution from monolayered slice cultures of rat hippocampus. *Neurosci. Lett.* **92**, 259–64.

Bonhoeffer, T., Staiger, V., and Aertsen, A. (1989). Synaptic plasticity in rat hippocampal slice cultures: local 'Hebbian' conjunction of pre- and postsynaptic stimulation leads to distributed synaptic enhancement. *Proc. Natl Acad. Sci. USA* **86**, 8113–17.

Chesi, A. J., Rucker, F., Tretter, Y., ten Bruggencate, G., and Alzheimer, C. (1998). Spread of excitation in chronically lesioned mouse hippocampus determined by laser scanning microscopy. *Exp. Neurol.* **152**, 177–87.

Grinvald, A., Manker, A., and Segal, M. (1982). Visualization of the spread of electrical activity in rat hippocampal slices by voltage-sensitive optical probes. *J. Physiol. (Lond.)* **333**, 269–91.

Iijima, T., Witter, M. P., Ichikawa, M., Tominaga, T., Kajiwara, R., and Matsumoto, G. (1996). Entorhinal–hippocampal interactions revealed by real-time imaging. *Science* **272**, 1176–9.

Inoue, M., Hashimoto, Y., Kudo, Y., and Miyakawa, H. (2001). Dendritic attenuation of synaptic potentials in the CA1 region of rat hippocampal slices detected with an optical method. *Eur. J. Neurosci.* **13**, 1711–21.

Jackson, M. B. and Scharfman, H. E. (1996). Positive feedback from hilar mossy cells to granule cells in the dentate gyrus revealed by voltage-sensitive dye and microelectrode recording. *J. Neurophysiol.* **76**, 601–16.

Kita, H., Yamada, H., Tanifuji, M., and Murase, K. (1995). Optical responses recorded after local stimulation in rat neostriatal slice preparations: effects of GABA and glutamate antagonists, and dopamine agonists. *Exp. Brain Res.* **106**, 187–95.

Momose-Sato, Y., Sato, K., Arai, Y., Yazawa, I., Mochida, H., and Kamino, K. (1999). Evaluation of voltage-sensitive dyes for long-term recording of neural activity in the hippocampus. *J. Membr. Biol.* **172**, 145–57.

Nakagami, Y., Saito, H., and Matsuki, N. (1996). Optical recording of rat entorhino-hippocampal system in organotypic culture. *Neurosci. Lett.* **216**, 211–13.

Nakagami, Y., Saito, H., and Matsuki, N. (1997). Optical recording of trisynaptic pathway in rat hippocampal slices with a voltage- sensitive dye. *Neuroscience* **81**, 1–8.

Orbach, H. S., Cohen, L. B., and Grinvald, A. (1985). Optical mapping of electrical activity in rat somatosensory and visual cortex. *J. Neurosci.* **5**, 1886–95.

Otsu, Y., Maru, E., Ohata, H., Takashima, I., Kajiwara, R., and Iijima, T. (2000). Optical recording study of granule cell activities in the hippocampal dentate gyrus of kainate-treated rats. *J. Neurophysiol.* **83**, 2421–30.

Plenz, D. and Aertsen, A. (1993). Current source density profiles of optical recording maps: a new approach to the analysis of spatio-temporal neural activity patterns. *Eur. J. Neurosci.* **5**, 437–48.

Saggau, P., Galvan, M., and Tenbruggencate, G. (1986). Longterm potentiation in guinea-pig hippocampal slices monitored by optical-recording of neuronal-activity. *Neurosci. Lett.* **69**, 53–8.

Sato, K., Matsuki, N., Ohno, Y., and Nakazawa, K. (2000). Extracellular ATP reduces optically monitored electrical signals in hippocampal slices through metabolism to adenosine. *Eur. J. Pharmacol.* **399**, 123–9.

Sekino, Y., Obata, K., Tanifuji, M., Mizuno, M., and Murayama, J. (1997). Delayed signal propagation via CA2 in rat hippocampal slices revealed by optical recording. *J. Neurophysiol.* **78**, 1662–8.

Tominaga, T., Tominaga, Y., Yamada, H., Matsumoto, G., and Ichikawa, M. (2000). Quantification of optical signals with electrophysiological signals in neural activities of Di-4-ANEPPS stained rat hippocampal slices. *J. Neurosci. Meth.* **102**, 11–23.

Glossary

ACSF   artificial cerebrospinal fluid
CNQX   6-cyano-7-nitroquinoxaline-2,3-dione
f EPSP   field excitatory postsynaptic potential
LTP   long-term potentiation
PS   population spike

13

Fusion pore modulation as a presynaptic mechanism contributing to expression of long-term potentiation

Sukwoo Choi, Jürgen Klingauf, and Richard W. Tsien

Working on the idea that postsynaptic and presynaptic mechanisms of long-term potentiation (LTP) expression are not inherently mutually exclusive, we have looked for the
existence and functionality of presynaptic mechanisms for augmenting transmitter release
in hippocampal slices. Specifically, we asked if changes in glutamate release might
contribute to the conversion of 'silent synapses' that show N-methyl-D-aspartate
(NMDA) responses but no detectable α-amino-3-hydroxy-5-methyl-4-isoxazolepropionic
acid (AMPA) responses, to ones that exhibit both. Here, we review experiments where
NMDA receptor responses provided a bioassay of cleft glutamate concentration, using
opposition between peak $[glu]_{cleft}$ and a rapidly reversible antagonist, L-AP5. We discuss
findings of a dramatic increase in peak $[glu]_{cleft}$ upon expression of pairing-induced LTP
(Choi). We present simulations with a quantitative model of glutamatergic synaptic
transmission that includes modulation of the presynaptic fusion pore, realistic cleft geometry and a distributed array of postsynaptic receptors and glutamate transporters. The
modelling supports the idea that changes in the dynamics of glutamate release can contribute to synaptic unsilencing. We review direct evidence from Renger *et al.*, in accord with
the modelling, that trading off the strength and duration of the glutamate transient can
markedly alter AMPA receptor responses with little effect on NMDA receptor responses.
An array of additional findings relevant to fusion pore modulation and its proposed
contribution to LTP expression are considered.

Keywords: fusion pore; silent synapse; long-term potentiation; presynaptic mechanism;
L-AP5

13.1 Introduction

There is wide if not universal consensus that activity-dependent changes in synaptic
efficacy such as LTP and LTD are critical for information storage in the brain and
the proper development of neural circuitry (McNaughton and Morris 1987; Bliss and
Collingridge 1993). However, uncertainty remains about the site or sites of LTP
expression. It is our belief that the possible coexistence of postsynaptic and presynaptic
expression mechanisms has not been fully explored, owing in part to an investigational
desire for conceptual simplicity, and in part to the difficulties of unambiguously distinguishing between various mechanisms.

One important observation, widely replicated at various central synapses (Isaac *et al.*
1995; Liao *et al.* 1995; Durand *et al.* 1996), is that a proportion of glutamatergic synaptic
connections exhibit no AMPAR-mediated currents, but show clear NMDAR-mediated
currents, particularly upon strong postsynaptic depolarization. These 'silent synapses'

can become fully functional upon induction of LTP (Isaac et al. 1995; Liao et al. 1995; Durand et al. 1996). The prevailing hypothesis to account for this conversion invokes a postsynaptic mechanism whereby silent synapses lack functionally active AMPARs but gain them as a result of the insertion of AMPAR-containing vesicles. A proportion of synapses (less than 20%) show no significant labelling by anti-AMPAR antibodies (Nüsser et al. 1998) and fluorescently tagged AMPARs can undergo externalization during the course of LTP (e.g. Shi et al. 1999, 2001; Hayashi et al. 2000).

None of the compelling evidence for postsynaptic changes at silent synapses excludes the possibility of concomitant changes in presynaptic function, as appears to occur in mossy fibre LTP. Indeed, previous work on synapses among cultured dissociated neurons provides unequivocal evidence for the existence of presynaptic mechanisms for expression of NMDAR-induced LTP. This is based on electrophysiological tests with hypertonic solution challenges (Malgaroli and Tsien 1992), the uptake of antibody markers of presynaptic vesicular turnover (Malgaroli et al. 1995), and the destaining of synaptic vesicles marked with the fluorescent dye FM1–43 (Ryan et al. 1996).

Although experiments in hippocampal cultures have provided proof of principle for the existence of presynaptic mechanisms, their extrapolation to brain tissue faces scepticism. Like others, we continue to explore basic synaptic mechanisms in cultured neurons, but have turned to hippocampal slices for critical tests of possible LTP expression mechanisms. We have contributed to two new developments: (i) the use of FM dyes to study vesicle turnover in brain slices (Pyle et al. 1999), and (ii) the application of NMDAR-based assays of cleft neurotransmitter concentration (Choi et al. 2000). In this paper, we summarize our experimental evidence for a presynaptically driven change in cleft neurotransmitter concentration at CA3 to CA1 hippocampal synapses (Choi et al. 2000). We present a quantitative framework for exploring the fusion pore hypothesis, of general interest beyond LTP, that models changes in fusion pore properties, the diffusion of glutamate within the synaptic cleft and surrounding tissues, and the interaction of glutamate with postsynaptic receptors and glutamate transporters. We then discuss the relationship between our results and data from others, particularly Renger et al. (2001), that supports the involvement of fusion pore modulation in synaptic maturation and plasticity.

13.2 Material and methods

(a) Modelling methods

The model of buffered diffusion of glutamate inside and outside the synaptic cleft was similar to that of Rusakov and Kullmann (1998). Release of glutamate from a vesicle was simulated by addition of two 'virtual' cylindrical compartments in the middle of the innermost cleft compartment, one representing the vesicle (40 nm in diameter and 40 nm in height), the other constituting the membrane-spanning fusion pore (variable diameter, 10 nm in length). We chose a value $D = 150 \, \mu m^2 \, s^{-1}$, the highest value that gives results comparable to estimates of the time-course of $[glu]_{cleft}$ (Clements 1996). The diffusion constant of glutamate within the 1–2 nm diameter fusion pore was reduced to $37.5 \, \mu m^2 \, s^{-1}$ to take account of the fact that dimensions of the diffusing species (0.7–0.8 nm) were close to the initial diameter of the permeation pathway (around 2 nm) (Spruce et al.

1990; Stiles *et al.* 1996). Transporters were incorporated in all compartments outside the cleft, at a concentration of 100 µM, using the kinetic description given by Wadiche and Kavanaugh (1998). To estimate the resulting AMPAR and NMDAR currents we used the kinetic schemes and rate constants published by Jonas *et al.* (1993) and Clements and Westbrook (1991), respectively. Binding of a second antagonist molecule was assumed to show a fourfold positive cooperativity, and the k_{off} of L-AP5 was adjusted in order to simulate the experimentally observed effects of L-AP5.

13.3 Results

(a) Experiments with a low-affinity NMDAR antagonist

To assess the peak $[glu]_{cleft}$ at 'silent synapses' that lacked detectable AMPAR-mediated responses, we employed a well-accepted pharmacological approach that relies on a rapidly unbinding antagonist for NMDARs (Clements 1996). The principle of the method (Fig. 13.1a) is that the degree of antagonist inhibition will depend upon the peak transmitter concentration during neurotransmission: the higher $[glu]_{cleft}$, the less the inhibition. L-AP5 (K_i ca. 40 µM; Olverman *et al.* 1988) was chosen as the low-affinity antagonist because its off-rate is faster than for other available NMDA antagonists. In the presence of this competitive antagonist, NMDAR becomes much more sensitive to *peak concentration* because the race with antagonist rebinding is a matter of on-rate, not equilibrium. The competition between glutamate and a fixed amount of L-AP5 can be likened to finding a seat in a crowded café. Those who are slow or infirm will be at a disadvantage, and may fail to get a seat even after many rounds of customers coming and going, because each competition for a vacancy is a winner-take-all contest. So it is for glutamate binding to the NMDAR in the presence of the competitive antagonist: if a receptor fails to bind neurotransmitter in the first place, it matters not that the ligand would have stayed bound for a long time.

Synaptic transmission was evoked by minimal stimulation of the Schaffer collateral-commissural pathway to hippocampal area CA1 (Figs 13.1b and 13.2a). At silent synapses that lacked detectable AMPAR currents but showed clear NMDAR responses, NMDA EPSCs were almost completely inhibited by 250 µM L-AP5 (12 out of 12 cells, mean inhibition = 99.7 ± 1.0%). Pairing of pre- and postsynaptic activity was imposed and was successful in inducing potentiation in 6 out of 12 cells; in these cases, failures of AMPAR responses sharply decreased after pairing as previously reported (Isaac *et al.* 1995; Liao *et al.* 1995; Durand *et al.* 1996). By contrast, no LTP was ever induced when the pairing procedure was carried out in the presence of 50 µM D-AP5 ($n = 8$ out of 8, $p < 0.004$), as expected for NMDAR-dependent plasticity.

We found a marked change when we tested the effects of L-AP5 on NMDAR currents in cases where silent synapses lacking AMPAR currents were converted into fully functional ones. Whereas L-AP5 reduced NMDAR currents by 99.2 ± 3.4% before pairing, the inhibition was much milder after pairing (50.2 ± 3.3%, $n = 6$, $p < 0.001$). The change from full inhibition to half inhibition was all the more convincing because each potentiated slice served as its own control. The reduction in the degree of L-AP5 inhibition indicated that the peak value of $[glu]_{cleft}$ was significantly increased along with the potentiation.

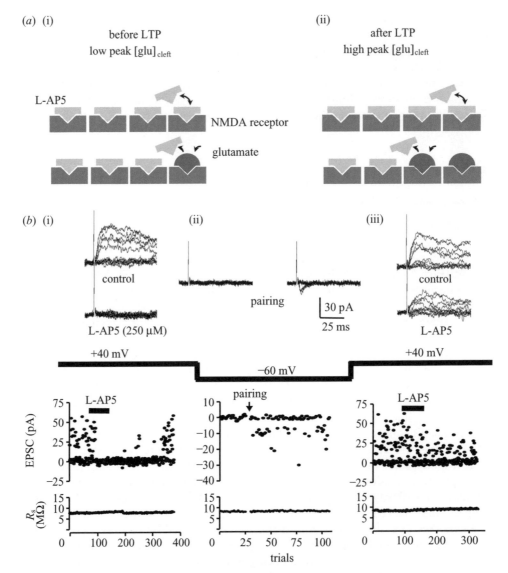

Fig. 13.1 Use of an NMDAR antagonist to probe cleft glutamate concentration. (*a*) Theoretical basis for assessment of [glu]$_{cleft}$ using the fast unbinding antagonist, L-AP5. At a given time, there are a fraction of unoccupied receptors owing to the fast unbinding rate of L-AP5. Then, the probability for glutamate to bind to unoccupied receptors is proportional to the ratio between the concentration of glutamate and L-AP5. The higher the peak glutamate concentration, the less the inhibition by L-AP5. Therefore, if LTP involves increases in peak [glu]$_{cleft}$, one would expect less inhibition by L-AP5 after LTP induction. (After Clements (1996).) (*b*) Representative experiment showing that the degree of inhibition of NMDA EPSCs by L-AP5 decreased during conversion of silent synapses into functional ones. EPSCs were elicited at a frequency of 0.5 Hz. (i) and (iii) Groups of 10 consecutive NMDAR-mediated current records, taken at +40 mV before and after exposure to 250 μM L-AP5. (ii) AMPAR EPSCs, taken at −60 mV, showing conversion from all-silent to non-silent transmission. Note sudden appearance of AMPAR EPSCs and lack of change of series resistance (R_s). (From Choi *et al.* (2000).)

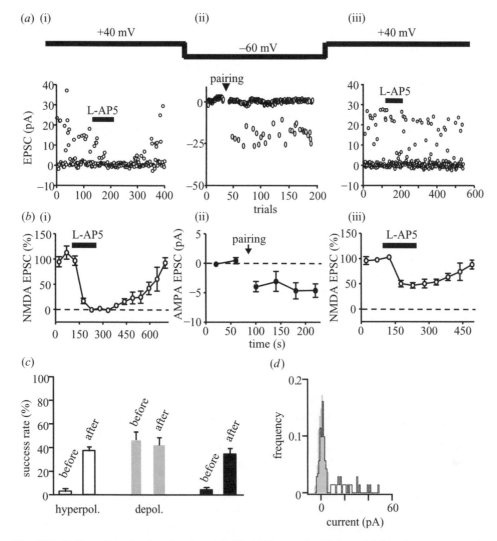

Fig. 13.2 Collected results showing the use of L-AP5 to probe [glu]$_{cleft}$. (*a*) Another representative experiment further illustrating the clearcut difference in L-AP5 responsiveness before and after switch-like expression of LTP. (*b*) Pooled data from silent synapses before pairing, showing that 250 µM L-AP5 completely inhibited NMDAR EPSCs (*n* = 12). L-AP5 was applied for 150 s. Pairing given within 800 s after the start of the whole-cell recording caused an immediate but stable recruitment of AMPAR responses (ii) as seen in data averaged without exclusion of failures. After pairing and successful potentiation, repeated application of L-AP5 (same concentration and duration) inhibited NMDAR EPSCs to a lesser extent ((iii), *n* = 6). (*c*) Summary showing rate of EPSC successes (non-failures) before and after pairing in cells in which pairing induced potentiation (*n* = 6). The proportion of synaptic failures was estimated by doubling the fraction of responses with amplitude less than zero. The success rate of NMDA EPSCs at +40 mV (shaded bars) did not change significantly during LTP (*p* > 0.05). (*d*) Amplitude distribution of NMDAR EPSCs during exposure to 250 µM L-AP5, before pairing (shaded histogram) and after pairing (open histogram). Note that the behaviour of NMDARs treated with 250 µM L-AP5 mimicked that of AMPARs at silent synapses. From Choi *et al.* (2000).

The interpretation of the findings with L-AP5 was clarified by control experiments that addressed several key questions.

Was the difference in antagonist sensitivity specific to the rapidly reversible antagonist? We performed control experiments using the slow unbinding antagonist, R-CPP. In contrast to L-AP5, R-CPP produced a degree of inhibition that did not significantly change during LTP expression. The proportion of current amplitude remaining in the presence of R-CPP was 0.580 ± 0.048 before pairing and 0.542 ± 0.043 after pairing ($p > 0.05$, $n = 4$). The finding that a blockade of NMDA receptor responses was specific to a fast unbinding antagonist but not a slow unbinding antagonist supported the idea that peak $[glu]_{cleft}$ increased during LTP.

(i) How stable were the recordings?
No significant changes in series resistance were found during our whole-cell recordings (Fig. 13.1*b*).

(ii) How was it possible to perform the L-AP5 test before washout of
the ability to induce LTP?
The lack of synaptic enhancement in half (6 out of 12) of the recordings can be attributed to washout of LTP under whole-cell recording (Malinow and Tsien 1990). We kept the time before LTP induction short by testing the antagonist on NMDA EPSCs first, without knowledge of whether the fixed stimulus would yield an all-silent connection at −60 mV. On average, the pairing protocol was applied 13.3 min after the initiation of whole-cell recording. In line with our 50% success in LTP induction around this time, previous work in acute slices has indicated that LTP could be induced with an acceptable rate of success 12–20 min after the initiation of whole-cell recording (Magee and Johnston 1997; Otmakhova *et al.* 2000). By contrast, organotypic slices exhibit more rapid washout, requiring that baseline recordings be restricted to 2–5 min before LTP induction (Hayashi *et al.* 2000; Montgomery *et al.* 2001), leaving insufficient time for a test with L-AP5 (Montgomery *et al.* 2001).

(iii) Do synapses displaying mixed AMPA/NMDA responses without induction
behave similarly to those that have subsequently undergone LTP?
Even if washout of the ability to induce LTP is a problem, one may test L-AP5 responsiveness at non-silent control synapses. When we studied such cases of mixed transmission (significant AMPA current at −60 mV as well as NMDAR current at +40 mV), we found that blockade of NMDAR currents by L-AP5 (250 μM) was always incomplete, even before any induction protocol (16 out of 16 cells, mean inhibition = 68.9 ± 3.7%). By contrast, at silent synapses, NMDA EPSCs were almost completely inhibited by L-AP5 (250 μM) (12 out of 12 cells, mean inhibition = 99.7 ± 1.0%).

(iv) Is there a credible postsynaptic explanation for the change in
antagonist sensitivity?
Incorporation of NMDARs is not part of the prevailing hypothesis. In any case, the drug-free NMDA current hardly increases on average, so the change in antagonist sensitivity cannot be attributed to the hypothetical incorporation of L-AP5-insensitive NMDARs.

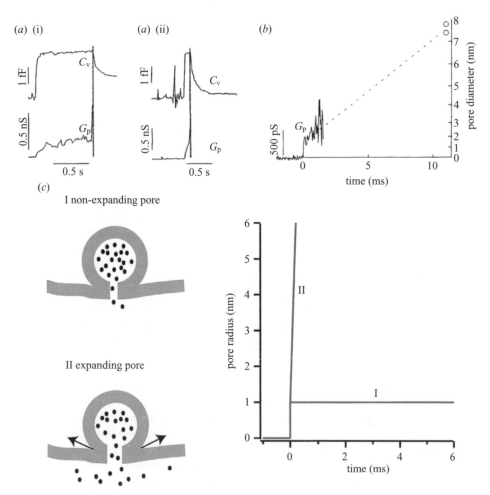

Fig. 13.3 Modes of fusion pore opening studied with capacitance measurements in neutrophils. (*a*) Variety of behaviour, including a long-lived plateau of pore conductance (G_p), followed by rapid expansion (i), or a brief plateau of G_p, followed by rapid expansion (ii) C_v, vesicular capacitance. (From Lollike *et al.* (1998).) (*b*) Capacitance measurement in neutrophil from Spruce *et al.* (1990) showing the genesis of increased pore conductance (alternatively expressed as pore radius, right). (*c*) Proposed fusion modes (see text), opening to a small, fixed level (2 nm pore diameter), labelled mode I; opening to the same level but undergoing immediate rapid expansion at a rate of 25 nm ms^{-1}, typical of that believed to support rapid exocytosis, labelled mode II.

(v) Can the competitive antagonist approach provide quantitative information about peak [glu]$_{cleft}$?

A more quantitative estimate of peak [glu]$_{cleft}$ sensed by NMDARs at silent synapses can be obtained on the basis of antagonist characteristics, empirically derived from outside-out patch recordings from hippocampal glutamate receptors (Choi *et al.* 2000). Because complete block of channel opening can only occur if antagonist binding greatly outraces neurotransmitter binding (Clements 1996), we estimated that the peak [glu]$_{cleft}$ at silent synapses was far less than 170 µM. This would be far lower than the approximate 2 mM estimated for conventionally active synapses (Clements *et al.* 1992; Diamond and Jahr 1997), and would be expected to produce negligible activation of AMPARs, given their highly cooperative [glu] dependence (Rosenmund *et al.* 1998).

(b) Modelling transmitter release and postsynaptic action

(i) Hypothetical explanations of the increased $[glu]_{cleft}$

How might the glutamate concentration sensed by NMDA receptors undergo such a sharp increase in association with potentiation? The switch-like nature of LTP expression weighs against cell biological mechanisms that would be expected to develop gradually, such as major changes in cleft width, transport buffer capacity, or alignment between presynaptic release sites and postsynaptic receptor clusters (Renger *et al.* 2001). Setting these aside as highly speculative, several additional hypotheses must be considered. First, the glutamate content of vesicles might increase (Pothos *et al.* 1998). Second, glutamate might 'spill over' to a postsynaptic site from near-neighbour synapses before pairing, only to be supplanted after potentiation by neurotransmitter release from the presynaptic terminal directly apposed to the site (Kullmann and Asztely 1998). Third, changes in $[glu]_{cleft}$ might arise from altered fusion pore dynamics (Choi *et al.* 2000). If this occurred as a result of LTP, vesicular glutamate at silent synapses might trickle out slowly enough to minimally activate AMPA receptors before induction, but produce easily detectable peak concentrations after LTP.

(ii) Precedents from other systems

Electrophysiological studies in non-neuronal secretory cells, mostly using capacitance measurements, have demonstrated that fusion pores can show multiple modes of operation (e.g. Spruce *et al.* 1990; Lollike *et al.* 1998). These modes can be distinguished as non-expanding and rapidly expanding (Fig. 13.3a), corresponding respectively to slow and incomplete secretion or a rapid spike of release as detected by amperometry (Bruns and Jahn 1995). Acceleration of fusion pore expansion has been inferred as a consequence of altered interactions between munc18 and the SNARE protein syntaxin (Fisher *et al.* 2001). The rate of fusion pore expansion can be sharply increased by PKC (Scepek *et al.* 1998; Graham *et al.* 2000), a kinase long ago implicated in LTP (Malinow *et al.* 1989). Our own findings with optical probes in cultured hippocampal synapses suggest the existence of transient fusion pore openings with lifetimes in the millisecond range (N. C. Harata, S. Choi, J. L. Pyle, A. M. Aravanis and R. W. Tsien, unpublished observation). Recent capacitance measurements have revealed the existence of non-expanding fusion pores in microvesicles similar to small synaptic vesicles (Klyachko and Jackson 2002). The conductance of the non-expanding fusion pore is 11 times smaller than that of large dense core vesicles, leaving open the possibility of even slower transmitter release than that which had been supposed. Taken together, these observations lend credence to the possibility that presynaptic fusion pores at hippocampal synapses may be under modulatory control.

(iii) Model of quantal responses at a glutamatergic synapse

To explore the implications of fusion pore modulation, we constructed a detailed model of glutamatergic transmission (Figs 13.3 and 13.4). Taking a lead from other secretory systems (Fig. 13.3a), we assumed that the fusion pore can switch between two

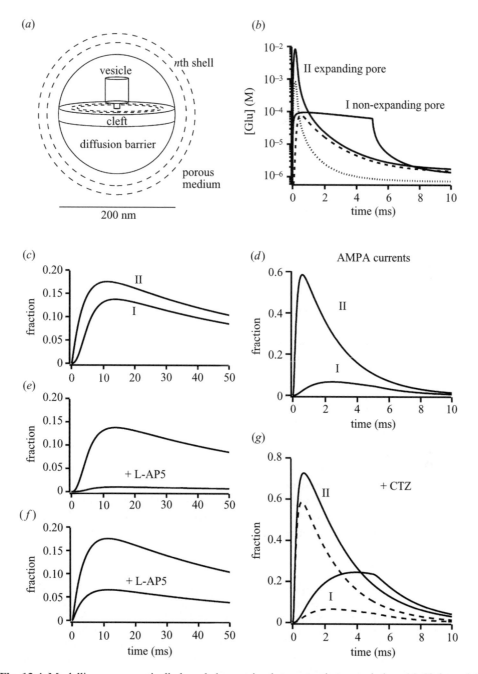

Fig. 13.4 Modelling presynaptically based changes in glutamatergic transmission. (a) Cleft model supplemented with simulation of glutamate efflux from presynaptic vesicle (see Section 13.2). A disc-shaped cleft was assigned a width of 20 nm and a radius of 100 nm. The glutamate diffusion coefficient (D_{glu}) was assumed to be 150 $\mu m^2 s^{-1}$. This value was chosen to allow the simulation of [glu]$_{cleft}$ to resemble experimental estimates with respect to the time-course of decay (Clements et al. 1992). (b) Calculated [glu]$_{cleft}$ for various scenarios: 'standard transmission', a vesicular content of 6000 glutamate molecules, escaping through a rapidly expanding fusion pore (mode II);

patterns, a non-expanding fusion pore with a small conductance (mode I) and a rapidly expanding fusion pore (mode II) (Fig. 13.3b). The expansion rate of 25 nm ms^{-1} was typical of that thought to support rapid exocytosis in other systems (Stiles $et\ al.$ 1996). We followed Rusakov and Kullmann (1998) in modelling the synaptic cleft and the porous extracellular space outside it (Fig. 13.4a). AMPA and NMDA receptors on the postsynaptic membrane were described by kinetics given respectively by Jonas $et\ al.$ (1993) and Clements and Westbrook (1991), with AMPAR desensitization rates set at a log midpoint between the estimates of Jonas and Sakmann (1992) and Raman and Trussell (1995). Figure 13.4b illustrates the calculated time-course of [glu]$_{cleft}$ for a vesicle containing 6000 transmitter molecules and a fusion pore undergoing the step-wise opening and immediate rapid expansion of mode II. The calculated [glu]$_{cleft}$ reached a peak value in the millimolar range, then decayed rapidly, in conformity with previous findings (Clements $et\ al.$ 1992; Diamond and Jahr 1997; Liu $et\ al.$ 1999). This standard transient may be compared with model predictions for the three scenarios for silent synapses. For a 10-fold reduction in vesicular transmitter contents, the calculated [glu]$_{cleft}$ was in essence a scaled-down version of the standard transient. For spillover, we calculated the glutamate concentration due to a neighbouring synapse positioned an average intersynaptic distance away (460 nm (Rusakov and Kullmann 1998)). The simulated [glu]$_{cleft}$ reached a lower peak, but then closely approximated the standard transient. Finally, for a non-expanding fusion pore (mode I, Fig. 13.2b), the predicted [glu]$_{cleft}$ also reached a peak near 100 nM, but then showed an extremely slow decay, owing to the extended time required for transmitter to escape the vesicle. The transient illustrated in Fig. 13.4b was based on the assumption that the fusion pore opened instantaneously to a fixed diameter of 1.8 nm, then closed again after 5 ms. The prolonged waveform of neurotransmitter is reminiscent of behaviour observed with amperometry in secretory cells (Bruns and Jahn 1995; Zhou $et\ al.$ 1996).

(iv) Distinguishing among expression scenarios
The simulated [glu]$_{cleft}$ transients for reduced vesicular content or 'spill-over' each satisfied the criterion of generating nearly undetectable AMPA currents. However, in both of these cases, the predicted NMDA currents were also much smaller than their counterparts during standard transmission (simulations not shown). Only for the non-expanding fusion pore did the transient in [glu]$_{cleft}$ result in relatively large NMDA and

---

similar to 'standard transmission' but with only 600 glutamate molecules (dotted line); similar to 'standard transmission' but assessed at a position 465 nm away from the centre of the cleft (dashed line); non-expanding fusion pore (mode I, see text). (c) fractional activation of NMDARs driven by [glu]$_{cleft}$ for modes I and II. Note that NMDARs show similar amplitudes because of combined influence of strength and duration of [glu]$_{cleft}$ transient. A small change in the time course of NMDAR activation was predicted but would be difficult to resolve because of sto-chastic channel gating. (d) Fractional activation of AMPARs for modes I and II. Differential between fractional activation of AMPARs would be further increased if AMPAR kinetics took account of binding of four glutamates (Rosenmund $et\ al.$ 1998). In contrast to changes in [glu]$_{cleft}$, increasing the number of AMPARs would not change activation kinetics significantly but would simply increase the amplitude of the current. (e), (f) Simulated effects of L-AP5 on NMDAR activation with scenarios I, non-expanding pore (e) and II, expanding pore (f). (g) Simulated effects of cyclothiazide on AMPAR activation with scenarios I and II.

relatively tiny AMPA components (Fig. 13.4c,d). Note that the fusion pore modelling provides a presynaptic rationale for the finding that LTP is associated with relatively little increase in NMDA current compared with the large potentiation of the AMPA current. Likewise, with appropriate assumptions about antagonist binding kinetics, it was possible within the non-expanding/expanding pore scenario to simulate the very different effects of 250 μM L-AP5 on silent synapses and standard transmission (Fig. 13.4e,f), whereas this was not feasible for the other cases (simulations not shown).

Another sharp distinction between scenarios hinges on the degree of AMPA receptor desensitization. Little desensitization arises from short-lived transients generated by 'spill-over' or by an expanding fusion pore, regardless of whether vesicular contents are normal or reduced. By contrast, the non-expanding fusion pore produced a prolonged, low-amplitude [glu]$_{cleft}$ transient that quickly drove AMPARs into a desensitized state. Accordingly, removal of desensitization has widely different consequences (Fig. 13.4g): only a modest (around 15%) increase of the simulated AMPA current in the case of a brief [glu]$_{cleft}$ transient (mode II), but a more than threefold increase in the amplitude of the tiny events associated with a non-expanding pore (mode I). Indeed, the modelling suggested that transmission by AMPARs might become detectable at 'silent synapses' if desensitization of the receptors were pharmacologically inhibited. Events revealed in this way should have a slow rise and a relatively abrupt decay, faster than the decline of 'standard' events. This set of predictions was borne out by our experiments with cyclothiazide in area CA1 (Choi *et al.* 2000; see also Gasparini *et al.* 2000).

13.4 Discussion

(a) Changes in glutamate dynamics and pairing-induced LTP at CA3–CA1 synapses

We have reviewed evidence that pairing-induced LTP in young hippocampal slices is associated with a dramatic increase in cleft neurotransmitter concentration. Our detection method relied on a local sensor, the NMDAR, that by definition must be present at synapses undergoing NMDAR-dependent, associative LTP. The use of a rapidly dissociating antagonist, L-AP5, is a well-accepted biophysical method for assaying peak cleft glutamate concentration (Clements 1996). By testing the method on NMDA receptors in outside-out patches of hippocampal membrane, we were able to set some quantitative limits. Before pairing, peak [glu]$_{cleft}$ at silent synapses was far below 170 μM, low enough to escape clear detection by postsynaptic AMPARs. After potentiation, peak [glu]$_{cleft}$ reached millimolar values, thus supporting NMDAR responses only partially blocked by 250 μM L-AP5, and yielding clearly detectable transmission via AMPARs (Choi *et al.* 2000). The use of NMDARs as reporters leaves open the possibility of concomitant changes in postsynaptic receptor properties, including incorporation of new AMPA receptors, phosphorylation of AMPARs, etc. Kinetic changes in the mode of gating of presynaptic fusion pores represent a precisely targeted action for which there is ample precedent in non-neuronal cells (Fig. 13.3a). The proposed mechanism offers considerable functional advantages for both synaptic plasticity and development. A basal state of local, NMDAR-only transmission would maximize the input-specificity of Hebb's rule, in contrast to the absence of proximal

NMDA transmission envisioned in the spillover hypothesis (Kullmann and Asztely 1998). It would also allow for rapid, stepwise increases in AMPAR transmission (e.g. Fig. 13.2a), difficult to achieve by other cell biological mechanisms (Liao et al. 1999).

(b) Insights from a model for glutamate dynamics in the synaptic cleft

We have presented a quantitative model of glutamatergic transmission that adheres closely to published information on fusion pore, cleft geometry and postsynaptic receptor kinetics. We were able to simulate an increase in $[glu]_{cleft}$ due to the conversion of presynaptic fusion pores from non-expanding to rapidly expanding. Modelling of this kind provides some useful lessons.

  (i) It dispels simple-minded calculations which estimate peak $[glu]_{cleft}$ by taking the transmitter content of a vesicle and dispersing it uniformly within the volume of the synaptic cleft, without consideration of rates of diffusion into and out of the cleft.
 (ii) It successfully simulates the finding that $[glu]_{cleft}$ decays with multiple exponential components (Clements 1996).
(iii) It provides a theoretical framework for understanding why neither AMPARs nor NMDARs are regularly saturated by quantal release of glutamate (Dube and Liu 1999; Liu et al. 1999; McAllister and Stevens 2000; Oertner et al. 2002).
 (iv) It provides perspective on the hypothesis that NMDA-only transmission reflects failures of release from the immediately apposed presynaptic terminal, amidst spillover of glutamate from neighbouring boutons (Kullmann and Asztely 1998). Simulation of the diffusion of glutamate from nearby synapses did not predict enough spillover to support full-blown NMDAR-only synaptic responses (Fig. 13.2); in addition, the incidence of NMDAR successes failed to increase after pairing (Fig. 13.1), excluding the predicted increase in the release probability of the immediately presynaptic terminal.
  (v) It focuses interest on the concept of 'kiss and run' fusion, and the possibility that a fusion pore might open up to a small, sustained conductance level, possibly shutting even before all the neurotransmitter had escaped.

(c) Complementary studies in hippocampal cultures and slices from other groups

The idea that the concentration profile of glutamate delivery governs AMPAR activation was directly tested by the group of Guosong Liu (Renger et al. 2001). Using iontophoretic application of various glutamate waveforms (Fig. 13.5), they demonstrated that 'fast' (1 ms, 100 nA) application of glutamate elicited both AMPAR and NMDAR currents, whereas 'slow' (10 ms, 10 nA) applications evoked very similar NMDAR currents but no detectable AMPAR response. Both kinds of responses were registered as inward currents near the normal resting potential, the NMDAR distinguished by its slow kinetics. Their results are in excellent accord with our modelling of the downstream responses to glutamate release from rapidly expanding and non-expanding fusion pores. Renger et al. (2001) went on to stimulate synaptic transmission, and found 'AMPA-quiet' as well as mixed synaptic responses. The 'AMPA-quiet' responses could be interleaved with clearcut AMPAR responses to 'fast' iontophoretic

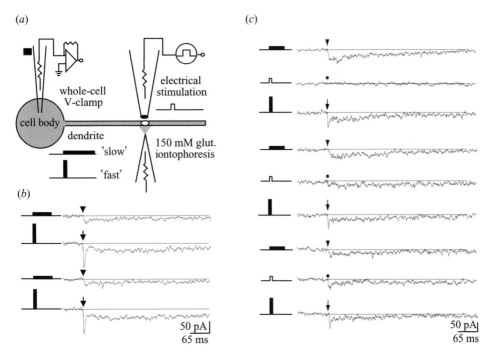

Fig. 13.5 Concentration profile of neurotransmitter delivery determines AMPAR activation. (*a*) Experimental design for alternately stimulating presynaptic release and iontophoretically probing postsynaptic receptors. Iontophoresis and stimulating electrodes are brought to within 1 µm of an isolated synapse. Filled vertical and horizontal bars represent 'fast' (1 ms, 100 nA) and 'slow' (10 ms, 10 nA) iontophoretic application parameters. (*b*) AMPA receptors are not significantly activated by a slow flux of glutamate. Slow pulses elicited NMDAR-only responses, while fast pulses elicited AMPAR and NMDAR responses from the same site. Because AMPAR activation was sensitive to sudden increases in neurotransmitter concentration, AMPA-quiet responses could be generated at synapses with functional AMPARs. (*c*) Silent synapses contain functional AMPARs. $EPSC_{AMPA\text{-quiet}}$ responses, resulting from endogenous transmitter release, were evoked by presynaptic electrical stimulation at a 9 DIV synapse (open vertical bars). Trials with synaptic stimulation were interleaved with iontophoretic applications of neurotransmitter. Presynaptically evoked $EPSC_{AMPA\text{-quiet}}$ responses were scattered among full-fledged AMPAR responses to fast iontophoretic pulses, indicating that AMPARs were functional despite the finding of AMPA-quiet synaptic events ($n = 4$). (From Renger *et al.* (2001), with permission.)

application. Thus, it was concluded that a 'silent synapse' can be generated by a fluctuating presynaptic mechanism, even under conditions where clearcut and steady AMPAR responsiveness already exists.

In another important experiment, Renger *et al.* (2001) showed that AMPA-quiet behaviour gradually disappears with development between 9 and 13 days *in vitro* (Fig. 13.6*a,b*). However, application of a well-known presynaptic toxin that cleaves SNARE proteins, TeNTx, converted the fully functional synapses back into ones that alternated between silent and non-silent behaviour (Fig. 13.6*c*). The effectiveness of TeNTx provides another indication that the presynaptic fusion machinery may be involved causing modulation of $[glu]_{cleft}$.

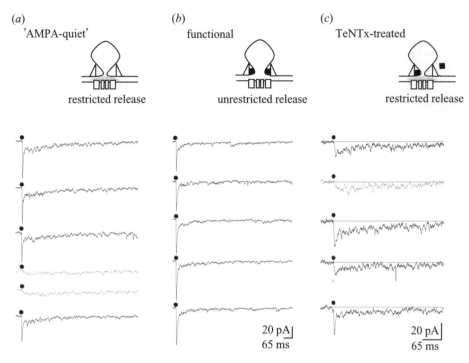

Fig. 13.6 Maturation of glutamate flux affects receptor activation. Neurotransmitter concentration could be altered through controlling the diffusion of glutamate into the synaptic cleft. For example, the synaptic vesicle pore conductance may be larger during a functional than a silent event. (*a*) AMPA-quiet events could be due to slow release through a non-expanding fusion pore. Current traces (bottom) show that series of evoked events varied between $EPSC_{dual}$ (black traces) and $EPSC_{AMPA\text{-}quiet}$ (grey traces) responses at single synapses. (*b*) Functional events could be due to fast release through rapidly expanding fusion pore. As shown in current traces (bottom), a higher proportion of evoked $EPSC_{dual}$ events was observed. (*c*) TeNtx treatment converts functional events to AMPA-quiet ones. Representative series of evoked EPSCs (bottom) from a single synapse (DIV 21) after 1 h TeNTx treatment (0 mM Mg^{2+}). Evoked EPSCs fluctuated between $EPSC_{AMPA\text{-}quiet}$ and $EPSC_{dual}$ among trials, reminiscent of evoked EPSCs from immature synapses. (From Renger *et al.* (2001), with permission.)

A change in the mode of opening of presynaptic fusion pores provides one way of explaining previous findings of an increased uptake of presynaptic markers such as the antibody against synaptotagmin I (Malgaroli *et al.* 1995), or accelerated destaining of the fluorescent vesicle marker FM1–43 (Ryan *et al.* 1996). The use of FM1–43 in slices by the Siegelbaum and Stanton groups has supported the idea that presynaptic vesicular dynamics are significantly altered during certain forms of LTP and LTD (Stanton *et al.* 2001; Zakharenko *et al.* 2001, 2002). Finally, imaging of EPSCaTs at single synapses by Fine, Bliss and colleagues (Emptage *et al.* 2003) has demonstrated an increase in the likelihood of these jointly NMDAR-, AMPAR-dependent events. One might interpret their data as a graded increase in the proportion of AMPA-unsilent events, from an initial nonzero value to a higher level after induction (see also Renger *et al.* 2001), thus providing an analogue increase in synaptic strength (Dixon *et al.* 2002). The EPSCaT imaging experiments inherently select for unitary connections that are not entirely AMPA-silent, whereas the experiments in Figs 13.1 and 13.2 were designed to probe 'all-silent' synapses. Nevertheless, both sets of results are compatible with scenarios wherein presynaptic terminals distribute their time among distinct fusion modes.

(d) Possible coexistence of postsynaptic and presynaptic mechanisms for unsilencing

It is important to note that a mechanism of fusion pore modulation and modification of postsynaptic receptor properties are not mutually exclusive. Perhaps both mechanisms coexist but unfold over somewhat different time domains. There is evidence that postsynaptically silent synapses containing only NMDARs might form first during early development, while AMPA receptors are added later by some mechanism akin to LTP (Gomperts *et al.* 1998; Liao *et al.* 1999; Nüsser *et al.* 1998). However, there is disagreement between the relatively low proportion of synapses that are immunochemically identifiable as potentially NMDA receptor-only synapses (17–28%; Nüsser *et al.* 1998) and the much higher proportion of physiologically silent events. This opens up the possibility that physiologically silent events do not represent one entity, but a mixture of pre- and postsynaptically silent synapses. One might even imagine the simultaneous coexistence of pre- and postsynaptic mechanisms for attenuating synaptic strength, a 'belt and braces' scenario, that would maximize the distinction between dormant and awakened synaptic connnections. Unsilencing might involve coordinated changes in the mode of release and an increase in postsynaptic receptivity. This has some teleological appeal, but it also calls for a case-by-case examination of the specific role of each mechanism in different brain regions at different stages of development. In one particular region of interest, the associational connections among CA3 neurons, Montgomery *et al.* (2001) have presented compelling evidence that postsynaptic unsilencing must occur. It would be interesting to look for presynaptic fusion pore modulation in the same region, under conditions in which the LAP5 approach is experimentally feasible.

We are grateful to D. Ramot for a careful reading of the manuscript. This work was supported by a Silvio Conte Center for Neuroscience Research (NIMH) to R.W.T. and by Korea Ministry of Science and Technology grant M1-0108-00-0051 under the neurobiology research programme to S.C.

References

Bliss, T. V. and Collingridge, G. L. (1993). A synaptic model of memory: long-term potentiation in the hippocampus. *Nature* **361**, 31–9.

Bruns, D. and Jahn, R. (1995). Real-time measurement of transmitter release from single synaptic vesicles. *Nature* **377**, 62–5.

Choi, S., Klingauf, J., and Tsien, R. W. (2000). Postfusional regulation of cleft glutamate concentration during LTP at 'silent synapses'. *Nature Neurosci.* **3**, 330–6.

Clements, J. D. (1996). Transmitter time course in the synaptic cleft: its role in central synaptic function. *Trends Neurosci.* **19**, 163–71.

Clements, J. D. and Westbrook, G. L. (1991). Activation kinetics reveal the number of glutamate and glycine binding sites on the N-methyl-D-aspartate receptor. *Neuron* **7**, 605–13.

Clements, J. D., Lester, R. A., Tong, G., Jahr, C. E., and Westbrook, G. L. (1992). The time course of glutamate in the synaptic cleft. *Science* **258**, 1498–501.

Diamond, J. S. and Jahr, C. E. (1997). Transporters buffer synaptically released glutamate on a submillisecond time-scale. *J. Neurosci.* **17**, 4672–87.

Dixon, D. B., Bliss, T. V. P., and Fine, A. (2002). Individual hippocampal synapses express incremental (analog) and bi-directional long-term plasticity. *Soc. Neurosci. Abstr.* **28**, 150.3.

Dube, G. R. and Liu, G. (1999). AMPA and NMDA receptors display similar affinity during rapid synaptic-like glutamate applications. *Soc. Neurosci. Abstr.* **25**, 992.

Durand, G. M., Kovalchuk, Y., and Konnerth, A. (1996). Long-term potentiation and functional synapse induction in developing hippocampus. *Nature* **381**, 71–5.

Emptage, N. J., Reid, C. A., Fine, A., and Bliss, T. V. P. (2003). Optical quantal analysis reveals a presynaptic component of LTP at hippocampal Schaffer-associational synapses. *Neuron* **38**, 797–804.

Fisher, R. J., Pevsner, J., and Burgoyne, R. D. (2001). Control of fusion pore dynamics during exocytosis by Munc18. *Science* **291**, 875–8.

Gasparini, S., Saviane, C., Voronin, L. L., and Cherubini, E. (2000). Silent synapses in the developing hippocampus: lack of functional AMPA receptors or low probability of glutamate release? *Proc. Natl Acad. Sci. USA* **97**, 9741–6.

Gomperts, S. N., Rao, A., Craig, A. M., Malenka, R. C., and Nicoll, R. A. (1998). Postsynaptically silent synapses in single neuron cultures. *Neuron* **21**, 1443–51.

Graham, M. E., Fisher, R. J., and Burgoyne, R. D. (2000). Measurement of exocytosis by amperometry in adrenal chromaffin cells: effects of clostridial neurotoxins and activation of protein kinase C on fusion pore kinetics. *Biochimie* **82**, 469–79.

Hayashi, Y., Shi, S. H., Esteban, J. A., Piccini, A., Poncer, J. C., and Malinow, R. (2000). Driving AMPA receptors into synapses by LTP and CaMKII: requirement for GluR1 and PDZ domain interaction. *Science* **287**, 2262–7.

Isaac, J. T., Nicoll, R. A., and Malenka, R. C. (1995). Evidence for silent synapses: implications for the expression of LTP. *Neuron* **15**, 427–34.

Jonas, P. and Sakmann, B. (1992). Glutamate receptor channels in isolated patches from CA1 and CA3 pyramidal cells of rat hippocampal slices. *J. Physiol. (Lond.)* **455**, 143–71.

Jonas, P., Major, G., and Sakmann, B. (1993). Quantal components of unitary EPSCs at the mossy fibre synapse on CA3 pyramidal cells of rat hippocampus. *J. Physiol. (Lond.)* **472**, 615–63.

Klyachko, V. A. and Jackson, M. B. (2002). Capacitance steps and fusion pores of small and large-dense-core vesicles in nerve terminals. *Nature* **418**, 89–92.

Kullmann, D. M. and Asztely, F. (1998). Extrasynaptic glutamate spillover in the hippocampus: evidence and implications. *Trends Neurosci.* **21**, 8–14.

Liao, D., Hessler, N. A., and Malinow, R. (1995). Activation of postsynaptically silent synapses during pairing-induced LTP in CA1 region of hippocampal slice. *Nature* **375**, 400–4.

Liao, D., Zhang, X., O'Brien, R., Ehler, M. D., and Huganir, R. L. (1999). Regulation of morphological postsynaptic silent synapses in developing hippocampal neurons. *Nature Neurosci.* **2**, 37–43.

Liu, G., Choi, S., and Tsien, R. W. (1999). Variability of neurotransmitter concentration and nonsaturation of postsynaptic AMPA receptors at synapses in hippocampal cultures and slices. *Neuron* **22**, 395–409.

Lollike, K., Borregaard, N., and Lindau, M. (1998). Capacitance flickers and pseudoflickers of small granules, measured in the cell-attached configuration. *Biophys. J.* **75**, 53–9.

McAllister, A. K. and Stevens, C. F. (2000). Nonsaturation of AMPA and NMDA receptors at hippocampal synapses. *Proc. Natl Acad. Sci. USA* **97**, 6173–8.

McNaughton, B. L. and Morris, R. G. M. (1987). Hippocampal synaptic enhancement and information storage within a distributed memory system. *Trends Neurosci.* **10**, 408–15.

Magee, J. C. and Johnston, D. (1997). A synaptically controlled, associative signal for Hebbian plasticity in hippocampal neurons. *Science* **275**, 209–13.

Malgaroli, A. and Tsien, R. W. (1992). Glutamate-induced long-term potentiation of the frequency of miniature synaptic currents in cultured hippocampal neurons. *Nature* **357**, 134–39.

Malgaroli, A., Ting, A. E., Wendland, B., Bergamaschi, A., Villa, A., Tsien, R. W., *et al.* (1995). Presynaptic component of long-term potentiation visualized at individual hippocampal synapses. *Science* **268**, 1624–8.

Malinow, R. and Tsien, R. W. (1990). Presynaptic enhancement shown by whole-cell recordings of long-term potentiation in hippocampal slices. *Nature* **346**, 177–80.

Malinow, R., Schulman, H., and Tsien, R. W. (1989). Inhibition of postsynaptic PKC or CaMKII blocks induction but not expression of LTP. *Science* **245**, 862–6.

Montgomery, J. M., Palvlidis, P., and Madison, D. V. (2001). Pair recordings reveal all-silent synaptic connections and the postsynaptic expression of long-term potentiation. *Neuron* **29**, 691–701.

Nüsser, Z., Lujan, R., O'Brien, R. J., Kamboj, S., Ehler, M. D., Rosen, K. R., *et al.* (1998). Cell type and pathway dependence of synaptic AMPA receptor number and variability in the hippocampus. *Neuron* **21**, 545–59.

Oertner, T. G., Sabatini, B. L., Nimchinsky, E. A., and Svoboda, K. (2002). Facilitation at single synapses probed with optical quantal analysis. *Nature Neurosci.* **5**, 657–64.

Olverman, H. J., Jones, A. W., Mewett, K. N., and Watkins, J. C. (1988). Structure/activity relations of N-methyl-D-aspartate receptor ligands as studied by their inhibition of [^{3}H]D-2-amino-5-phosphonopentanoic acid binding in rat brain membranes. *Neuroscience* **26**, 17–31.

Otmakhova, N. A., Otmakhov, N., Mortenson, L. H., and Lisman, J. E. (2000). Inhibition of the cAMP pathway decreases early long-term potentiation at CA1 hippocampal synapses. *J. Neurosci.* **20**, 4446–51.

Pothos, E. N., Przedborski, S., Davila, V., Schmitz, Y., and Sulzer, D. (1998). D2-Like dopamine autoreceptor activation reduces quantal size in PC12 cells. *J. Neurosci.* **18**, 4106–18.

Pyle, J. L., Kavalali, E. T., Choi, S., and Tsien, R. W. (1999). Visualization of synaptic activity in hippocampal slices with FM1–43 enabled by fluorescence quenching. *Neuron* **24**, 803–8.

Raman, I. M. and Trussell, L. O. (1995). The mechanism of alpha-amino-3-hydroxy-5-methyl-4-isoxazolepropionate receptor desensitization after removal of glutamate. *Biophys. J.* **68**, 137–46.

Renger, J. J., Egles, C., and Liu, G. (2001). A developmental switch in neurotransmitter flux enhances synaptic efficacy by affecting AMPA receptor activation. *Neuron* **29**, 469–84.

Rosenmund, C., Stern-Bach, Y., and Stevens, C. F. (1998). The tetrameric structure of a glutamate receptor channel. *Science* **280**, 1596–9.

Rusakov, D. A. and Kullmann, D. M. (1998). Extrasynaptic glutamate diffusion in the hippocampus: ultrastructural constraints, uptake, and receptor activation. *J. Neurosci.* **18**, 3158–70.

Ryan, T. A., Ziv, N. E., and Smith, S. J. (1996). Potentiation of evoked vesicle turnover at individually resolved synaptic boutons. *Neuron* **17**, 125–34.

Scepek, S., Coorssen, J. R., and Lindau, M. (1998). Fusion pore expansion in horse eosinophils is modulated by Ca^{2+} and protein kinase C via distinct mechanisms. *EMBO J.* **17**, 4340–6.

Shi, S. H., Hayashi, Y., Petralia, R. S., Zaman, S. H., Wenthold, R. J., Svoboda, K., *et al.* (1999). Rapid spine delivery and redistribution of AMPA receptors after synaptic NMDA receptor activation. *Science* **284**, 1811–6.

Shi, S. H., Hayashi, Y., Esteban, J. A., and Malinow, R. (2001). Subunit-specific rules governing AMPA receptor trafficking to synapses in hippocampal pyramidal neurons. *Cell* **105**, 331–43.

Spruce, A. E., Breckenridge, L. J., Lee, A. K., and Almers, W. (1990). Properties of the fusion pore that forms during exocytosis of a mast cell secretory vesicle. *Neuron* **4**, 643–54.

Stanton, P. K., Heinemann, U., and Muller, W. (2001). FM1–43 imaging reveals cGMP-dependent long-term depression of presynaptic transmitter release. *J. Neurosci.* **21**, RC167.

Stiles, J. R., Van Helden, D., Bartol Jr, T. M., Salpeter, E. E., and Salpeter, M. M. (1996). Miniature endplate current rise times less than 100 microseconds from improved dual recordings can be modeled with passive acetylcholine diffusion from a synaptic vesicle. *Proc. Natl Acad. Sci. USA* **93**, 5747–52.

Wadiche, J. I. and Kavanaugh, M. P. (1998). Macroscopic and microscopic properties of a cloned glutamate transporter/chloride channel. *J. Neurosci.* **18**, 7650–61.

Zakharenko, S. S., Zablow, L., and Siegelbaum, S. A. (2001). Visualization of changes in presynaptic function during longterm synaptic plasticity. *Nature Neurosci.* **4**, 711–17.

Zakharenko, S. S., Zablow, L., and Siegelbaum, S. A. (2002). Altered presynaptic vesicle release and cycling during mGluR-dependent LTD. *Neuron* **35**, 1099–110.

Zhou, Z., Misler, S., and Chow, R. H. (1996). Rapid fluctuations in transmitter release from single vesicles in bovine adrenal chromaffin cells. *Biophys. J.* **70**, 1543–52.

Glossary

AMPA	α-amino-3-hydroxy-5-methyl-4-isoxazolepropionic acid
AMPAR	AMPA receptor
CA1 and CA3	anatomical regions of the hippocampal formation (CA stands for '*cornu Ammon* or Ammon's horn)
EPSCaT	excitatory postsynaptic Ca^{2+} transient
FM1-43	*N*-(3-triethylammoniumpropyl)-4-(4-(dibutylamino)styryl)pyridinium dibromide, a fluorescent dye used to monitor vesicular traffic
LTD	long-term depression
LTP	long-term potentiation
NMDA	*N*-methyl-D-aspartate
NMDAR	NMDA receptor
PKC	protein kinase C
R-CPP	3-(*R*)-(2-carboxypiperazin-4-yl)-propyl-1-phosphonic acid
SNARE	soluble *N*-ethylmaleimide-sensitive-factor attachment protein
TeNTx	tetanus neurotoxin

14

AMPA receptor trafficking and long-term potentiation

Roberto Malinow

Activity-dependent changes in synaptic function are believed to underlie the formation of memories. A prominent example is long-term potentiation (LTP), whose mechanisms have been the subject of considerable scrutiny over the past few decades. I review studies from our laboratory that support a critical role for AMPA receptor trafficking in LTP and experience-dependent plasticity.

Keywords: excitatory; transmission; memory; long-term potentiation; experience-dependent plasticity

14.1 Introduction

There is general belief that a long-lasting change in synaptic function is the cellular basis of learning and memory (Eccles 1964; Hebb 1949; Alkon and Nelson 1990; Kandel 1997). The most thoroughly characterized example of such synaptic plasticity is LTP. While many neuroscientists like to disparage LTP, and even gain notoriety by their attempts to diminish its importance, this phenomenon continues to hold the interest of most scientists interested in the cellular basis of learning and memory. History will tell who has misspent energies.

A remarkable feature of LTP is that a short period of synaptic activity can trigger persistent changes of synaptic transmission lasting at least several hours and often longer. This property led investigators to suggest that LTP is the cellular correlate of learning (Bliss and Gardner-Medwin 1973; Bliss and Lømo 1973). Work over the past 25 years that has elucidated many properties of LTP reinforces this view and suggests its involvement in various other adult and developmental physiological as well as pathological processes (Martin *et al.* 2000; Zoghbi *et al.* 2000; Cline 2001).

Much effort has been directed towards understanding the detailed molecular mechanisms that account for the change in synaptic efficacy. For many years, studies often yielded conflicting conclusions (Kullmann and Siegelbaum 1995). Although many studies suggested primarily postsynaptic modifications (Davies *et al.* 1989; Kauer *et al.* 1988; Manabe *et al.* 1992; Muller *et al.* 1988), a consistent finding was a change in synaptic failures after LTP (Malinow and Tsien 1990; Kullmann and Nicoll 1992; Stevens and Wang 1994; Isaac *et al.* 1996). Because synaptic failures were assumed to be due to failure to release transmitter (a presynaptic property), these results were in apparent contradiction. A resolution arrived with the identification of postsynaptically 'silent synapses' and the demonstration that they could be converted to active synapses by a postsynaptic modification (Kullmann 1994; Isaac *et al.* 1995; Liao *et al.* 1995; Durand *et al.* 1996). Synapses are postsynaptically silent if they show an NMDA but no AMPA receptor response. Thus, at resting potentials NMDARs are minimally opened, and transmitter release at such a synapse is recorded as a failure. The appearance of an AMPA response at such synapses during LTP, with no change in the NMDA response, suggests a post-synaptic modification consisting of a functional recruitment of AMPARs. One potential mechanism envisioned was the rapid delivery of AMPARs from non-synaptic sites to the synapse. An increase in NMDA responses following some LTP-inducing stimuli (Asztely *et al.* 1992) could represent the formation of new silent synapses (Engert and Bonhoeffer 1999; Maletic-Savatic *et al.* 1999). The role of silent synapses in LTP provided strong motivation for the development of cellular and molecular techniques that could monitor and perturb trafficking of AMPARs to and away from synapses.

14.2 Molecular interactions of AMPA receptors

AMPARs are hetero-oligomeric proteins made of the subunits GluR1–GluR4 (also known as GluRA–D) (Wisden and Seeburg 1993; Hollmann and Heinemann 1994). Each receptor complex contains four subunits (Rosenmund *et al.* 1998). In the adult hippocampus two species of AMPAR appear to predominate: receptors made of GluR1 and GluR2 or those composed of GluR3 and GluR2 (Wenthold *et al.* 1996). Immature hippocampus, as well as other mature brain regions, express GluR4, which also com-plexes with GluR2 to form a receptor (Zhu *et al.* 2000). The intracellular cytoplasmic tails of AMPARs are either long or short. GluR1, GluR4 and an alternative splice form of GluR2 (GluR2L) have longer cytoplasmic tails and are homologous. By contrast, the predominant splice form of GluR2, GluR3 and an alternative splice form of GluR4 that is primarily expressed in the cerebellum (GluR4c) have shorter, homologous cyto-plasmic tails. Through their C-terminal tails, each subunit interacts with specific cyto-plasmic proteins. Many of these AMPAR-interacting proteins thus far identified have single or multiple PDZ domains, which are well-characterized protein–protein inter-action motifs that often interact with the extreme C-terminal tails of target proteins (Sheng and Sala 2001). GluR1 forms a group I PDZ ligand whereas GluR2, GluR3 and GluR4c form group II PDZ ligands. GluR4 and GluR2L have variant C-terminal tails, and it is unclear if they interact with classical PDZ-domain proteins. In a variety of cell types, proteins containing PDZ-domains have been implicated in playing important roles in the targeting and clustering of membrane proteins to specific subcellular domains (Sheng and Sala 2001).

GluR1 interacts with the PDZ-domain regions of SAP97 (Leonard *et al.* 1998) and RIL (Schulz *et al.* 2001). SAP97 is closely related to a family of proteins (SAP90/ PSD95, chapsyn110/PSD93 and SAP102) that interact with NMDAR subunits. RIL, on the other hand, may link AMPARs to actin. GluR2 and GluR3 interact with GRIP (Dong *et al.* 1997, 1999) and AMPAR-binding protein (ABP)/GRIP2 (Srivastava *et al.* 1998; Dong *et al.* 1999), proteins with six or seven PDZ domains. GluR2 and GluR3 as well as GluR4c also interact with protein interacting with C-kinase (Dev *et al.* 1999; Xia *et al.* 1999), which contains a single PDZ domain that interacts with both PKCα and GluR2. Other group II PDZ-domain-containing proteins that interact with GluR2, GluR3 and GluR4c have recently been identified and include rDLG6 (Inagaki *et al.* 1999) and afadin (Rogers *et al.* 2001). No binding partners have yet been reported for GluR4 and GluR2L.

Some additional proteins interact with the cytoplasmic tails of AMPAR subunits at regions that are not at the exact C terminus. GluR1 interacts with band 4.1 N and is linked through it to actin (Shen *et al.* 2000). The interaction occurs at a region on GluR1 that is homologous with all other subunits, and thus band 4.1 N may also interact with other AMPAR subunits. There are, however, two residues in this region where different subunits contain serines (GluR1) or alanines (GluR2 and GluR4) or one of each (GluR3). This could confer differential binding to proteins such as 4.1, and could be modulated by phosphorylation. A surprising finding is that the cytoplasmic tail of GluR2, in addition to interacting with PDZ proteins, also binds to NSF (Nishimune *et al.* 1998; Osten *et al.* 1998; Song *et al.* 1998), an ATPase known to play an essential role in the membrane fusion processes that underlie intracellular protein trafficking and presynaptic vesicle exocytosis (Rothman 1994). Another key component of membrane fusion machinery, α and β soluble NSF attachment proteins, can also be co-immunoprecipitated with AMPARs containing GluR2 (Osten *et al.* 1998).

Because these AMPAR-interacting proteins contain PDZ domains, are proteins implicated in membrane fusion, or interact with the actin cytoskeleton, they have been suggested to play important roles in controlling the trafficking of AMPARs and/or their stabilization at synapses. The proposed specific functions of each of these proteins in controlling AMPAR behaviour are discussed in greater detail in the following sections.

14.3 AMPAR Delivery to synapses and long-term potentiation

(a) Subcellular steady-state distribution of AMPARs

Several studies over the past few years have tested the notion that silent synapses lack AMPARs and that AMPARs are rapidly delivered to synapses during LTP. An important requirement for this model is that there be a pool of non-synaptic AMPARs near synapses available for delivery. Several studies have used microscopic techniques to examine the distribution of glutamate receptors at and near synapses in rat brains (Petralia and Wenthold 1992; Martin *et al.* 1993; Molnar *et al.* 1993; Baude *et al.* 1995; Kharazia *et al.* 1996; Nusser *et al.* 1998; Petralia *et al.* 1999; Takumi *et al.* 1999). Although the concentration of AMPARs is normally higher at synapses, these studies generally find ample amounts of non-synaptic AMPARs on both surfaces and intracellular regions of dendrites. Indeed, given the much larger space occupied by non-synaptic regions, non-synaptic AMPARs appear to outnumber synaptic AMPARs by quite a large margin (Shi *et al.* 1999). The distance between these non-synaptic receptors and synaptic regions is a few microns, a distance that could be traversed in seconds by membrane trafficking processes. Importantly, recent studies using postembedding immunogold techniques (Nusser *et al.* 1998; Petralia *et al.* 1999; Takumi *et al.* 1999) found that a sizeable fraction of synapses in CA1 hippocampus lacks or has very few AMPARs, whereas most synapses have NMDARs. The fraction of synapses lacking AMPARs is greater earlier in development, consistent with the electrophysiological observations that silent synapses are more prevalent at these ages (Durand *et al.* 1996; Liao and Malinow 1996; Rumpel *et al.* 1998; Wu *et al.* 1996; Isaac *et al.* 1997). A recent study, employing two-photon uncagion of glutamate

(Matsuzaki *et al.* 2001) demonstrated a close correlation between AMPAR responsivity and size of spine. Small spines and filopodia were largely devoid of AMPAR responses. These structures did contain NMDAR responses. Although some studies in dissociated cultured neurons support these views (Gomperts *et al.* 2000; Liao *et al.* 1999) others do not (Renger *et al.* 2001) possibly owing to different culture conditions.

(b) Optical detection of recombinant AMPAR trafficking during long-term potentiation

To monitor AMPAR trafficking in living tissue, we generated and acutely expressed GFP-tagged GluR1 receptors in organotypic hippocampal slices (Shi *et al.* 1999). Although slices of tissue provide a more challenging experimental preparation to examine receptor trafficking, this tissue was used, rather than dissociated neurons, because there had been little success in generating LTP using standard electrophysiological protocols in dissociated neurons. These recombinant GluR1-GFP receptors are functional and their cellular distribution can be monitored with two-photon laser scanning microscopy. Upon expression, these receptors distribute diffusely throughout the dendritic tree. Interestingly, they remain in the dendritic shaft regions, with little encroachment into dendritic spines, which are the sites of excitatory contacts. This restriction from synapses is in contrast with what is found in dissociated cultured neurons in which expression of recombinant GluR1 concentrates at synapses (Lissin *et al.* 1998; Shi *et al.* 1999). In slices, little movement of GluR1-GFP was detected in the absence of stimulation. However, high-frequency synaptic activation, which generated LTP, induced movement of GFP-tagged receptors to the surface of the dendritic shaft as well as to dendritic spines. These movements of GFP-tagged receptors were detected over the course of around 15–30 min and were prevented by blockade of NMDARs. The tagged receptors remained in at least some of the spines for at least 50 min. This study concluded that GuR1-containing receptors are maintained in reserve at the dendritic shaft and can be delivered to synapses during LTP.

Several studies have produced findings that strengthen these conclusions. Adult knockout mice lacking GluR1 cannot generate LTP, indicating that this subunit plays a critical role (Zamanillo *et al.* 1999). In a follow-up study, GluR1-GFP was genetically inserted into these GluR1 knockout mice and GFP fluorescence was detected in dendritic spines (Mack *et al.* 2001). This distribution differs from what is observed when GluR1-GFP is acutely expressed in hippocampal slices before LTP, but resembles the distribution after LTP. These observations are consistent with the view that an LTP-like process drives the genetically expressed GluR1-GFP into synapses when the animals are alive. This study also found that LTP was rescued by expression of only around 10% of the normal amount of GluR1. This further supports the view that normally there is an overabundance of GluR1 available for generating LTP.

(c) Electrophysiological tagging to monitor synaptic delivery of recombinant AMPARs

Although optical studies provide important information about receptor distribution, the location of a receptor (even with electron microscopic resolution) cannot unambiguously reveal its contribution to synaptic transmission. To address this issue we developed electrophysiologically tagged recombinant AMPARs. Such receptors differ in their rectification from endogenous receptors. Rectification is an intrinsic biophysical property of a receptor that can be detected as the ratio of the response observed at -60 mV to that at $+40$ mV. Most endogenous AMPARs contain the GluR2 subunit and can pass current equally well in both inward and outward directions. In contrast, AMPARs lacking GluR2 (or containing GluR2 that is genetically modified) exhibit profound inward rectification such that they can pass minimal current in the outward direction when the cell is depolarized to $+40$ mV. Thus, incorporation of recombinant AMPARs into synapses and their contribution to synaptic transmission can be monitored functionally. With this assay for AMPAR delivery, it has been possible to show that LTP and overexpression of active CaMKII induce delivery of GluR1-containing receptors into synapses (Hayashi *et al.* 2000). An interaction between GluR1 and a PDZ-domain protein is necessary for LTP or CaMKII to drive synaptic delivery of GluR1, as point mutations in the PDZ-binding region of GluR1 prevent its synaptic delivery. The identity of the GluR1-interacting PDZ-domain protein(s) responsible for LTP is not known. It appears, however, that an interaction between GluR1 and a PDZ-domain protein is required for GluR1 to reach dendritic spines (Piccini and Malinow 2002).

An important role for GluR1 in LTP is supported by studies with mice lacking GluR1, which show no LTP in adults (Zamanillo *et al.* 1999). Interestingly, LTP is neither absent in all brain regions (e.g. LTP in dentate gyrus is present; Zamanillo *et al.* (1999)) nor in all ages (e.g. LTP in CA1 is present in juvenile animals; Mack *et al.* (2001)). This suggests that AMPAR subunits other than GluR1 may play critical roles in activity-dependent synaptic plasticity. Indeed, the CA1 hippocampal region in immature animals, as well as the dentate gyrus in older animals, contain GluR4, a subunit with considerable homology to GluR1. Studies using electrophysiological assays to monitor the synaptic delivery of recombinant GluR4 indicate that this subunit mediates activity-dependent AMPAR delivery in immature hippocampus (Zhu *et al.* 2000). Interestingly, this delivery of recombinant GluR4 to synapses required NMDAR activity (i.e. delivery was blocked by APV) but not CaMKII activity.

As expression of GluR4 in hippocampus decreases to near undetectable levels by postnatal day 10, the LTP observed in CA1 hippocampus of juvenile (approximately postnatal day 28) animals that lack GluR1 may be mediated by other AMPAR subunits. It is possible that this role is played by GluR2L, the alternative splice form of GluR2 with a cytoplasmic tail that resembles GluR1 and GluR4 (Wisden and Seeburg 1993; Hollmann and Heinemann 1994). Indeed, recent results indicate activity-driven synaptic delivery of recombinant GluR2L (Zhu *et al.* 2002).

(d) Synaptic delivery of endogenous receptors

Although the studies described above monitored synaptic delivery of recombinant AMPARs, other studies have tested if such a process occurs for endogenous receptors. One study expressed the cytoplasmic tail of GluR1 to block the trafficking of GluR1. This construct is known to bind to cytoplasmic proteins that interact with GluR1, and thus it should compete with endogenous GluR1 with such binding. As such, interactions are important for LTP (for instance, mutations of GluR1 at its PDZ interaction site, or PKA phosphorylation site, see below, can block LTP). When expressed in organotypic slices for 2–3 days, the GluR1 cytoplasmic tail had no effect on the amplitude of AMPAR-mediated transmission. This supports the view that GluR1-containing receptors are not constitutively delivered to synapses in the absence of strong (LTP-like) stimuli. This construct also had no effect on the amplitude of NMDA-mediated responses. These results indicate that this construct is not generally perturbing protein trafficking; even those mediated by type I PDZ interactions (which are important for NMDA-R trafficking; Barria and Malinow (2002)). However, cells expressing this construct showed no LTP after a pairing protocol (Shi et al. 2001). This construct thus prevents endogenous GluR1 from interacting with critical cytoplasmic proteins required for synaptic incorporation of GluR1.

Another study (Zhu et al. 2000) tested the endogenous synaptic delivery of GluR4 during early postnatal hippocampal development. Again, GluR4 cytoplasmic tail was expressed in neurons. Expression of this construct in neurons of age postnatal day 11 or older had no effect on transmission. Expression of this construct in neurons at postnatal day 6 for 24 h led to a large decrease in synaptic transmission relative to nearby non-infected neurons. However, this depression was not observed if sponta-neous activity was blocked in the slices during the expression period. This indicates that spontaneous activity drives GluR4-containing receptors into synapses during early postnatal development, and the GluR4 cytoplasmic tail can block this. In these experiments, the GluR4 cytoplasmic tail had no effect on the NMDAR responses, supporting the specific actions of cytoplasmic tail constructs.

In contrast to the expression of cytoplasmic tails from long-tailed receptors, expression of the GluR2 cytoplasmic tail depressed transmission, even when slices were incubated in conditions that blocked spontaneous activity (Shi et al. 2001). Trans-mission was reduced to approximately 50% of that seen in nearby non-infected neurons, suggesting that around 50% of receptors are continually undergoing replacement. This is consistent with numerous reports indicating that GluR2-containing receptors are continually cycling into and out of the synapse (Nishimune et al. 1998; Luscher et al. 1999; Lü thi et al. 1999; Noel et al. 1999; Ehlers 2000; Lin et al. 2000; Kim and Lisman 2001; Shi et al. 2001; Zhou et al. 2001). A recent report indicates that the critical pore residue, R586Q in GluR2 can affect its exit from the endoplasmic reticulum and surface expression in dissociated cultured neurons (Greger et al. 2002). However, in cultured slices and in in vivo systems (see below), the synaptic incorporation of GluR2 appears not to be affected by this residue. For instance, in slices, the same synaptic incorporation is seen by a pore-dead mutant (GluR2(R586E), around 50% synaptic depression), rectification mutant (GluR2(R586Q), around 50% depression at +40 mV) and endo-genous GluR2 (depression of approximately 50% by GluR2 cytoplasmic tail) (Shi et al. 2001). In addition, an in vivo study shows the same synaptic incorporation by GluR2 (R586Q) mutant (around 50% increased rectification) and endogenous GluR2 (as deter-mined by expression of GluR2 cytoplasmic tail, approximately 50% depression) in vivo.

LTP in cells expressing the GluR2 cytoplasmic tail was not reduced, supporting the view that interactions by GluR2 are not critical for the generation of LTP. This is supportive of earlier findings with mice lacking GluR2 that showed LTP (Jia et al. 1996). Indeed, LTP was observed to be quite large, although this may simply be due to the fact that transmission began at a depressed level, and a normal level of GluR1 delivery would produce potentiation that appears large.

Some studies in dissociated cultured neurons have supported the view that LTP produces delivery of AMPARs to synapses (Liao et al. 2001; Lu et al. 2001).

(e) Role of AMPA receptor phosphorylation in synaptic delivery

There has been considerable evidence indicating that protein kinases play critical roles in the generation of LTP (Madison *et al.* 1991; Bliss and Collingridge 1993; Malenka and Nicoll 1999). Some kinases (e.g. CaMKII; Lisman *et al.* (1997)) are thought to mediate directly the signals leading to LTP, whereas others (e.g. PKA; Blitzer *et al.* (1995)) may 'gate' (i.e. modulate) its generation. The targets of these kinases responsible for mediating or gating LTP have been the source of considerable investigation. During LTP the CaMKII-phosphorylation site on GluR1, Ser831, is phosphorylated (Barria *et al.* 1997*a,b*; Mammen *et al.* 1997). Such phosphorylation can increase conductance through GluR1 receptors (Derkach *et al.* 1999), and AMPARS show increased conductance during LTP (Benke *et al.* 1998) and following expression of constitutively active CaMKII (Poncer *et al.* 2002). Thus, it was of considerable interest to determine if phosphorylation of Ser831 is required for synaptic delivery of GluR1-containing receptors. However, mutations on GluR1-Ser831 that prevent its phosphorylation by CaMKII do not prevent delivery of the receptor to synapses by active CaMKII (Hayashi *et al.* 2000) or by LTP (S.-H. Shi and R. Malinow, unpublished observations). Thus, CaMKII must be acting on a different target to effect synaptic delivery of GluR1. Recent studies indicate that CaMKII can phosphorylate a synaptic rasGAP (Chen *et al.* 1998; Kim *et al.* 1998) and potentially control levels of ras activity. Ras activity appears to be necessary to generate LTP and is the downstream effector of CaMKII that drives synaptic delivery of AMPARs (Zhu *et al.* 2002). This conforms with results indicating a critical role for MAP kinase, a downstream effector for ras, in LTP (English and Sweatt 1996, 1997).

Interestingly, mutations at Ser845, the PKA phosphorylation site of GluR1 (Roche *et al.* 1996), do prevent delivery of GluR1 to synapses by active CaMKII or LTP (Shi and Malinow 2001). Phosphorylation at this site of GluR1 also accompanies surface reinsertion of receptors (Ehlers 2000) and LTP induction after prior LTD (Lee *et al.* 2000). Phosphorylation at this site by exogenous application of drugs that raise cAMP does not induce delivery of recombinant GluR1 (Shi and Malinow 2001). Thus, PKA phosphorylation of GluR1 is necessary, but not sufficient, for its synaptic delivery; that is, phosphorylation of Ser845 acts as a gate. Of note, the PKA-scaffolding molecule, AKAP, binds to SAP97 and thereby effectively brings PKA to GluR1 (Colledge *et al.* 2000). Thus, it is possible that the PDZ mutation on GluR1 blocks its synaptic delivery, at least in part, because it prevents PKA phosphorylation at Ser845. Of note, SAP97 associates with GluR1 primarily in intracellular sites (Sans *et al.* 2001), consistent with its playing a role in making GluR1 competent for synaptic delivery.

Recent studies indicate that activity-driven phosphorylation of GluR4 by PKA is necessary and sufficient for delivery of these recombinant AMPARs to synapses during early development (Esteban *et al.* 2003). Such phosphorylation relieves a retention interaction that, in the absence of synaptic activity, maintains GluR4-containing receptors away from the synapse. Thus, a mechanism (PKA phosphorylation of AMPARs) that mediates plasticity early in development (with GluR4) becomes a gate for plasticity (with GluR1) later in development. Increasing requirements over development may be one way that plasticity becomes more specific and also recalcitrant with age.

14.4 General trafficking mechanisms

A key question has been if plasticity acts by directly modulating a process that is responsible for turning over receptors at synapses (e.g. increasing rate of delivery or decreasing rate of removal) or if there are distinct processes responsible for plasticity and receptor turnover. One recent study (Shi *et al.* 2001) examined this question and argues for distinct AMPARs responsible for LTP and receptor turnover. AMPARs composed of GluR1 and GluR2 (or any receptor with a long cytoplasmic tail together with GluR2) participates in regulated delivery. In the absence of electrical activity, these receptors are restricted from accessing synapses. LTP (for GluR1-containing receptors) or spontaneous activity (for GluR4-containing receptors) drives these receptors (along with associated scaffolding) into synapses. The long cytoplasmic tails, and not the short cytoplasmic tails, of GluR1/GluR2 heteromers are critical for this activity-dependent synaptic delivery. Receptors composed of GluR2 and GluR3 continuously replace synaptic GluR2/GluR3 receptors in a manner that maintains constant transmission. How can this model explain long-term changes in synaptic receptor number following plasticity that enhances transmission? At some point after their synaptic delivery, receptors containing GluR1 or GluR4 become replaceable by GluR2/GluR3 receptors. The scaffolding associated with GluR1 or GluR4 (called 'slot' complexes; Shi *et al.* (2001)) must somehow control this. One study provides evidence for replacement of synaptic GluR4-containing receptors by GluR2/GluR3 receptors (Zhu *et al.* 2000). This occurs over the course of days after the activity-driven delivery of GluR4-containing receptors.

(a) Role of trafficking in experience-dependent plasticity

Considerable progress has been made in uncovering the cellular and molecular mechanisms underlying activity-dependent synaptic plasticity *in vitro*. However, although LTP is a leading contender as a mechanism to encode experience in brain circuits, there are few reports (cf. Finnerty *et al.* 1999; Rogan *et al.* 1997; Rioult-Pedotti *et al.* 2000) suggesting that LTP occurs *in vivo* in response to natural stimuli. We have recently tested if synaptic modifications identified to occur during LTP *in vitro* are also driven by experience in the intact brain (Takahashi *et al.* 2003). We examined excitatory transmission between layer 4 and layer 2/3 neurons in barrel cortex during a period when considerable experience-dependent plasticity occurs (Micheva and Beaulieu 1996; Lendvai *et al.* 2000; Stern *et al.* 2001). For instance, between PND12 and PND14 there is a twofold increase in the number of synapses in barrel cortex (Micheva and Beaulieu 1996). While synapse numbers appear not affected by sensory deprivation (Winfield 1981; Vees *et al.* 1998), other aspects of synaptic function, such as receptor content, could be dependent on experience.

In agreement with *in vitro* models of AMPAR trafficking, we find that recombinant GluR1 is driven into synapses by experience. Furthermore, GluR1-ct, which can block LTP *in vitro* (Hayashi *et al.* 2000), prevents experience-driven synaptic potentiation. These results indicate a large (e.g. around 2.5-fold) increase in transmission at synapses between layer 4 and layer 2/3 neurons between PND 12 and PND 14 that is driven by experience and mediated by synaptic delivery of GluR1-containing AMPARs. The increase in rectification in neurons expressing homomeric GluR1 is considerably smaller (around 1.3-fold). This is consistent with transient delivery of GluR1-containing receptors with subsequent replacement by GluR2-containing receptors. In accordance with *in vitro* studies (Noel *et al.* 1999; Scannevin and Huganir 2000; Sheng and Lee 2001; Shi *et al.* 2001; Tomita *et al.* 2001; Malinow and Malenka 2002), we find that replacement of synaptic receptors depends on interactions by the GluR2 cytoplasmic tail and that it can occur in the absence of experience. Our results indicate that the rules of AMPAR trafficking identified *in vitro* apply to behaviourally driven plasticity. Thus, the presence of AMPARs with long cytoplasmic tails at a synapse may represent the signature of recent experience-dependent plasticity.

14.5 Conclusions

Lynch and Baudry (1984) proposed almost two decades ago that LTP is due to an increase in the number of synaptic glutamate receptors. However, the idea did not gain universal favour and a vigorous exchange over the ensuing decades debated the pre- and postsynaptic contributions to the expression of LTP. Thus, the general acceptance of postsynaptic silent synapses and AMPAR trafficking as playing important roles in synaptic plasticity represents a significant advance in the field. It provides a clear conceptual framework that should facilitate studies aimed at determining which molecules play critical roles in LTP and exactly what role they play.

A molecular blueprint of LTP should allow us to begin probing experience-driven plasticity. Several issues should be experimentally approachable. What brain regions show experience-dependent receptor trafficking, and what experiences drive this? Does experience-dependent trafficking show a 'critical period'? Are there specific patterns of activity at different ages that drive experience-dependent trafficking for each age? Is the trafficking of each glutamate receptor with a long cytoplasmic tail, driven by specific types of experiences? What signalling pathways are activated and required for plasticity *in vivo*? One can hope that gains from *in vitro* studies will aid in elucidating the nature of synaptic modifications driven by experience.

References

Alkon, D. L. and Nelson, T. J. (1990). Specificity of molecular changes in neurons involved in memory storage. *FASEB J.* **4**, 1567–76.

Asztely, F., Wigstrom, H., and Gustafsson, B. (1992). The relative contribution of nmda receptor channels in the expression of long-term potentiation in the hippocampal CA1 region. *Eur. J. Neurosci.* **4**, 681–90.

Barria, A. and Malinow, R. (2002). Subunit-specific NMDA receptor trafficking to synapses. *Neuron* **35**, 345–53.

Barria, A., Derkach, V., and Soderling, T. (1997a). Identification of the Ca^{2+}/calmodulin-dependent protein kinase II regulatory phosphorylation site in the alpha-amino-3-hydroxyl-5-methyl-4-isoxazole-propionate-type glutamate receptor. *J. Biol. Chem.* **272**, 32 727–30.

Barria, A., Muller, D., Derkach, V., Griffith, L. C., and Soderling, T. R. (1997b). Regulatory phosphorylation of AMPA-type glutamate receptors by CaM-KII during long-term potentiation (see comments). *Science* **276**, 2042–5.

Baude, A., Nusser, Z., Molnar, E., McIlhinney, R. A. J., and Somogyi, P. (1995). High-resolution immunogold localization of AMPA type glutamate receptor subunits at synaptic and non-synaptic sites in rat hippocampus. *Neurosci.* **69**, 1031–55.

Benke, T. A., Luthi, A., Isaac, J. T., and Collingridge, G. L. (1998). Modulation of AMPA receptor unitary conductance by synaptic activity. *Nature* **393**, 793–7.

Bliss, T. V. and Collingridge, G. L. (1993). A synaptic model of memory: long-term potentiation in the hippocampus. *Nature* **361**, 31–9.

Bliss, T. V. and Gardner-Medwin, A. R. (1973). Long-lasting potentiation of synaptic transmission in the dentate area of the unanaestetized rabbit following stimulation of the perforant path. *J. Physiol. (Lond.)* **232**, 357–74.

Bliss, T. V. and Lømo, T. (1973). Long-lasting potentiation of synaptic transmission in the dentate area of the anaesthetized rabbit following stimulation of the perforant path. *J. Physiol. (Lond.)* **232**, 331–56.

Blitzer, R. D., Wong, T., Nouranifar, R., Iyengar, R., and Landau, E. M. (1995). Postsynaptic cAMP pathway gates early LTP in hippocampal CA1 region. *Neuron* **15**, 1403–14.

Chen, H. J., Rojas-Soto, M., Oguni, A., and Kennedy, M. B. (1998). A synaptic Ras-GTPase activating protein (p135 SynGAP) inhibited by CaM kinase II. *Neuron* **20**, 895–904.

Cline, H. T. (2001). Dendritic arbor development and synaptogenesis. *Curr. Opin. Neurobiol.* **11**, 118–26.

Colledge, M., Dean, R. A., Scott, G. K., Langeberg, L. K., Huganir, R. L., and Scott, J. D. (2000). Targeting of PKA to glutamate receptors through a MAGUK–AKAP complex. *Neuron* **27**, 107–19.

Davies, S. N., Lester, R. A., Reymann, K. G., and Collingridge, G. L. (1989). Temporally distinct pre- and post-synaptic mechanisms maintain long-term potentiation. *Nature* **338**, 500–3.

Derkach, V., Barria, A., and Soderling, T. R. (1999). Ca^{2+}/calmodulin-kinase II enhances channel conductance of alpha-amino-3-hydroxy-5-methyl-4-isoxazolepropionate type glutamate receptors. *Proc. Natl Acad. Sci. USA* **96**, 3269–74.

Dev, K. K., Nishimune, A., Henley, J. M., and Nakanishi, S. (1999). The protein kinase C alpha binding protein PICK1 interacts with short but not long form alternative splice variants of AMPA receptor subunits. *Neuropharmacology* **38**, 635–44.

Dong, H., O'Brien, R. J., Fung, E. T., Lanahan, A. A., Worley, P. F., and Huganir, R. L. (1997). GRIP: a synaptic PDZ domain-containing protein that interacts with AMPA receptors. *Nature* **386**, 279–84.

Dong, H., Zhang, P., Song, I., Petralia, R. S., Liao, D., and Huganir, R. L. (1999). Characterization of the glutamate receptor-interacting proteins GRIP1 and GRIP2. *J. Neurosci.* **19**, 6930–41.

Durand, G. M., Kovalchuk, Y., and Konnerth, A. (1996). Long-term potentiation and functional synapse induction in developing hippocampus. *Nature* **381**, 71–5.

Eccles, J. C. (1964). *The physiology of synapses*. New York: Academic Press.

Ehlers, M. D. (2000). Reinsertion or degradation of AMPA receptors determined by activity-dependent endocytic sorting. *Neuron* **28**, 511–25.

Engert, F. and Bonhoeffer, T. (1999). Dendritic spine changes associated with hippocampal long-term synaptic plasticity. *Nature* **399**, 66–70.

English, J. D. and Sweatt, J. D. (1996). Activation of p42 mitogen-activated protein kinase in hippocampal long term potentiation. *J. Biol. Chem.* **271**, 24 329–32.

English, J. D. and Sweatt, J. D. (1997). A requirement for the mitogen-activated protein kinase cascade in hippocampal long term potentiation. *J. Biol. Chem.* **272**, 19 103–6.

Esteban, J. A., Shi, S. H., Wilson, C., Nuriya, M., Huganir, R. L., and Malinow, R. (2003). PKA phosphorylation of AMPA receptor subunits controls synaptic trafficking underlying plasticity. *Nature Neurosci.* **6**, 136–43.

Finnerty, G. T., Roberts, L. S., and Connors, B. W. (1999). Sensory experience modifies the short-term dynamics of neocortical synapses. *Nature* **400**, 367–71.

Gomperts, S. N., Carroll, R., Malenka, R. C., and Nicoll, R. A. (2000). Distinct roles for ionotropic and metabotropic glutamate receptors in the maturation of excitatory synapses. *J. Neurosci.* **20**, 2229–37.

Greger, I. H., Khatri, L., and Ziff, E. B. (2002). RNA editing at arg607 controls AMPA receptor exit from the endoplasmic reticulum. *Neuron* **34**, 759–72.

Hayashi, Y., Shi, S.-H., Esteban, J. A., Piccini, A., Poncer, J. C., and Malinow, R. (2000). Driving AMPA receptors into synapses by LTP and CaMKII: requirement for GluR1 and PDZ domain interaction. *Science* **287**, 2262–7.

Hebb, D. (1949). *The organization of behavior.* New York: Wiley.

Hollmann, M. and Heinemann, S. (1994). Cloned glutamate receptors. *A. Rev. Neurosci.* **17**, 31–108.

Inagaki, H., Maeda, S., Lin, K. H., Shimizu, N., and Saito, T. (1999). rDLG6: a novel homolog of Drosophila DLG expressed in rat brain. *Biochem. Biophys. Res. Commun.* **265**, 462–8.

Isaac, J. T., Nicoll, R. A., and Malenka, R. C. (1995). Evidence for silent synapses: implications for the expression of LTP. *Neuron* **15**, 427–34.

Isaac, J. T., Hjelmstad, G. O., Nicoll, R. A., and Malenka, R. C. (1996). Long-term potentiation at single fiber inputs to hippocampal CA1 pyramidal cells. *Proc. Natl Acad. Sci. USA* **93**, 8710–15.

Isaac, J. T., Crair, M. C., Nicoll, R. A., and Malenka, R. C. (1997). Silent synapses during development of thalamocortical inputs. *Neuron* **18**, 269–80.

Jia, Z. (and 11 others) (1996). Enhanced LTP in mice deficient in the AMPA receptor GluR2. *Neuron* **17**, 945–56.

Kandel, E. R. (1997). Genes, synapses, and long-term memory. *J. Cell. Physiol.* **173**, 124–5.

Kauer, J. A., Malenka, R. C., and Nicoll, R. A. (1988). A persistent postsynaptic modification mediates long-term potentiation in the hippocampus. *Neuron* **1**, 911–17.

Kharazia, V. N., Wenthold, R. J., and Weinberg, R. J. (1996). GluR1-immunopositive interneurons in rat neocortex. *J. Comp. Neurol.* **368**, 399–412.

Kim, C. H. and Lisman, J. E. (2001). A labile component of AMPA receptor-mediated synaptic transmission is dependent on microtubule motors, actin and N-ethylmaleimide-sensitive factor. *J. Neurosci.* **21**, 4188–94.

Kim, J. H., Liao, D., Lau, L. F., and Huganir, R. L. (1998). SynGAP: a synaptic RasGAP that associates with the PSD-95/SAP90 protein family. *Neuron* **20**, 683–91.

Kullmann, D. M. (1994). Amplitude fluctuations of dual-component EPSCs in hippocampal pyramidal cells: implications for long-term potentiation. *Neuron* **12**, 1111–20.

Kullmann, D. M. and Nicoll, R. A. (1992). Long-term potentiation is associated with increases in quantal content and quantal amplitude. *Nature* **357**, 240–4.

Kullmann, D. M. and Siegelbaum, S. A. (1995). The site of expression of NMDA receptor-dependent LTP: new fuel for an old fire. *Neuron* **15**, 997–1002.

Lee, H.-K., Barbarosie, M., Kameyama, K., Bear, M. F., and Huganir, R. L. (2000). Regulation of distinct AMPA receptor phosphorylation sites during bidirectional synaptic plasticity. *Nature* **405**, 955–9.

Lendvai, B., Stern, E. A., Chen, B., and Svoboda, K. (2000). Experience-dependent plasticity of dendritic spines in the developing rat barrel cortex *in vivo. Nature* **404**, 876–81.

Leonard, A. S., Davare, M. A., Horne, M. C., Garner, C. C., and Hell, J. W. (1998). SAP97 is associated with the alpha-amino-3-hydroxy-5-methylisoxazole-4-propionic acid receptor GluR1 subunit. *J. Biol. Chem.* **273**, 19 518–24.

Liao, D. and Malinow, R. (1996). Deficiency in induction but not expression of LTP in hippocampal slices from young rats. *Learn. Mem.* **3**, 138–49.

Liao, D., Hessler, N. A., and Malinow, R. (1995). Activation of postsynaptically silent synapses during pairing-induced LTP in CA1 region of hippocampal slice. *Nature* **375**, 400–4.

Liao, D., Zhang, X., O'Brien, R., Ehlers, M. D., and Huganir, R. L. (1999). Regulation of morphological postsynaptic silent synapses in developing hippocampal neurons. *Nature Neurosci.* **2**, 37–43.

Liao, D., Scannevin, R. H., and Huganir, R. (2001). Activation of silent synapses by rapid activity-dependent synaptic recruitment of AMPA receptors. *J. Neurosci.* **21**, 6008–17.

Lin, J. W., Ju, W., Foster, K., Lee, S. H., Ahmadian, G., Wyszynski, M., *et al.* (2000). Distinct molecular mechanisms and divergent endocytotic pathways of AMPA receptor internalization. *Nature Neurosci.* **3**, 1282–90.

Lisman, J., Malenka, R. C., Nicoll, R. A., and Malinow, R. (1997). Learning mechanisms: the case for CaM-KII. *Science* **276**, 2001–2.

Lissin, D. V., Gomperts, S. N., Carroll, R. C., Christine, C. W., Kalman, D., Kitamura, M., *et al.* (1998). Activity differentially regulates the surface expression of synaptic AMPA and NMDA glutamate receptors. *Proc. Natl Acad. Sci. USA* **95**, 7097–102.

Lu, W., Man, H., Ju, W., Trimble, W. S., MacDonald, J. F., and Wang, Y. T. (2001). Activation of synaptic NMDA receptors induces membrane insertion of new AMPA receptors and LTP in cultured hippocampal neurons. *Neuron* **29**, 243–54.

Luscher, C., Xia, H., Beattie, E. C., Carroll, R. C., von Zastrow, M., Malenka, R. C., *et al.* (1999). Role of AMPA receptor cycling in synaptic transmission and plasticity. *Neuron* **24**, 649–58.

Lüthi, A., Chittajallu, R., Duprat, F., Palmer, M. J., Benke, T. A., Kidd, F. L., *et al.* (1999). Hippocampal LTD expression involves a pool of AMPARs regulated by the NSF-GluR2 interaction. *Neuron* **24**, 389–99.

Lynch, G. and Baudry, M. (1984). The biochemistry of memory: a new and specific hypothesis. *Science* **224**, 1057–63.

Mack, V., Burnashev, N., Kaiser, K. M., Rozov, A., Jensen, V., Hvalby, O., *et al.* (2001). Conditional restoration of hippocampal synaptic potentiation in Glur-A-deficient mice. *Science* **292**, 2501–4.

Madison, D. V., Malenka, R. C., and Nicoll, R. A. (1991). Mechanisms underlying long-term potentiation of synaptic transmission. *A. Rev. Neurosci.* **14**, 379–97.

Malenka, R. C. and Nicoll, R. A. (1999). Long-term potentiation—a decade of progress? *Science* **285**, 1870–4.

Maletic-Savatic, M., Malinow, R., and Svoboda, K. (1999). Rapid dendritic morphogenesis in CA1 hippocampal dendrites induced by synaptic activity. *Science* **283**, 1923–7.

Malinow, R. and Malenka, R. C. (2002). AMPA receptor trafficking and synaptic plasticity. *A. Rev. Neurosci.* **25**, 103–26.

Malinow, R. and Tsien, R. W. (1990). Presynaptic enhancement shown by whole-cell recordings of long-term potentiation in hippocampal slices. *Nature* **346**, 177–80.

Mammen, A. L., Kameyama, K., Roche, K. W., and Huganir, R. L. (1997). Phosphorylation of the alpha-amino-3-hydroxy-5-methylisoxazole4-propionic acid receptor GluR1 subunit by calcium/calmodulin-dependent kinase II. *J. Biol. Chem.* **272**, 32 528–33.

Manabe, T., Renner, P., and Nicoll, R. A. (1992). Postsynaptic contribution to long-term potentiation revealed by the analysis of miniature synaptic currents. *Nature* **355**, 50–5.

Martin, L. J., Blackstone, C. D., Levey, A. I., Huganir, R. L., and Price, D. L. (1993). AMPA glutamate receptor subunits are differentially distributed in rat brain. *Neurosci.* **53**, 327–58.

Martin, S. J., Grimwood, P. D., and Morris, R. G. (2000). Synaptic plasticity and memory: an evaluation of the hypothesis. *A. Rev. Neurosci.* **23**, 649–711.

Matsuzaki, M., Ellis-Davies, G. C., Nemoto, T., Miyashita, Y., Iino, M., and Kasai, H. (2001). Dendritic spine geometry is critical for AMPA receptor expression in hippocampal CA1 pyramidal neurons. *Nature Neurosci.* **4**, 1086–92.

Micheva, K. D. and Beaulieu, C. (1996). Quantitative aspects of synaptogenesis in the rat barrel field cortex with special reference to GABA circuitry. *J. Comp. Neurol.* **373**, 340–54.

Molnar, E., Baude, A., Richmond, S. A., Patel, P. B., Somogyi, P., and McIlhinney, R. A. J. (1993). Biochemical and immunocytochemical characterization of antipeptide antibodies to a cloned GluR1 glutamate receptor subunit: cellular and subcellular distribution in the rat forebrain. *Neurosci.* **53**, 307–26.

Muller, D., Joly, M., and Lynch, G. (1988). Contributions of quisqualate and NMDA receptors to the induction and expression of LTP. *Science* **242**, 1694–7.

Nishimune, A., Isaac, J. T., Molnar, E., Noel, J., Nash, S. R., Tagaya, M., *et al.* (1998). NSF binding to GluR2 regulates synaptic transmission. *Neuron* **21**, 87–97.

Noel, J., Ralph, G. S., Pickard, L., Williams, J., Molnar, E., Uney, J. B., *et al.* (1999). Surface expression of AMPA receptors in hippocampal neurons is regulated by an NSF-dependent mechanism. *Neuron* **23**, 365–76.

Nusser, Z., Lujan, R., Laube, G., Roberts, J. D., Molnar, E., and Somogyi, P. (1998). Cell type and pathway dependence of synaptic AMPA receptor number and variability in the hippocampus. *Neuron* **21**, 545–59.

Osten, P., Srivastava, S., Inman, G. J., Vilim, F. S., Khatri, L., Lee, L. M., *et al.* (1998). The AMPA receptor GluR2 C terminus can mediate a reversible, ATP-dependent interaction with NSF and alpha- and beta-SNAPs. *Neuron* **21**, 99–110.

Petralia, R. S. and Wenthold, R. J. (1992). Light and electron immunocytochemical localization of AMPA-selective glutamate receptors in the rat brain. *J. Comp. Neurol.* **318**, 329–54.

Petralia, R. S., Esteban, J. A., Wang, Y. X., Partridge, J. G., Zhao, H. M., Wenthold, R. J., *et al.* (1999). Selective acquisition of AMPA receptors over postnatal development suggests a molecular basis for silent synapses. *Nature Neurosci.* **2**, 31–6.

Piccini, A. and Malinow, R. (2002). Critical postsynaptic density 95/disc large/zonula occludens-1 interactions by glutamate receptor 1 (GluR1) and GluR2 required at different subcellular sites. *J. Neurosci.* **22**, 5387–92.

Poncer, J. C., Esteban, J. A., and Malinow, R. (2002). Multiple mechanisms for the potentiation of AMPA receptor-mediated transmission by alpha-Ca^{2+}/calmodulin-dependent protein kinase II. *J. Neurosci.* **22**, 4406–11.

Renger, J. J., Egles, C., and Liu, G. (2001). A developmental switch in neurotransmitter flux enhances synaptic efficacy by affecting AMPA receptor activation. *Neuron* **29**, 469–84.

Rioult-Pedotti, M. S., Friedman, D., and Donoghue, J. P. (2000). Learning-induced LTP in neocortex. *Science* **290**, 533–6.

Roche, K. W., O'Brien, R. J., Mammen, A. L., Bernhardt, J., and Huganir, R. L. (1996). Characterization of multiple phosphorylation sites on the AMPA receptor GluR1 subunit. *Neuron* **16**, 1179–88.

Rogan, M. T., Staubli, U. V., and LeDoux, J. E. (1997). Fear conditioning induces associative long-term potentiation in the amygdala. *Nature* **390**, 604–7. (Erratum appears in *Nature* (1998). **391**, 818.)

Rogers, C. A., Maron, C., Schulteis, C., Allen, W.-R., and Heinemann, S.-F. (2001). Afadin, a link between AMPA receptors and the actin cytoskeleton. In *Society for Neuroscience Annual Meeting*. San Diego, CA: Society for Neuroscience.

Rosenmund, C., Stern-Bach, Y., and Stevens, C. F. (1998). The tetrameric structure of a glutamate receptor channel. *Science* **280**, 1596–9.

Rothman, J. E. (1994). Mechanisms of intracellular protein transport. *Nature* **372**, 55–63.

Rumpel, S., Hatt, H., and Gottmann, K. (1998). Silent synapses in the developing rat visual cortex: evidence for postsynaptic expression of synaptic plasticity. *J. Neurosci.* **18**, 8863–74.

Sans, N., Racca, C., Petralia, R. S., Wang, Y. X., McCallum, J., and Wenthold, R. J. (2001). Synapse-associated protein 97 selectively associates with a subset of AMPA receptors early in their biosynthetic pathway. *J. Neurosci.* **21**, 7506–16.

Scannevin, R. H. and Huganir, R. L. (2000). Postsynaptic organization and regulation of excitatory synapses. *Nature Rev. Neurosci.* **1**, 133–41.

Schulz, W., Nakagawa, T., Kim, J.-H., Sheng, M., Seeburg, P. H., and Osten, P. (2001). Novel interaction of the GluR-A AMPA receptor subuint with the PDZ-LIM domain protein RIL. In *Society for Neuroscience Annual Meeting*. San Diego, CA: Society for Neuroscience.

Shen, L., Liang, F., Walensky, L. D., and Huganir, R. L. (2000). Regulation of AMPA receptor GluR1 subunit surface expression by a 4.1N-linked actin cytoskeletal association. *J. Neurosci.* **20**, 7932–40.

Sheng, M. and Lee, S. H. (2001). AMPA receptor trafficking and the control of synaptic transmission. *Cell* **105**, 825–8.

Sheng, M. and Sala, C. (2001). PDZ domains and the organization of supramolecular complexes. *A. Rev. Neurosci.* **24**, 1–29.

Shi, S., Hayashi, Y., Esteban, J. A., and Malinow, R. (2001). Subunit-specific rules governing ampa receptor trafficking to synapses in hippocampal pyramidal neurons. *Cell* **105**, 331–43.

Shi, S.-H. and Malinow, R. (2001). Synaptic trafficking of AMPARs containing GluR1 is gated by PKA phosphorylation at Ser845. In *Society for Neuroscience Annual Meeting*. San Diego, CA: Society for Neuroscience.

Shi, S.-H., Hayashi, Y., Petralia, R. S., Zaman, S. H., Wenthold, R. J., Svoboda, K., *et al.* (1999). Rapid spine delivery and redistribution of AMPA receptors after synaptic NMDA receptor activation (see comments). *Science* **284**, 1811–16.

Song, I., Kamboj, S., Xia, J., Dong, H., Liao, D., and Huganir, R. L. (1998). Interaction of the N-ethylmaleimide-sensitive factor with AMPA receptors. *Neuron* **21**, 393–400.

Srivastava, S., Osten, P., Vilim, F. S., Khatri, L., Inman, G., States, B., *et al.* (1998). Novel anchorage of GluR2/3 to the postsynaptic density by the AMPA receptor-binding protein ABP. *Neuron* **21**, 581–91.

Stern, E. A., Maravall, M., and Svoboda, K. (2001). Rapid development and plasticity of layer 2/3 maps in rat barrel cortex *in vivo*. *Neuron* **31**, 305–15.

Stevens, C. F. and Wang, Y. (1994). Changes in reliability of synaptic function as a mechanism for plasticity. *Nature* **371**, 704–7.

Takahashi, T., Svoboda, K., and Malinow, R. (2003). Experience enhances transmission by driving AMPA receptors into synapses. *Science* **299**. (In the press.)

Takumi, Y., Ramírez-León, V., Laake, P., Rinvik, E., and Ottersen, O. P. (1999). Different modes of expression of AMPA and NMDA receptors in hippocampal synapses. *Nature Neurosci.* **2**, 618–24.

Tomita, S., Nicoll, R. A., and Bredt, D. S. (2001). PDZ protein interactions regulating glutamate receptor function and plasticity. *J. Cell Biol.* **153**, F19–F24.

Vees, A. M., Micheva, K. D., Beaulieu, C., and Descarries, L. (1998). Increased number and size of dendritic spines in ipsilateral barrel field cortex following unilateral whisker trimming in postnatal rat. *J. Comp. Neurol.* **400**, 110–24.

Wenthold, R. J., Petralia, R. S., Blahos, J. II and Niedzielski, A. S. (1996). Evidence for multiple AMPA receptor complexes in hippocampal CA1/CA2 neurons. *J. Neurosci.* **16**, 1982–9.

Winfield, D. A. (1981). The postnatal development of synapses in the visual cortex of the cat and the effects of eyelid closure. *Brain Res.* **206**, 166–71.

Wisden, W. and Seeburg, P. H. (1993). Mammalian ionotropic glutamate receptors. *Curr. Opin. Neurobiol.* **3**, 291–8.

Wu, G., Malinow, R., and Cline, H. T. (1996). Maturation of a central glutamatergic synapse. *Science* **274**, 972–6.

Xia, J., Zhang, X., Staudinger, J., and Huganir, R. L. (1999). Clustering of AMPA receptors by the synaptic PDZ domain-containing protein PICK1. *Neuron* **22**, 179–87.

Zamanillo, D., Sprengel, R., Hvalby, O., Jensen, V., Burnashev, N., Rozov, A., *et al.* (1999). Importance of AMPA receptors for hippocampal synaptic plasticity but not for spatial learning. *Science* **284**, 1805–11.

Zhou, Q., Xiao, M., and Nicoll, R. A. (2001). Contribution of cytoskeleton to the internalization of AMPA receptors. *Proc. Natl Acad. Sci. USA* **98**, 1261–6.

Zhu, J. J., Esteban, J. A., Hayashi, Y., and Malinow, R. (2000). Postnatal synaptic potentiation: delivery of GluR4-containing AMPA receptors by spontaneous activity. *Nature Neurosci.* **3**, 1098–106.

Zhu, J. J., Qin, Y., Zhao, M., Van Aelst, L., and Malinow, R. (2002). Ras and Rap control AMPA receptor trafficking during synaptic plasticity. *Cell* **110**, 443–55.

Zoghbi, H. Y., Gage, F. H., and Choi, D. W. (2000). Neurobiology of disease. *Curr. Opin. Neurobiol.* **10**, 655–60.

Glossary

AMPA	α-amino-3-hydroxy-5-methyl-4-isoxazole propionate
AMPAR	AMPA receptor
GFP	green fluorescent protein
GRIP	glutamate receptor-interacting protein
LTP	long-term potentiation
NSF	N-ethylmaleimide-sensitive-factor
NMDA	N-methyl-D-aspartate
NMDAR	N-methyl-D-aspartate receptor

15

GluR2 protein–protein interactions and the regulation of AMPA receptors during synaptic plasticity

Fabrice Duprat, Michael Daw, Wonil Lim, Graham Collingridge, and John Isaac

AMPA-type glutamate receptors mediate most fast excitatory synaptic transmissions in the mammalian brain. They are critically involved in the expression of long-term potentiation and long-term depression, forms of synaptic plasticity that are thought to underlie learning and memory. A number of synaptic proteins have been identified that interact with the intracellular C-termini of AMPA receptor subunits. Here, we review recent studies and present new experimental data on the roles of these interacting proteins in regulating the AMPA receptor function during basal synaptic transmission and plasticity.

Keywords: AMPA receptor; GluR2; interacting proteins; N-ethylmaleimide-sensitive fusion protein; protein interacting with C-kinase 1

15.1 Proteins interacting with GluR2

AMPARs interact with a variety of synaptic proteins through the intracellular C-termini of their constituent subunits (Braithwaite *et al.* 2000; Sheng and Lee 2001). These interactions have been the subject of intense study because they are believed to have critical roles in the trafficking, targeting, anchoring and functional regulation of receptors at synapses in the mammalian brain (Braithwaite *et al.* 2000; Lüscher *et al.* 2000; Sheng and Lee 2001). Recent studies show that AMPARs are rapidly inserted into synapses during hippocampal LTP (Hayashi *et al.* 2000; Lu *et al.* 2001; Pickard *et al.* 2001) and are rapidly removed during hippocampal LTD (e.g. Carroll *et al.* 1999; Beattie *et al.* 2000). This has led to considerable interest in determining whether proteins interacting with AMPARs are involved in the expression mechanisms of these forms of synaptic plasticity.

Interactions with the GluR2 subunit are of particular interest because GluR2 (in its edited form) controls the key biophysical properties of AMPAR function: Ca^{2+} permeability, single channel conductance and rectification (e.g. Burnashev *et al.* 1992; Bowie and Mayer 1995; Kamboj *et al.* 1995). The critical importance of the appropriate physiological regulation of GluR2 has been demonstrated in mutant mice that either lack GluR2 (Jia *et al.* 1996) or lack GluR2 editing (e.g. Brusa *et al.* 1995). Furthermore, there is now accumulating evidence that during certain pathological conditions there is a decrease in the GluR2 content of AMPARs which causes increased Ca^{2+} influx through AMPARs and which has been implicated in the subsequent

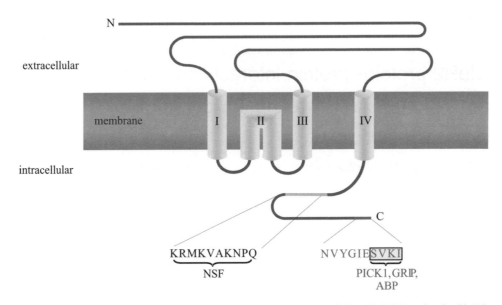

Fig. 15.1 Protein–protein interaction sites on the C-terminus of the AMPAR subunit GluR2. The sites of interaction are shown together with the sequence of each binding domain: the NSF site, and the extreme C-terminal PDZ protein binding site (PDZ motif highlighted).

neurotoxicity (Weiss and Sensi 2000). Thus, proteins that specifically bind to GluR2 are candidate mechanisms for the pathophysiological regulation of AMPAR function.

To date, two distinct interaction domains have been identified for the GluR2 C-terminus (Fig. 15.1). NSF protein interacts at a site proximal to the fourth transmembrane domain ('the NSF site'; Nishimune *et al.* 1998; Osten *et al.* 1998; Song *et al.* 1998), while at the extreme C-terminus there is a PDZ motif that binds ABP (Srivastava *et al.* 1998), GRIP (Dong *et al.* 1997) and PICK1 (Dev *et al.* 1999; Xia *et al.* 1999). In addition, recent work has shown that the clathrin adaptor complex protein AP2 associates with GluR2 via interactions at the NSF site (Lee *et al.* 2002). Interacting proteins at both the NSF and PDZ sites are involved in a rapid regulation of AMPAR function during synaptic plasticity.

15.2 The *N*-ethylmaleimide-sensitive fusion protein site

Most extensively studied is the role of interactions at the NSF site. Blocking these interactions with a peptide, 'pep2m' (KRMKVAKNAQ), causes a rapid run-down in AMPAR-mediated EPSCs at hippocampal CA1 synapses (Nishimune *et al.* 1998; Song *et al.* 1998). Immunocytochemical analyses show that this reduction in transmission is due to a loss of surface-expressed AMPARs (Lüscher *et al.* 1999; Noel *et al.* 1999). A recent study has found that AP2 interacts with AMPARs via this site and has identified distinct roles for NSF and AP2 in the regulation of AMPARs (Lee *et al.* 2002). Collectively these studies show that AMPARs rapidly recycle between intracellular and

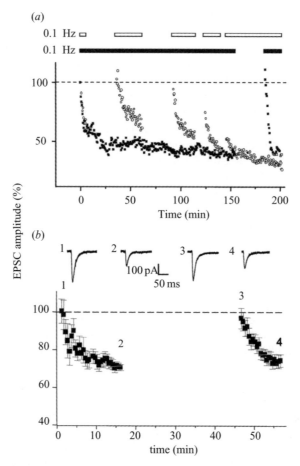

Fig. 15.2 The run-down of AMPAR-mediated synaptic transmission in the presence of pep2m is activity dependent. (*a*) Data from a single experiment showing EPSC amplitude versus time for a whole-cell patch-clamp recording from a CA1 neuron in a hippocampal slice (see Lüthi *et al.* (1999) for methods). AMPAR-mediated EPSCs were evoked by electrical stimulation of two independent pathways onto the same cell (data for one pathway represented by filled, one by open circles; inset top shows the patterns of activity at each pathway). Interruption of stimulation at the 'open' pathway allowed a recovery of EPSC amplitude, while continuous stimulation of the 'filled' pathway produced a stable depression. The use of different time intervals for the interruption of stimulation of the 'open' pathway reveals the time-course of this recovery. A subsequent pause in stimulation of the 'filled' pathway also allows recovery of EPSC amplitude at this pathway. (*b*) Pooled data (*n* = 14) from experiments with intracellular pep2m showing the consistent effect of pausing stimulation for 30 min on EPSC amplitude following the initial run-down.

postsynaptic membranes and, furthermore, that interactions at the NSF site are involved in this rapid regulation.

Although it is known that AMPARs rapidly recycle during basal transmission, it is not clear what process drives the rapid recycling of AMPARs. To investigate this we studied whether the run down of AMPAR-mediated EPSCs observed in the presence of pep2m is dependent on synaptic activity (Fig. 15.2). As previously shown, infusion of pep2m (100–1000 μM) into CA1 pyramidal neurons in hippocampal slices (Nishimune *et al.* 1998; Lüthi *et al.* 1999) caused a rapid reduction in EPSC amplitude in two independent pathways. Here, we show that the interruption of stimulation at one pathway caused a recovery of EPSC amplitude while continuous stimulation at the other pathway yielded a sustained depression of EPSC amplitude (Fig. 15.2*a*). The time-course of this recovery, as estimated by varying the period of stimulation interruption, was slower than the depression caused by pep2m. The activity-dependent depression of transmission by pep2m was consistently observed in a number of cells (Fig. 15.2*b*). However, in interleaved control experiments using the inactive peptide pep4c (KRMKVAKSAQ; Nishimune *et al.* 1998) that differs from pep2m by a single amino acid, EPSC amplitude showed no run down in transmission (EPSC amplitude after 10 min of stimulation = $106 \pm 4\%$ initial baseline, $n = 10$), and little activity-dependent recovery (EPSC amplitude following 30 min interruption of stimulation = $119 \pm 6\%$ of amplitude before stimulus interruption; $n = 10$). These data, together with similar data from another study (Lüscher *et al.* 1999), indicate that synaptic activity drives the rapid recycling of AMPARs. One possible mechanism for this is that binding of glutamate to AMPARs causes a ligand-induced internalization that drives the insertion of replacement AMPARs via a mechanism involving interactions at the NSF site on GluR2. When this mechanism is blocked this reveals a second slower component for the delivery of AMPARs to synapses which is independent of interactions at the NSF site. The mechanism for this is at present unknown; however, one possibility is that this reflects insertion of AMPARs involving a GluR1-dependent process (Passafaro *et al.* 2001).

In addition to regulating AMPAR function during basal synaptic transmission there is also good evidence that interactions at the NSF site are important for the expression of hippocampal NMDA receptor-dependent LTD. This form of LTD involves the rapid internalization of AMPARs (e.g. Carroll *et al.* 1999; Beattie *et al.* 2000). Acute blockade of interactions at the NSF site with pep2m prevents LTD (Lüscher *et al.* 1999; Lüthi *et al.* 1999; Lee *et al.* 2002). Since pep2m also causes a run down in synaptic transmission, one explanation for this is that there is a pool of mobile AMPARs regulated by interactions at the NSF site that are specifically involved in LTD. However, a recent study (Lee *et al.* 2002) has provided evidence that the NSF–GluR2 interaction is primarily involved in the regulation of AMPARs during basal synaptic transmission while the newly identified AP2 interaction at this site is important for AMPAR regulation during NMDA receptor-dependent LTD. Since AP2 is directly involved in clathrin-dependent endocytosis this provides a simple mechanism by which AMPARs are internalized during LTD and indicates that the NSF–GluR2 interaction is primarily involved in the insertion or stabilization of AMPARs.

15.3 The PDZ site

There has also been much interest in the role of ABP/GRIP and PICK1, proteins that interact at the PDZ binding motif at the extreme C-terminus of GluR2. Interactions at this site have been shown to regulate the surface expression of the GluR2 subunit in cultured hippocampal neurons (e.g. Dong *et al.* 1997; Osten *et al.* 2000; Passafaro *et al.* 2001; Braithwaite *et al.* 2002). At hippocampal CA1 synapses, acute blockade of these interactions by infusing peptides that mimic the extreme C-terminus of GluR2 into neurons causes a PKC-dependent increase in AMPAR-mediated synaptic transmission in a third of neurons and blocks hippocampal NMDA receptor-dependent LTD in all cells (Daw *et al.* 2000; Kim *et al.* 2001). This indicates that GRIP/ABP and/or PICK1 are important for the PKC-dependent regulation of AMPARs during basal transmission and that these interactions regulate receptors during LTD. Furthermore, our data indicated a role for these interacting proteins in LTP of synapses that had previously undergone LTD, so-called 'de-depression' (Daw *et al.* 2000). Based on our findings we proposed a model in which GRIP/ABP binds AMPARs sub-synaptically and together with PICK1/PKC dynamically regulates their surface expression during LTD, and in an LTP-like mechanism during de-depression (Daw *et al.* 2000).

Recent studies have focused on determining the precise roles of each of these PDZ domain-containing proteins in the regulation of AMPAR expression at synapses. In particular there has been a lot of interest in PICK1 since it was originally identified as an interactor for PKCα (Staudinger *et al.* 1995, 1997). In addition, to PKCα and GluR2, PICK1 also interacts with a number of other proteins including mGluR7 (Boudin *et al.* 2000; Dev *et al.* 2000; El Far *et al.* 2000), non-voltage-gated Na^+ channels (Baron *et al.* 2002; Duggan *et al.* 2002; Hruska-Hageman *et al.* 2002) and ephrin receptors (Torres *et al.* 1998). Although PICK1 contains only a single PDZ domain, it can also dimerize via a coiled-coil domain (Perez *et al.* 2001) providing the possibility that PICK1 dimers could target other proteins such as PKCα to AMPARs. Indeed, evidence for such a mechanism is provided by the finding that PKC activators cause the translocation of PICK1 and PKCα to synapses which is accompanied by an increase in the phosphorylation of GluR2 (Chung *et al.* 2000; Perez *et al.* 2001). PICK1 therefore may function as a chaperone bringing activated PKC to AMPARs.

Other studies have now started to address the functional role of PICK1 in regulating AMPARs during synaptic transmission and plasticity. At cerebellar parallel fibre–Purkinje cell synapses, peptides and other reagents that interfere with the PICK1–GluR2 interaction have no effect on basal synaptic transmission, but block cerebellar LTD (Xia *et al.* 2000). This is consistent with previous studies showing that this form of LTD involves the PKC phosphorylation of GluR2 (Matsuda *et al.* 2000) and the internalization of AMPARs (Wang and Linden 2000). This leads to the hypothesis that PICK1 mediates this PKC-dependent internalization (Xia *et al.* 2000).

The functional role of PICK1 at hippocampal CA1 synapses, however, is less clear. Immunocytochemical studies show that overexpression of PICK1 in cultured hippocampal neurons causes a profound loss of surface-expressed recombinant GluR2 (Perez *et al.* 2001) or endogenous GluR2 subunits (L. Cotton, K. Dev and J. Henley, personal communication). This indicates that PICK1 can downregulate AMPAR function at hippocampal synapses. The acute role of PICK1 has also been studied using C-terminal GluR2 peptides in which serine[880] is phosphorylated or has been substituted for a glutamate. Phosphorylation of serine[880], or glutamate substitution that mimics phosphorylation, prevents GRIP/ABP but not PICK1 binding (Chung *et al.* 2000), making these peptides selective inhibitors of the PICK1–GluR2 interaction (Li *et al.* 1999; Daw *et al.* 2000; Kim *et al.* 2001). One study reported that either of these PICK1 selective inhibitors caused an increase in basal synaptic transmission and partially blocked LTD at hippocampal synapses (Kim *et al.* 2001). Based on these and other immunocytochemical findings it has been proposed that PICK1 causes AMPAR

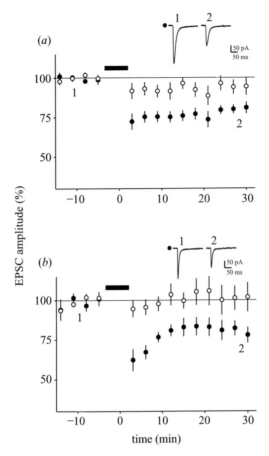

Fig. 15.3 Pep2-EVKI, a peptide that blocks the PICK1–GluR2 interaction, does not block hippocampal LTD (data re-plotted from Daw *et al.* (2000)). (*a*) Pooled data (*n*=8) from experiments in which 100 M pep2-EVKI was infused into CA1 hippocampal neurons during whole-cell patchclamp recordings. EPSC amplitude at two independent pathways was monitored and LTD induced (black bar) in one pathway (black circles) using 300 stimuli at 0.5 Hz paired with a holding potential of − 40 mV (peptide was infused into neurons for at least 30 min before applying the induction protocol; see Daw *et al.* (2000) for methods). Inset shows EPSCs from the LTD pathway for an example experiment taken at the times indicated. (*b*) Pooled data (*n* = 10) for similar experiments (interleaved with experiments in (*a*)) in which the inactive control peptide pep2-SVKE was infused into the neurons.

internalization during hippocampal LTD (Perez *et al.* 2001; Kim *et al.* 2001), in an analogous mechanism to that proposed for cerebellar LTD (Xia *et al.* 2000). However, we have reported that a C-terminal GluR2 peptide in which serine[880] is substituted for a glutamate ('pep2- EVKI' [YNVYGIEEVKI]), had no effect on basal synaptic transmission and did not block hippocampal LTD (Daw *et al.* 2000). Figure 15.3 shows data from this study re-plotted to illustrate the effects of pep2-EVKI infusion on LTD. In two pathway experiments using whole-cell patch-clamp recordings from CA1 neurons in hippocampal slices we compared the effect of the intracellular infusion of pep2-EVKI, which blocks the PICK1–GluR2 interaction, with that of an inactive control peptide pep2-SVKE (YNVYGIESVKE). In the presence of either pep2-EVKI (Fig. 15.3a) or pep2-SVKE (Fig. 15.3b) LTD could be reliably induced. These data indicate therefore that PICK1 is not involved in LTD under our experimental conditions, but rather that the GRIP/ABP interaction is important in regulating AMPARs. The reasons for these discrepancies in the acute effects of blocking PICK1–GluR2 interactions are not clear, and therefore at present the role of PICK1 in hippocampal NMDA receptor-dependent LTD remains a matter for debate. Clearly, considerable work is required to fully elucidate the role of PICK1 in hippocampal synaptic plasticity. This will require electrophysiological studies on the effects of long-term manipulations of PICK1 function on synaptic transmission and plasticity, as well as a more detailed characterization of the effects of PICK1 overexpression on AMPAR subunit surface expression. In addition, the role of PKC in hippocampal LTD and in the regulation of AMPAR surface expression also needs to be clarified. Finally, PICK1 is a promiscuous interactor and the consequences of this multi-functionality need to be addressed when considering the mechanism(s) of AMPAR regulation by PICK1.

The study of the roles of protein–protein interaction involving AMPAR subunits in the dynamic regulation of fast excitatory synaptic transmission is an exciting and emerging area. Although ever-increasing numbers of interacting proteins are being identified, elucidating their individual roles in the processes underlying the expression of LTP and LTD is proving to be a challenging task. Much further work is required to achieve a detailed understanding of the precise functions of these interactions.

The authors thank Dr W. Anderson for supplying the data acquisition software. This work was supported by the Wellcome Trust (F.D., W.L., J.T.R.I.), BBSRC (M.I.D.), and MRC (G.L.C.).

References

Baron, A., Deval, E., Salinas, M., Lingueglia, E., Voilley, N., and Lazdunski, M. (2002). Protein kinase C stimulates the acid-sensing ion channel ASIC2a via the PDZ domain-containing protein PICK1. *J. Biol. Chem.* **277**, 50 463–8.

Beattie, E. C., Carroll, R. C., Yu, X., Morishita, W., Yasuda, H., von Zastrow, M., *et al.* (2000). Regulation of AMPA receptor endocytosis by a signaling mechanism shared with LTD. *Nature Neurosci.* **3**, 1291–300.

Boudin, H., Doan, A., Xia, J., Shigemoto, R., Huganir, R. L., Worley, P., *et al.* (2000). Pre-synaptic clustering of mGluR7a requires the PICK1 PDZ domain binding site. *Neuron* **28**, 485–97.

Bowie, D. and Mayer, M. L. (1995). Inward rectification of both AMPA and kainate subtype glutamate receptors generated by polyamine-mediated ion channel block. *Neuron* **15**, 453–62.

Braithwaite, S. P., Meyer, G., and Henley, J. M. (2000). Interactions between AMPA receptors and intracellular proteins. *Neuropharmacology* **39**, 919–30.

Braithwaite, S. P., Xia, H., and Malenka, R. C. (2002). Differential roles for NSF and GRIP/ABP in AMPA receptor cycling. *Proc. Natl Acad. Sci. USA* **99**, 7096–101.

Brusa, R., Zimmermann, F., Koh, D. S., Feldmeyer, D., Gass, P., Seeburg, P. H., *et al.* (1995). Early-onset epilepsy and postnatal lethality associated with an editing-deficient GluR-B allele in mice. *Science* **270**, 1677–80.

Burnashev, N., Monyer, H., Seeburg, P. H., and Sakmann, B. (1992). Divalent ion permeability of AMPA receptor channels is dominated by the edited form of a single subunit. *Neuron* **8**, 189–98.

Carroll, R. C., Lissin, D. V., von Zastrow, M., Nicoll, R. A., and Malenka, R. C. (1999). Rapid redistribution of glutamate receptors contributes to long-term depression in hippocampal cultures. *Nature Neurosci.* **2**, 454–60.

Chung, H. J., Xia, J., Scannevin, R. H., Zhang, X., and Huganir, R. L. (2000). Phosphorylation of the AMPA receptor subunit GluR2 differentially regulates its interaction with the PDZ domain-containing proteins. *J. Neurosci.* **20**, 7258–67.

Daw, M. I., Chittajallu, R., Bortolotto, Z. A., Dev, K. K., Duprat, F., Henley, J. M., *et al.* (2000). PDZ proteins interacting with C-terminal GluR2/3 are involved in a PKC-dependent regulation of AMPA receptors at hippocampal synapses. *Neuron* **28**, 873–86.

Dev, K. K., Nishimune, A., Henley, J. M., and Nakanishi, S. (1999). The protein kinase Cα binding protein PICK1 interacts with short but not long form alternative splice variants of AMPA receptor subunits. *Neuropharmacology* **38**, 635–44.

Dev, K. K., Nakajima, Y., Kitano, J., Braithwaite, S. P., Henley, J. M., and Nakanishi, S. (2000). PICK1 interacts with and regulates PKC phosphorylation of mGLUR7. *J. Neurosci.* **20**, 7252–7.

Dong, H., O'Brien, R. J., Fung, E. T., Lanahan, A. A., Worley, P. F., and Huganir, R. L. (1997). GRIP: a synaptic PDZ-containing protein that interacts with AMPA receptors. *Nature* **386**, 279–84.

Duggan, A., Garcia-Anoveros, J., and Corey, D. P. (2002). The PDZ domain protein PICK1 and the sodium channel BNaC1 interact and localize at mechanosensory terminals of dorsal root ganglion neurons and dendrites of central neurons. *J. Biol. Chem.* **277**, 5203–8.

El Far, O., Airas, J., Wischmeyer, E., Nehring, R. B., Karschin, A., and Betz, H. (2000). Interaction of the C-terminal tail region of the metabotropic glutamate receptor 7 with the protein kinase C substrate PICK1. *Eur. J. Neurosci.* **12**, 4215–21.

Hayashi, Y., Shi, S.-H., Esteban, J. A., Piccini, A., Poncer, J.-C., and Malinow, R. (2000). Driving AMPA receptors into synapses by LTP and CaMKII: requirement for GluR1 and PDZ domain interaction. *Science* **287**, 2262–7.

Hruska-Hageman, A. M., Wemmie, J. A., Price, M. P., and Welsh, M. J. (2002). Interaction of the synaptic protein PICK1 (protein interacting with C kinase 1) with the non-voltage gated sodium channels BNC1 (brain Na+ channel 1) and ASIC (acid-sensing ion channel). *Biochem. J.* **361**, 443–50.

Jia, Z., Agopyan, N., Miu, P., Xiong, Z., Henderson, J., Gerlai, R., *et al.* (1996). Enhanced LTP in mice deficient in the AMPA receptor GluR2. *Neuron* **17**, 945–56.

Kamboj, S. K., Swanson, G. T., and Cull-Candy, S. G. (1995). Intracellular spermine confers rectification on rat calcium-permeable AMPA and kainate receptors. *J. Physiol. (Lond.)* **486**, 297–303.

Kim, C. H., Chung, H. J., Lee, H. K., and Huganir, R. L. (2001). Interaction of the AMPA receptor subunit GluR2/3 with PDZ domains regulates hippocampal long-term depression. *Proc. Natl Acad. Sci. USA* **98**, 11 725–30.

Lee, S. H., Liu, L., Wang, Y. T., and Sheng, M. (2002). Clathrin adaptor AP2 and NSF interact with overlapping sites of GluR2 and play distinct roles in AMPA receptor trafficking and hippocampal LTD. *Neuron* **36**, 661–74.

Li, P., Kerchner, G. A., Sala, C., Wei, F., Huettner, J. E., Sheng, M. *et al.* (1999). AMPA receptor-PDZ interactions in facilitation of spinal sensory synapses. *Nature Neurosci.* **2**, 972–7.

Lu, W.-Y., Man, H.-Y., Ju, W., Trimble, W. S., MacDonald, J. F., and Wang, Y. T. (2001). Activation of synaptic NMDA receptors induces membrane insertion of new AMPA receptors and LTP in cultured hippocampal neurons. *Neuron* **29**, 243–4.

Lüscher, C., Xia, H., Beattie, E. C., Carroll, R. C., Von Zastrow, M., Malenka, R. C., *et al.* (1999). Role of AMPA receptor cycling in synaptic transmission and plasticity. *Neuron* **24**, 649–58.

Lüscher, C., Nicoll, R. A., Malenka, R. C., and Muller, D. (2000). Synaptic plasticity and dynamic modulation of the postsynaptic membrane. *Nature Neurosci.* **3**, 545–50.

Lüthi, A., Chittajallu, R., Duprat, F., Palmer, M. J., Benke, T. A., Kidd, F. L., *et al.* (1999). Hippocampal LTD expression involves a pool of AMPARs regulated by the NSF-GluR2 interaction. *Neuron* **24**, 389–99.

Matsuda, S., Launey, T., Mikawa, S., and Hirai, H. (2000). Disruption of AMPA receptor GluR2 clusters following long-term depression induction in cerebellar Purkinje neurons. *EMBO J.* **9**, 2765–74.

Nishimune, A., Isaac, J. T. R., Molnar, E., Noel, J., Nash, S. R., Tagaya, M., *et al.* (1998). NSF binding to GluR2 regulates synaptic transmission. *Neuron* **21**, 87–97.

Noel, J., Ralph, G. S., Pickard, L., Willimans, J., Molnar, E., Uney, J. B., *et al.* (1999). Surface expression of AMPA receptors in hippocampal neurons is regulated by an NSF-dependent mechanism. *Neuron* **23**, 365–76.

Osten, P., Srivastava, S., Inman, G. J., Vilim, F. S., Khatri, L., Lee, L. M., *et al.* (1998). The AMPA receptor GluR2 C terminus can mediate a reversible, ATP-dependent interaction with NSF and α- and β-SNAPs. *Neuron* **21**, 99–110.

Osten, P., Khatri, L., Kohr, G., Giese, G., Daly, C., Schulz, T. W., *et al.* (2000). Mutagenesis reveals a role for ABP/GRIP binding to GluR2 in synaptic surface accumulation of the AMPA receptor. *Neuron* **27**, 313–25.

Passafaro, M., Piech, V., and Sheng, M. (2001). Subunit-specific temporal and spatial patterns of AMPA receptor exocytosis in hippocampal neurons. *Nature Neurosci.* **4**, 917–26.

Perez, J. L., Khatri, L., Chang, C., Srivastava, S., Osten, P., and Ziff, E. B. (2001). PICK1 targets activated protein kinase Cα to AMPA receptor clusters in spines of hippocampal neurons and reduces surface levels of the AMPA-type glutamate receptor subunit 2. *J. Neurosci.* **21**, 5417–28.

Pickard, L., Noel, J., Duckworth, J. K., Fitzjohn, S. M., Henley, J. M., Collingridge, G. L., *et al.* (2001). Transient synaptic activation of NMDA receptors leads to the insertion of native AMPA receptors at hippocampal neuronal plasma membranes. *Neuropharmacology* **41**, 700–13.

Sheng, M. and Lee, S. H. (2001). AMPA receptor trafficking and the control of synaptic transmission. *Cell* **105**, 825–8.

Song, I., Kamboj, S., Xia, J., Dong, H., Liao, D., and Huganir, R. L. (1998). Interaction of the N-ethylmaleimide-sensitive factor with AMPA receptors. *Neuron* **21**, 393–400.

Srivastava, S., Osten, P., Vilim, F. S., Khatri, L., Inman, G., States, B., *et al.* (1998). Novel anchorage of GluR2/3 to the postsynaptic density by AMPA receptorbinding protein ABP. *Neuron* **21**, 581–91.

Staudinger, J., Zhou, J., Burgess, R., Elledge, S. J., and Olson, E. N. (1995). PICK1: a perinuclear binding protein and substrate for protein kinase C isolated by the yeast two-hybrid system. *J. Biol. Chem.* **128**, 263–71.

Staudinger, J., Lu, J., and Olson, E. N. (1997). Specific interaction of the PDZ domain protein PICK1 with the COOH terminus of protein kinase C-α. *J. Biol. Chem.* **272**, 32019–24.

Torres, R., Firestein, B. L., Dong, H., Staudinger, J., Olson, E. N., Huganir, R. L., *et al.* (1998). PDZ proteins bind, cluster and synaptically colocalise with Eph receptors and their ephrin ligands. *Neuron* **21**, 1453–63.

Wang, Y. T. and Linden, D. J. (2000). Expression of cerebellar long-term depression requires postsynaptic clathrin-mediated endocytosis. *Neuron* **25**, 635–47.

Weiss, J. H. and Sensi, S. L. (2000). Ca^{2+}–Zn^{2+} permeable AMPA or kainate receptors: possible key factors in selective neuro-degeneration. *Trends Neurosci.* **23**, 365–71.

Xia, J., Zhang, X., Staudinger, J., and Huganir, R. L. (1999). Clustering of AMPA receptors by the synaptic PDZ domain-containing protein PICK1. *Neuron* **22**, 179–87.

Xia, J., Chung, H. J., Wihler, C., Huganir, R. L., and Linden, D. J. (2000). Cerebellar long-term depression requires PKC-regulated interactions between GluR2/3 and PDZ domain-containing proteins. *Neuron* **28**, 499–510.

Glossary

ABP	AMPAR-binding protein
AMPA	α-amino-3-hydroxy-5-methyl-4-isoxazolepropionate
AMPAR	AMPA receptor
AP2	adaptor protein 2
CA1	Cornu Ammonis 1
EPSC	excitatory postsynaptic current
GluR2	glutamate receptor subunit 2
GRIP	glutamate receptor interacting protein
LTD	long-term depression
LTP	long-term potentiation
NMDA	*N*-methyl-D-aspartate
NSF	*N*-ethylmaleimide-sensitive fusion protein
PDZ	postsynaptic density-95/discs large/zona occludens-1
PICK1	protein interacting with C-kinase 1
PKC	protein kinase C

16

Expression mechanisms underlying long-term potentiation: a postsynaptic view

Roger A. Nicoll

This review summarizes the various experiments that have been carried out to determine if the expression of long-term potentiation (LTP), in particular N-methyl-D-aspartate (NMDA) receptor-dependent LTP, is presynaptic or postsynaptic. Evidence for a pre-synaptic expression mechanism comes primarily from experiments reporting that glutamate overflow is increased during LTP and from experiments showing that the failure rate decreases during LTP. However, other experimental approaches, such as monitoring synaptic glutamate release by recording astrocytic glutamate transporter currents, have failed to detect any change in glutamate release during LTP. In addition, the discovery of silent synapses, in which LTP rapidly switches on α-amino-3-hydroxy-5-methyl-4-isoxazolepropionic acid (AMPA) receptor function at NMDA-receptor-only synapses, provides a postsynaptic mechanism for the decrease in failures during LTP. It is argued that the preponderance of evidence favours a postsynaptic expression mechanism, whereby NMDA receptor activation results in the rapid recruitment of AMPA receptors as well as a covalent modification of synaptic AMPA receptors.

Keywords: long-term potentiation; plasticity; hippocampus; postsynaptic density; AMPA receptor; NMDA receptor

16.1 Introduction

It is remarkable that the debate over whether LTP is expressed presynaptically or postsynaptically persists after approximately 20 years. Such a protracted battle has indicated to some that a solution may never be found (Sanes and Lichtman 1999). While it is difficult not to get frustrated over the seemingly intractable nature of the problem, I believe that progress has been made and, perhaps more importantly, that the debate has stimulated a great deal of research into the fundamental mechanisms controlling transmitter release and postsynaptic responsiveness. This paper covers:

(i) the origins of the controversy;
(ii) the various types of experiments that have been designed to address the issue of whether the expression of LTP is pre- or postsynaptic;
(iii) the evidence for silent synapses; and
(iv) the mechanisms involved in the control of synaptic AMPA receptor trafficking.

16.2 Some caveats

It has been proposed that some of the confusion exists because LTP at different types of synapses might differ mechanistically. This is certainly the case for LTP at hippocampal mossy fibre synapses, which, unlike LTP at most other synapses, is independent of NMDA receptor activation (Nicoll and Malenka 1995). It also remains possible that differences exist for NMDA receptor-dependent LTP at different classes of synapse. In addition, there is considerable evidence that LTP at the same set of synapses may have different properties at different time-points following induction. While both of these points are valid, even if observations are limited to LTP at CA1 hippocampal excitatory synapses, where much of the research has been carried out, and limited to the first hour following induction, much of the controversy remains. Thus, this review will primarily focus on studies performed in the CA1 region of the hippocampal slice and on the first hour following induction. Anyone who has studied LTP knows that the magnitude varies considerably from slice to slice, despite apparent control of all established variables. Thus, it is clear that we still have limited knowledge of this phenomenon, which opens the possibility that the precise conditions influence not only the magnitude of LTP but also perhaps some of the underlying mechanisms.

16.3 Origins of the debate

The mid-1980s witnessed a great outpouring of papers addressing the induction of LTP. These include the demonstration that:

(i) NMDA-receptor activation is required (Collingridge et al. 1983);
(ii) a rise in postsynaptic calcium is required (Lynch et al. 1983); and
(iii) depolarization of the postsynaptic cell is required (Malinow and Miller 1986; Wigstrom et al. 1986).

In addition, it was found that Mg^{2+} causes a voltage-dependent block of the NMDA receptor (Nowak et al. 1984), and the NMDA receptor is highly permeable to Ca^{2+} (MacDermott et al. 1986; Jahr and Stevens 1987; Ascher and Nowak 1988). Based on these observations a simple postsynaptic model for the induction of LTP emerged, in which activation of NMDA receptors, coupled with strong postsynaptic depolarization, causes a large rise in Ca^{2+} in the postsynaptic spine. The rise in Ca^{2+} initiates a series of steps that ultimately results in a persistent enhancement in synaptic transmission. This model is universally agreed upon. It is the site at which the persistent change resides that has been so difficult to resolve.

Shortly before the elucidation of the induction mechanism, Dolphin et al. (1982) measured extracellular glutamate in vivo from the dentate gyrus and reported that LTP is associated with an increase in glutamate overflow. Given that the induction is clearly postsynaptic this finding required the involvement of a retrograde messenger, which remains to be identified. A provocative and, in retrospect, prescient proposal advanced by Lynch and Baudry (1984) was that the expression of LTP is due to the 'insertion of glutamate receptors in the postsynaptic membranes'.

One of the first physiological studies (McNaughton 1982) to address the issue of whether the expression of LTP is pre- or postsynaptic examined paired pulse facilitation (PPF), in which the response to the second of two closely spaced stimuli is enhanced. This is a presynaptic phenomenon and manipulations that alter presynaptic release probability invariably alter PPF. As LTP of perforant path synapses was not associated with a change in PPF, a postsynaptic expression mechanism was proposed (McNaughton 1982). This finding has subsequently been confirmed in numerous studies (e.g. Manabe *et al.* 1993; Asztely *et al.* 1996), but also challenged (e.g. Schulz *et al.* 1994). The inability to reach a strong consensus on whether LTP is associated with a change in PPF is emblematic of the problem associated with virtually all observations made concerning the expression of LTP.

Another early physiological experiment examined the relative effects of LTP on the AMPA and NMDA components of the EPSC. The logic was quite simple: the NMDA receptors would serve as a separate bioassay for measuring the amount of glutamate release. If only the AMPA component changed this would be strong evidence for a selective postsynaptic modification, whereas if both changed to the same degree, this would be more consistent with a presynaptic modification. LTP was associated primarily with an enhancement in the AMPA component (Kauer *et al.* 1988; Muller *et al.* 1988; Perkel and Nicoll 1993). This finding was quickly challenged (e.g. Bashir *et al.* 1991) and a great deal has been published subsequently about this. However, recent studies have emphasized the selectivity in the enhancement of the AMPA component (e.g. Liao *et al.* 1995; Durand *et al.* 1996; Choi *et al.* 2000; Montgomery *et al.* 2001).

Within 2 years of the initial experiments that examined the effect of LTP on the NMDA component, two papers, one by Malinow and Tsien (1990) and the other by Bekkers and Stevens (1990), appeared concluding that LTP is expressed presynaptically. These authors found that LTP was associated with a decrease in the coefficient of variation and in the failure rate. Based on classical work at the neuromuscular junction, such changes were very powerful evidence for a presynaptic expression mechanism. Both the change in the coefficient of variation (Manabe *et al.* 1993) and the change in failure rate (Kullmann and Nicoll 1992) associated with LTP were readily confirmed. Indeed, there is little debate concerning these two observations and it is fair to say that these two papers swayed public opinion overwhelmingly to accepting a presynaptic expression mechanism.

16.4 Experiments designed to test whether LTP is associated with an increase in transmitter release

However, a number of observations did not fit comfortably with a presynaptic expression mechanism. These experiments fell into two broad categories: those designed to test whether release increases during LTP and those designed to test whether the sensitivity and/or number of AMPA receptors increases during LTP. I begin by discussing the first category.

(i) The PPF data discussed in Section 16.3 are not consistent with an increase in the probability of transmitter release, although it should be noted that interactions between release probability and LTP have been reported (Schulz 1997).

(ii) If LTP were due to an increase in the probability of transmitter release, then it should be possible to occlude LTP by maximally increasing the probability of release. This has been accomplished by applying the K^+ channel blocker 4-AP, which markedly enhances transmitter release by broadening the presynaptic action potential (Muller and Lynch 1989; Hjelmstad *et al.* 1997). In the presence of 4-AP other manipulations that enhance the probability of release, such as elevating Ca^{2+}, fail to further increase transmission, confirming that the probability of release is close to saturation. However, the magnitude of LTP evoked under these conditions is no different from that evoked under normal conditions (Hjelmstad *et al.* 1997). A tenfold change in transmitter release induced by blocking or activating presynaptic adenosine receptors also failed to alter LTP (Asztely *et al.* 1994).

(iii) The rate at which use-dependent antagonists block glutamate receptors can be used to measure the probability of glutamate release. The rate of receptor blockade during synaptic stimulation is directly related to the probability of transmitter release. Two types of experiments have been carried out. First, the irreversible NMDA receptor antagonist MK-801 has been used (Manabe and Nicoll 1994). The rate of block of NMDA EPSCs, upon repeated stimulation, was simultaneously compared in the same cell for control synapses and synapses expressing LTP. No difference was observed. Mimicking the change in synaptic strength seen with LTP by increasing the probability of transmitter release (e.g. PPF), demonstrated that this MK-801 assay had the necessary sensitivity to detect a change in release, if it had occurred. However, these results were later challenged and a presynaptic mechanism proposed (Kullmann *et al.* 1996). Second, a similar set of experiments was carried out using polyamine compounds in the GluR2-lacking mouse (Mainen *et al.* 1998). GluR2-lacking AMPA receptors are reversibly blocked in a use-dependent manner by polyamine compounds. LTP had no effect on the rate of block, implying that no change in glutamate release occurred during LTP.

(iv) Astrocytic glutamate transporter currents have been used to monitor synaptically released glutamate during LTP (Diamond *et al.* 1998; Luscher *et al.* 1998). Astrocytes surround excitatory synapses, and Bergles and Jahr (1997) convincingly showed that astrocytic glutamate transporter currents are remarkably sensitive to synaptically released glutamate. Changing the probability of release or the number of activated synapses demonstrated that glial transporter currents have the necessary sensitivity to detect a change in release if occurring during LTP. However, LTP produced no change in the currents (Diamond *et al.* 1998; Luscher *et al.* 1998).

(v) FM1–43 has been used to examine directly the effects of LTP on presynaptic vesicle recycling (Zakharenko *et al.* 2001). The fluorescent marker FM1–43 reversibly binds to membranes and is taken up into endocytosed vesicles. After loading the vesicle pool and washing away the extracellular FM1–43, the probability of vesicle release can be assayed by measuring the rate of destaining of synaptic boutons during presynaptic stimulation. Standard NMDA receptor-dependent LTP (50 or 100 Hz tetanus) was not associated with any change in the rate of destaining and yet control experiments demonstrated that this technique had the necessary sensitivity to detect a change if it had occurred during LTP. This finding argues strongly that there is no presynaptic increase in release probability during NMDA receptor-dependent LTP. In this same paper the authors did find a change in the destaining curve for another form of LTP that is induced by 200 Hz stimulation and depends on both NMDA receptors and L-type Ca^{2+} channels.

Taken as a whole, the body of evidence reviewed here is very difficult to reconcile with a presynaptic expression mechanism. However, it must be acknowledged that there is not unanimous agreement among the experimental findings or in their interpretation. In addition, it can be argued that this conclusion is based on negative results, which typically are not as convincing as positive results. Nevertheless, in all cases the necessary controls were conducted to calibrate the sensitivity of the particular assay and thus ensure that the required sensitivity was present.

16.5 Experiments designed to test whether LTP is associated with an increase in the sensitivity and/or number of AMPA receptors

I now turn to experiments designed to test whether the sensitivity and/or number of AMPA receptors increase during LTP.

(i) An early experiment reported a delayed increase in the response to ionto-phoretically applied AMPA following the induction of LTP (Davies *et al.* 1989). This is a rather surprising result, given the large area of tissue that would be exposed to the 20 s application of AMPA used in most of this study compared with the very small number of synapses that would undergo LTP. Nevertheless, if we accept this finding, it not only establishes a delayed postsynaptic contribution to LTP, but also rules out a postsynaptic contribution early in LTP, because the late change establishes that the necessary sensitivity is present in this experiment to detect an early postsynaptic change. More recently, a rapid increase in the size of responses to exogenous AMPA has been reported (Montgomery *et al.* 2001) during LTP. Another approach to overcome the small fraction of synapses expressing LTP is to load pyramidal cells with a constitutively active CaMKII. A great deal of evidence exists to indicate that activation of CaMKII is sufficient for LTP (Soderling and Derkach 2000). By loading pyramidal cells with a constitutively active form of CaMKII (Lledo *et al.* 1995) all synapses would be exposed to the loaded CaMKII and potentiated. CaMKII not only enhanced EPSCs, as expected, but also enhanced the responses to iontophoretically applied AMPA. Furthermore, the enhancement of AMPA EPSCs occluded with LTP and CaMKII no longer enhanced synaptic transmission at synapses already expressing LTP.

(ii) Experiments have used quantitative autoradiography to measure the binding properties of AMPA and NMDA receptors in the dentate gyrus after inducing LTP in the perforant path *in vivo* (Maren *et al.* 1993). A selective increase in AMPA binding was observed and this was due to an increase in the number of AMPA binding sites. It is unclear if this increase in binding reflects AMPA receptor trafficking, assembly or synthesis.

(iii) Experiments have been designed to examine the effect of LTP on mEPSCs (Manabe *et al.* 1992; Oliet *et al.* 1996). Studies at the neuromuscular junction have shown that a change in size of miniature synaptic responses is due to a change in postsynaptic responsiveness. Analysis of quantal events in central nervous system neurons is complicated by the fact that an individual neuron receives thousands of synapses, whereas LTP is induced in only a tiny fraction of synapses. To circumvent this problem, extracellular Ca^{2+} was replaced with Sr^{2+}, which causes the asynchronous release of quanta only from activated synapses. Under these conditions a clear increase in size of mEPSCs was recorded (Oliet *et al.* 1996). An increase in apparent frequency was also observed which could be due to:

(1) an increase in the detection of events that were previously below threshold;
(2) the turning on of silent synapses; or
(3) an increase in the probability of transmitter release.

(iv) Another method for estimating quantal size relies on recording synaptic responses to minimal stimulation, in which a single or a few presynaptic fibres are activated.Responses to such stimulation are composed of a mixture of failures and responses. If one removes the failures and averages together the trials in which a response is evoked, the average quantal size can be estimated, assuming that only a single synapse is being recorded. The average size of the successes is also referred to as potency (Stevens and Wang 1994). Isaac *et al.* (1996) and Stricker *et al.* (1996) have found that LTP is invariably associated with an increase in potency and this can occur in the complete absence of a change in failure rate. However, this finding contrasts with two other studies in which no change in potency was associated with LTP (Stevens and Wang 1994; Bolshakov and Siegelbaum 1995). The basis for this difference is unclear, but resolution of this disagreement is of critical importance, because a lack of change in potency is incompatible with a postsynaptic contribution to LTP.

(v) Nonstationary noise analysis has been used to estimate the single-channel conductance of AMPA receptors before and after LTP (Benke *et al.* 1998). LTP was often associated with an increase in single channel conductance, indicating and postsynaptic change in AMPA receptor function during LTP.

(vi) Mice in which the GluRA/GluR1 AMPA receptor subunit has been deleted exhibit a striking deficit in LTP in the CA1 region (Zamanillo *et al.* 1999). This finding strongly implicates the AMPA receptor in the expression of LTP.

16.6 Evidence for silent synapses

The results summarized in Section 16.5 turned the spotlight directly on the change in synaptic failures; a unanimously agreed upon result and the single most compelling finding for a presynaptic expression mechanism. Might the change in synaptic failures have a postsynaptic explanation? A comparison of the coefficient of variation of the AMPA and NMDA component found that the variation was substantially higher for the AMPA component and that this difference decreased during LTP (Kullmann 1994). To account for these results Kullmann suggested that there might be a population of synapses that lacked functional AMPA receptors, while having the normal complement of NMDA receptors, and that during LTP these synapses would acquire AMPA receptor function. (Kullmann later emphasized the role of glutamate spillover, rather than differences in AMPA receptor composition, to account for these results (Kullmann *et al.* 1996).) A series of experiments were designed to test more directly for the existence of silent synapses (Isaac *et al.* 1995). Indeed, using minimal stimulation techniques a population of synapses was found that contained no detectable AMPA component, but had a normal NMDA component. Furthermore, an LTP-inducing protocol rapidly switched on these silent synapses. Liao *et al.* (1995) obtained virtually identical results. Numerous investigators have confirmed these findings. However, a recent study (Choi *et al.* 2000) indicated that silent synapses are due to the incomplete emptying of synaptic vesicles, so that the concentration of glutamate in the synaptic cleft is insufficient to activate AMPA receptors, but does activate NMDA receptors. LTP would result in more complete vesicle fusion. However, some of the results upon which this interpretation is based have been challenged (Montgomery *et al.* 2001) and such an increase in glutamate release should be detected by astrocytic glutamate transporter currents (see Section 16.4).

16.7 Regulation of synaptic AMPA receptors

The demonstration of silent synapses and their rapid upregulation by LTP raised a host of questions. For instance, what is a silent synapse? Are AMPA receptors present at the synapse but functionally inactive? Or are AMPA receptors actually missing from the synapse? To answer these and many related questions on receptor localization and trafficking, a more cellular and molecular biological approach was needed. A number of immunocytochemical studies in neuronal cultures have analysed the distribution of synaptic glutamate receptors. While virtually all excitatory synapses contained NMDA receptors, only a portion of synapses stained for AMPA receptors (Rao and Craig 1997; Gomperts *et al.* 1998; Liao *et al.* 1999). Furthermore, using single cell cultures these anatomical results could be correlated to the presence of NMDA receptor only miniature synaptic currents (Gomperts *et al.* 1998). Immunogold ultrastructural localization studies have found that, by contrast to the uniform synaptic distribution of NMDA receptors, the number of AMPA receptors varies widely and some excitatory synapses appear to lack AMPA receptors (Nusser *et al.* 1998; Petralia *et al.* 1999; Takumi *et al.* 1999).

Much of the recent work on excitatory synapses has focused on the mechanisms involved in the trafficking of synaptic AMPA receptors and the role of activity in this process (Malenka and Nicoll 1999; Braithwaite *et al.* 2000; Scannevin and Huganir 2000; Malinow *et al.* 2000; Sheng 2001; Malinow and Malenka 2002; Barry and Ziff 2002; Bredt and Nicoll 2003). Perhaps the most elegant experiments have used electrophysiologically tagged AMPA receptors to dissect out the mechanisms involved in the delivery of AMPA receptors to the synapse (Malinow *et al.* 2000; Shi *et al.* 2001). Our own recent studies have concentrated on two synaptic proteins, stargazin and PSD-95, which play important roles in controlling the number of synaptic AMPA receptors. Stargazin, the protein deleted in the mutant mouse stargazer, is essential, not only for the localization of AMPA receptors to the synapse, but also for the surface expression of these receptors in cerebellar granule cells (Chen *et al.* 2000). Overexpression of PSD-95 in dissociated neuronal cultures enhances synapse maturation, increasing synaptic size and enhancing AMPA receptor synaptic responses (El-Husseini *et al.* 2000). In slice cultures PSD-95 causes a rapid and selective increase in AMPA EPSCs (Schnell *et al.* 2002). This enhancement is mediated by the direct binding of stargazin to both AMPA receptors and PSD- 95 which then rapidly delivers AMPA receptors to the synapse (Schnell *et al.* 2002).

While attention has focused primarily on the trafficking of AMPA receptors during LTP, there is also considerable evidence that covalent modification of AMPA receptors by CaMKII can increase the single channel conductance of the receptor (Benke *et al.* 1998; Soderling and Derkach 2000).

16.8 Conclusions

In this brief review I have summarized the history of the controversy of whether the expression of LTP is pre- or postsynaptic. Although I have tried to be as objective as possible, there is, nevertheless, an unmistakable postsynaptic bias in terms of the data selected for inclusion and in the interpretation of these data. I believe that I speak for many researchers in the field when I say that the study of LTP has been a humbling experience. LTP is vastly more complex than anyone could have imagined. However, I do feel strongly that, fuelled by the LTP debate, our basic understanding of the properties of excitatory synapses has progressed enormously during the past decade and that with this knowledge the detailed molecular mechanisms underlying LTP will inevitably emerge.

The author thanks Dr D. S. Bredt for his helpful comments on the manuscript. Research in the author's laboratory is supported by the NIH and the Bristol-Meyers Squibb Co. The author is a member of the Keck Center for Integrative Neuroscience and the Silvio Conte Center for Neuroscience Research.

References

Ascher, P. and Nowak, L. (1988). The role of divalent cations in the N-methyl-D-aspartate responses of mouse central neurones in culture. *J. Physiol. (Lond.)* **399**, 247–66.

Asztely, F., Xiao, M. Y., Wigstrom, H., and Gustafsson, B. (1994). Effect of adenosine-induced changes in presynaptic release probability on long-term potentiation in the hippocampal CA1 region. *J. Neurosci.* **14**, 6707–14.

Asztely, F., Xiao, M. Y., and Gustafsson, B. (1996). Long-term potentiation and paired-pulse facilitation in the hippocampal CA1 region. *NeuroReport* **7**, 1609–12.

Barry, M. F. and Ziff, E. B. (2002). Receptor trafficking and the plasticity of excitatory synapses. *Curr. Opin. Neurobiol.* **12**, 279–86.

Bashir, Z. I., Alford, S., Davies, S. N., Randall, A. D., and Collingridge, G. L. (1991). Long-term potentiation of NMDA receptor-mediated synaptic transmission in the hippocampus. *Nature* **349**, 156–8.

Bekkers, J. M. and Stevens, C. F. (1990). Presynaptic mechanism for long-term potentiation in the hippocampus. *Nature* **346**, 724–9.

Benke, T. A., Luthi, A., Isaac, J. T., and Collingridge, G. L. (1998). Modulation of AMPA receptor unitary conductance by synaptic activity. *Nature* **393**, 793–7.

Bergles, D. E. and Jahr, C. E. (1997). Synaptic activation of glutamate transporters in hippocampal astrocytes. *Neuron* **19**, 1297–308.

Bolshakov, V. Y. and Siegelbaum, S. A. (1995). Regulation of hippocampal transmitter release during development and long-term potentiation. *Science* **269**, 1730–4.

Braithwaite, S. P., Meyer, G., and Henley, J. M. (2000). Interactions between AMPA receptors and intracellular proteins. *Neuropharmacology* **39**, 919–30.

Bredt, D. S. and Nicoll, R.A. (2003). AMPA receptor trafficking at excitatory synapses, *Neuron*, **40**, 361–79.

Chen, L., Chetkovich, D. M., Petralia, R. S., Sweeney, N. T., Kawasaki, Y., Wenthold, R. J., *et al.* (2000). Stargazin regulates synaptic targeting of AMPA receptors by two distinct mechanisms. *Nature* **408**, 936–43.

Choi, S., Klingauf, J., and Tsien, R. W. (2000). Postfusional regulation of cleft glutamate concentration during LTP at 'silent synapses'. *Nature Neurosci.* **3**, 330–6.

Collingridge, G. L., Kehl, S. J., and McLennan, H. (1983). Excitatory amino acids in synaptic transmission in the Schaffer collateral-commissural pathway of the rat hippocampus. *J. Physiol. (Lond.)* **334**, 33–46.

Davies, S. N., Lester, R. A., Reymann, K. G., and Collingridge, G. L. (1989). Temporally distinct pre- and post-synaptic mechanisms maintain long-term potentiation. *Nature* **338**, 500–3.

Diamond, J. S., Bergles, D. E., and Jahr, C. E. (1998). Glutamate release monitored with astrocyte transporter currents during LTP. *Neuron* **21**, 425–33.

Dolphin, A. C., Errington, M. L., and Bliss, T. V. (1982). Long-term potentiation of the perforant path *in vivo* is associated with increased glutamate release. *Nature* **297**, 496–8.

Durand, G. M., Kovalchuk, Y., and Konnerth, A. (1996). Long-term potentiation and functional synapse induction in developing hippocampus. *Nature* **381**, 71–5.

El-Husseini, A. E., Schnell, E., Chetkovich, D. M., Nicoll, R. A., and Bredt, D. S. (2000). PSD-95 involvement in maturation of excitatory synapses. *Science* **290**, 1364–8.

Gomperts, S. N., Rao, A., Craig, A. M., Malenka, R. C., and Nicoll, R. A. (1998). Post-synaptically silent synapses in single neuron cultures. *Neuron* **21**, 1443–51.

Hjelmstad, G. O., Nicoll, R. A., and Malenka, R. C. (1997). Synaptic refractory period provides a measure of probability of release in the hippocampus. *Neuron* **19**, 1309–18.

Isaac, J. T., Nicoll, R. A., and Malenka, R. C. (1995). Evidence for silent synapses: implications for the expression of LTP. *Neuron* **15**, 427–34.

Isaac, J. T., Hjelmstad, G. O., Nicoll, R. A., and Malenka, R. C. (1996). Long-term potentiation at single fiber inputs to hippocampal CA1 pyramidal cells. *Proc. Natl Acad. Sci. USA* **93**, 8710–15.

Jahr, C. E. and Stevens, C. F. (1987). Glutamate activates multiple single channel conductances in hippocampal neurons. *Nature* **325**, 522–5.

Kauer, J. A., Malenka, R. C., and Nicoll, R. A. (1988). A persistent postsynaptic modification mediates long-term potentiation in the hippocampus. *Neuron* **1**, 911–17.

Kullmann, D. M. (1994). Amplitude fluctuations of dual-component EPSCs in hippocampal pyramidal cells: implications for long-term potentiation. *Neuron* **12**, 1111–20.

Kullmann, D. M. and Nicoll, R. A. (1992). Long-term potentiation is associated with increases in quantal content and quantal amplitude. *Nature* **357**, 240–4.

Kullmann, D. M., Erdemli, G., and Asztely, F. (1996). LTP of AMPA and NMDA receptor-mediated signals: evidence for presynaptic expression and extrasynaptic glutamate spillover. *Neuron* **17**, 461–74.

Liao, D., Hessler, N. A., and Malinow, R. (1995). Activation of postsynaptically silent synapses during pairing-induced LTP in CA1 region of hippocampal slice. *Nature* **375**, 400–4.

Liao, D., Zhang, X., O'Brien, R., Ehlers, M. D., and Huganir, R. L. (1999). Regulation of morphological postsynaptic silent synapses in developing hippocampal neurons. *Nature Neurosci.* **2**, 37–43.

Lledo, P. M., Hjelmstad, G. O., Mukherji, S., Soderling, T. R., Malenka, R. C., and Nicoll, R. A. (1995). Calcium/calmodulin-dependent kinase II and long-term potentiation enhance synaptic transmission by the same mechanism. *Proc. Natl Acad. Sci. USA* **92**, 11 175–9.

Luscher, C., Malenka, R. C., and Nicoll, R. A. (1998). Monitoring glutamate release during LTP with glial transporter currents. *Neuron* **21**, 435–41.

Lynch, G., and Baudry, M. (1984). The biochemistry of memory: a new and specific hypothesis. *Science* **224**, 1057–63.

Lynch, G., Larson, J., Kelso, S., Barrionuevo, G., and Schottler, F. (1983). Intracellular injections of EGTA block induction of hippocampal long-term potentiation. *Nature* **305**, 719–21.

MacDermott, A. B., Mayer, M. L., Westbrook, G. L., Smith, S. J., and Barker, J. L. (1986). NMDA-receptor activation increases cytoplasmic calcium concentration in cultured spinal cord neurones. *Nature* **321**, 519–22.

McNaughton, B. L. (1982). Long-term synaptic enhancement and short-term potentiation in rat fascia dentata act through different mechanisms. *J. Physiol. (Lond.)* **324**, 249–62.

Mainen, Z. F., Jia, Z., Roder, J., and Malinow, R. (1998). Use-dependent AMPA receptor block in mice lacking GluR2 suggests postsynaptic site for LTP expression. *Nature Neurosci.* **1**, 579–86.

Malenka, R. C. and Nicoll, R. A. (1999). Long-term potentiation— a decade of progress? *Science* **285**, 1870–4.

Malinow, R. and Malenka, R. C. (2002). AMPA receptor trafficking and synaptic plasticity. *A. Rev. Neurosci.* **25**, 103–26.

Malinow, R. and Miller, J. P. (1986). Postsynaptic hyperpolarization during conditioning reversibly blocks induction of long-term potentiation. *Nature* **320**, 529–30.

Malinow, R. and Tsien, R. W. (1990). Presynaptic enhancement shown by whole-cell recordings of long-term potentiation in hippocampal slices. *Nature* **346**, 177–80.

Malinow, R., Mainen, Z. F., and Hayashi, Y. (2000). LTP mechanisms: from silence to four-lane traffic. *Curr. Opin. Neurobiol.* **10**, 352–7.

Manabe, T. and Nicoll, R. A. (1994). Long-term potentiation: evidence against an increase in transmitter release probability in the CA1 region of the hippocampus. *Science* **265**, 1888– 92.

Manabe, T., Renner, P., and Nicoll, R. A. (1992). Postsynaptic contribution to long-term potentiation revealed by the analysis of miniature synaptic currents. *Nature* **355**, 50–5.

Manabe, T., Wyllie, D. J., Perkel, D. J., and Nicoll, R. A. (1993). Modulation of synaptic transmission and long-term potentiation: effects on paired pulse facilitation and EPSC variance in the CA1 region of the hippocampus. *J. Neurophysiol.* **70**, 1451–9.

Maren, S., Tocco, G., Standley, S., Baudry, M., and Thompson, R. F. (1993). Postsynaptic factors in the expression of long-term potentiation (LTP): increased glutamate receptor binding following LTP induction *in vivo. Proc. Natl Acad. Sci. USA* **90**, 9654–8.

Montgomery, J. M., Pavlidis, P., and Madison, D. V. (2001). Pair recordings reveal all-silent synaptic connections and the postsynaptic expression of long-term potentiation. *Neuron* **29**, 691–701.

Muller, D. and Lynch, G. (1989). Evidence that changes in presynaptic calcium currents are not responsible for long-term potentiation in hippocampus. *Brain Res.* **479**, 290–9.

Muller, D., Joly, M., and Lynch, G. (1988). Contributions of quisqualate and NMDA receptors to the induction and expression of LTP. *Science* **242**, 1694–7.

Nicoll, R. A. and Malenka, R. C. (1995). Contrasting properties of two forms of long-term potentiation in the hippocampus. *Nature* **377**, 115–18.

Nowak, L., Bregestovski, P., Ascher, P., Herbet, A., and Prochiantz, A. (1984). Magnesium gates glutamate-activated channels in mouse central neurones. *Nature* **307**, 462–5.

Nusser, Z., Lujan, R., Laube, G., Roberts, J. D., Molnar, E., and Somogyi, P. (1998). Cell type and pathway dependence of synaptic AMPA receptor number and variability in the hippo-campus. *Neuron* **21**, 545–59.

Oliet, S. H., Malenka, R. C., and Nicoll, R. A. (1996). Bidirectional control of quantal size by synaptic activity in the hippocampus. *Science* **271**, 1294–7.

Perkel, D. J. and Nicoll, R. A. (1993). Evidence for all-or-none regulation of neurotransmitter release: implications for long-term potentiation. *J. Physiol. (Lond.)* **471**, 481–500.

Petralia, R. S., Esteban, J. A., Wang, Y. X., Partridge, J. G., Zhao, H. M., Wenthold, R. J., *et al.* (1999). Selective acquisition of AMPA receptors over postnatal development suggests a molecular basis for silent synapses. *Nature Neurosci.* **2**, 31–6.

Rao, A. and Craig, A. M. (1997). Activity regulates the synaptic localization of the NMDA receptor in hippocampal neurons. *Neuron* **19**, 801–12.

Sanes, J. R. and Lichtman, J. W. (1999). Can molecules explain long-term potentiation? *Nature Neurosci.* **2**, 597–604.

Scannevin, R. H. and Huganir, R. L. (2000). Postsynaptic organization and regulation of excitatory synapses. *Nature Rev. Neurosci.* **1**, 133–41.

Schnell, E., Sizemore, M., Karimzadegan, S., Chen, L., Bredt, D. S., and Nicoll, R. A. (2002). Direct interactions between PSD-95 and stargazin control synaptic AMPA receptor number. *Proc. Natl Acad. Sci. USA* **99**, 13 902–7.

Schulz, P. E. (1997). Long-term potentiation involves increases in the probability of neuro-transmitter release. *Proc. Natl Acad. Sci. USA* **94**, 5888–93.

Schulz, P. E., Cook, E. P., and Johnston, D. (1994). Changes in paired-pulse facilitation suggest presynaptic involvement in long-term potentiation. *J. Neurosci.* **14**, 5325–37.

Sheng, M. (2001). Molecular organization of the postsynaptic specialization. *Proc. Natl Acad. Sci. USA* **98**, 7058–61.

Shi, S., Hayashi, Y., Esteban, J. A., and Malinow, R. (2001). Subunit-specific rules governing AMPA receptor trafficking to synapses in hippocampal pyramidal neurons. *Cell* **105**, 331–43.

Soderling, T. R. and Derkach, V. A. (2000). Postsynaptic protein phosphorylation and LTP. *Trends Neurosci.* **23**, 75–80.

Stevens, C. F. and Wang, Y. (1994). Changes in reliability of synaptic function as a mechanism for plasticity. *Nature* **371**, 704–7.

Stricker, C., Field, A. C., and Redman, S. J. (1996). Changes in quantal parameters of EPSCs in rat CA1 neurones *in vitro* after the induction of long-term potentiation. *J. Physiol. (Lond.)* **490**, 443–54.

Takumi, Y., Ramirez-Leon, V., Laake, P., Rinvik, E., and Ottersen, O. P. (1999). Different modes of expression of AMPA and NMDA receptors in hippocampal synapses. *Nature Neurosci.* **2**, 618–24.

Wigstrom, H., Gustafsson, B., Huang, Y. Y., and Abraham, W. C. (1986). Hippocampal long-term potentiation is induced by pairing single afferent volleys with intracellularly injected depolarizing current pulses. *Acta Physiol. Scand.* **126**, 317–19.

Zakharenko, S. S., Zablow, L., and Siegelbaum, S. A. (2001). Visualization of changes in pre-synaptic function during long-term synaptic plasticity. *Nature Neurosci.* **4**, 711–17.

Zamanillo, D., Sprengel, R., Hvalby, O., Jensen, V., Burashev, N., Rozor, A., *et al.* (1999). Importance of AMPA receptors for hippocampal synaptic plasticity but not for spatial learning. *Science* **284**, 1805–11.

Glossary

AMPA   α-amino-3-hydroxy-5-methyl-4-isoxazolepropionic acid
4-AP   4-aminopyridine
CaMKII   calcium/calmodulin-dependent protein kinase II
EPSC   excitatory postsynaptic current
LTP   long-term potentiation
mEPSC   miniature excitatory postsynaptic current
NMDA   *N*-methyl-D-aspartate
PPF   paired pulse facilitation

17

Silent synapses: what are they telling us about long-term potentiation?

Dimitri M. Kullmann

At several cortical synapses glutamate release events can be mediated exclusively by NMDA receptors, with no detectable contribution from AMPA receptors. This observation was originally made by comparing the trial-to-trial variability of the two components of synaptic signals evoked in hippocampal neurons, and was subsequently confirmed by recording apparently pure NMDA receptor-mediated EPSCs with stimulation of small numbers of axons. It has come to be known as the 'silent synapse' phenomenon, and is widely assumed to be caused by the absence of functional AMPA receptors, which can, however, be recruited into the postsynaptic density by long-term potentiation (LTP) induction. Thus, it provides an important impetus for relating AMPA receptor trafficking mechanisms to the expression of LTP, a theme that is taken up elsewhere in this issue. This article draws attention to several findings that call for caution in identifying silent synapses exclusively with synapses without AMPA receptors. In addition, it attempts to identify several missing pieces of evidence that are required to show that unsilencing of such synapses is entirely accounted for by insertion of AMPA receptors into the postsynaptic density. Some aspects of the early stages of LTP expression remain open to alternative explanations.

Keywords: silent synapses; AMPA; NMDA; expression; spillover

17.1 The silent synapse phenomenon

Numerous experimental observations have been used to shed light on the early steps of NMDA receptor-dependent LTP expression. About 10 years ago, among the more robust findings (that is, reproduced in several laboratories) were two results that, at first sight, led to opposing conclusions. First, LTP was found to be associated with an increase in the average number of quanta of glutamate detected by the postsynaptic neuron in response to a presynaptic action potential (Bekkers and Stevens 1990; Malinow and Tsien 1990; Kullmann and Nicoll 1992; Larkman *et al.* 1992; Liao *et al.* 1992; Voronin 1994). By analogy with many other synapses in the nervous system, an increase in quantal content implies a presynaptic increase in transmitter release probability. Second, LTP was reported to be accompanied by a relatively selective increase in the signal mediated by AMPA receptors, with little change in the NMDA receptor-mediated component (Kauer *et al.* 1988; Muller and Lynch 1988; Perkel and Nicoll 1993). This finding, by contrast, is most easily explained by an enhancement in the function of AMPA receptors at the postsynaptic membrane. An important step towards a resolution of this paradox came with several observations that have become known as the 'silent synapse' phenomenon: evoked monoquantal events can be detected in a postsynaptic neuron, which are apparently exclusively mediated by NMDA receptors (Kullmann and Siegelbaum 1995). After LTP induction, these events are replaced by dual-component (AMPA and NMDA receptor-mediated) signals.

Initial evidence for silent synapses came from a comparison of the trial-to-trial variability of the AMPA and NMDA receptor-mediated components of EPSCs in CA1 pyramidal neurons (Kullmann 1994; Selig *et al.* 1995). Briefly, the argument goes as follows. Because the CV (a dimensionless measure of variability) is principally determined by the stochastic release of different numbers of vesicles from presynaptic afferents, it can be used to compare the probabilistic behaviour of signals mediated by the different receptors. Before LTP induction, the CV of the AMPA component evoked by a stimulus repeatedly delivered to a population of afferent fibres is consistently larger than that of the NMDA component. Because the CV varies inversely with the quantal content, this observation implies that, on average, fewer AMPA receptor-mediated quanta mediate the EPSC than NMDA receptor-mediated quanta. (Differences in the stochastic behaviour of channels themselves can be shown not to affect this conclusion (Kullmann 1994).) After LTP, the CV of the AMPA component decreases to become more similar to that of the NMDA component.

An alternative approach to demonstrate more graphically the existence of silent synapses was subsequently reported. This relied on minimal stimulation to excite a small number of presynaptic axons (Fig. 17.1). Exclusively NMDA receptor-mediated EPSCs could be shown to occur, and AMPA receptor-mediated quanta emerged following LTP induction (Isaac *et al.* 1995; Liao *et al.* 1995; Durand *et al.* 1996). An even more direct demonstration of silent synapses comes from paired recordings of synaptically coupled pyramidal neurons, which removes residual uncertainty about the number of axons stimulated under different recording conditions (Montgomery *et al.* 2001).

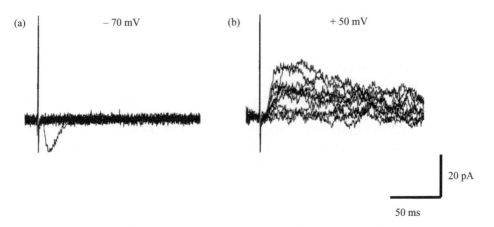

Fig. 17.1 The silent synapse phenomenon. An example of synaptic transmission mediated by AMPA and NMDA receptors. A granule cell was recorded at room temperature, initially voltage clamped at −70 mV to block the NMDA receptors (*a*), and then depolarized to +50 mV (*b*). The stimulation of a few lateral perforant path axons evoked AMPA receptor-mediated EPSCs with a high failure rate (*a*). The failure rate for the NMDA receptor-mediated component was much lower (*b*). Data from M.-Y. Min and D. M. Kullmann.

17.2 Possible underlying phenomena

The first, and still most compelling, interpretation of silent synapses is that, under baseline conditions, functional AMPA receptors are absent at a subset of synapses (Kullmann 1994) (Fig. 17.2*a*). This view has received important support from immunogold labelling of AMPA and NMDA receptors in the hippocampus: although AMPA receptors are undetectable at a proportion of synapses, NMDA receptors are more uniformly distributed (Nusser *et al.* 1998; Racca *et al.* 2000). Although this approach is sensitive to assumptions about the sensitivity of antibodies, it is qualitatively consistent with the existence of postsynaptically silent ('deaf') synapses. LTP is assumed to be accompanied by the appearance of such clusters, either by insertion into the postsynaptic density from a cytoplasmic store, or by translocation from an extrasynaptic location (Malenka and Nicoll 1999). The evidence for AMPA receptor trafficking mechanisms, both constitutive and in response to LTP induction stimuli, is overwhelming (Malinow and Malenka 2002). However, before assessing how completely this model accounts for the phenomenology of LTP, it is worth considering several alternative possibilities. These all rely on the fact that NMDA receptors have very different kinetics than AMPA receptors (Lester *et al.* 1990; Patneau and Mayer 1990; Jonas *et al.* 1993).

With prolonged application of glutamate, the apparent affinity of NMDA receptors is approximately 100-fold higher than that of AMPA receptors (Patneau and Mayer 1990). This does not mean that they are necessarily 100-fold more sensitive to glutamate transients such as occur in response to presynaptic exocytosis, because the occupancy and opening probability of receptors also depend on the time course of the glutamate transient. At one extreme, if NMDA and AMPA receptors are exposed to an

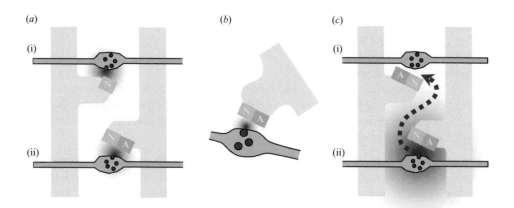

Fig. 17.2 Possible explanations of silent synapses. (*a*) A 'deaf' synapse (i) expresses NMDA but not functional AMPA receptors. By contrast, a 'vocal' synapse (ii) expresses both receptors. (*b*) The slow exocytosis of glutamate at a 'whispering' synapse reaches a concentration in the cleft that is sufficient to activate high-affinity NMDA receptors but not AMPA receptors. (*c*) glutamate spillover activates NMDA but not AMPA receptors at an 'eaves-dropping' and presynaptically silent synapse (i). The releasing varicosity (ii) is likely to be in synaptic contact with a different neuron, explaining why no AMPA receptor-mediated component is detected.

extremely brief glutamate transient, they might even have similar occupancies, because in this situation their opening probabilities are principally determined by their binding rates, which are generally thought to be similar for the two receptors (Kullmann 1999). This may account for some studies that have yielded similar estimates for AMPA and NMDA receptor occupancy at hippocampal synapses (McAllister and Stevens 2000). However, as the glutamate transient becomes slower, the unbinding and ultimately desensitization rates take on a greater importance. If the glutamate wave is relatively slow, NMDA receptors might be relatively selectively activated by glutamate, because their unbinding and desensitization rates are considerably slower than those of AMPA receptors. This could occur through at least two mechanisms.

First, slow release of glutamate through a fusion pore might allow the agonist to reach a relatively low concentration, which activates NMDA receptors relatively selectively (giving rise to a 'whispering' synapse, Fig. 17.2b). The evidence that such slow release occurs at hippocampal synapses *in situ* is incomplete (Choi *et al.* 2000). Nevertheless, some findings argue that different modes of vesicle cycling do occur (Murthy and Stevens 1998), and that a slow mode of release can be converted to a faster mode (Renger *et al.* 2001). For such a mechanism to occur in LTP (Choi *et al.* 2000) a signal would need to travel to the presynaptic terminal from the postsynaptic spine, which is agreed to be the site of coincidence detection.

Second, a slow wave of glutamate might activate NMDA receptors relatively selectively if the latter are relatively remote from the release site. Diffusion of glutamate could result in sufficient dilution and slowing of the transient to ensure that NMDA receptors are relatively selectively activated, even if AMPA receptors are also present. The evidence for extrasynaptic glutamate escape is overwhelming:

(i) Several subtypes of glutamate receptor (including metabotropic and kainate receptors) are present on axons relatively far from the site of release, and can detect synaptically released glutamate in the hippocampus (Yokoi *et al.* 1996; Shigemoto *et al.* 1996, 1997; Semyanov and Kullmann 2000, 2001; Cossart *et al.* 2001; Jiang *et al.* 2001).

(ii) The principal transporters that clear glutamate from the extracellular space are extrasynaptic (Danbolt 2001).

(iii) The time course of the astrocytic currents associated with their action indicates that glutamate persists in the extracellular space for a relatively long time, therefore allowing the neurotransmitter to diffuse a relatively long distance from the site of release (Bergles *et al.* 1999).

These considerations lead to the expectation that NMDA receptors relatively far from the release sites may be activated. Numerical simulations, moreover, show that, as the distance from the release site increases, the occupancy of NMDA receptors decreases more slowly than that of AMPA receptors (Rusakov and Kullmann 1998; Barbour 2001). This raises the possibility that synaptic signals mediated by NMDA receptors, with little activation of AMPA receptors, may arise from such a spillover (Fig. 17.2c). A potential interpretation of this finding is that cross-talk among neighbouring glutamatergic synapses might even account for much of the silent synapse phenomenon (Kullmann *et al.* 1996; Kullmann and Asztely 1998). Thus, synapses may not be as private as previously assumed, at least for the activation of NMDA receptors. In support of this hypothesis, manipulations of glutamate uptake with changes in temperature and uptake blockers alter the proportion of silent synapses in a pattern that agrees with changes in the extent of glutamate spillover (Asztely *et al.* 1997).

These findings have prompted a re-evaluation of the spatial extent of spillover signalling. Considerable uncertainty surrounds several parameters underlying the release, diffusion and uptake of glutamate (Rusakov and Kullmann 1998; Barbour 2001). Nevertheless, some degree of cross-talk at 'eavesdropping' synapses that occur in close proximity (< 200 nm) is inescapable. This is especially so for those not-infrequent cases where there is no interposed astrocytic process (Spacek 1985; Lehre and Danbolt 1998; Ventura and Harris 1999). Another situation where NMDA receptor-mediated cross-talk is likely to occur is where a single bouton makes two synapses onto different spines (Sorra and Harris 1993): stochastic release at one of the release sites may well result in significant activation of NMDA receptors at both synapses. Finally, abundant extrasynaptic NMDA receptors also occur, many of which are likely to detect extrasynaptic glutamate escape (Charton *et al.* 1999). Whether some of these occur at nascent synapses is open to debate.

17.3 Unsilencing with long-term potentiation

It must be pointed out that the explanations listed in Section 17.2 for silent synapses are not mutually exclusive: it is highly likely that several, if not all, of these possibilities coexist. Nevertheless, how can each model be related to the increase in quantal content that occurs with NMDA receptor-dependent LTP? (All of the following interpretations coexist happily with an increase in quantal amplitude mediated by phosphorylation and/or recruitment of additional AMPA receptors into existing clusters at synapses.)

17.4 AMPA receptor insertion

In the postsynaptically silent synapse model ('deaf synapses') the simplest explanation for unsilencing with LTP is the insertion of AMPA receptor clusters into postsynaptic densities where they are initially absent (Kullmann 1994) (Fig. 17.3*a*). An abundance of evidence for both constitutive and regulated AMPA receptor trafficking to and from the membrane now exists (reviewed by Malinow and Malenka (2002)). Although there is little doubt that AMPA receptor insertion takes place during LTP, and that newly functional receptors contribute to synaptic transmission, there are several apparent discrepancies and missing pieces of evidence.

First, close attention to the pattern of distribution of AMPA receptors among synapses studied with immunogold labelling reveals that only relatively small synapses are devoid of these receptors (Nusser *et al.* 1998; Takumi *et al.* 1999). It has been argued that small synapses (assessed by the dimensions of the postsynaptic density, spine or bouton) have relatively low release probabilities (Harris and Sultan 1995; Schikorski and Stevens 1997). Thus, it is puzzling that silent synapses as identified by electrophysiological recordings are so abundant.

Second, where is the store of latent AMPA receptors? For the quantal content to increase, it is not sufficient for individual receptors to be recruited in a graded manner.

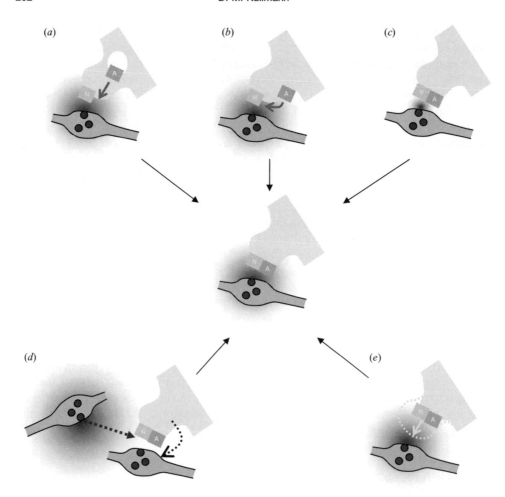

Fig. 17.3 Unsilencing with LTP induction: the possible mechanisms. (*a*) The insertion of a vesicle of AMPA receptors into a deaf synapse. (*b*) Movement of a raft of perisynaptic AMPA receptors into the synaptic cleft. (*c*) A change in the mode of exocytosis could increase the occupancy of AMPA receptors. (*d*) Conversion of a mute eavesdropping synapse by an increase in presynaptic release probability. (*e*) A structural change in a postsynaptic spine could cause it to approach a release site.

This leads to the prediction that vesicles containing multiple receptors (approximately the same number as present in already 'vocal' synapses) should occur under baseline conditions. As yet, no such vesicles have been convincingly revealed with immunogold methods, even though multiple AMPA receptors can be reliably detected in serial sections of the postsynaptic density itself. Some evidence for clustering of AMPA receptors within dendrites has been reported with fluorescent microscopy (Shi *et al.* 1999), but this approach lacks the spatial resolution to determine whether they are pre-packaged in an organelle suited for rapid all-or-none delivery to the synapse. The alternative possibility, that latent receptors are actually loosely scattered in multiple cytoplasmic vesicles before assembly into a cluster, is obviously less attractive, but it

PLATES

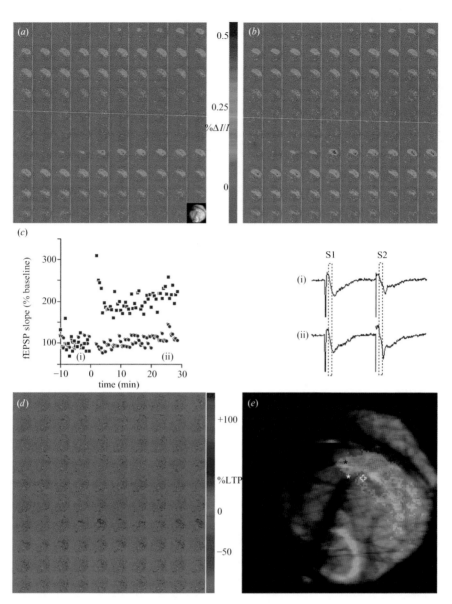

Plate 1. Optical imaging of synaptic responses and potentiation in a hippocampal slice. (*a*) Optical signals in response to two stimuli at 100 ms intervals, just prior to high-frequency stimulation. Images were obtained at 0.6 ms intervals; every third image is shown in this montage, i.e. at intervals of 1.8 ms, reading left to right and top to bottom. (An ordinary image of the slice is visible in the last element of the montage, and at higher magnification in part (*e*), where the positions of the stimulating and recording electrodes are indicated.) The false-colour scale indicates the fractional change in intensity in per cent, %$\Delta I/I$. (*b*) Optical signals recorded as in (*a*), 20 min after high-frequency stimulation applied via the second stimulating electrode. The response to the second stimulus is increased. (*c*) Electrical responses to two-pathway stimulation, recorded prior to, and after, potentiation of the second stimulated pathway. On the left is plotted the fEPSP slope in response to 0.033 Hz stimuli applied to electrode 1 (blue circles) and electrode 2 (red squares). At time 0, a brief high-frequency stimulus was applied via electrode 2, resulting in potentiation of the synaptic response. The traces on the right were obtained at the times labelled (i) and (ii) on the left; the dashed regions correspond to the intervals over which the EPSP slopes were measured. (*d*) Optical image of synaptic potentiation, obtained by frame-by-frame digital subtraction of the series shown in (*a*) from the series in (*b*). The false-colour scale shows the percentage change in the optical signal, %LTP. (*e*) The spatial extent of significant LTP (post-tetanus optical signal more than two standard deviations different from the pretetanus level) is indicated by coloured areas, superimposed on the grey-scale reference image of the slice. False colours correspond to the scale in (*d*). Black and white stars indicate positions of S1 and S2 stimulating electrodes, respectively; the white cross indicates the position of the recording electrode. The filamentous shadows are cast by lens paper on which the slice is mounted in the perfusion chamber. The field of view is 1.7 mm on each side.
(See Chapter 12, p. 136.)

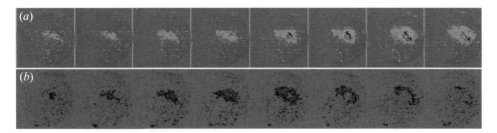

Plate 2. The spatio-temporal pattern of potentiation is not predictable from the pattern of the baseline synaptic response. (*a*) All frames, at 0.6 ms intervals, are now shown of the portion of the optical recording (%$\Delta I/I$) in Fig. 12.1*a* covering the onset of the response to S2. The colour scale is as in Fig. 12.1*a*. (*b*) The equivalent frames at 0.6 ms intervals from the %LTP series of Fig. 12.1(*d*). The potentiation appears as an expanding wavefront. The colour scale is as in Fig. 12.1(*d*). (See Chapter 12, p. 138.)

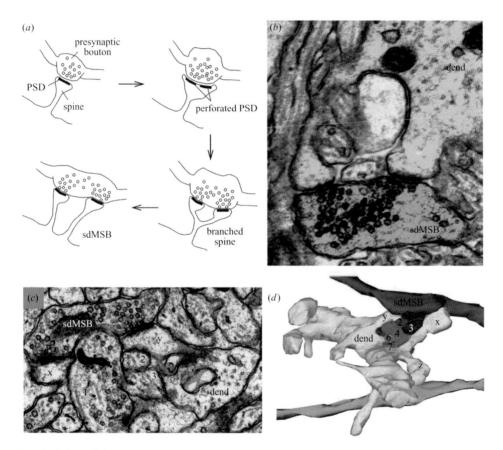

Plate 3. Spine splitting and LTP. (*a*) Model of spine splitting to enhance connectivity between hippocampal neurons. (*b*) Fortuitous longitudinal section through two spines arising from the same dendrite (yellow, dend) to synapse on a multiple synapse bouton (green, sdMSB). (*c,d*) Example section and reconstruction of sdMSB, dendritic spines and parent dendrite that synapse with the sdMSB, and axons (numbered) that pass between the spines that synapse on the sdMSB. One of the spines on the sdMSB is itself branched (x, z) but the two heads synapse on different axons, so that it does not represent synapse splitting. (See Chapter 19, p. 230.)

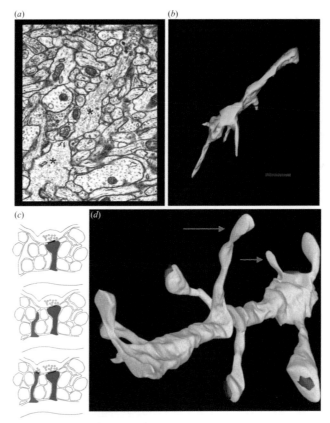

Plate 4. Spine outgrowth to form sdMSBs. (*a*) Axonal growth cone (red asterisks). (*b*) Reconstruction of the axonal growth cone illustrated in (*a*). Scale bar, 0.5 μm. (*c*) Model of spine outgrowth to form sdMSBs. (*d*) Reconstruction of dendritic segment with two non-synaptic dendritic protrusions (yellow arrows). (See Chapter 19, p. 231.)

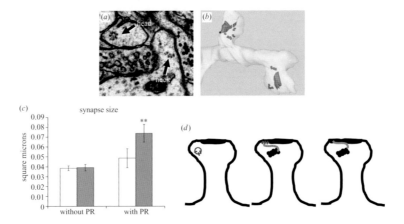

Plate 5. Protein-synthesis-dependent synapse enlargement during LTP. (*a*) Polyribosomes in a dendritic spine head and a different spine neck. (*b*) Three-dimensional reconstruction of dendritic spines containing polyribosomes (grey spheres) and having large synapses (red). (*c*) Spines without polyribosomes had synapses of the same size under both LTP (grey bars) and control (open bars) conditions. Spines with polyribosomes had larger synapses under the LTP condition only (**$p < 0.02$). (*d*) Model illustrating how glutamatergic receptors (blue) located in postsynaptic vesicles (red) are inserted into the plasma membrane soon after induction of LTP. The new protein synthesis then adds postsynaptic density proteins to stabilize these receptors in the membrane. (See Chapter 19, p. 233.)

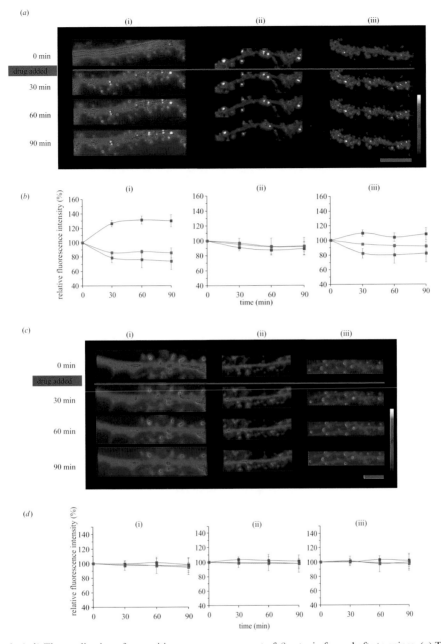

Plate 6. (*a,b*) The application of roscovitine causes a movement of β-catenin from shafts to spines. (*a*) Time-lapse images of EGFP-β-catenin pre- and post-treatment. (i) EGFP–β-catenin treated with roscovitine; (ii) pre-depolarized then treated with roscovitine; and (iii) pre-treated with roscovitine then depolarized. Neurons were treated immediately after *t* = 0. Scale bar, 10 μm. (*b*) Relative fluorescence intensities. Spine region (violet), shaft region (orange) and total (blue). (i) Roscovitine (*n* = 3); (ii) roscovitine (pre-depolarized, *n* = 5); and (iii) depolarization (pre-treated with roscovitine, *n* = 6). (*c,d*) Point mutations at Tyr-654 block roscov-itine-induced EGFP–β-catenin redistribution. (*c*) Time-lapse images of EGFP–β-catenin pre- and post-treatment. (i) EGFP–β-catenin treated with roscovitine in the presence of sodium orthovanadate; (ii) EGFP–Y654E–β-catenin treated with roscovitine; and (iii) EGFP–Y654F–β-catenin treated with roscovitine. Neurons were treated immediately after *t* = 0. Scale bar, 10 μm. (*d*) Relative fluorescence intensities. Spine region (violet), shaft region (orange), and total (blue). (i) EGFP–β-catenin treated with roscovitine in the presence of sodium orthovanadate, *n* = 5; (ii) EGFP–Y654E–β-catenin treated with roscovitine, *n* = 4; and (iii) EGFP–Y654F–β-catenin treated with roscovitine, *n* = 4. (See Chapter 20, p. 242.)

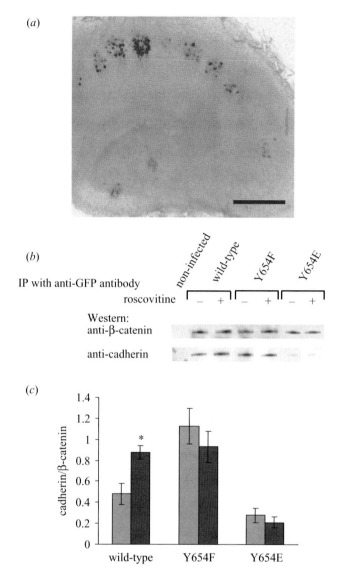

Plate 7. Point mutation at Tyr-654 block roscovitine-induced affinity increase for cadherin. (*a*) An organotypic hippocampal slice expressing EGFP–β-catenin. The DIC and fluorescence images were overlaid. EGFP–β-catenin was introduced via the microinjection of sindbis virus. Scale bar, 500 μm. (*b*) Immunoprecipitation analysis of roscovitine effect on cadherin–β-catenin affinity. Cell lysates from either the wild-type, Y654F- or Y654E-expressing slices were immunoprecipitated with an anti-GFP antibody, and blotted with either anti-β-catenin or anti-cadherin antibodies. Slices were pretreated for 3 hours with either the control medium or medium containing roscovitine. (*c*) Ratios of cadherin : β-catenin band intensities. The wild-type β-catenin showed a significantly increased ratio after roscovitine treatment, whereas Tyr-654 mutants do not (mean±s.e.m., $n = 3$, wildtype; $p < 0.05$, Y654F and Y654E; n.s.). Dark shading, control; light shading, roscovitine. (See Chapter 20, p. 244.)

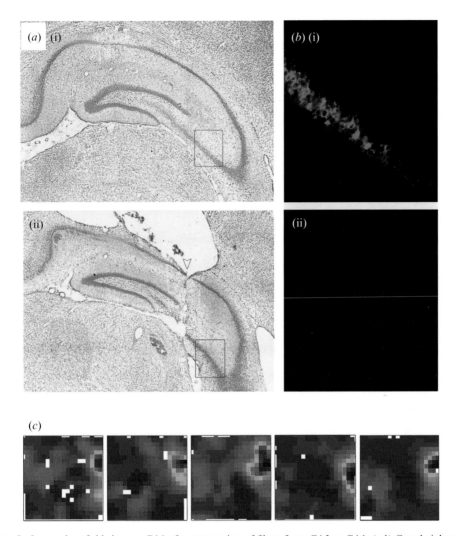

Plate 8. Intact place fields in area CA1 after transection of fibres from CA3 to CA1. (*a,b*) Cresyl violet and fluorescence images from an unlesioned control rat (*a*(i) and *b*(i)) and a rat with CA1 isolated from CA3 by a longitudinal cut (arrowhead) at the border between these subfields (*a*(ii) and *b*(ii)). A retrograde tracer (aminostilbamidine) was infused at the recording position in dorsal CA1 (green). Fluorescence images in (*b*) correspond to red boxes in adjacent left sections in (*a*). (*c*) Colour-coded firing rate map for a cell from the lesioned rat in ((*a*) and (*b*)). The cell was recorded for 5 consecutive days (left to right). Dark red indicates maximum rate (left to right: 8, 12, 12, 17 and 11 Hz). (See Chapter 23, p. 287.)

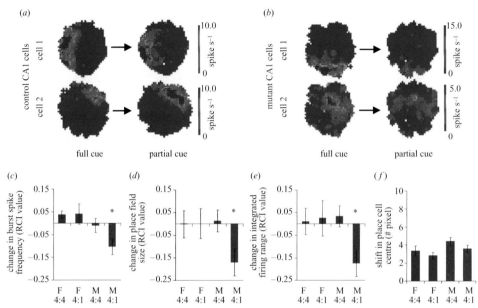

Plate 9. CA1 place cell activity in CA3-NR1 KO mice. (*a,b*) Examples of place fields that are representative of cells that showed no reduction (*fNR1*; (*a*)) and a reduction of field size (mutant; (*b*)) before and after partial cue removal. (*c–e*) Relative change in the place field properties for each cell recorded across two conditions quantified with a relative change index (RCI, defined as the difference between the cell's firing between two conditions divided by the sum of the cell's firing across the two conditions). Among the cells that were identified as the same cells throughout the two recording sessions, the average burst spike frequency ((*c*) $F_{3,140} = 4.16$, $p < 0.007$; Fisher's *post hoc* comparison (mutant 4 : 1 versus all the other three paradigms), *$p < 0.05$), place field size over 1 Hz ((*d*) $F_{3,140} = 2.68$, $p < 0.049$; Fisher's *post hoc* comparison (mutant 4 : 1 versus all the other three paradigms), *$p < 0.05$) and the integrated firing rate ((*e*) $F_{3,140} = 3.20$, $p < 0.025$; Fisher's *post hoc* comparison (mutant 4 : 1 versus all the other three paradigms), *$p < 0.05$) were significantly reduced in the mutant animals (red bars) only after partial cue removal (4 : 1). By contrast, partial cue removal did not affect the CA1 place cell activity in the control mice (blue bars). (*f*) Location of the CA1 place field centre between the two recording sessions was not shifted regardless of genotype and cue manipulation ($F_{3,140} = 2.15$, $p = 0.097$). F, *fNR1* control mice; M, mutant mice. (See Chapter 24, p. 309.)

may be necessary to meet the challenge presented by this model if cytoplasmic clusters continue to evade detection.

Third, a similar argument can be made about intracellular membrane specializations that might be suited for trafficking receptors to the synapse. Although a spine apparatus that might be involved in such trafficking has been reported at some synapses, this is preferentially found at large synapses, that is, those that probably already have AMPA receptors, and not at small synapses that may lack AMPA receptors (Spacek and Harris 1997).

An alternative possibility, that latent clusters of AMPA receptors are already in the membrane, but in an extrasynaptic location (Fig. 17.3b), suffers from similar problems: why have such extrasynaptic clusters not been revealed by immunogold methods?

Finally, methods that have been used to reveal activity-dependent incorporation of AMPA receptors (either physiological or anatomical) have a limited temporal resolution. This leaves open the possibility that AMPA receptor insertion requires several minutes to take place. However, LTP induction takes place only over a few seconds (Gustafsson and Wigstrom 1990). It is difficult to argue that receptor phosphorylation accounts for the very earliest stages of LTP (seconds–minutes), only later being supplemented or replaced by receptor insertion, because the increase in quantal content appears to take place extremely rapidly (Petersen *et al.* 1998).

In summary, although AMPA receptor insertion no doubt occurs during LTP induction, the subcellular location of the reserve store of such receptors remains to be identified unambiguously, and it will be important to narrow the time window during which the phenomenon occurs. Nevertheless, insertion of receptors does not rule out other mechanisms taking place during the earliest stages of LTP.

17.5 Other possible explanations for unsilencing

Compared with the abundance of evidence for receptor trafficking, alternative models for LTP expression that can also explain why synapses become unsilenced are relatively less well supported by experimental data. One simple hypothesis is that a retrograde signal switches on presynaptically silent ('mute') synapses (Fig. 17.3d). NMDA receptors at such synapses may initially be activated by the spillover of glutamate from neighbouring synapses. The coincidence of such NMDA receptor activation with postsynaptic depolarization would cause a retrograde signal (chemical or mechanical) to switch on the presynaptic synapse. This model, although supported by some indirect evidence (Kullmann and Siegelbaum 1995; Kullmann *et al.* 1996), is difficult to reconcile with the finding that synaptic glutamate transporter currents recorded in astrocytes do not change after LTP (Diamond *et al.* 1998; Luscher *et al.* 1998). Another method to detect changes in transmitter release by monitoring presynaptic vesicle cycling also failed to reveal an alteration following LTP induction by conventional stimuli (Zakharenko *et al.* 2001). Surprisingly, an increase was seen after a more intense induction protocol, implying that recruitment of vesicles and/or an increase in release probability at releasing synapses may occur under some special circumstances.

Overall, thus, the evidence that unsilencing normally arises from a presynaptic increase in release probability is not favoured by the balance of evidence. What other explanations remain? One possibility is that the mode of release changes from slow escape of glutamate from a fusion pore to rapid all-or-none release (Fig. 17.3c). This could change the shape of the glutamate transient within the synaptic cleft, and therefore increase the activation of AMPA receptors, without altering significantly either the activation of NMDA receptors or the total amount of glutamate released into the extracellular space. Some indirect evidence for such a phenomenon has been reported (Choi et al. 2000).

Another model that has, thus far, been relatively overlooked, is that LTP is accompanied by a rapid structural modification of the spine and/or presynaptic varicosity that changes the time course of the glutamate transient sensed by the postsynaptic NMDA receptors (Fig. 17.3e). This could occur, for instance, by bringing the pre- and postsynaptic parts of the synapse closer together, or by reducing the escape of glutamate from the synaptic cleft. Growth of a spine or filopodial extension expressing receptors towards an existing release site would give a similar result. A cluster of receptors at such a nascent synapse could, under appropriate conditions initially detect glutamate release exclusively via NMDA receptors, and would therefore behave as a silent synapse. As the distance between the postsynaptic process and release site decreased, the AMPA receptors would begin to respond to glutamate. This model does not require changes in either the amount or mode or presynaptic transmitter release, neither does it depend on alterations in AMPA receptor expression. Interestingly, it could account for the observation that LTP is not exclusively expressed by AMPA receptors: a consistent, albeit smaller, increase in the NMDA receptor-mediated component has been reported to occur with either tetanus- or pairing-induced LTP (Asztely et al. 1992; Kullmann et al. 1996). LTP of isolated NMDA receptor-mediated EPSCs has, moreover, been reported by several groups (Tsien and Malinow 1990; Bashir et al. 1991). A simple explanation of this is that NMDA receptors are brought physically closer to the site of release by the structural changes. However, alternative possibilities such as changes in their phosphorylation state or insertion into postsynaptic densities cannot be ruled out.

Although there is evidence for structural rearrangements accompanying LTP, these have generally been detected over tens of minutes (Hosokawa et al. 1995; Engert and Bonhoeffer 1999; Toni et al. 1999). Nevertheless, this may reflect a trade-off of spatial and temporal resolution: large changes in receptor occupancy occur over sub-micrometre distances in the neuropil, which may fall below the threshold for detection with available methods.

17.6 Conclusion

The silent synapse phenomenon is a major impetus for studying the mechanisms that deliver receptors to synapses. Although the evidence for AMPA receptor insertion during LTP is overwhelming, several steps in this cascade remain to be documented, including the identity and location of the store of reserve receptors and the speed by which this is achieved. Moreover, the absence of AMPA receptors at synapses is not the only possible explanation for silent synapses: the very distinct kinetics of NMDA receptors raise the possibility that glutamate spillover and/or fusion-pore release give rise to selective activation of these receptors at synapses that contain both species.

These models also prompt the possibility of some alternative mechanisms for LTP expression, which rely on alterations in the mode of transmitter release or structural changes in the vicinity of release sites, which result in the functional recruitment of AMPA receptors that are insufficiently sensitive to detect glutamate under baseline conditions. Ultimately, silent synapses may result from multiple mechanisms. The relative importance of these mechanisms, and their implications for the earliest steps in LTP expression, remain to be elucidated.

References

Asztely, F., Wigstrom, H., and Gustafsson, B. (1992). The relative contribution of NMDA receptor channels in the expression of long-term potentiation in the hippocampal CA1 region. *Eur. J. Neurosci.* **4**, 681–90.

Asztely, F., Erdemli, G., and Kullmann, D. M. (1997). Extrasynaptic glutamate spillover in the hippocampus: dependence on temperature and the role of active glutamate uptake. *Neuron* **18**, 281–93.

Barbour, B. (2001). An evaluation of synapse independence. *J. Neurosci.* **21**, 7969–84.

Bashir, Z. I., Alford, S., Davies, S. N., Randall, A. D., and Collingridge, G. L. (1991). Long-term potentiation of NMDA receptor-mediated synaptic transmission in the hippocampus. *Nature* **349**, 156–8.

Bekkers, J. M. and Stevens, C. F. (1990). Presynaptic mechanism for long-term potentiation in the hippocampus. *Nature* **346**, 724–9.

Bergles, D. E., Diamond, J. S., and Jahr, C. E. (1999). Clearance of glutamate inside the synapse and beyond. *Curr. Opin. Neurobiol.* **9**, 293–8.

Charton, J. P., Herkert, M., Becker, C. M., and Schroder, H. (1999). Cellular and subcellular localization of the 2B-subunit of the NMDA receptor in the adult rat telencephalon. *Brain Res.* **816**, 609–17.

Choi, S., Klingauf, J., and Tsien, R. W. (2000). Postfusional regulation of cleft glutamate concentration during LTP at 'silent synapses'. *Nature Neurosci.* **3**, 330–6.

Cossart, R., Tyzio, R., Dinocourt, C., Esclapez, M., Hirsch, J. C., Ben-Ari, Y., *et al.* (2001). Presynaptic kainate receptors that enhance the release of GABA on CA1 hippocampal interneurons. *Neuron* **29**, 497–508.

Danbolt, N. C. (2001). Glutamate uptake. *Prog. Neurobiol.* **65**, 1–105.

Diamond, J. S., Bergles, D. E., and Jahr, C. E. (1998). Glutamate release monitored with astrocyte transporter currents during LTP. *Neuron* **21**, 425–33.

Durand, G. M., Kovalchuk, Y., and Konnerth, A. (1996). Long-term potentiation and functional synapse induction in developing hippocampus. *Nature* **381**, 71–5.

Engert, F. and Bonhoeffer, T. (1999). Dendritic spine changes associated with hippocampal long-term synaptic plasticity. *Nature* **399**, 66–70.

Gustafsson, B. and Wigstrom, H. (1990). Long-term potentiation in the hippocampal CA1 region: its induction and early temporal development. *Prog. Brain Res.* **83**, 223–32.

Harris, K. M. and Sultan, P. (1995). Variation in the number, location and size of synaptic vesicles provides an anatomical basis for the nonuniform probability of release at hippocampal CA1 synapses. *Neuropharmacology* **34**, 1387–95.

Hosokawa, T., Rusakov, D. A., Bliss, T. V., and Fine, A. (1995). Repeated confocal imaging of individual dendritic spines in the living hippocampal slice: evidence for changes in length and orientation associated with chemically induced LTP. *J. Neurosci.* **15**, 5560–73.

Isaac, J. T., Nicoll, R. A., and Malenka, R. C. (1995). Evidence for silent synapses: implications for the expression of LTP. *Neuron* **15**, 427–34.

Jiang, L., Xu, J., Nedergaard, M., and Kang, J. (2001). A kainate receptor increases the efficacy of gabaergic synapses. *Neuron* **30**, 503–13.

Jonas, P., Major, G., and Sakmann, B. (1993). Quantal components of unitary EPSCs at the mossy fibre synapse on CA3 pyramidal cells of rat hippocampus. *J. Physiol.* (*Lond.*) **472**, 615–63.

Kauer, J. A., Malenka, R. C., and Nicoll, R. A. (1988). A persistent postsynaptic modification mediates long-term potentiation in the hippocampus. *Neuron* **1**, 911–17.

Kullmann, D. M. (1994). Amplitude fluctuations of dual-component EPSCs in hippocampal pyramidal cells: implications for long-term potentiation. *Neuron* **12**, 1111–20.

Kullmann, D. M. (1999). Excitatory synapses. Neither too loud nor too quiet. *Nature* **399**, 111–12.

Kullmann, D. M. and Asztely, F. (1998). Extrasynaptic glutamate spillover in the hippocampus: evidence and implications. *Trends Neurosci.* **21**, 8–14.

Kullmann, D. M. and Nicoll, R. A. (1992). Long-term potentiation is associated with increases in quantal content and quantal amplitude. *Nature* **357**, 240–4.

Kullmann, D. M. and Siegelbaum, S. A. (1995). The site of expression of NMDA receptor-dependent LTP: new fuel for an old fire. *Neuron* **15**, 997–1002.

Kullmann, D. M., Erdemli, G., and Asztely, F. (1996). LTP of AMPA and NMDA receptor-mediated signals: evidence for presynaptic expression and extrasynaptic glutamate spillover. *Neuron* **17**, 461–74.

Larkman, A., Hannay, T., Stratford, K., and Jack, J. (1992). Presynaptic release probability influences the locus of long-term potentiation. *Nature* **360**, 70–3.

Lehre, K. P. and Danbolt, N. C. (1998). The number of glutamate transporter subtype molecules at glutamatergic synapses: chemical and stereological quantification in young adult rat brain. *J. Neurosci.* **18**, 8751–7.

Lester, R. A., Clements, J. D., Westbrook, G. L., and Jahr, C. E. (1990). Channel kinetics determine the time course of NMDA receptor-mediated synaptic currents. *Nature* **346**, 565–7.

Liao, D., Jones, A., and Malinow, R. (1992). Direct measurement of quantal changes underlying long-term potentiation in CA1 hippocampus. *Neuron* **9**, 1089–97.

Liao, D., Hessler, N. A., and Malinow, R. (1995). Activation of postsynaptically silent synapses during pairing-induced LTP in CA1 region of hippocampal slice. *Nature* **375**, 400–4.

Luscher, C., Malenka, R. C., and Nicoll, R. A. (1998). Monitoring glutamate release during LTP with glial transporter currents. *Neuron* **21**, 435–41.

McAllister, A. K. and Stevens, C. F. (2000). Nonsaturation of AMPA and NMDA receptors at hippocampal synapses. *Proc. Natl Acad. Sci. USA* **97**, 6173–8.

Malenka, R. C. and Nicoll, R. A. (1999). Long-term potentiation—a decade of progress? *Science* **285**, 1870–4.

Malinow, R. and Malenka, R. C. (2002). AMPA receptor trafficking and synaptic plasticity. *A. Rev. Neurosci.* **25**, 103–26.

Malinow, R. and Tsien, R. W. (1990). Presynaptic enhancement shown by whole-cell recordings of long-term potentiation in hippocampal slices. *Nature* **346**, 177–80.

Montgomery, J. M., Pavlidis, P., and Madison, D. V. (2001). Pair recordings reveal all-silent synaptic connections and the postsynaptic expression of long-term potentiation. *Neuron* **29**, 691–701.

Muller, D. and Lynch, G. (1988). Long-term potentiation differentially affects two components of synaptic responses in hippocampus. *Proc. Natl Acad. Sci. USA* **85**, 9346–50.

Murthy, V. N. and Stevens, C. F. (1998). Synaptic vesicles retain their identity through the endocytic cycle. *Nature* **392**, 497–501.

Nusser, Z., Lujan, R., Laube, G., Roberts, J. D., Molnar, E., and Somogyi, P. (1998). Cell type and pathway dependence of synaptic AMPA receptor number and variability in the hippocampus. *Neuron* **21**, 545–59.

Patneau, D. K. and Mayer, M. L. (1990). Structure–activity relationships for amino acid transmitter candidates acting at N-methyl-d-aspartate and quisqualate receptors. *J. Neurosci.* **10**, 2385–99.

Perkel, D. J. and Nicoll, R. A. (1993). Evidence for all-or-none regulation of neurotransmitter release: implications for longterm potentiation. *J. Physiol.* **471**, 481–500.

Petersen, C. C., Malenka, R. C., Nicoll, R. A., and Hopfield, J. J. (1998). All-or-none potentiation at CA3-CA1 synapses. *Proc. Natl Acad. Sci. USA* **95**, 4732–7.

Racca, C., Stephenson, F. A., Streit, P., Roberts, J. D., and Somogyi, P. (2000). NMDA receptor content of synapses in stratum radiatum of the hippocampal CA1 area. *J. Neurosci.* **20**, 2512–22.

Renger, J. J., Egles, C., and Liu, G. (2001). A developmental switch in neurotransmitter flux enhances synaptic efficacy by affecting AMPA receptor activation. *Neuron* **29**, 469–84.

Rusakov, D. A. and Kullmann, D. M. (1998). Extrasynaptic glutamate diffusion in the hippocampus: ultrastructural constraints, uptake, and receptor activation. *J. Neurosci.* **18**, 3158–70.

Schikorski, T. and Stevens, C. F. (1997). Quantitative ultra-structural analysis of hippocampal excitatory synapses. *J. Neurosci.* **17**, 5858–67.

Selig, D. K., Hjelmstad, G. O., Herron, C., Nicoll, R. A., and Malenka, R. C. (1995). Independent mechanisms for long-term depression of AMPA and NMDA responses. *Neuron* **15**, 417–26.

Semyanov, A. and Kullmann, D. M. (2000). Modulation of GABAergic signaling among interneurons by metabotropic glutamate receptors. *Neuron* **25**, 663–72.

Semyanov, A. and Kullmann, D. M. (2001). Kainate receptor-dependent axonal depolarization and action potential initiation in interneurons. *Nature Neurosci.* **4**, 718–23.

Shi, S. H., Hayashi, Y., Petralia, R. S., Zaman, S. H., Wenthold, R. J., Svoboda, K., *et al.* (1999). Rapid spine delivery and redistribution of AMPA receptors after synaptic NMDA receptor activation. *Science* **284**, 1811–16.

Shigemoto, R., Kulik, A., Roberts, J. D., Ohishi, H., Nusser, Z., Kaneko, T., *et al.* (1996). Target-cell-specific concentration of a metabotropic glutamate receptor in the presynaptic active zone. *Nature* **381**, 523–5.

Shigemoto, R., Kinoshita, A., Wada, E., Nomura, S., Ohishi, H., Takada, M., *et al.* (1997). Differential presynaptic localization of metabotropic glutamate receptor subtypes in the rat hippocampus. *J. Neurosci.* **17**, 7503–22.

Sorra, K. E. and Harris, K. M. (1993). Occurrence and three-dimensional structure of multiple synapses between individ- *Phil. Trans. R. Soc. Lond.* B (2003) ual radiatum axons and their target pyramidal cells in hippocampal area CA1. *J. Neurosci.* **13**, 3736–48.

Spacek, J. (1985). Three-dimensional analysis of dendritic spines. III. Glial sheath. *Anat. Embryol.* **171**, 245–52.

Spacek, J. and Harris, K. M. (1997). Three-dimensional organization of smooth endoplasmic reticulum in hippocampal CA1 dendrites and dendritic spines of the immature and mature rat. *J. Neurosci.* **17**, 190–203.

Takumi, Y., Ramirez-Leon, V., Laake, P., Rinvik, E., and Ottersen, O. P. (1999). Different modes of expression of AMPA and NMDA receptors in hippocampal synapses. *Nature Neurosci.* **2**, 618–24.

Toni, N., Buchs, P. A., Nikonenko, I., Bron, C. R., and Muller, D. (1999). LTP promotes formation of multiple spine synapses between a single axon terminal and a dendrite. *Nature* **402**, 421–5.

Tsien, R. W. and Malinow, R. (1990). Long-term potentiation: presynaptic enhancement following postsynaptic activation of Ca(+ +)-dependent protein kinases. *Cold Spring Harbor Symp. Quantitative Biol.* **55**, 147–59.

Ventura, R. and Harris, K. M. (1999). Three-dimensional relationships between hippocampal synapses and astrocytes. *J. Neurosci.* **19**, 6897–906.

Voronin, L. L. (1994). Quantal analysis of hippocampal long-term potentiation. *Rev. Neurosci.* **5**, 141–70.

Yokoi, M., Kobayashi, K., Manabe, T., Takahashi, T., Sakaguchi, I., Katsuura, G., *et al.* (1996). Impairment of hippocampal mossy fiber LTD in mice lacking mGluR2. *Science* **273**, 645–7.

Zakharenko, S. S., Zablow, L., and Siegelbaum, S. A. (2001). Visualization of changes in presynaptic function during longterm synaptic plasticity. *Nature Neurosci.* **4**, 711–17.

Glossary

AMPA	α-amino-3-hydroxy-5-methyl-4-isoxazole propionic acid
CV	coefficient of variation
EPSC	excitatory postsynaptic current
LTP	long-term potentiation
NMDA	N-methyl-D-aspartate

Persistence

18

How long will long-term potentiation last?

Wickliffe C. Abraham

The paramount feature of long-term potentiation (LTP) as a memory mechanism is its characteristic persistence over time. Although the basic phenomenology of LTP persistence was established 30 years ago, new insights have emerged recently about the extent of LTP persistence and its regulation by activity and experience. It is now evident that LTP, at least in the dentate gyrus, can either be decremental, lasting from hours to weeks, or stable, lasting months or longer. Although mechanisms engaged during the induction of LTP regulate its subsequent persistence, the maintenance of LTP is also governed by activity patterns post-induction, whether induced experimentally or generated by experience. These new findings establish dentate gyrus LTP as a useful model system for studying the mechanisms governing the induction, maintenance and interference with long-term memory, including very long-term memory lasting months or longer. The challenge is to study LTP persistence in other brain areas, and to relate, if possible, the properties and regulation of LTP maintenance to these same properties of the information that is actually stored in those regions.

Keywords: long-term potentiation; hippocampus; maintenance mechanisms; enriched environment; neurogenesis; metaplasticity

Since the pioneering studies performed 30 years ago by Tim Bliss, Terje Lømo, and Tony Gardner-Medwin (Bliss and Lømo 1973; Bliss and Gardner-Medwin 1973), LTP has generated enormous interest as a potential memory mechanism. This is because LTP exhibits numerous properties expected of an associative memory mechanism, such as rapid induction, input specificity, associative interactions, persistence, and dependence on correlated pre- and postsynaptic activity. The close similarity between these features and those of the learning rule of Hebb (1949) has added lustre to the LTP phenomenon. In addition, there is important yet complex regulation of LTP by prior synaptic activity (metaplasticity), neighbouring afferents (e.g. synaptic tagging), and state variables such as levels of stress hormones and activity in neuromodulatory transmitter systems (see Martin *et al.* (2000) for a review of these properties of LTP). It can be argued, however, that among all these intriguing and important characteristics, the paramount feature that defines LTP as a potential memory mechanism is its persistence over time. Thus, although short-lasting frequency potentiation of synaptic potentials was described in the hippocampus many years ago, it was not until the discovery of LTP that researchers seriously considered that a model system for studying synaptic mechanisms of mammalian memory had been established. It is curious, therefore, that despite the fundamental importance of LTP maintenance over days and weeks, relatively few studies have addressed its mechanisms and regulation. The purpose of this review is to summarize the data from experiments charting how long LTP can last, and then to address the factors that regulate how long LTP will in fact persist under various conditions. Finally, I briefly discuss the relation of LTP persistence to memory retention, and pose some key questions for future research on the mechanisms and behavioural relevance of the maintenance of LTP.

18.1 How long *can* LTP persist?

(a) Early studies of LTP persistence

Bliss and Gardner-Medwin (1973) pioneered the use of field potential recordings in the dentate gyrus of awake animals to investigate the persistence of LTP. This preparation remains the method of choice for studying LTP in freely moving animals, probably because the large iso-potential region in the dentate hilus allows a certain tolerance of recording electrode movement over time without significantly affecting the stability of the field recordings. The principal finding of this early report was that one bout of stimulation could induce LTP in the rabbit dentate gyrus lasting up to 3 days. However, it was noted that this might not be the limit, because in one animal, repeated episodes of stimulation resulted in LTP of the population spike lasting 16 weeks. Subsequent studies from several laboratories confirmed in rats that LTP can indeed last from less than a day to many weeks, depending on the stimulation protocol (Barnes 1979; Racine *et al.* 1983; Barnes and McNaughton 1985; de Jonge and Racine 1985; Staubli and Lynch 1987; Jeffery *et al.* 1990; Abraham *et al.* 1993).

More mechanistic studies of LTP persistence, occurring in parallel with the descriptive ones above, showed that LTP has at least two stages of maintenance: early-LTP which is dependent on post-translational modifications and lasts for, at most, a few hours, followed by a late LTP which is dependent on *de novo* gene expression and protein synthesis and which lasts for many hours (Krug *et al.* 1984; Otani *et al.* 1989; Nguyen *et al.* 1994). However, studies in chronically recorded animals where negative exponential functions have been fitted to the LTP decay data have revealed that, in addition to the early LTP which decays with a time constant of 2–3 h (Racine *et al.* 1983; Abraham and Otani 1991), there are at least two distinct families of late-LTP decay functions, with average decay time constants of around 3.5 and 25 days, respectively (Abraham and Otani 1991; Abraham *et al.* 1993; Fig. 18.1). For convenience, these families of decay functions were termed LTP1, LTP2, and LTP3 (Racine *et al.* 1983; Abraham and Otani 1991), with the suggestion that LTP3 may be more dependent on transcription than the other forms. Regardless of how LTP persistence is best categorized, an important conclusion from these studies, after the first two decades of research, was that LTP in the dentate gyrus was decremental, that is, it eventually returned to baseline even if it took many weeks to do so (Fig. 18.1; Abraham and Otani 1991; Abraham *et al.* 1995; Abraham 2000). An identical conclusion was reached for heterosynaptic LTD in the dentate gyrus, which decays in parallel with the LTP induced simultaneously on the stimulated pathway (Abraham *et al.* 1994). Furthermore, the fact that control recordings in non-tetanized pathways could be stably maintained for the same period of time, and that LTP could be reinstated to the original level with a second bout of HFS meant that the decline of recorded LTP over time was in fact due to its decay, and not due to recording instabilities that sometimes occur during long-term recordings (de Jonge and Racine 1985; Abraham *et al.* 1995).

(b) Recent developments

The relatively simple view of LTP persistence outlined above has been challenged in recent years in two ways. First, two forms of LTP intermediate between the early and

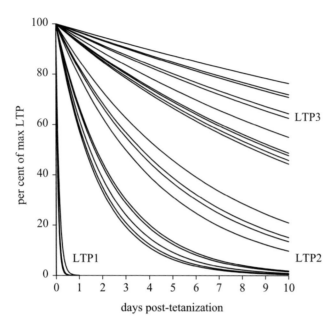

per cent of max LTP

days post-tetanization

Fig. 18.1 Dentate gyrus LTP decay curves obtained from a survey of the literature by Abraham and Otani (1991). Three families of curves were identified and calculated to have average decay time constants of 2.1 h, 3.5 days and 20.3 days. They were termed LTP1, LTP2 and LTP3, respectively. LTP1 is protein-synthesis independent, and corresponds to early-phase LTP in the more commonly used terminology. LTP2 and LTP3 both fall in the category of late-phase LTP. These and other data indicate that late LTP may involve more than one set of mechanisms that determine its persistence. (Curves were redrawn from the table of decay constants reported by Abraham and Otani (1991).)

late phases have been described: one protein synthesis-independent (Winder *et al.* 1998), the other dependent on translational but not transcriptional processes (Raymond *et al.* 2000). The latter study confirmed a previous finding made in anaesthetized animals (Otani *et al.* 1989).

Second, there is evidence that LTP may not necessarily be decremental. Staubli and Lynch (1987) first described non-decremental LTP lasting at least several weeks in area CA1 of the hippocampus. More recently, we have shown that even dentate gyrus synapses, under the right conditions, have the capacity for stable LTP lasting at least many months, and in one case up to a year (Abraham *et al.* 2002; Fig. 18.2). These latter studies are particularly important because they demonstrate that LTP has the capacity to be extremely stable, thus expanding the temporal range of memories that can, in principle, be supported by this mechanism (see below for further discussion). Another implication of this growing diversity of LTP persistence functions, however, is that multiple mechanisms undoubtedly contribute to the maintenance of LTP, thus complicating studies of its regulation and its molecular or anatomical expression mechanisms.

(c) LTP across brain regions

Although dentate gyrus synapses provide a useful model system for studying LTP properties, it seems likely that the persistence of LTP will vary across brain regions,

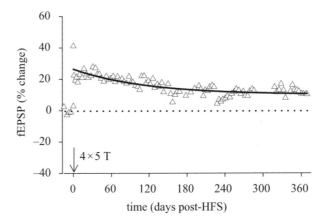

Fig. 18.2 One year LTP in the dentate gyrus of a single animal given four bouts of five trains (4 × 5 T) of high-frequency stimulation, spaced 5 min apart. The fEPSP slope values have been normalized with respect to the values obtained in the control non-tetanized hemisphere. The solid line describes the single negative exponential function fitted to the LTP maintenance data. The asymptote of this function was 10% above the original baseline value. (Data were taken, with permission, from Abraham *et al.* (2002).)

perhaps according to the information processing requirements of those regions. For example, it has been proposed from computational models that learning-related LTP in the dentate gyrus should be relatively transient under normal circumstances, owing to erasure by heterosynaptic LTD or depotentiation as elicited by subsequent experiences (Rolls 1996*b*). In agreement with this idea, most studies have observed decremental LTP in the dentate gyrus, as reviewed above, and heterosynaptic LTD can indeed readily erase LTP in the dentate gyrus of awake animals (cf. Fig. 18.3). In contrast, it has been suggested that memory storage, and thus LTP, should be longer lasting in areas CA3 and CA1 of the hippocampus (Granger *et al.* 1996). Furthermore, neo-cortical LTP is predicted to be even more persistent than hippocampal LTP, because cortically based memories that are dependent on the hippocampus consolidate and lose that dependence over time, presumably because the relevant neocortical representations become sufficiently integrated and stable to permit accurate retrieval without assistance from the hippocampus (Milner 1989; McClelland *et al.* 1995).

Unfortunately, there are few studies of LTP persistence outside the dentate gyrus by which to test the above predictions. The Schaffer collateral synapses in area CA1 have generally been reported to show decremental LTP (Buzsáki 1980; Leung and Shen 1995), but they do appear to have the capacity for stable LTP lasting for weeks (Staubli and Lynch 1987), even when induced by relatively mild HFS such as theta-burst stimulation. Interestingly, in our investigations, such stimulation fails to elicit any LTP at all in the dentate gyrus of awake animals (Abraham and Logan 2000). It is possible, therefore, that CA1 has a lower threshold for exhibiting stable LTP, and this may reflect differences in the normal information storage functions of these regions. Curiously, there have been no studies of LTP persistence in area CA3 of the hippo-campus, despite its prominence as an auto-associative memory store in many models (McClelland *et al.* 1995; Rolls 1996*a,b*).

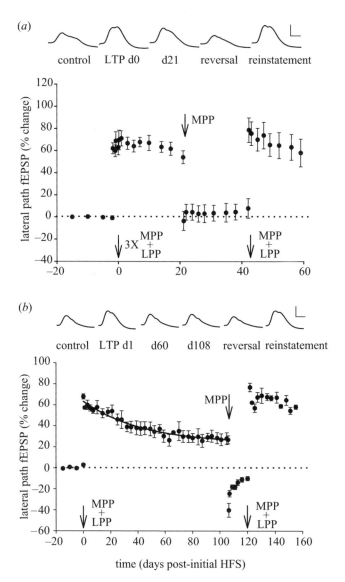

Fig. 18.3 Induction, reversal and reinstatement of stable LTP. (*a*) LTP at lateral perforant path synapses was induced by combined medial and lateral HFS on three consecutive days (to saturate LTP). The LTP met our criteria for stability (Abraham *et al.* 2002) in all six cases. LTP was completely reversed by heterosynaptic HFS of the medial path alone, but could be reinstated to its original level 2 weeks later by another combined HFS. Lateral path waveforms are averages of 30 sweeps taken before the initial HFS (control), 60 min following the third combined HFS (d0), day 21 post-HFS (d21), 2 weeks following LTP reversal, and 60 min following LTP reinstatement, for an individual animal. Data are mean ± s.e.m. Scale bars: 5 mV, 5 ms. (*b*) Lateral path data for four animals that showed stable LTP following a single combined HFS. At 108 days post-HFS, tetanization of the medial path alone caused reversal of the lateral path LTP. Two weeks later, stable LTP was reinstated by combined stimulation of the medial and lateral paths. Lateral path waveforms are averages of 30 sweeps taken from an individual animal. Averages were taken just prior to tetanization (control), and on days 1, 60 and 108 post-HFS, day 1 post-reversal and day 14 post-reinstatement. Data are mean ± s.e.m. Scale bars: 5 mV, 5 ms.

The persistence of neocortical LTP has been studied by Racine and colleagues, using callosal projections to sensorimotor cortex in awake animals as a model system. In this preparation, persistent LTP appears to require multiple stimulation episodes delivered across many days (Racine *et al.* 1995). This LTP, once established, lasts for many weeks, although the full scope of its persistence has not yet been charted (Trepel and Racine 1998). None the less, the data are at least superficially consistent with views that the neocortex is a slow learner, requiring repeated training or stimulation episodes for long-term synaptic change (Marr 1971; Milner 1989; McClelland *et al.* 1995). It is notable too, that visual cortical synapses can utilize LTP-like mechanisms to adapt to altered visual experience during early development, and that these synaptic connections then become relatively 'hard-wired' and resistant to change once the developmental sensitive period finishes (Olson and Freeman 1980; Wiesel 1982). Insofar as LTP indeed contributes to such experience-dependent plasticity, the extreme persistence of the changes suggests that LTP in the neocortex has a remarkable capacity for durability. One caveat of the LTP studies, however, is that white matter stimulation is less efficacious at inducing neocortical synaptic plasticity *in vitro* than intracortical stimulation, which can generate robust LTP after a single HFS (Kirkwood *et al.* 1993). Thus, neocortical synapses may also have the capacity for rapid plasticity, and therefore rapid learning. Verifying whether rapid LTP occurs *in vivo* may require the development of new stimulation protocols in this preparation, although evidence from other conditioning paradigms already suggests this is indeed the case (Frégnac *et al.* 1998).

18.2 How Long *will* LTP persist?

The diversity of LTP persistence across protocols and brain areas indicates that this key property of LTP is likely to be under complex regulation. Indeed, despite what the capacity for LTP maintenance may be under optimal conditions, the actual persistence of LTP is in fact sensitive to a host of regulatory events occurring not only during the induction protocol, but also preceding and following LTP establishment. Those regulatory events that specifically affect the late phase(s) of LTP will be reviewed below, and where known, the mechanisms underlying this regulation will be outlined.

(a) Protocol and state variables affecting the induction of persistent LTP

One key protocol variable that determines how long LTP in the dentate gyrus will persist is the number of HFS trains delivered. Repetition of trains on one day, or across consecutive days, increases the persistence of LTP (Bliss and Gardner-Medwin 1973; Barnes 1979; Jeffery *et al.* 1990; Abraham *et al.* 1993; Abraham *et al.* 2002), although there may be a limit to the duration of LTP that can be generated by repetition of a particular HFS protocol (Abraham *et al.* 1995). The frequency at which multiple trains are delivered is another key variable, as delivery of the trains spaced at 5–10 min intervals generates more persistent LTP than massed delivery (Huang and Kandel 1994; Abraham *et al.* 2002). Repetition of the HFS prolongs LTP maintenance by promoting activation of the protein synthesis processes for late-phase LTP (Huang and Kandel 1994), but the reason why these processes are sensitive to the number and timing of the stimulus trains remains unclear.

A protocol variable that appears to regulate whether stable LTP will last stably over months is the amount of time the animal spends in the recording chamber before and after HFS. As far as can be ascertained, the previous studies reporting decremental LTP in the dentate gyrus, including our own, kept animals in the recording chambers for around 10–20 min before and after HFS. By contrast, in a recent study of stable LTP carried out in my laboratory, animals were given at least 30 min in the recording chamber before HFS, and 60 min after, before being returned to their home cage (Abraham et al. 2002). A direct comparison of such short- and long-baseline protocols revealed this to be an important factor determining whether stable LTP was generated. This comparison also revealed that HFS in the longer baseline protocol was more efficient at causing phosphorylation of CREB on serine133, although the expression of another LTP-related inducible transcription factor, Zif268, was not affected (Abraham et al. 2002). This finding is consistent with other evidence that CREB phosphorylation is a key intermediate step in activating the transcriptional processes necessary for late-phase LTP (Bourtchouladze et al. 1994; Davis et al. 2000). Unfortunately, it is not yet clear why the length of time in the recording chamber should make such a difference to CREB phosphorylation and the maintenance of LTP. It is tempting to speculate that, despite the animals being well habituated to the handling and movement associated with making recordings, the small stress or behavioural arousal associated with these procedures was enough to affect the mechanisms of LTP consolidation when experienced shortly before, or after, HFS. However, further investigation is required before deciding whether this is the critical intervening variable.

A key state variable at the time of induction that affects subsequent LTP persistence is the level of activity in neuromodulatory inputs to the hippocampus, such as the dopaminergic and noradrenergic afferents. Several studies have shown that generation of the late-phase of CA1 LTP is critically dependent on activation of D1/D5 dopamine receptors, both in vitro and in vivo (Frey et al. 1990; Swanson-Park et al. 1999). Whether activation of D1/D5 receptors is sufficient to induce late-phase LTP is more debatable (Huang and Kandel 1995; Swanson-Park et al. 1999), and it is likely that late-phase LTP requires coactivation of both dopamine and NMDA receptors. Because D1/D5 receptors couple to G_s-proteins, one such coincidence detector could be Type I adenylyl cyclase, which is activated by both calcium and G_s-proteins. Gene transcription and protein synthesis could then be triggered through the cAMP, protein kinase A, phosphoCREB pathway. Interestingly, D1/D5 receptors do not regulate LTP persistence in the dentate gyrus. Instead this role appears to be played by β-adrenergic receptors, although this action can be obscured by the fact that β-adrenergic receptors also regulate the induction of early-phase LTP (Swanson-Park et al. 1999). None the less, treatments that specifically lead to more persistent LTP in the dentate gyrus, such as stimulation of the basolateral amygdala and the behavioural access to reinforcing or punishing stimuli, have been shown to act through stimulation of β-adrenergic receptors (Seidenbecher et al. 1997; Frey et al. 2001). This activation needs to occur within a fairly narrow time-window flanking the induction of LTP. It is possible that it is through downregulation of these neuromodulatory transmitter systems that the general anaesthetic pentobarbital, when administered just during the time of HFS, reduces both gene expression and LTP maintenance (Jeffery et al. 1990).

(b) Anterograde regulation of LTP persistence

Both positive and negative regulation of LTP persistence can be generated by synaptic activation occurring before the induction of LTP. For example, activation of synapses by a low-frequency (5 Hz) train of 900 pulses has been shown, in CA1 slices, to inhibit the subsequent induction of late-phase LTP by multi-train HFS, without affecting the early phase (Woo and Nguyen 2002). This represents an interesting form of meta-plasticity, i.e., the regulation of plasticity by prior activity (Abraham and Bear 1996), in that it selectively downregulates the late-phase. This regulation requires activation of NMDA receptors during the LFS followed by upregulation of protein phosphatase 1/2a activity (Woo and Nguyen 2002). The downstream effect of increased phosphatase activity may be to prevent or reverse CREB phosphorylation, which is PP1 sensitive (Hagiwara *et al.* 1992), although phosphatase modulation of other key signalling molecules such as extracellular signal-related kinase ERK or protein kinase C may also be important.

Heterosynaptic upregulation of LTP persistence by prior activity has also been reported. Thus, when strong HFS sufficient to induce late-phase LTP is delivered to one afferent pathway in CA1, the induction of late-phase LTP is then primed for all other synapses on the same cell. This means that subsequent delivery to a second pathway of a weak HFS that normally generates only early-phase LTP will elicit late-phase LTP instead (Frey and Morris 1997). The priming effect can persist for at least 30 min, and the postulated mechanism is that the weakly activated synapses are tagged in such a way that they can somehow capture the proteins previously synthesized in response to strong activation of other synapses for use in establishing their own late-phase LTP. This interpretation has been termed the synaptic tag hypothesis (Frey and Morris 1997).

(c) Retrograde regulation of LTP persistence

Once triggered, the induction process for LTP occurs within seconds (Gustafsson *et al.* 1989). However, the biochemical and morphological processes that render LTP persistent continue for hours and possibly days post-induction (Abraham *et al.* 1993; Meberg *et al.* 1993; Frey and Morris 1997; Williams *et al.* 1998). Several studies have shown that, early after induction, LTP is rather sensitive to reversal (depotentiation) when studied *in vitro*. Treatments such as hypoxia and adenosine receptor activation readily reverse LTP, particularly in the first few minutes after its induction (Arai *et al.* 1990; Huang *et al.* 1999). Prolonged LFS will also readily reverse LTP up to an hour post-HFS, but after that depotentiation appears to be harder to obtain (Fujii *et al.* 1991; O'Dell and Kandel 1994; Staubli and Chun 1996; but see Bashir and Collingridge 1994). This time dependence may reflect a particular resistance by late-phase LTP to reversal by homosynaptic stimulation (Woo and Nguyen 2002). Intriguingly, a selective disruption of late-phase LTP can be caused by soluble amyloid-β peptide (Chen *et al.* 2002), an effect that may underlie some of the memory deficits observed in Alzheimer's disease. In freely moving animals, LTP in the dentate gyrus is also resistant to reversal by homosynaptic stimulation (Errington *et al.* 1995; Abraham *et al.* 1996; but see Kulla *et al.* 1999), but it can be readily reversed by heterosynaptic stimulation (Doyère *et al.* 1997). Interestingly, soon after its induction, LTP in CA1 is sensitive to reversal by experience. Thus, exposure to a stressful novel environment will promote LTP reversal, when experienced at 1 h post-HFS but not at 24 h (Xu *et al.* 1998; Manahan-Vaughan and Braunewell 1999). The mechanisms underlying these diverse means of reversing LTP may be equally diverse, but it is interesting to note that a block of memory retention by exposure to novel stimuli shortly after training was associated with a reduction in subsequent CREB phosphorylation (Viola *et al.* 2000).

An important but relatively unstudied issue is whether the maintenance of late-phase LTP is actively regulated or whether it passively follows a time-course set by the initial processes of induction and consolidation. Two recent studies indicate that LTP persistence over days is in fact subject to ongoing regulation. In one study, LTP that was normally decremental over 7 days post-HFS was made stable when the NMDA receptor antagonist (RS)-3-(2-carboxypiperazin-4-yl)-propyl-1-phosphonic acid (CPP) was injected once daily (Villarreal *et al.* 2001). This treatment also prevented forgetting a learned spatial task. It is not certain, unfortunately, whether the LTP reversal in control animals was due to normal behavioural experiences or whether it was induced by the daily injection procedure, as a non-injected control group was not included. Nonetheless, the data do appear to support the view that LTP can be caused to decay by an active NMDA receptor-dependent process in the days following induction.

The fact that LTP can be stably maintained (Staubli and Lynch 1987; Abraham *et al.* 2002) indicates that decay is not obligatory, although it should be cautioned that the LTP in these studies may simply have exhibited a very slow time-course of decay. Even if such LTP is in fact non-decremental, it does not reflect a permanent synaptic change because it is still subject to regulation. For example, an otherwise stable LTP can be actively reversed by heterosynaptic stimulation given 3 weeks post-induction. In these experiments, we induced robust and saturated stable LTP in lateral perforant path synapses of freely moving animals by combined medial and lateral path HFS, repeated on three consecutive days. Three weeks later, medial path HFS alone caused an immediate and dramatic heterosynaptic reversal of lateral path LTP (from 54% LTP to -4% below original baseline $n = 6$; Fig. 18.3*a*). LTP remained stably reversed for 2 weeks, after which it was reinstated to its original level by one bout of combined medial and lateral HFS.

To test whether stable LTP is also sensitive to behavioural activation of hippocampal pathways, we induced stable LTP in perforant path synapses and then 2 weeks later we gave the animals, which are normally singly housed under stimulus-poor conditions, repeated exposures to a complex environment (CE) that involved a novel larger cage containing multiple objects and 1–2 other animals (Abraham *et al.* 2002). Significant, albeit incomplete, reversal of LTP gradually occurred as a result of 1 h per day of CE for 3 weeks, beginning 2 weeks post-HFS (Fig. 18.4*a*). When the 'dose' of exposure to the CE was increased to 14 h per day (i.e. overnight exposure), complete depotentiation rapidly occurred within a week (Fig. 18.4*b*). It remains to be determined whether the depotentiation of LTP by CE is due to homosynaptic activity at the potentiated synapses, heterosynaptic activity in neighbouring synapses, or both. Interestingly, reversal of LTP by CE did not occur when exposure commenced 90 days post-induction (Abraham *et al.* 2002), suggesting that there is a long-term consolidation process that takes weeks to complete. Nevertheless, this does not mean that LTP becomes so stabilized that it is completely impervious to new patterns of

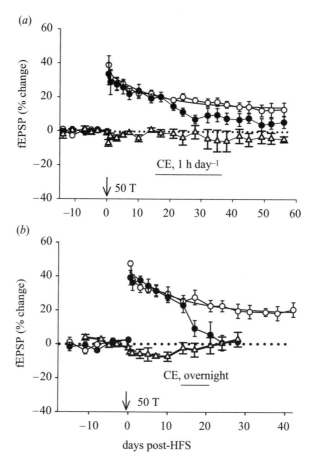

Fig. 18.4 Reversal of dentate gyrus LTP by exposure to complex environments (CE). (*a*) Comparison of LTP maintenance for two groups: home cage controls (HC, $n = 5$) and animals receiving CE exposure for 1 h day^{-1} for 3 weeks (CE, $n = 5$). The CE group showed a lasting partial reversal of LTP. Data are corrected for changes in the control hemisphere, which have also been plotted for the CE group ($n = 4$). The smooth curve is the fitted negative exponential function to the HC data; asymptote = 13% LTP. (*b*) Comparison of LTP maintenance for two groups: HC controls ($n = 6$) and animals receiving CE exposure overnight for 7 days beginning 14 days post-HFS (CE, $n = 5$). The HC group showed LTP with an average asymptote of 18%, but the CE group showed a rapid and lasting reversal of LTP, confirming the sensitivity of LTP maintenance in the dentate gyrus to behavioural experiences. Data are corrected for changes in the control hemisphere, which have also been plotted for the CE group ($n = 5$). Key: open circles, HC; filled circles, CE; open triangles, CE control hemisphere. 50 T, 50 trains of high-frequency stimulation. (Data are taken with permission from Abraham *et al.* (2002).)

activity. Thus, LTP that is allowed to stabilize over 120 days can still be rapidly reversed by heterosynaptic HFS of the medial perforant path (Fig. 18.3*b*).

Taken together, the above data indicate that LTP is only maintained stably in the hippocampus under particular induction and maintenance conditions. Establishment of the late-phase does not fully protect the LTP against subsequent reversal, even though it may render it more resistant to certain depotentiating stimuli. Instead, there are patterns of neural activity, such as heterosynaptic stimulation and the activity generated by repeated exposure to novel and complex environments, which can efficiently reverse the LTP, possibly working via NMDA receptor-dependent mechanisms. Such LTP reversal paradigms may provide useful model systems for studying the biological mechanisms underlying the psychological phenomenon of retrograde interference, i.e. the impairment of memory recall by newly learned information.

18.3 Neurogenesis and LTP

It is an odd twist of fate that the dentate gyrus has been the focus of most LTP persistence studies, yet it is also one of the few brain regions that shows a significant degree of ongoing neurogenesis (Kaplan and Hinds 1977; Van Praag et al. 1999). In most studies, neurogenesis is probably not a major complicating factor for the tracking of LTP maintenance because animals are singly housed in impoverished environments, and under these conditions the birth of new neurons occurs at a slow rate. The fact that stable recordings of both potentiated and non-potentiated synapses can be made for months under these conditions supports this view (Abraham et al. 1995, 2002). But what of the reversal of LTP by exposure to complex environments? Under these conditions, both the neurogenesis rate and the survival rate of neurons should be high, potentially leading to a net accumulation of granule cells (Gould et al. 1999; Young et al. 1999). Such architecture changes could distort the field potential recordings and degrade the measurements of LTP. It is interesting to note, therefore, that exposure of adult animals to complex environments does not affect the fEPSP measurement for non-potentiated pathways (Sharp et al. 1987; Abraham et al. 2002; Fig. 18.4). Furthermore, the reversal of LTP by complex environments is time dependent, and occurs within days of exposure to the complex environment, at a time before the new neurons could have fully differentiated and formed viable synapses. Thus, although it is conceivable that an increase in new neurons and overall synaptic number could dilute the contribution of potentiated synapses to the overall field potential recording, and make a stable LTP appear to decline, the timing of the neurogenesis process does not appear to be able to account for a rapid and complete loss of LTP. None the less, it is still important to note that the dentate gyrus has a much greater range of ages among its neurons than elsewhere in the brain, and thus the properties of LTP observed in this region may be heterogeneous and not easily extrapolated (Wang et al. 2000).

18.4 LTP maintenance as a model for memory

Most studies have shown that late-phase LTP decrements over days or weeks. This has been a more than sufficient duration to warrant extensive molecular and behavioural studies of LTP as a putative memory mechanism. But is such plasticity persistent enough to account for long-term information storage? This remains a pertinent question despite the demonstrations of stable or very slowly decrementing LTP, because such persistent LTP may be an artefact of having the experimental animals live in an impoverished environment (Fig. 18.4). Thus, there remain lingering doubts about the usefulness of LTP as a mechanism underlying very long-term memory storage (Abraham 2000), because memories can persist longer than a few weeks, even in rats (Maren *et al.* 1999; Kubie *et al.* 1999; Clark *et al.* 2002). However, there are several theoretical and experimental considerations that can reconcile differences between LTP maintenance and memory retention. First, memories can be subject to reactivation and rehearsal, and these processes may preserve that memory by refreshing what would otherwise be decaying synaptic weight changes. By contrast, the maintenance of one-shot LTP may not be subject to such reactivation effects because of its artificial nature, and thus its persistence may not accurately model the maintenance of real memories. Secondly, LTP persistence may vary between brain regions, and conclusions drawn from one brain region may not be generalizable to others. At the present time, LTP persistence has only been extensively studied in the hippocampus, a structure that does not store information for long periods of time, according to many experimental studies and computational models (Squire 1986; McClelland *et al.* 1995; but see Nadel and Moscovitch 1997; Cipolotti *et al.* 2000). Thus, structures that are believed to store very long-term memories, such as the neocortex, may be capable of showing much longer-lasting LTP. Third, in certain neural network models of sequential learning, synaptic weights at individual synapses can shift dramatically as a result of new learning and yet the network can retain an originally stored memory (Robins and Frean 1998). Thus, memories may outlast LTP, or LTD, at any particular set of synapses under study.

18.5 Questions for the future

Despite the above caveats about the persistence of LTP *vis à vis* memory, the physiological properties of LTP continue to play a critical role in bridging the molecular and behavioural levels of analysis. A thorough understanding of the basic properties of LTP persistence and how it is regulated will help inform the thinking and experimental planning at these other levels of analysis. However, despite the recent progress that has been made, there is still a sense that we are chipping away at the tip of the iceberg of factors controlling LTP maintenance. Below some key questions requiring future study, are raised.

(a) Do NMDA receptor-dependent and receptor-independent LTP have different maintenance mechanisms and persistence properties?

So far, studies of LTP have focused on NMDA receptor-dependent LTP (Jeffery *et al.* 1990; Abraham *et al.* 2002). However, it has been suggested that LTP induced by activation of VDDCs may have different underlying induction and early-phase maintenance mechanisms (Grover and Teyler 1990, 1995), although this view is not easily reconciled with reports that the late-phase of NMDA receptor-dependent LTP requires VDCC activation, at least in hippocampal slices (Impey *et al.* 1996). It is important therefore to establish for how long VDCC-specific LTP can last, and whether the mechanisms of maintaining this LTP overlap with those for NMDA receptor-dependent LTP.

(b) Does LTD last as long as LTP, and is it regulated by the same factors?

Because many groups have found homosynaptic LTD difficult to observe *in vivo*, little is known about this issue. Homosynaptic LTD can persist across days (Doyère *et al.* 1996), and is protein-synthesis dependent (Manahan-Vaughan *et al.* 2000), but it is not known how long it can be maintained. Also, as for LTP, there may be important differences between NMDA receptor-dependent and receptor-independent LTD that have not yet been explored. By contrast, heterosynaptic LTD in the dentate gyrus lasts for as long as simultaneously induced LTP, and their decay rates are highly correlated (Abraham *et al.* 1994). Whether LTD maintenance is as sensitive to behavioural variables as LTP is an important question that is currently under investigation.

(c) Does LTP or LTD vary in its persistence across brain regions, as predicted by theoretical models?

Based on the retrograde amnesia gradients that are commonly observed after hippocampal lesions, it is the conventional view that the hippocampus is involved only transiently in the representation of episodic information until the representations in neocortex become sufficiently elaborated to independently sustain long-term retention (Marr 1971; Squire 1986; Milner 1989; McClelland *et al.* 1995). One key issue then is how persistent is neocortical LTP? The prediction based on these conventional theories is that neocortical LTP should be capable of stable expression. Furthermore, it should be much more resistant to behavioural interference than hippocampal LTP. Racine and colleagues have begun to address these issues, as noted above, but a fuller description of LTP persistence properties is still required. Of course, as LTP can be observed in most areas of the brain, these same issues are pertinent to many other brain regions.

(d) How long can synaptic plasticity persist in animals living continuously in a complex environment?

Most experiments on LTP persistence are conducted in animals living in stimulus-poor environments, including individual housing. Despite being adult animals, their synapses may be in an immature state through lack of stimulation, and thus show different LTP induction and maintenance properties than synapses of animals living in more complex or naturalistic environments. We may get a very different view of the properties of plasticity in various brain regions if studies are done in animals living constantly in enriched environments. Such studies, if combined with behavioural experiments, may modify our views of the contributions made by different brain regions to long-term memory consolidation and storage.

(e) Do the factors that regulate the maintenance of LTP or LTD equally regulate the persistence of long-term memory?

It is an underlying assumption, or perhaps merely hope, that understanding the regulation of LTP maintenance will help us understand the properties of long-term memory storage in the corresponding brain regions. Although it is potentially misleading to compare the properties of monosynaptic LTP with the properties of memory stored in a network of synapses, none the less the theory has a certain appeal that will seed experimental tests. Indeed, a recent study reported that a treatment that prolonged LTP retention in the dentate gyrus also prolonged memory retention for a hippocampus-dependent spatial memory task (Villarreal *et al.* 2001). Conversely, reduction of LTP maintenance in *zif268*-knock out mice was associated with reduced retention on several diverse memory tasks (Jones *et al.* 2001). Another approach would be to focus on those brain areas in which experience-dependent LTP can be observed, such as the amygdala or neocortex (Rogan *et al.* 1997; Rioult-Pedotti *et al.* 2000). Regulation of LTP persistence in these models should be directly correlated with the maintenance of the associated memory.

18.6 Summary and conclusions

Although most properties of a network-based memory do not need to be reflected in the plasticity properties of individual synapses in the network, the retention of memory appears to require a certain stability of the underlying synaptic plasticity. Studies of LTP persistence have shown that it has the capacity, in principle, to underlie memories ranging from short-term to very long-term. Stable LTP is of particular interest given the brain's capacity to retain memories over very long periods of time, but our understanding of the factors regulating its induction, maintenance and distribution in the brain is at a very early stage, and it is vital that these issues are addressed. Ultimately, rodent models may not be able to address key issues regarding very long-term memory in humans, given the differences in lifespan between species. Thus it is still pertinent to ask, as in the title of this paper: 'how long will LTP last?' At this stage in our research efforts, perhaps the response is to adapt a sentiment expressed by Tim Bliss some time ago: 30 years and going strong.

This research, and the preparation of the manuscript, were supported by the Health Research Council of New Zealand. Dr B. Mockett and Dr D. Ireland made valuable criticisms of earlier drafts of the manuscript.

References

Abraham, W. C. (2000). Persisting with LTP as a memory mechanism: clues from variations in LTP maintenance. In *Neuronal mechanisms of memory formation: concepts of long-term potentiation and beyond* (ed. C. Hölscher), pp. 37–57. Cambridge University Press.

Abraham, W. C. and Bear, M. F. (1996). Metaplasticity: the plasticity of synaptic plasticity. *Trends Neurosci.* **19**, 126–30.

Abraham, W. C. and Logan, B. (2000). Stability of hippocampal LTP: the never-ending story. *Soc. Neurosci. Abstr.* **26**, 361.

Abraham, W. C. and Otani, S. (1991). Macromolecules and the maintenance of long-term potentiation. In *Kindling and synaptic plasticity* (ed. F. Morrell), pp. 92–109. Boston: Birkhäuser.

Abraham, W. C., Demmer, J., Richardson, C., Williams, J., Lawlor, P., Mason, S. E., *et al.* (1993). Correlations between immediate early gene induction and the persistence of long-term potentiation. *Neuroscience* **56**, 717–27.

Abraham, W. C., Christie, B. R., Logan, B., Lawlor, P., and Dragunow, M. (1994). Immediate early gene expression associated with the persistence of heterosynaptic long-term depression in the hippocampus. *Proc. Natl Acad. Sci. USA* **91**, 10 049–53.

Abraham, W. C., Mason-Parker, S. E., Williams, J., and Dragunow, M. (1995). Analysis of the decremental nature of LTP in the dentate gyrus. *Mol. Brain Res.* **30**, 367–72.

Abraham, W. C., Mason-Parker, S. E., and Logan, B. (1996). Low-frequency stimulation does not readily cause long-term depression or depotentiation in the dentate gyrus of awake rats. *Brain Res.* **722**, 217–22.

Abraham, W. C., Greenwood, J. M., Logan, B. L., Mason-Parker, S. E., and Dragunow, M. (2002). Induction and experience-dependent reversal of stable LTP lasting months in the hippocampus. *J. Neurosci.* **22**, 9626–34.

Arai, A., Larson, J., and Lynch, G. (1990). Anoxia reveals a vulnerable period in the development of long-term potentiation. *Brain Res.* **511**, 353–7.

Barnes, C. A. (1979). Memory deficits associated with senescence: a behavioral and neurophysiological study in the rat. *J. Comp. Physiol. Psychol.* **93**, 74–104.

Barnes, C. A. and McNaughton, B. L. (1985). An age comparison of the rates of acquisition and forgetting of spatial information in relation to long-term enhancement of hippocampal synapses. *Behav. Neurosci.* **99**, 1040–8.

Bashir, Z. I. and Collingridge, G. L. (1994). An investigation of depotentiation of long-term potentiation in the CA1 region of the hippocampus. *Exp. Brain Res.* **100**, 437–43.

Bliss, T. V. P. and Gardner-Medwin, A. R. (1973). Long-lasting potentiation of synaptic transmission in the dentate area of the unanaesthetized rabbit following stimulation of the perforant path. *J. Physiol.* **232**, 357–74.

Bliss, T. V. P. and Lømo, T. (1973). Long-lasting potentiation of synaptic transmission in the dentate area of the anaesthetized rabbit following stimulation of the perforant path. *J. Physiol.* **232**, 331–56.

Bourtchouladze, R., Frenguelli, B., Blendy, J., Cioffi, D., Schutz, G., and Silva, A. J. (1994). Deficient long-term memory in mice with a targeted mutation of the cAMP-responsive element-binding protein. *Cell* **79**, 59–68.

Buzsáki, G. (1980). Long-term potentiation of the commissural path-CA1 pyramidal cell synapse in the hippocampus of the freely moving rat. *Neurosci. Lett.* **19**, 293–6.

Chen, Q. S., Wei, W. Z., Shimahara, T., and Xie, C. W. (2002). Alzheimer amyloid beta-peptide inhibits the late phase of long-term potentiation through calcineurin-dependent mechanisms in the hippocampal dentate gyrus. *Neurobiol. Learn. Mem.* **77**, 354–71.

Cipolotti, L., Shallice, T., Chan, D., Fox, N., Scahill, R., Harrison, G., *et al.* (2000). Long-term retrograde amnesia... the crucial role of the hippocampus. *Neuropsychologia* **39**, 151–72.

Clark, R. E., Broadbent, N. J., Zola, S. M., and Squire, L. R. (2002). Anterograde amnesia and temporally graded retrograde amnesia for a nonspatial memory task after lesions of hippocampus and subiculum. *J. Neurosci.* **22**, 4663–9.

Davis, S., Vanhoutte, P., Pagès, C., Caboche, J., and Laroche, S. (2000). The MAP/ERK cascade targets both Elk-1 and cAMP response element-binding protein to control long-term potentiation-dependent gene expression in the dentate gyrus *in vivo*. *J. Neurosci.* **20**, 4563–72.

de Jonge, M. and Racine, R. J. (1985). The effects of repeated induction of long-term potentiation in the dentate gyrus. *Brain Res.* **328**, 181–5.

Doyère, V., Errington, M. L., Laroche, S., and Bliss, T. V. P. (1996). Low-frequency trains of paired stimuli induce long-term depression in area CA1 but not in dentate gyrus of the intact rat. *Hippocampus* **6**, 52–7.

Doyère, V., Srebro, B., and Laroche, S. (1997). Heterosynaptic LTD and depotentiation in the medial perforant path of the dentate gyrus in the freely moving rat. *J. Neurophysiol.* **77**, 571–8.

Errington, M. L., Bliss, T. V. P., Richter-Levin, G., Yenk, K., Doyère, V., and Laroche, S. (1995). Stimulation at 1–5 Hz does not produce long-term depression or depotentiation in the hippocampus of the adult rat *in vivo*. *J. Neurophysiol.* **74**, 1793–9.

Frégnac, Y., Schulz, D., Thorpe, S., and Bienenstock, E. (1998). A cellular analogue of visual cortical plasticity. *Nature* **333**, 367–70.

Frey, S., Bergado-Rosado, J., Seidenbecher, T., Pape, H.-C., and Frey, J. U. (2001). Reinforcement of early long-term potentiation (early-LTP) in dentate gyrus by stimulation of the basolateral amygdala: heterosynaptic induction mechanisms of late-LTP. *J. Neurosci.* **21**, 3697–703.

Frey, U. and Morris, R. G. M. (1997). Synaptic tagging and long-term potentiation. *Nature* **385**, 533–6.

Frey, U., Schroeder, H., and Matthies, H. (1990). Dopaminergic antagonists prevent long-term maintenance of posttetanic LTP in the CA1 region of rat hippocampal slices. *Brain Res.* **522**, 69–75.

Fujii, S., Saito, K., Miyakawa, H., Ito, K.-I., and Kato, H. (1991). Reversal of long-term potentiation (depotentiation) induced by tetanus stimulation of the input to CA1 neurons of guinea pig hippocampal slices. *Brain Res.* **555**, 112–22.

Gould, E., Beylin, A., Tanapat, P., Reeves, A., and Shors, T. J. (1999). Learning enhances adult neurogenesis in the hippocampal formation. *Nature Neurosci.* **2**, 260–5.

Granger, R., Wiebe, S. P., Taketani, M., and Lynch, G. (1996). Distinct memory circuits composing the hippocampal region. *Hippocampus* **6**, 567–78.

Grover, L. M. and Teyler, T. J. (1990). Two components of long-term potentiation induced by different patterns of afferent activation. *Nature* **347**, 477–9.

Grover, L. M. and Teyler, T. J. (1995). Different mechanisms may be required for maintenance of NMDA receptor-dependent and independent forms of long-term potentiation. *Synapse* **19**, 121–33.

Gustafsson, B., Asztely, F., Hanse, E., and Wigstrom, H. (1989). Onset characteristics of long-term potentiation in the guinea-pig hippocampal CA1 region *in vitro*. *Eur. J. Neurosci.* **1**, 382–94.

Hagiwara, M., Alberts, A., Brindle, P., Meinkoth, J., Feramisco, J., Deng, T., *et al.* (1992). Transcriptional attenuation following cAMP induction requires PP-1-mediated dephosphorylation of CREB. *Cell* **70**, 105–13.

Hebb, D. O. (1949). *The organization of behavior*. New York: Wiley.

Huang, C.-C., Liang, Y.-C., and Hsu, K.-S. (1999). A role for extracellular adenosine in time-dependent reversal of long-term potentiation by low-frequency stimulation at hippocampal CA1 synapses. *J. Neurosci.* **19**, 9728–38.

Huang, Y.-Y. and Kandel, E. R. (1994). Recruitment of long-lasting and protein kinase A-dependent long-term potentiation in the CA1 region of hippocampus requires repeated tetanization. *Learn. Mem.* **1**, 74–82.

Huang, Y.-Y. and Kandel, E. R. (1995). D1/D5 receptor agonists induce a protein synthesis-dependent late potentiation in the CA1 region of the hippocampus. *Proc. Natl Acad. Sci. USA* **92**, 2446–50.

Impey, S., Mark, M., Villacres, E. C., Poser, S., Chavkin, C., and Storm, D. R. (1996). Induction of CRE-mediated gene expression by stimuli that generate long-lasting LTP in area CA1 of the hippocampus. *Neuron* **16**, 973–82.

Jeffery, K. J., Abraham, W. C., Dragunow, M., and Mason, S. E. (1990). Induction of fos-like immunoreactivity and the maintenance of long-term potentiation in the dentate gyrus of unanesthetized rats. *Mol. Brain Res.* **8**, 267–74.

Jones, M. W., Errington, M. L., French, P. J., Fine, A., Bliss, T. V. P., Garel, S., *et al.* (2001). A requirement for the immediate early gene *Zif268* in the expression of late LTP and long-term memories. *Nature Neurosci.* **4**, 289–96.

Kaplan, M. S. and Hinds, J. H. (1977). Neurogenesis in the adult rat: electron microscopic analysis of light radioautographs. *Science* **197**, 1092–4.

Kirkwood, A., Dudek, S. M., Gold, J. T., Aizenman, C. D., and Bear, M. F. (1993). Common forms of synaptic plasticity in the hippocampus and neocortex *in vitro*. *Science* **260**, 1518–21.

Krug, M., Lössner, B., and Ott, T. (1984). Anisomycin blocks the late phase of long-term potentiation in the dentate gyrus of freely moving rats. *Brain Res. Bull.* **13**, 39–42.

Kubie, J. L., Sutherland, R. J., and Miller, R. U. (1999). Hippocampal lesions produce a temporally graded retrograde amnesia on a dry version of the Morris swimming task. *Psychobiology* **27**, 313–30.

Kulla, A., Reymann, K. G., and Manahan-Vaughan, D. (1999). Time-dependent induction of depotentiation in the dentate gyrus of freely moving rats: involvement of group 2 metabotropic glutamate receptors. *Eur. J. Neurosci.* **11**, 3864–72.

Leung, S. T. and Shen, B. (1995). Long-term potentiation at the apical and basal dendritic synapses of CA1 after local stimulation in behaving rats. *J. Neurophysiol.* **73**, 1938–46.

McClelland, J. L., McNaughton, B. L., and O'Reilly, R. C. (1995). Why there are complementary learning systems in the hippocampus and neocortex: insights from the successes and failures of connectionist models of learning and memory. *Psychol. Rev.* **102**, 419–57.

Manahan-Vaughan, D. and Braunewell, K.-H. (1999). Novelty acquisition is associated with induction of hippocampal long-term depression. *Proc. Natl Acad. Sci. USA* **96**, 8739–44.

Manahan-Vaughan, D., Kulla, A., and Frey, J. U. (2000). Requirement of translation but not transcription for the maintenance of long-term depression in the CA1 region of freely moving rats. *J. Neurosci.* **20**, 8572–6.

Maren, S., Aharonov, G., and Fanselow, M. S. (1999). Neurotoxic lesions of the dorsal hippocampus and Pavlovian fear conditioning in rats. *Behav. Brain Res.* **110**, 436–42.

Marr, D. (1971). Simple memory: a theory for archicortex. *Phil. Trans. R. Soc. Lond.* B **262**, 23–81.

Martin, S. J., Grimwood, P. D., and Morris, R. G. M. (2000). Synaptic plasticity and memory: an evaluation of the hypothesis. *A. Rev. Neurosci.* **23**, 649–711.

Meberg, P. J., Barnes, C. A., McNaughton, B. L., and Routtenberg, A. (1993). Protein kinase C and F1/GAP-43 gene expression in hippocampus inversely related to synaptic enhancement lasting 3 days. *Proc. Natl Acad. Sci. USA* **90**, 12 050–4.

Milner, P. (1989). A cell assembly theory of hippocampal amnesia. *Neuropsychologia* **27**, 23–30.

Nadel, L. and Moscovitch, M. (1997). Memory consolidation, retrograde amnesia and the hippocampal complex. *Curr. Opin. Neurobiol.* **7**, 217–27.

Nguyen, P. V., Abel, T., and Kandel, E. R. (1994). Requirement of a critical period of transcription for induction of a late phase of LTP. *Science* **265**, 1104–7.

O'Dell, T. J. and Kandel, E. R. (1994). Low-frequency stimulation erases LTP through an NMDA receptor-mediated activation of protein phosphatases. *Learn. Mem.* **1**, 129–39.

Olson, C. R. and Freeman, R. D. (1980). Profile of the sensitive period for monocular deprivation in kittens. *Exp. Brain Res.* **39**, 17–21.

Otani, S., Marshall, C. J., Tate, W., Goddard, G. V., and Abraham, W. C. (1989). Maintenance of long-term potentiation in rat dentate gyrus requires protein synthesis but not mRNA synthesis immediately post-tetanization. *Neuroscience* **28**, 519–26.

Racine, R. J., Milgram, N. W., and Hafner, S. (1983). Long-term potentiation phenomena in the rat limbic forebrain. *Brain Res.* **260**, 217–31.

Racine, R. J., Chapman, C. A., Trepel, C., Teskey, G. C., and Milgram, N. W. (1995). Postactivation potentiation in the neocortex. IV. Multiple sessions required for induction of long-term potentiation in the chronic preparation. *Brain Res.* **702**, 87–93.

Raymond, C. R., Thompson, V., Tate, W. P., and Abraham, W. C. (2000). Metabotropic glutamate receptors trigger homosynaptic protein synthesis to prolong LTP. *J. Neurosci.* **20**, 969–76.

Rioult-Pedotti, M.-S., Friedman, D., and Donoghue, J. P. (2000). Learning-induced LTP in neocortex. *Science* **290**, 533–6.

Robins, A. and Frean, M. (1998). Local learning algorithms for sequential tasks in neural networks. *Adv. Comput. Intell.* **2**, 221–7.

Rogan, M. T., Stäubli, U. V., and LeDoux, J. E. (1997). Fear conditioning induces associative long-term potentiation in the amygdala. *Nature* **390**, 604–7.

Rolls, E. T. (1996*a*). A theory of hippocampal function in memory. *Hippocampus* **6**, 601–20.

Rolls, E. T. (1996*b*). Roles of LTP and LTD in neuronal network operations in the brain. In *Cortical plasticity* (ed. M. S. Fazeli and G. L. Collingridge), pp. 223–250. Oxford: BIOS Scientific Publishers Ltd.

Seidenbecher, T., Reymann, K. G., and Balschun, D. (1997). A post-tetanic time window for the reinforcement of long-term potentiation by appetitive and aversive stimuli. *Proc. Natl Acad. Sci. USA* **94**, 1449–99.

Sharp, P. E., Barnes, C. A., and McNaughton, B. L. (1987). Effects of aging on environmental modulation of hippocampal evoked responses. *Behav. Neurosci.* **101**, 170–8.

Squire, L. R. (1986). Mechanisms of memory. *Science* **232**, 1612–19.

Staubli, U. and Chun, D. (1996). Factors regulating the reversibility of long-term potentiation. *J. Neurosci.* **16**, 853–60.

Staubli, U. and Lynch, G. (1987). Stable hippocampal long-term potentiation elicited by 'theta' pattern stimulation. *Brain Res.* **435**, 227–34.

Swanson-Park, J. L., Coussens, C. M., Mason-Parker, S. E., Raymond, C. R., Hargreaves, E. L., Dragunow, M., *et al.* (1999). A double dissociation within the hippocampus of dopamine D1/D5 receptor and β-adrenergic receptor contributions to the persistence of long-term potentiation. *Neuroscience* **92**, 485–97.

Trepel, C. and Racine, R. J. (1998). Long-term potentiation in the neocortex of the adult, freely moving rat. *Cereb. Cortex* **8**, 719–29.

Van Praag, H., Kempermann, G., and Gage, F. H. (1999). Running increases cell proliferation and neurogenesis in the adult mouse dentate gyrus. *Nature Neurosci.* **2**, 266–70.

Villarreal, D. M., Do, V., Haddad, E., and Derrick, B. E. (2001). NMDA receptor antagonists sustain LTP and spatial memory: active processes mediate LTP decay. *Nature Neurosci.* **5**, 48–52.

Viola, H. E., Furman, M., Izquierdo, L. A. I., Alonso, M., Barros, D. M., De Souza, M. M., *et al.* (2000). Phosphorylated cAMP response element-binding protein as a molecular marker of memory processing in rat hippocampus: effect of novelty. *J. Neurosci.* **20**, RC112, 1–5.

Wang, S., Scott, B. W., and Wojtowicz, J. M. (2000). Heterogenous properties of dentate granule neurons in the adult brain. *J. Neurobiol.* **42**, 248–57.

Wiesel, T. (1982). Postnatal development of the visual cortex and the influence of the environment. *Nature* **299**, 583–92.

Williams, J. W., Mason-Parker, S. E., Abraham, W. C., and Tate, W. P. (1998). Biphasic changes in the levels of N-methyl-D-aspartate receptor-2 subunits correlate with the induction and persistence of long-term potentiation. *Mol. Brain Res.* **60**, 21–27.

Winder, D. G., Mansuy, I. M., Osman, M., Moallem, T. M., and Kandel, E. R. (1998). Genetic and pharmacological evidence for a novel, intermediate phase of long-term potentiation suppressed by calcineurin. *Cell* **92**, 25–37.

Woo, N. H. and Nguyen, P. V. (2002). 'Silent' metaplasticity of the late phase of long-term potentiation requires protein phosphatases. *Learn. Mem.* **9**, 202–13.

Xu, L., Anwyl, R., and Rowan, M. J. (1998). Spatial exploration induces a persistent reversal of long-term potentiation in rat hippocampus. *Nature* **394**, 891–4.

Young, D., Lawlor, P., Leone, P., Dragunow, M., and During, M. J. (1999). Environmental enrichment inhibits spontaneous apoptosis, prevents seizures and is neuroprotective. *Nature Med.* **5**, 448–53.

Glossary

CE	complex environment
CREB	cyclic AMP response element binding protein
fEPSP	field excitatory postsynaptic potential
HFS	high-frequency stimulation
LFS	low-frequency stimulation
LTD	long-term depression
LTP	long-term potentiation
NMDA	N-methyl-D-aspartate
VDCC	voltage-dependent calcium channels

19

Structural changes at dendritic spine synapses during long-term potentiation

Kristen M. Harris, John C. Fiala, and Linnaea Ostroff

Two key hypotheses about the structural basis of long-term potentiation (LTP) are evaluated in light of new findings from immature rat hippocampal slices. First, it is shown why dendritic spines do not split during LTP. Instead a small number of spine-like dendritic protrusions may emerge to enhance connectivity with potentiated axons. These 'same dendrite multiple synapse boutons' provide less than a 3% increase in connectivity and do not account for all of LTP or memory, as they do not accumulate during maturation. Second, polyribosomes in dendritic spines served to identify which of the existing synapses enlarged to sustain more than a 30% increase in synaptic strength. Thus, both enhanced connectivity and enlarged synapses result during LTP, with synapse enlargement being the greater effect.

Keywords: synapse; serial electron microscopy; three-dimensional reconstruction; dendritic spine; plasticity; development

19.1 No spine splitting

Dendritic spines are tiny protrusions that stud the surface of neurons and form the postsynaptic component of most of the excitatory synaptic connections in the brain (Harris and Kater 1994). It has long been suggested that increasing the size and/or number of dendritic spines would enhance the strength of connections between neurons. This process is thought to underlie cellular mechanisms of learning and memory such as LTP in the hippocampus and elsewhere. Splitting existing synapses has been an attractive model for increasing synaptic coupling between neurons (Lusher *et al.* 2000), because input specificity would be preserved if the daughter spines retain synaptic connections with the parent axon.

Despite the simplicity and elegance of this model, little has been done to test its accuracy. A three-dimensional analysis of interconnectivity in hippocampal neuropil was needed to determine whether spine splitting is a viable mechanism. Dendrites, axons and synapses were reconstructed from hippocampal CA1 neurons with a special emphasis on detecting the various steps that would be required for spines and synapses to split (Fig. 19.1a). The first step in the proposed sequence is perforation of the synapse. Second, the dendritic spine begins to divide, thereby transiently forming a branched spine with two heads synapsing on the same presynaptic axon. Finally, the spine completes its division, resulting in two or more spines from the same dendrite synapsing with the same presynaptic axon, the so-called sdMSB.

Perforated synapses occur on mushroom-shaped dendritic spines that synapse with a single presynaptic bouton in support of step one. They represent around 10–15% of

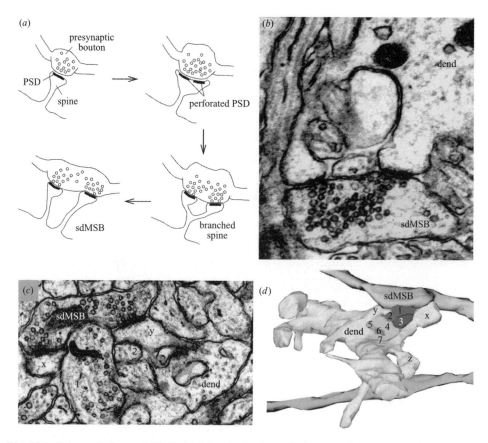

Fig. 19.1 Spine splitting and LTP. (*a*) Model of spine splitting to enhance connectivity between hippocampal neurons. (*b*) Fortuitous longitudinal section through two spines arising from the same dendrite (yellow, dend) to synapse on a multiple synapse bouton (green, sdMSB). (*c,d*) Example section and reconstruction of sdMSB, dendritic spines and parent dendrite that synapse with the sdMSB, and axons (numbered) that pass between the spines that synapse on the sdMSB. One of the spines on the sdMSB is itself branched (x, z) but the two heads synapse on different axons, so that it does not represent synapse splitting. (See Plate 3 of the Plate Section, at the centre of this book.)

mature synapses in hippocampal area CA1 (Harris and Stevens 1989). To test the second step in the spine-splitting hypothesis more than 100 branched dendritic spines have been reconstructed on mature hippocampal CA1 neurons (Sorra *et al.* 1998) and subsequently on immature PN15 and PN21 neurons (unpublished reconstructions). In no case did two or more heads of branched spines synapse with the same presynaptic axon. The different heads of a single branched spine had simple, perforated or segmented synapses. These findings provide morphological evidence that spine branches are not simple daughter spines arising from the splitting of an existing synapse. If sdMSBs arise during synaptic plasticity they do so by a mechanism that leaves no trace of splitting spines associated with an existing presynaptic bouton.

Under control conditions in perfusion fixed brain sdMSBs are rarely observed (Sorra and Harris 1993). Following LTP, we and other researchers have identified a small (less

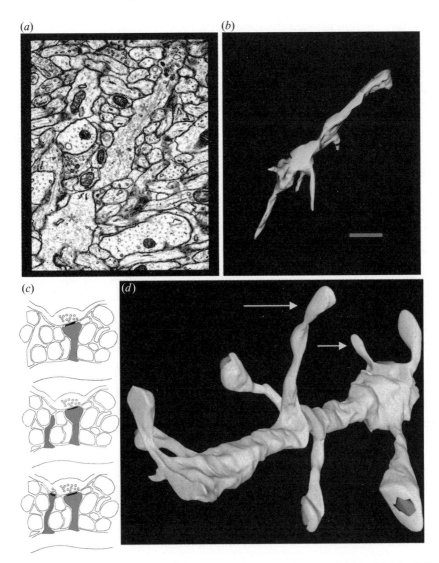

Fig. 19.2 Spine outgrowth to form sdMSBs. (*a*) Axonal growth cone (red asterisks). (*b*)Reconstruction of the axonal growth cone illustrated in (*a*). Scale bar, 0.5 μm. (*c*) Model of spine outgrowth to form sdMSBs. (*d*) Reconstruction of dendritic segment with two non-synaptic dendritic protrusions (yellow arrows). (See Plate 4 of the Plate Section, at the centre of this book.)

than 3% of all synapses) number of spines from a single dendrite that formed synapses on sdMSBs (Fig. 19.1*b*; Toni *et al.* 1999; Fiala *et al.* 2002). However, reconstructions revealed that long, mature axons and dendrites always passed between the neighbouring spines, apparently precluding their formation via splitting (Fig. 19.1*b,c*).

These results were obtained in acute hippocampal slices from postnatal day 15 rats (Fiala *et al.* 2002) or organotypic slices from immature rats (Toni *et al.* 1999). In these immature preparations, synaptogenesis is ongoing, so it could be argued that axons and dendrites passing between the spines grew there after the spines split. To test this hypothesis we measured the gap between the neighbouring spines and compared it with the dimensions of axonal growth cones found in the same slices (Fig. 19.2*a*). Seven sdMSBs were detected in the LTP condition in slices, and in addition, 10 sdMSBs were reconstructed from postnatal day 21 hippocampus, *in vivo*. The gap between the spines averaged 0.6 μm at both ages, and the average number of mature axons traversing the gap was 3.1 at PN15 and 3.7 at PN21. A growth cone was reconstructed from one of the PN15 slices demonstrating the typically large dimensions with a diameter greater than the width of the gap (Fig. 19.2*b*). Other gaps had spiny dendrites passing through them. These observations suggest that it is unlikely that axons and dendrites grew through the gap after the spines had split, via the mechanisms outlined in Fig. 19.1*a*.

19.2 Spine outgrowth

How then do sdMSBs form if not by spine splitting? An alternative mechanism is via spine outgrowth (Fig. 19.2*c*). During LTP, spine-like dendritic protrusions without synapses were discovered that could weave through the neuropil to encounter presynaptic axons already synapsing with their neighbouring spines (Fig. 19.2*d*). This mechanism would not require spine splitting, yet input specificity could be preserved if the potentiated presynaptic axons were more attractive to the emerging spines.

The formation of sdMSBs does not seem to account for the magnitude of LTP. Even during LTP less than 3% of synapses are of this type. LTP can involve a 100% increase in synaptic efficacy suggesting that some additional mechanism might be involved. Furthermore, if the formation of sdMSBs were a major mechanism to enhance connectivity between neurons and store memories, one would expect sdMSBs to accumulate with maturation. Instead, less than 2% of mature synapses occur on dendritic spines arising from the same dendrite and sharing the same presynaptic axon (Sorra and Harris 1993).

19.3 Protein synthesis-mediated synapse enlargement

Enlargement of existing synapses is another favoured model for enhancing synaptic efficacy during LTP (Yuste and Bonhoeffer 2001). This hypothesis has also eluded an unequivocal answer because it has been impossible to distinguish potentiated synapses from neighbouring synapses that were not potentiated (Sorra and Harris 1998). Even approaches labelling sites of calcium accumulation (Toni *et al*. 1999) have been inadequate because the calcium precipitate is only detected above background in SER, hence only the 10–15% of spines that contain SER could be labelled though a larger percentage may have undergone LTP.

Results from many studies indicate that enduring LTP requires new protein synthesis (Nguyen *et al*. 1994; Frey and Morris 1997), and recent studies suggest that translation will occur near the specific synapses that undergo LTP (Steward and Worley 2001). Polyribosomes are distinctive ultrastructural features that are required for new protein synthesis. In fact, they are clear indicators of exactly where translation is occurring at

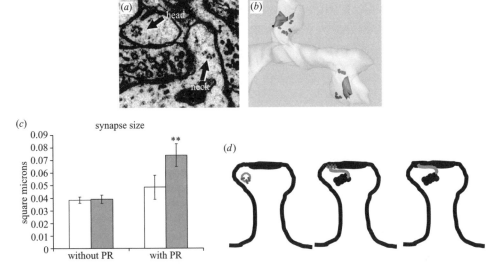

Fig. 19.3. Protein-synthesis-dependent synapse enlargement during LTP. (*a*) Polyribosomes in a dendritic spine head and a different spine neck. (*b*) Three-dimensional reconstruction of dendritic spines containing polyribosomes (grey spheres) and having large synapses (red). (*c*) Spines without polyribosomes had synapses of the same size under both LTP (grey bars) and control (open bars) conditions. Spines with polyribosomes had larger synapses under the LTP condition only (**$p < 0.02$). (*d*) Model illustrating how glutamatergic receptors (blue) located in postsynaptic vesicles (red) are inserted into the plasma membrane soon after induction of LTP. The new protein synthesis then adds postsynaptic density proteins to stabilize these receptors in the membrane. (See Plate 5 of the Plate Section, at the centre of this book.)

the time of fixation (Steward and Schuman 2001). It is thus reasonable to assume that the presence of polyribosomes in particular dendritic spines would be an accurate marker of which spines had recently undergone protein-synthesis-dependent LTP.

Hippocampal dendrites were examined in three-dimensional reconstructions to determine the precise location of every polyribosome (Fig. 19.3*a,b*; Ostroff *et al.* 2002). Only $12 \pm 4\%$ of dendritic spines contained polyribosomes under control conditions whereas $39 \pm 4\%$ of spines contained them during LTP. A commensurate loss of polyribosomes from dendritic shafts accompanied this increase in spines with poly-ribosomes during LTP. Postsynaptic densities on dendritic spines that contained polyribo-somes were larger during LTP (Fig. 19.3*c*), suggesting that local changes in protein synthesis serve to stabilize stimulation-induced growth of the synapse (Fig. 19.3*d*). This coincidence in polyribosomes and synapse enlargement suggests they mark the specific spines that are expressing LTP.

19.4 Summary

Together these findings support the hypothesis that LTP uses two structural mechanisms to strengthen synaptic connections. The primary mechanism is a protein-synthesis-dependent enlargement of existing synapses. A few non-synaptic dendritic protrusions may also be captured to form additional synapses with potentiated boutons.

This work was supported by NIH grants NS21184, NS33574 and MH/DA57351 funded jointly by NIMH and NIDA.

References

Fiala, J. C., Allwardt, B., and Harris, K. M. (2002). Dendritic spines do not split during hippocampal LTP or maturation. *Nature Neurosci.* **5**, 297–8.

Frey, U. and Morris, R. G. M. (1997). Synaptic tagging and long-term potentiation. *Nature* **385**, 533–6.

Harris, K. M. and Stevens, J. K. (1989). Dendritic spines of CA1 pyramidal cells in the rat hippocampus: serial electron microscopy with reference to their biophysical characteristics. *J. Neurosci.* **9**, 2982–97.

Harris, K. M. and Kater, S. B. (1994). Dendritic spines: cellular specializations imparting both stability and flexibility to synaptic function. *A. Rev. Neurosci.* **17**, 341–71.

Lusher, C., Nicoll, R. A., Malenka, R. C., and Muller, D. (2000). Synaptic plasticity and dynamic modulation of the postsynaptic membrane. *Nature Neurosci.* **3**, 545–50.

Nguyen, P. V., Abel, T., and Kandel, E. R. (1994). Requirement of a critical period of transcription for induction of a late phase of LTP. *Science* **265**, 1104–7.

Ostroff, L. E., Fiala, J. C., Allwardt, B., and Harris, K. M. (2002). Polyribosomes redistribute from dendritic shafts into spines with enlarged synapses during LTP in developing rat hippocampal slices. *Neuron* **35**, 535–45.

Sorra, K. E. and Harris, K. M. (1993). Occurrence and three-dimensional structure of multiple synapses between individual radiatum axons and their target pyramidal cells in hippocampal area CA1. *J. Neurosci.* **13**, 3736–48.

Sorra, K. E. and Harris, K. M. (1998). Stability in synapse number and size at 2 hr after long-term potentiation in hippocampal area CA1. *J. Neurosci.* **18**, 658–71.

Sorra, K. E., Fiala, J. C., and Harris, K. M. (1998). Critical assessment of the involvement of perforations, spinules, and spine branching in hippocampal synapse formation. *J. Comp. Neurol.* **398**, 225–40.

Steward, O. and Schuman, E. M. (2001). Protein synthesis at synaptic sites on dendrites. *A. Rev. Neurosci.* **24**, 299–325.

Steward, O. and Worley, P. F. (2001). Selective targeting of newly synthesized *Arc* RNA to active synapses requires NMDA receptor activation. *Neuron* **30**, 227–40.

Toni, N., Buchs, P. A., Nikonenko, I., Bron, C. R., and Muller, D. (1999). LTP promotes formation of multiple spine synapses between a single axon terminal and a dendrite. *Nature* **402**, 421–5.

Yuste, R. and Bonhoeffer, T. (2001). Morphological changes in dendritic spines associated with long-term synaptic plasticity. *A. Rev. Neurosci* **24**, 1071–89.

Glossary

LTP   long-term potentiation
sdMSB   same dendrite multiple synapse bouton
SER   smooth endoplasmic reticulum

20

Cadherins and synaptic plasticity: activity-dependent cyclin-dependent kinase 5 regulation of synaptic β-catenin–cadherin interactions

Erin M. Schuman and Sachiko Murase

Cyclin-dependent kinase 5 (Cdk5)/p35 kinase activity is known to decrease the affinity of β-catenin for cadherin in developing cortical neurons. Our recent work demonstrated that depolarization causes an increased affinity between β-catenin and cadherin. Here, we examine whether Cdk5/p35 regulates β-catenin–cadherin affinity in response to neural activity. In hippocampal neurons depolarization caused a significant decrease in Cdk5 kinase activity, without changing the protein levels of either Cdk5 or p35, suggesting that the proteasome pathway is not involved. Decreasing Cdk5 kinase activity with the inhibitor roscovitine increased the amount of β-catenin that was co-immunoprecipitated with cadherin. Inhibiting Cdk5 activity also resulted in a redistribution of EGFP–β-catenin from the dendritic shaft to the spines, where cadherins are highly concentrated. The redistribution of β-catenin induced by roscovitine is similar to that induced by depolarization. Interestingly, the redistribution induced by the Cdk5 inhibitor was completely blocked by either a tyrosine phosphatase inhibitor, orthovanadate or by point mutations of β-catenin Tyr-654 to Glu or Phe. Immunoprecipitation studies further revealed that roscovitine increases the affinity of the wild-type, but not mutated, EGFP–β-catenin for cadherin. These results suggest that Cdk5 activity regulates the affinity of β-catenin for cadherin by changing the phosphorylation level of β-catenin Tyr-654.

Keywords: cadherin; β-catenin; cyclin-dependent kinase 5; tyrosine phosphorylation; depolarization; synaptic remodelling

20.1 Introduction

Synapses can undergo dynamic changes in their strength that last from minutes to hours to days. Activity-induced changes in synaptic proteins probably underlie long-term synaptic plasticity in the brain. Although cell adhesion molecules are thought to participate in synaptic remodelling, the links between neural activity and subsequent structural modifications are unknown. In addition to serving as recognition markers for synaptogenesis, the presence of adhesion molecules in or near the synaptic cleft raises the possibility that they may participate in initiating and maintaining synaptic changes (Murase and Schuman 1999). Cadherins are a family of proteins that mediate Ca^{2+}-dependent homophilic cell adhesion (Takeichi 1990). Cadherins are located at synaptic sites (Fannon and Colman 1996; Uchida *et al.* 1996; Tang *et al.* 1998) and biochemical studies have demonstrated that cadherins associate with core synaptic proteins both pre- and post-synaptically (Husi *et al.* 2000; Phillips *et al.* 2001), suggesting that cadherins regulate synaptic function.

Several recent studies support a role for the classic cadherins in synaptic plasticity (Tang *et al.* 1998; Benson and Tanaka 1998; Tanaka *et al.* 2000; Bozdagi *et al.* 2000). We previously reported (Tang *et al.* 1998) that either cadherin function-blocking antibodies or inhibitory peptides blocked LTP in area CA1 of rat hippocampal slices. Using a different stimulation protocol designed to elicit L-LTP, Benson and colleagues showed that an antibody to N-cadherin blocked early-phase but not L-LTP. The same study documented an increase in the number of cadherin-positive synaptic sites during L-LTP (Bozdagi *et al.* 2000). These observations suggest that cadherins may initiate and/or maintain the synaptic changes that occur during LTP. In contrast, another study found that the magnitude of LTP was enhanced in hippocampal slices prepared from mice that express a truncated version of a specific cadherin, cadherin-11 (Manabe *et al.* 2000), suggesting that, under some conditions, cadherins may also limit the formation of plasticity. A recent study also demonstrated that expression of a dominant negative cadherin perturbed spine morphology in developing neurons (Togashi *et al.* 2002).

The cytoplasmic domain of cadherin interacts with F-actin via proteins called catenins: β-catenin binds directly to the C-terminal part of cadherin, and also binds to α-catenin, which in turn interacts with F-actin (Ozawa *et al.* 1990; Hirano *et al.* 1992). The interaction with actin filaments is required for the adhesive activity of cadherin (Nagafuchi *et al.* 1994). Thus, changes in β-catenin–cadherin affinity may regulate cadherin adhesion. Phosphorylation of β-catenin Tyr-654 significantly decreases the affinity for cadherin (Roura *et al.* 1999). Several tyrosine kinases (Matsuyoshi *et al.* 1992; Behrens *et al.* 1993; Hamaguchi *et al.* 1993; Hazan and Norton 1998; Roura *et al.* 1999; Bonvini *et al.* 2001) and tyrosine phosphatases (Balsamo *et al.* 1996; Fuchs *et al.* 1996; Kypta *et al.* 1996; Balsamo *et al.* 1998; Müller *et al.* 1999) are known to regulate β-catenin tyrosine phosphorylation levels. High levels of β-catenin Tyr phosphorylation result in a loss of cadherin adhesion (Ozawa and Kemler 1998), promoting cell migration (Sommers *et al.* 1994; Müller *et al.* 1999) and neurite outgrowth (Pathre *et al.* 2001).

We recently demonstrated that, in adult hippocampal neurons, synaptic activity increases the affinity of β-catenin for cadherin in an NMDAR-dependent manner (Murase *et al.* 2002). Synaptic activity also increases the concentration of β-catenin at dendritic spines where cadherin mediates synaptic connections (Murase *et al.* 2002). The redistribution of β-catenin is probably driven by decreased levels of Tyr phosphorylation. Point mutations of β-catenin Tyr-654 to Glu or Phe cause dramatic alterations in both synaptic structure and function (Murase *et al.* 2002). These results suggest that phosphorylation of β-catenin Tyr-654 plays an important role in activity-induced synaptic remodelling.

Cdk5/p35 is a neuron-specific Ser/Thr kinase whose activity regulates important developmental events such as neural migration (Chae *et al.* 1997) and neurite outgrowth (Nikolic *et al.* 1996). Cdk5 interacts with β-catenin through its regulatory subunit, p35, and regulates the affinity of β-catenin for cadherin in developing cortical neurons (Kwon *et al.* 2000). Although β-catenin can be a substrate for Cdk5 (Kesavapany *et al.* 2001), it is unknown whether β-catenin Ser/Thr phosphorylation affects the affinity for cadherin. Here, we show in adult hippocampal neurons that depolarization inhibits Cdk5 activity, which increases the affinity of β-catenin for cadherin. Inhibition of Cdk5 by roscovitine results in a redistribution of β-catenin from dendritic shaft to spines. A point mutation of Tyr-654 completely blocks the redistribution effect of roscovitine, suggesting that Cdk5 activity regulates the affinity of β-catenin by altering the phosphorylation level of Tyr-654.

20.2 Material and methods

(a) Generation of sindbis virus expressing wild-type and point mutant EGFP-β-catenin

The details that follow were described previously in Murase *et al.* (2002). Briefly, full length chicken β-catenin cDNA was subcloned into BspEI–EcoRI sites of the pEGFPC1 vector (Clontech). Point mutations were created from EGFP-β-catenin using a QuickChange site-directed mutagenesis kit (Stratagene). The NheI–ApaI fragment was then subcloned into XbaI–ApaI sites of pSindRep5. The recombinants of sindbis virus were prepared by using a sindbis expression system (Invitrogen). The plasmid was linearized by PacI digestion, and was used to perform *in vitro* transcription. The virus was generated in BHK cells. All results were confirmed by DNA sequencing.

(b) Cultured neurons

Dissociated hippocampal neurons from postnatal 2 day rat pups were plated at a density of 15 000–45 000 cells cm^{-2} onto polylysine and laminin-coated cover-slips. Cultures were maintained in growth medium (Neurobasal-A supplemented with B27 and GlutaMax-1) for 18–28 days before use. Recombinant DNA was introduced by sindbis virus infection in the growth medium 18–24 hours before imaging. To block protein synthesis, 40 μM anisomycin was added to the growth medium 1–2 hours before imaging.

(c) Imaging

HBS containing 110 mM NaCl, 5.4 mM KCl, 1.8 mM CaCl$_2$, 0.8 mM MgCl$_2$, 10 mM D-glucose, and 10 mM HEPES-NaOH (pH 7.4) (osmolarity adjusted to 290 mOsmol with sucrose) was used for imaging. Roscovitine, U0126 (Calbiochem) and sodium orthovanadate were used at final concentrations of 50 μM, 50 μM and 1 mM, respectively. It was confirmed that incubation in 0.2% DMSO from stock solutions did not affect the EGFP–β-catenin distribution in neurons. No cell death was observed after incubation for 3 hours with 50 μM roscovitine as assessed by propidium iodide staining ($n = 9$). To evaluate the effect of orthovanadate, the neurons were incubated with 40 μM anisomycin for more than 1 hour before $t = 0$ to arrest protein synthesis. Images were acquired by an Olympus AX70 CCD microscope with a water emersion objective lens at room temperature (magnification, × 63). A mercury lamp was used for excitation, excitation filter: 480 ± 40 nm; emission filter: 535 ± 50 nm (Chroma 41001). Each image was taken with a 2 s exposure.

(d) Immunoprecipitation

Hippocampal slices (300 μm) from 5- to 6-week-old male Sprague–Dawley rats were recovered at room temperature for 1.5 hours on filter paper placed over a tissue culture dish containing oxygenated ACSF (119 mM NaCl, 2.5 mM KCl, 1.3 mM MgSO$_4$, 2.5 mM CaCl$_2$, 1.0 mM NaH$_2$PO$_4$, 26.2 mM NaHCO$_3$, and 11.0 mM D-glucose). The slices were incubated in oxygenated ACSF, in some cases containing 50 μM roscovitine, for 3 hours. For the point mutation analysis, the sindbis virus was microinjected with quartz micropipettes prepared from microfilaments (1 mm OD, 0.7 mm OD, 10 cm length, Sutter Instrument) into hippocampal slices (300 μm) from 9-day-old rat pups. The slices were then cultured for 24–36 hours (Stoppini *et al.* 1991). The slices were homogenized in 300 μl lysis buffer (150 mM NaCl, 1% NP-40, and 50 mM Tris–HCl (pH 8.0)) containing a protease inhibitor cocktail (Roche) on ice, and centrifuged at 12 000*g* for 10 min at 4 °C. Monoclonal anti-cadherin, CH-19 (pancadherin) antibody (Sigma), was used for immunoprecipitation. For EGFP–β-catenins, monoclonal anti-GFP antibody (Clontech) was used. Western blot analysis was performed with monoclonal anti-β-catenin antibody, 15B8 (Sigma) or pancadherin CH-19 antibody as primary antibodies, and with peroxidase labelled anti-mouse IgG antibody (Amersham Pharmacia Biotech) as a secondary antibody.

(e) Kinase assay for Cdk5

Dissociated hippocampal neuron cultures were used for the kinase assay as described by Nickolic *et al.* (1998). After washing three times with HBS, the neurons were incubated with high KCl–HBS for 5–7 min. The neurons were then recovered in HBS for 30 min before incubating in lysis buffer (ELB), containing 250 mM NaCl, 0.1% NP-40, 50 mM HEPES–KOH (pH 7.0), 5 mM EDTA, protease inhibitor cocktail, on ice for 20 min. The lysate was collected and centrifuged at 12 000*g* for 10 min at 4 °C. Rabbit polyclonal anti-Cdk5 antibody, C-8 (Santa Cruz) was used for immunoprecipitation. The Cdk5 kinase assay was done in the presence of 1 mM ATP, 2 μ Ciγ^{32}P-ATP, 0.5 mg histone H1 (Calbiochem) and kinase buffer containing 50 mM HEPES (pH 7.5) and 10 mM MgCl$_2$ (Nikolic *et al.* 1998). For Western blot, monoclonal anti-Cdc2 p34 (17), anti-Cdk2 (D-12) and anti-Cdk5 (DC 17) antibodies and rabbit polyclonal anti-p35 antibody, C-19 (Santa Cruz) were used as primary antibodies, and peroxidase labelled anti-mouse or anti-rabbit IgG antibodies (Amersham Pharmacia Biotech) as secondary antibodies. The bands were visualized using ECL system (Amersham Pharmacia Biotech). Statistical significance was assessed with the Student's *t*-test. *p* values of 0.05 were considered significant and higher values are designated as not significant (n.s.).

(f) Time-lapse image analysis

The details were described previously in Murase *et al.* (2002). Briefly, areas containing dendrites of around 50 μm in length were selected for analysis with Image J software. The m.p.v. of each area was used to calculate the total fluorescence intensity. Every dendritic spine within the area (typically 10–20 spines) was analysed by measuring the m.p.v. within a circle (around 1.4 m in diameter) surrounding it. The m.p.v. of the dendritic shaft was also measured to calculate the fluorescence intensity of the shaft region. The background was subtracted from each measurement. The photobleaching effect was removed by normalizing with a photobleaching curve (Murase *et al.* 2002).

20.3 Results

(a) Cdk5 activity is inhibited by neural activity

Both Cdk5 and its activator protein, p35, are enriched at synaptic sites in hippocampal neurons (Tomizawa *et al.* 2002). To investigate whether Cdk5 is regulated by neural activity, the phosphorylation of histone H1 protein, a substrate for Cdk5, was measured with immunoprecipitates from dissociated cultured hippocampal neurons. When the neuronal cell lysate was immunoprecipitated with an anti-Cdk5 antibody, an abundant amount of ^{32}P was incorporated into H1, indicating high Cdk5 activity (Fig. 20.1*a*). The activity level of Cdk5 was, however, significantly reduced when the neurons were briefly depolarized by the application of high KCl–HBS (Fig. 20.1*a*). Although the degradation of p35 is known to regulate the activity of Cdk5 (Patrick *et al.* 1998), the protein levels of Cdk5 and p35 were not changed by KCl stimulation (Fig. 20.1*b*). These results indicate that neural activity causes an inhibition of Cdk5 activity by a mechanism that does not involve the degradation of p35.

In developing cortical neurons, the affinity of β-catenin for cadherin is regulated by Cdk5 activity (Kwon *et al.* 2000). Therefore, we next examined whether Cdk5 also regulates the affinity between β-catenin and cadherin in adult hippocampal neurons. When hippocampal slices were incubated with the Cdk inhibitor roscovitine, the amount of β-catenin co-immunoprecipitated with an anti-cadherin antibody was significantly increased compared with that co-immunoprecipitated from the control slices (Fig. 20.1*c*). Although roscovitine is also known to inhibit MAPKs (Meijer *et al.* 1997), no significant change was observed in the amount of β-catenin when the slices were incubated with an MEK inhibitor, U0126, indicating that the roscovitine-induced affinity increase is not due to the inhibition of MAPKs (Fig. 20.1*c*). Although roscovitine is known to inhibit Cdk1 and Cdk2, as well as Cdk5 (Rudolph *et al.* 1996; Meijer *et al.* 1997), the expression of neither Cdk1 nor Cdk2 was detected from hippocampal cell lysates by Western blot analysis (Fig. 20.1*d*), suggesting the effect of roscovitine on cadherin–β-catenin affinity is specifically due to the inhibition of Cdk5. Taken together, these results suggest that the downregulation of β-catenin–cadherin association mediated by Cdk5 is inhibited by neural activity.

(b) Cdk5 regulates β-catenin distribution

Our recent study (Murase *et al.* 2002) demonstrated that depolarization increased the affinity between neuronal β-catenin and cadherin, and caused a redistribution of β-catenin from dendritic shafts to spines in a tyrosine-phosphorylation-dependent manner (Murase *et al.* 2002). To investigate whether Cdk5 is involved in this redistribution, time-lapse images were taken of neurons expressing EGFP–β-catenin. As shown in Fig. 20.2*a,b*(i), the application of roscovitine induced a redistribution of EGFP–β-catenin from dendritic shafts to spines, similar to that induced by KCl stimulation (Murase *et al.* 2002). To test if the redistribution induced by these two treatments shares similar mechanisms, we performed occlusion experiments. We first examined whether a single depolarization event produces a saturated level of redistribution. We depolarized neurons and then 90 min later depolarized them again. No further redistribution was evoked by the second depolarization (mean per cent

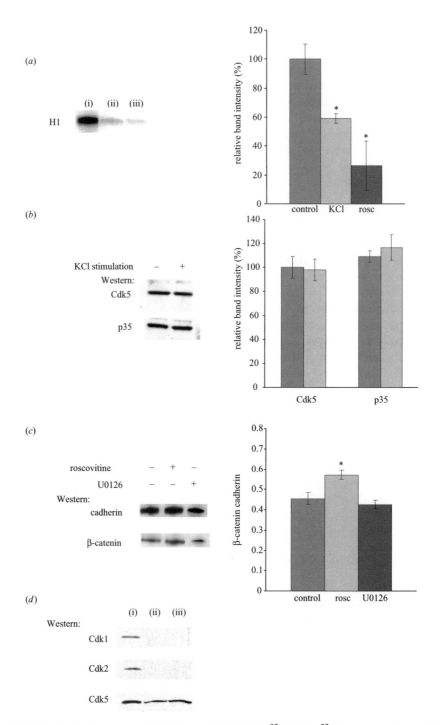

Fig. 20.1 Depolarization causes inhibition of Cdk5. (*a*) γ^{32}P-ATP: ^{32}P incorporation to histone H1 protein. Compared with the control (lane (i)), the Cdk5 kinase activity of KCl-stimulated neurons (lane (ii)) is significantly reduced ($59.3 \pm 3.2\%$ of control, $n = 3$, $p < 0.05$). Roscovitine,

fluorescence $\pm$ s.e.m. at 90 min after the second depolarization: total, $100.0 \pm 5.9\%$; spine, $103.5 \pm 8.1\%$; shaft, $97.9 \pm 2.3\%$, $n = 4$), indicating that the redistribution induced by the first depolarization is maximal and saturated. As shown in Fig. 20.2a,b(ii), a prior depolarization completely blocked the redistribution induced by a subsequent application of roscovitine. By contrast, neurons pre-incubated with roscovitine exhibited additional significant redistribution by depolarization (Fig. 20.2a,b(iii)). These results suggest that Cdk5 inhibition contributes to depolarization-induced β-catenin redistribution, but depolarization can also invoke Cdk5-independent pathways to bring about redistribution.

(c) Point mutations of β-catenin Tyr-654 block regulation of cadherin–β-catenin affinity by Cdk5

The redistribution of β-catenin induced by depolarization is completely prevented by the general tyrosine phosphatase inhibitor, orthovanadate (Murase *et al.* 2002). Although, orthovanadate has other enzymatic inhibitory effects (Cantley *et al.* 1977; Sargeant and Stinson 1979), an increased level of phosphorylated β-catenin is observed after incubation with orthovanadate (Ozawa and Kemler 1998), suggesting a direct effect on β-catenin phosphotyrosine levels. To determine initially whether the regulation of tyrosine phosphorylation is also involved in roscovitine-induced redistribution, we again used orthovanadate. The effect of roscovitine was completely blocked by orthovanadate, suggesting Tyr phosphorylation is critical for roscovitine-induced redistribution (Fig. 20.2c,d(i)). Because the phosphorylation of β-catenin Tyr-654 is known to regulate the affinity between β-catenin and cadherin (Roura *et al.* 1999), we tested the effect of two different point mutations of Tyr-654, one in which phosphorylation is mimicked (Y654E) and another in which phosphorylation is prevented (Y654F). Neither Y654E– nor Y654F–β-catenin–GFP mutants were redistributed after the application of roscovitine (Fig. 20.2c,d(ii,iii)). Together, these results strongly suggest that decreasing the phosphorylation level of Tyr-654 is a necessary step in the redistribution of EGFP–β-catenin caused by inhibiting Cdk5.

To test if the mutation of β-catenin Tyr-654 blocks the roscovitine-induced affinity increase between cadherin and β-catenin, we microinjected sindbis virus containing cDNA of either the wild-type, Y654E or Y654F mutant β-catenin into organotypic hippocampal slices. After 24–36 hours, the slices exhibited abundant expression of

---

a specific Cdk5 inhibitor largely inhibits ^{32}P incorporation (lane (iii), $16.7 \pm 10.8\%$ of control, $n = 3$, $p < 0.05$). Abbreviation: rosc, roscovitine. (*b*) Cell lysate: total amounts of Cdk5 and p35 from control and depolarized neurons. The inhibition of Cdk5 by depolarization is not caused by degradation of p35 (Cdk5: $98.1 \pm 9.1\%$ of control, $n = 3$, n.s.; p35: $107.0 \pm 10.7\%$, $n = 3$, n.s.). Dark shading, control; light shading, KCl stimulated. (*c*) IP with anti-cadherin: inhibition of Cdk5 increases the affinity between β-catenin and cadherin in adult hippocampal neurons. Cell lysate from control and roscovitine-treated neurons was used for immunoprecipitation with an anti-cadherin antibody. The amount of β-catenin co-immunoprecipitated with anti-cadherin antibody from roscovitine-treated neurons was significantly larger than control ($p < 0.05$, $n = 3$). Abbreviation: rosc, roscovitine. (*d*) Western blot analysis with anti-Cdk1, anti-Cdk2 and anti-Cdk5 antibodies. Lane (i), cell lysate from PC12 cells; lane (ii), cell lysate from DIV18 cultured hippocampal neurons; lane (iii), cell lysate from P10 hippocampal neurons. Both DIV18 and P10 hippocampal neurons showed an abundant expression of Cdk5, but not Cdk1 or Cdk2.

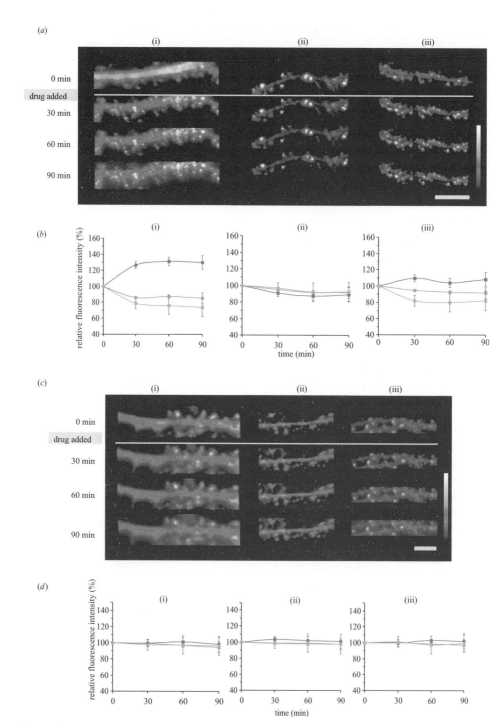

Fig. 20.2 (*a,b*) The application of roscovitine causes a movement of β-catenin from shafts to spines. (*a*) Time-lapse images of EGFP-β-catenin pre- and post-treatment. (i) EGFP–β-catenin treated with roscovitine; (ii) pre-depolarized then treated with roscovitine; and (iii) pre-treated

EGFP–β-catenin (Fig. 20.3*a*). The cell lysate from the infected slices was immuno-precipitated with an anti-GFP antibody, and blotted with either anti-β-catenin or anticadherin antibodies (Fig. 20.3*b*). No β-catenin or cadherin bands were observed from lysate prepared from non-infected slices (Fig. 20.3*b*, first lane). As expected, both the EGFP–β-catenin fusion proteins showed higher molecular weights (around 115 kDa) than the endogenous β-catenin (90 kDa). The amount of EGFP–β-catenin immuno-precipitated with anti-GFP was not affected by roscovitine treatment (Fig. 20.3*b*). In the case of the wild-type EGFP–β-catenin, the cadherin/EGFP–β-catenin ratio was significantly increased by roscovitine treatment (Fig. 20.3*b,c*). As expected, the Y654F mutant showed a higher basal affinity for cadherin when compared with the wild-type (compare the control bars in Fig. 20.3*c*). The affinity of the Y654F mutant was not further increased by the inhibition of Cdk5 (Fig. 20.3*b,c*). Alternatively, the Y654E mutant showed a lower basal affinity for cadherin (compare the control bars in Fig. 20.3*c*), which was also unaffected by roscovitine (Fig. 20.3*b,c*). These results are consistent with the redistribution studies and suggest that the action of the Cdk5 occurs upstream of the β-catenin Tyr-654 regulation.

20.4 Discussion

(a) Cdk5 regulates the affinity between cadherin and β-catenin in an activity-dependent manner

Our results indicate that Cdk5 activity is significantly inhibited by synaptic activity. The mechanism by which neural activity regulates Cdk5 remains to be investigated. Here, we show that the degradation of the Cdk5 activator is not involved. It is known that phosphorylation of Cdk5 by a Tyr kinase, Abl, can increase Cdk5 activity (Zukerberg *et al.* 2000). However, very low levels of tyrosine phosphorylation of Cdk5 were detected in hippocampal neurons incubated with Tyr phosphatase inhibitor, and the amount of phosphorylation was not changed by depolarization (data not shown). A recent study has shown the interaction of an inhibitor protein with the Cdk5/p35 complex (Ching *et al.* 2002). One can speculate that such a protein is a synaptically regulated target.

Incubation of hippocampal slices with roscovitine caused a significant increase in QJ;β-catenin's affinity for cadherin. The association of β-catenin with cadherin is

---

with roscovitine then depolarized. Neurons were treated immediately after $t = 0$. Scale bar, 10 μm. (*b*) Relative fluorescence intensities. Spine region (violet), shaft region (orange) and total (blue). (i) Roscovitine ($n = 3$); (ii) roscovitine (pre-depolarized, $n = 5$); and (iii) depolarization (pre-treated with roscovitine, $n = 6$). (*c,d*) Point mutations at Tyr-654 block roscovitine-induced EGFP–β-catenin redistribution. (*c*) Time-lapse images of EGFP–β-catenin pre- and post-treat-ment. (i) EGFP–β-catenin treated with roscovitine in the presence of sodium orthovanadate; (ii) EGFP–Y654E–β-catenin treated with roscovitine; and (iii) EGFP–Y654F–β-catenin treated with roscovitine. Neurons were treated immediately after $t = 0$. Scale bar, 10 μm. (*d*) Relative fluorescence intensities. Spine region (violet), shaft region (orange), and total (blue). (i) EGFP–β-catenin treated with roscovitine in the presence of sodium orthovanadate, $n = 5$; (ii) EGFP–Y654E–β-catenin treated with roscovitine, $n = 4$; and (iii) EGFP–Y654F–β-catenin treated with roscovitine, $n = 4$. (See Plate 6 of the Plate Section, at the centre of this book.)

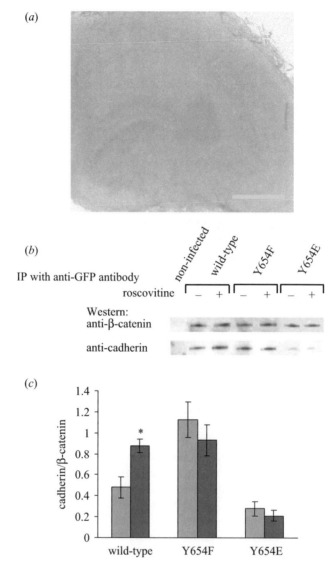

Fig. 20.3. Point mutation at Tyr-654 block roscovitine-induced affinity increase for cadherin. (*a*) An organotypic hippocampal slice expressing EGFP–β-catenin. The DIC and fluorescence images were overlaid. EGFP–β-catenin was introduced via the microinjection of sindbis virus. Scale bar, 500 μm. (*b*) Immunoprecipitation analysis of roscovitine effect on cadherin–β-catenin affinity. Cell lysates from either the wild-type, Y654F- or Y654E-expressing slices were immuno-precipitated with an anti-GFP antibody, and blotted with either anti-β-catenin or anti-cadherin antibodies. Slices were pretreated for 3 hours with either the control medium or medium containing roscovitine. (*c*) Ratios of cadherin : β-catenin band intensities. The wild-type β-catenin showed a significantly increased ratio after roscovitine treatment, whereas Tyr-654 mutants do not (mean ± s.e.m., $n = 3$, wildtype; $p < 0.05$, Y654F and Y654E; n.s.). Dark shading, control; light shading, roscovitine. (See Plate 7 of the Plate Section, at the centre of this book.)

important for cadherin to achieve high adhesive activity. Therefore, our result suggests a role for Cdk5 in the regulation of cadherin activity in adult hippocampal neurons. Our recent study demonstrated that changes in affinity between β-catenin and cadherin can alter synaptic structure and function (Murase *et al.* 2002). Together with the inhibition of Cdk5 by depolarization, our results suggest an important role for Cdk5 in neural activity-induced synaptic modulation or synaptic plasticity. In fact, a recent study has shown that a transient increase of Cdk5 activity is required for associative learning (Fischer *et al.* 2002).

(b) Phosphorylation of β-catenin Tyr-654 is a potential target of the affinity regulation by Cdk5

Cdk5 is known to phosphorylate β-catenin Ser/Thr and regulate the association of β-catenin with presenilin 1 (Kesavapany *et al.* 2001). However, phosphorylation of β-catenin Ser/Thr itself does not appear to change cadherin–β-catenin affinity, because the roscovitine-induced redistribution can be blocked by orthovanadate in the absence of any Ser/Thr phosphatase inhibitors. It is more likely that Cdk5 activity promotes β-catenin Tyr phosphorylation. Because the effect of roscovitine is blocked by mutations of Tyr-654, it is possible that Cdk5 regulates cadherin–β-catenin affinity through the activity of a Tyr kinase or phosphatase, whose target is β-catenin Tyr-654. The detailed molecular mechanism for how Cdk5 modulates phosphorylation of β-catenin Tyr-654 remains to be investigated. It is possible that phosphorylation of β-catenin Ser/Thr by Cdk5 induces the association of Tyr kinases to β-catenin (or the dissociation of Tyr phosphatases from β-catenin). Taken together, our results suggest that the depolarization-induced enhancement of cadherin–β-catenin affinity is at least partly achieved by Cdk5 inhibition, which results in the decreased phosphorylation level of QJ;β-catenin Tyr-654. Future studies will determine the contribution of β-catenin's localization to synaptic plasticity in hippocampal slices.

The authors thank G. Patrick for helpful discussions, and H. Weld for making beautiful cultured hippocampal neurons. E.M.S. is an Associate Investigator of the Howard Hughes Medical Institute.

References

Balsamo, J., Leung, T., Ernst, H., Zanin, M. K. B., and Hoffman, S. (1996). Regulated binding of a PTP1B-like phosphatase to *N*-cadherin: control of cadherin-mediated adhesion by dephosphorylation of beta-catenin. *J. Cell Biol.* **134**, 801–13.

Balsamo, J., Arregui, C., Leung, T., and Lilien, J. (1998). The non-receptor protein tyrosine phosphatase PTP1B binds to the cytoplasmic domain of *N*-cadherin and regulates the cadherin-actin linkage. *J. Cell Biol.* **143**, 523–32.

Behrens, J., Vakaet, L., Friis, R., Winterhager, E., van Roy, F., Mareel, M. M., *et al.* (1993). Loss of epithelial differentiation and gain of invasiveness correlates with tyrosine phosphorylation of the E-cadherin/beta-catenin complex in cells transformed with a temperature-sensitive v-SRC gene. *J. Cell Biol.* **120**, 757–66.

Benson, D. L. and Tanaka, H. (1998). N-cadherin distribution during synaptogenesis in hippocampal neurons. *J. Neurosci.* **18**, 6892–904.

Bonvini, P., An, W. G., Rosolen, A., Nguyen, P., Trepel, J., Garcia de Herreros, A., et al. (2001). Geldanamycin abrogates ErbB2 association with proteosome-resistant β-catenin in melanoma cells, increases β-catenin-E-cadherin association, and decreases β-cateninsensitive transcription. Cancer Res. **61**, 1671–7.

Bozdagi, O., Shan, W., Tanaka, H., Benson, D. L., and Huntley, G. W. (2000). Increasing numbers of synaptic puncta during late-phase LTP, N-cadherin is synthesized, recruited to synaptic sites, and required for potentiation. Neuron **28**, 245–59.

Cantley Jr, L. C., Josephson, L., Warner, R., Yanagisawa, M., Lechene, C., and Guidotti, G. (1977). Vanadate is a potent (Na,K)-ATPase inhibitor found in ATP derived from muscle. J. Biol. Chem. **252**, 7421–3.

Chae, T., Kwon, Y. T., Bronson, R., Dikkes, P., Li, E., and Tsai, L. H. (1997). Mice lacking p35, a neuronal specific activator of Cdk5, display cortical lamination defects, seizures, and adult lethality. Neuron **18**, 29–42.

Ching, Y. P., Pang, A. S., Lam, W.H., Qi, R. Z., and Wang, J.H. (2002). Identification of a Neuronal Cdk5 activator-binding protein as Cdk5 inhibitor. J. Biol. Chem. **277**, 15 237–40.

Fannon, A.M. and Colman, D. R. (1996). A model for central synaptic junctional complex formation based on the differential adhesive specificities of the cadherins. Neuron **17**, 423–34.

Fischer, A., Sananbenesi, F., Schrick, C., Spiess, J., and Radulovic, J. (2002). Cyclin-dependent kinase 5 is required for associative learning. J. Neurosci. **22**, 3700–3707.

Fuchs, M., Muller, T., Lerch, M. M., and Ullrich, A. (1996). Association of human protein-tyrosine phosphatase k with members of the armadillo family. J. Biol. Chem. **271**, 16 712–19.

Hamaguchi, M., Matsuyoshi, N., Ohnishi, Y., Gotoh, B., Takeichi, M., and Nagai, Y. (1993). p60v-src causes tyrosine phosphorylation and inactivation of the N-cadherin-catenin cell adhesion system. EMBO J. **12**, 307–14.

Hazan, R. B. and Norton, L. (1998). The epidermal growth factor receptor modulates the interaction of E-cadherin with the actin cytoskeleton. J. Biol. Chem. **273**, 9078–9084.

Hirano, S., Kimoto, N., Shimoyama, Y., Hirohashi, S., and Takeichi, M. (1992). Identification of a neural alpha-catenin as a key regulator of cadherin function and multicellular organization. Cell **70**, 293–301.

Husi, H., Ward, M. A., Choudhary, J. S., Blackstock, W. P., and Grant, S. G. N. (2000). Proteomic analysis of NMDA receptor-adhesion protein signaling complexes. Nature Neurosci. **3**, 661–9.

Kesavapany, S., Lau, K. F., McLoughlin, D. M., Brownlees, J., Ackerley, S., Leigh, P. N., et al. (2001). p35/cdk5 binds and phosphorylates beta-catenin and regulates beta-catenin/presenilin-1 interaction. Eur. J. Neurosci. **13**, 241–7.

Kwon, Y. T., Gupta, A., Zhou, Y., Nikolic, M., and Tsai, L.-H. (2000). Regulation of N-cadherin-mediated adhesion by the p35-Cdk5 kinase. Curr. Biol. **10**, 363–372.

Kypta, R. M., Su, H., and Reichardt, L. F. (1996). Association between a transmembrane protein tyrosine phosphatase and the cadherin-catenin complex. J. Cell Biol. **134**, 1519–29.

Manabe, T., Togashi, H., Uchida, N., Suzuki, S. C., Hayakawa, Y., Yamamoto, M., et al. (2000). Loss of cadherin-11 receptor enhances plastic changes in hippocampal synapses and modifies behavioral responses. Mol. Cell. Neurosci. **15**, 534–46.

Matsuyoshi, N., Hamaguchi, M., Taniguchi, S., Nagafuchi, A., Tsukita, S., and Takeichi, M. (1992). Cadherin-mediated cell-cell adhesion is perturbed by v-src tyrosine phosphorylation in metastatic fibroblasts. J. Cell Biol. **118**, 703–14.

Meijer, L., Borgne, A., Mulner, O., Chong, J. P., Blow, J. J., Inagaki, N., et al. (1997). Biochemical and cellular effects of roscovitine, a potent and selective inhibitor of the cyclin-dependent kinases cdc2, cdk2 and cdk5. Eur. J. Biochem. **243**, 527–36.

Müller, T., Cohidas, A., Reichmann, E., and Ullrich, A. (1999). Phosphorylation and free pool of β-catenin are regulated by tyrosine kinases and tyrosine phosphatases during epithelial cell migration. J. Biol. Chem. **274**, 10 173–83.

Murase, S. and Schuman, E. M. (1999). The role of cell adhesion molecules in synaptic plasticity and memory. *Curr. Opin. Cell Biol.* **11**, 549–53.

Murase, S., Mosser, E., and Schuman, E.M. (2002). Depolarization drives β-catenin into neuronal spines promoting changes in synaptic structure and function. *Neuron* **35**, 91–105.

Nagafuchi, A., Ishihara, S., and Tsukita, S. (1994). The roles of catenins in the cadherin-mediated cell adhesion functional analysis of E-cadherin-α catenin fusion molecules. *J. Cell Biol.* **127**, 235–45.

Nikolic, M., Chou, M. M., Lu, W., Mayer, B. J., and Tsai, L. H. (1998). The p35/Cdk5 kinase is a neuron-specific Rac effector that inhibits Pak1 activity. *Nature* **395**, 194–8.

Nikolic, M., Dudek, H., Kwon, Y. T., Ramos, Y. F., and Tsai, L. H. (1996). The cdk5/p35 kinase is essential for neurite outgrowth during neuronal differentiation. *Genes Dev.* **10**, 816–25.

Ozawa, M. and Kemler, R. (1998). Altered cell adhesion activity by pervanadate due to the dissociation of β-catenin from the E cadherin–catenin complex. *J. Biol. Chem.* **273**, 6166–70.

Ozawa, M., Ringwald, M., and Kemler, R. (1990). Uvomorulin-catenin complex formation is regulated by a specific domain in the cytoplasmic region of the cell adhesion molecule. *Proc. Natl Acad. Sci. USA* **87**, 4246–50.

Pathre, P., Arregui, C., Wampler, T., Kue, I., Leung, T. C., Lilien, J., et al. (2001). PTP1B regulates neurite extension mediated by cell–cell and cell–matrix adhesion molecules. *J. Neurosci. Res.* **63**, 143–50.

Patrick, G. N., Zhou, P., Kwon, Y. T., Howley, P. M., and Tsai, L. H. (1998). p35, the neuronal-specific activator of cyclindependent kinase 5 (Cdk5) is degraded by the ubiquitinproteasome pathway. *J. Biol. Chem.* **273**, 24 057–64.

Phillips G. R., Huang, J. K., Wang, Y., Tanaka, H., Shapiro, L., Zhang, W., et al. (2001). The presynaptic particle web, ultrastructure, composition, dissolution, and reconstitution. *Neuron* **32**, 63–77.

Roura, S., Miravet, S., Piedra, J., de Harreors, A. G., and Muñach, M. (1999). Regulation of E-cadherin/catenin association by tyrosine phosphorylation. *J. Biol. Chem.* **274**, 36 734–40.

Rudolph, B., Saffrich, R., Zwicker, J., Henglein, B., Muller, R., Ansorge, W., et al. (1996). Activation of cyclindependent kinases by Myc mediates induction of cyclin A, but not apoptosis. *EMBO J.* **15**, 3065–76.

Sargeant, L. E., and Stinson, R. A. (1979). Inhibition of human alkaline phosphatases by vanadate. *Biochem. J.* **181**, 247–50.

Sommers, C. L., Gelmann, E. P., Kemler, R., Cowin, P., and Byers, S. W. (1994). Alterations in β-catenin phosphorylation and plakoglobin expression in human breast cancer cells. *Cancer Res.* **54**, 3544–52.

Stoppini, L., Buchs, P. A., and Muller, D. (1991). A simple method for organotypic cultures of nervous tissue. *J. Neurosci. Meth.* **37**, 173–82.

Takeichi, M. (1990). Cadherins, a molecular family important in selective cell–cell adhesion. *A. Rev. Biochem.* **59**, 237–52.

Tanaka, H., Shan, W., Phillips, G. R., Arndt, K., Bozdagi, O., Shapiro, L., et al. (2000). Molecular modification of N-cadherin in response to synaptic activity. *Neuron* **25**, 93–107.

Tang, L., Hung, C. P., and Schuman, E. M. (1998). A role for the cadherin family of cell adhesion molecules in hippocampus long-term potentiation. *Neuron* **20**, 1165–75.

Togashi, H., Abe, K., Mizoguchi, A., Takaoka, K., Chisaka, O., and Takeichi, M. (2002). Cadherin regulates dendritic spine morphogenesis. *Neuron* **35**, 77–89.

Tomizawa, K., Ohta, J., Matsushita, M., Moriwaki, A., Li, S. T., Takei, K., et al. (2002). Cdk5/p35 regulates neurotransmitter release through phosphorylation and downregulation of P/Q-type voltage-dependent calcium channel activity. *J Neurosci.* **22**, 2590–7.

Uchida, N., Honjo, Y., Johnson, K. R., Wheelock, M. J., and Takeichi, M. (1996). The catenin/cadherin adhesion system is located in synaptic junctions bordering transmitter release zones. *J. Cell Biol.* **135**, 767–79.

Zukerberg, L. R., Patrick, G. N., Nicolic, M., Humbert, S., Wu, C.-L., Lanier, L. M., *et al.* (2000). Cables links Cdk5 and c-Abl and facilitates Cdk5 tyrosine phosphorylation, kinase upregulation, and neurite outgrowth. *Neuron* **26**, 633–46.

Glossary

ACSF   artificial cerebral spinal fluid
Cdk5   cyclin-dependent kinase 5
DIC   differential interference contrast
EGFP   enhanced green fluorescent protein
GFP   green fluorescent protein
HBS   HEPES buffered saline
L-LTP   late-phase long-term potentiation
LTP   long-term potentiation
m.p.v.   mean pixel value

21

In search of general mechanisms for long-lasting plasticity: *Aplysia* and the hippocampus

Christopher Pittenger and Eric R. Kandel

Long-term synaptic plasticity is thought to underlie many forms of long-lasting memory. Long-lasting plasticity has been most extensively studied in the marine snail *Aplysia* and in the mammalian hippocampus, where Bliss and Lømo first described long-term potentiation 30 years ago. The molecular mechanisms of plasticity in these two systems have proven to have many similarities. Here, we briefly describe some of these areas of overlap. We then summarize recent advances in our understanding of the mechanisms of long-lasting synaptic facilitation in *Aplysia* and suggest that these may prove fruitful areas for future investigation in the mammalian hippocampus and at other synapses in the mammalian brain.

Keywords: long-term potentiation; facilitation; hippocampus; *Aplysia*; long-term plasticity

21.1 Introduction

Memory formation requires the long-term storage of information in the brain, and long-lasting synaptic plasticity is thought to be a principal mechanism by which this information is stored. Learning-related synaptic plasticity has been most thoroughly studied in the marine snail *Aplysia* and in the mammalian hippocampus, where Bliss and Lømo (1973) first described the phenomenon of LTP 30 years ago. The relationship between behavioural change and plasticity at a particular set of synapses is necessarily complex in a neural system as complicated as the mammalian brain, especially in hippocampus-based explicit memory. In spatial memory involving the hippocampus, the synaptic changes that contribute to a given behavioural change are likely to be distributed across many synapses. Even an apparently unitary behavioural change may require changes in different populations of synapses, such as the different synapses in the hippocampal circuit and elsewhere in the medial temporal lobe. Finally, several dissociable forms of plasticity can coexist at the same synapse, potentially obscuring the relationship between learning and experimentally observed synaptic change. Nevertheless, a number of instances in which molecules and pathways involved in LTP have independently been implicated in learning has validated LTP as a useful model of the plasticity underlying hippocampus-dependent memory.

The mechanisms of memory can be divided into two parts: the molecular mechanisms and the systems properties of storage. Study of the molecular mechanisms of plasticity in the hippocampus has been complemented and counterbalanced by studies in simpler model systems, such as the marine snail *Aplysia*. While there will, of course, be aspects of the systems properties of hippocampus-based memory that cannot be recapitulated in a simple invertebrate, these molecular mechanisms are proving to be remarkably well conserved. In many instances, synergy between the two systems has advanced our understanding more quickly than would have been possible with either alone. In a complex area, such as the mechanisms of learning-related synaptic plasticity, results from any single model must be accepted with caution. When similar or identical molecules and mechanisms are implicated in two such different model systems, as has been the case in many instances, we can be much more confident of their validity and importance.

Studies of the late phase of synaptic plasticity illustrate this point. Persistence of both memory and plasticity requires regulated gene induction and the production of new proteins. When these processes are blocked pharmacologically in various model systems, both memory (Flexner *et al.* 1965; Agranoff 1967; Castellucci *et al.* 1986; Freeman *et al.* 1995; Bourtchouladze *et al.* 1998) and synaptic plasticity (Castellucci *et al.* 1986; Huang *et al.* 1996) are truncated to a short period of time after training or stimulation. Many behaviourally relevant memories, including those that we hold most dear and that define our individuality, must persist in the long term. Long-lasting, transcription-dependent plasticity therefore merits close investigation. Recently, there have been three major developments in the study of hippocampal L-LTP, all of which have been encountered independently in *Aplysia*.

(i) A consensus is emerging as to the mechanisms of communication between the synapse and the nucleus (Impey *et al.* 1999).

(ii) We are beginning to better understand the transcriptional regulators involved in L-LTP (Barco *et al.* 2002; Pittenger *et al.* 2002).

(iii) The discovery of synaptic capture and synaptic tagging has given us new insight into the targeting of newly synthesized macromolecules to potentiated synapses (Frey and Morris 1997; Barco *et al.* 2002; Dudek and Fields 2002).

Aplysia was introduced for the study of learning and memory precisely because it allows a relatively straightforward mapping of learned behaviour onto synaptic change and because it allows a cell and molecular biological analysis of these changes (Kandel 1979; see Antonov *et al.* 2003). Here, we briefly review instances where molecular and cellular mechanisms of long-lasting plasticity in *Aplysia* recapitulate those in the more behaviourally interesting, but more complicated, mammalian brain. In discussing L-LTP we focus on the Schaffer collateral synapse in the rodent hippocampus, because this is where the most detailed work has been done. However, there is no *a priori* reason to believe that results from the *Aplysia* system, or any other model system, should be better recapitulated at the Schaffer collateral synapse than at other plastic synapses in the mammalian brain. We then describe some new developments in the study of *Aplysia* plasticity, with the hope that these may point the way to fruitful areas for investigation of L-LTP and learning in mammals.

21.2 Molecular mechanisms of memory in *Aplysia* and the mammalian hippocampus: parallel lives

(a) Communication between synapses and the nucleus

For a synaptic trigger to lead to gene induction in the nucleus requires the transmission of a signal along the length of the dendrite—often a considerable distance. In *Aplysia*, synaptic stimulation activates several kinases, which can physically move into the nucleus to act on nuclear substrates. After sufficiently robust and repeated synaptic stimulation with the modulatory transmitter serotonin, the catalytic subunit of the cAMP-dependent PKA moves to the nucleus, where it can participate in late phase processes (Bacskai *et al.* 1993). PKA activates the p42 MAPK, which can likewise move to the nucleus and phosphorylate nuclear targets (Martin *et al.* 1997*a*). The activation of kinases, by repetitive synaptic stimulation or by the action of modulatory transmitters such as dopamine, also mediates signalling to the nucleus during Schaffer collateral LTP. PKA is involved in L-LTP (Frey *et al.* 1993; Abel *et al.* 1997), but current data more strongly support a role in gating inhibition by phosphatases than a direct role in phosphorylating nuclear substrates (Blitzer *et al.* 1995; Winder *et al.* 1998). The role of the MAPK cascade, however, is clearly conserved; MAPK is activated by robust, repeated synaptic stimulation, is necessary for L-LTP, and appears to gain access to nuclear substrates by physically moving into the nucleus upon activation (English and Sweatt 1996, 1997; Martin *et al.* 1997*a*; Patterson *et al.* 2001). Mammals thus recapitulate at least some aspects of the signalling from synapse to nucleus seen in *Aplysia*.

(b) Transcriptional regulation for LTP and long-term memory

Once the inducing signal has been transmitted to the nucleus, regulated transcription factors must be activated. In *Aplysia*, early evidence indicated that the CRE was a critical enhancer for this gene induction (Dash *et al.* 1990). Later cloning of the *Aplysia* CREB gene allowed confirmation that this inducible transcription factor is a central early element of the cascade of gene activation required for the establishment of long-lasting synaptic facilitation (Bartsch *et al.* 1998). In mammals the situation is complicated by the existence of several alternatively spliced and heterodimerizing CREB-like transcription factors, but CREB and CRE-driven transcription appear to have a similarly central role (Bourtchouladze *et al.* 1994; Pittenger *et al.* 2002).

(c) Inhibitory constraints: memory suppressor genes

Recent studies in both *Aplysia* and the hippocampus have revealed the importance of memory suppressor genes, genes whose function is to limit synaptic strengthening in the short or the long term. Interference with such molecules enhances synaptic plasticity, and in some cases enhances learning and memory (Abel *et al.* 1998). In *Aplysia*, this was first shown with the inhibitory transcription factor CREB2. Interference with CREB2 enhances long-lasting facilitation, such that weaker synaptic stimulation can lead to long-lasting change (Bartsch *et al.* 1995). In the mouse hippocampus, recent results from our laboratory suggest that interference with ATF4, the mammalian homologue of *Aplysia* CREB2, can likewise enhance LTP and can potentiate hippocampus-dependent learning (Chen *et al.* 2003).

A better-studied memory suppressor in rodents is the phosphatase calcineurin. Calcineurin (or PP2B) is the first step in a phosphatase cascade that parallels and antagonizes signalling by kinases. These phosphatases remove phosphate groups from various regulatory molecules, including substrates of PKA, and thereby gate communication between the synapse and the nucleus in the induction of lasting potentiation (Blitzer *et al.* 1995; Mansuy *et al.* 1998). Reduction in calcineurin activity enhances LTP *in vitro* and *in vivo* and improves animals' learning in a number of hippocampus-dependent tasks (Malleret *et al.* 2001). The importance of memory suppressor genes in multiple forms of lasting plasticity identifies them as important, and perhaps conserved, regulators.

(d) Targeting of newly synthesized proteins to activated synapse

Once genes have been induced and new gene products produced, they must be targeted to the appropriate synapses for long-term plastic processes to take hold. This is a difficult sorting problem, because each mammalian hippocampal neuron has around 10 000 synapses for its one nucleus. The prevailing model of how this might occur is the 'synaptic tagging' hypothesis. Plasticity-inducing synaptic activity is proposed to initiate three processes: local events that lead to immediate (but labile) synaptic changes; a synaptic mark that tags the synapse as an appropriate target for long-term strengthening; and a signal back to the nucleus, as described in Section 21.2a, to induce the genes that are required for that strengthening to take place. As newly produced proteins and RNAs are transported from the cell body, the synaptic tag controls which synapses they reinforce. This process can be demonstrated, even though we do not yet know the specific nature of the synaptic tag, through the phenomenon of 'synaptic capture': a synapse tagged with a relatively weak stimulus can 'capture' the products of transcription induced by stronger stimulation at a different synapse, acquiring L-LTP with a stimulation normally only sufficient for E-LTP.

Synaptic capture has been demonstrated in both mammals (Frey and Morris 1997) and *Aplysia* (Martin *et al.* 1997*b*; Casadio *et al.* 1999). The experiments in *Aplysia* revealed a requirement for local synthesis of proteins in the establishment of long-lasting plasticity. While mRNA targeting and local protein synthesis have long been studied in mammals, it is only more recently that their importance in synaptic plasticity has become clear (Steward and Schuman 2001).

21.3 New directions from *Aplysia*

In light of these similarities, other aspects of the mechanisms of long-lasting plasticity in *Aplysia* bear investigation in mammalian systems. The cell biological simplicity of the *Aplysia* system continues to allow levels of analysis that are not yet feasible in mammalian systems; this is particularly true since the development of techniques that allow isolation of two synapses from the same presynaptic neuron (Martin *et al.* 1997*b*). Here, we review several recent findings in *Aplysia* that we hope will illuminate productive avenues of exploration in the hippocampus and other mammalian systems.

(a) Transcriptional regulators: CREB and its partners

In *Aplysia*, it has been clear for some time that CREB does not act alone to activate the genes required for long-lasting facilitation. CREB is merely a central component of an interacting group of related transcription factors—both activators and repressors— which together may be better able to orchestrate an appropriate transcriptional response than a single factor could. CREB cooperates with several different categories of regulators. A repressor, ApCREB2, antagonizes CREB's actions; alleviating this repression in cell culture reduces the threshold for producing long-lasting synaptic facilitation (Bartsch et al. 1995). (As we will discuss in a moment, CREB2 also has a more active role in regulating long-lasting synaptic depression.) Aplysia CREB itself provides a splice variant that also acts as a repressor (ApCREB-1B, which is similar to mammalian ICER (inducible cAMP element repressor, a short splice variant of the CREB gene)) as well as an isoform that acts in the cytoplasm to modulate CREB activity (Bartsch et al. 1998). A constitutively expressed activator, ApAF, acts downstream of CREB to contribute to facilitation (Bartsch et al. 2000), and another activator, ApC/EBP, also contributes to facilitation; but it is itself induced by CREB and thus represents the next level in a cascade of transcriptional regulators (Alberini et al. 1994).

Experiments in cell culture clearly show that CREB cannot by itself achieve all gene induction required for long-lasting facilitation. Injection of phosphorylated CREB can produce facilitation independent of any synaptic stimulation; but this facilitation is only 50% of that achieved through more conventional induction, showing that other contributors are required. Interference with transcription factors that act downstream of CREB can disrupt facilitation despite presumably normal CREB function, showing that these downstream regulators have a similarly critical role (Alberini et al. 1994; Bartsch et al. 2000). Findings such as these confirm that CREB does not operate as a unitary transcriptional switch but rather as an important component of a more complex machinery.

It will be fascinating to investigate whether similar complexity attends CREB-mediated gene regulation in the hippocampus and other mammalian brain regions; indeed, since the CREB gene itself is so much more complicated in mammals, it would be surprising if attendant factors were not similarly elaborated. Some early data support this prediction. Interference with CREB produces compensation by the related CREM gene in the hippocampus and elsewhere, suggesting that they cooperate in transcriptional regulation (Hummler et al. 1994). C/EBP is upregulated by learning in mice (Taubenfeld et al. 2001), and interference with inhibitory isoforms of C/EBP and with ATF4 (the mammalian homologue of Aplysia CREB2) leads to improved learning in some hippocampus-dependent behavioural tasks (Chen et al. 2003). These initial findings suggest that in mammals, as in Aplysia, CREB cooperates with a constellation of other factors in the consolidation of memory.

(b) Induced genes

While many genes have been shown to be regulated by neuronal activity, we have as yet a relatively poor understanding of the downstream genes induced by CREB and other regulators, specifically in the consolidation of memory. Several candidates come from investigations in Aplysia and may bear investigation in mammalian systems.

The first induced gene identified in Aplysia was C/EBP (Alberini et al. 1994). As noted above, mammalian C/EBP has recently been shown to be induced in the hippocampus after learning; this induction correlates with CREB activation, further supporting the notion that at least this aspect of the Aplysia machinery is conserved in mammals (Taubenfeld et al. 2001).

Induced degradation of the PKA regulatory subunit in *Aplysia* extends PKA's activity and contributes to long-lasting facilitation (Chain *et al.* 1995). This is achieved by CREB-mediated induction of a neuron-specific ubiquitin C-terminal hydrolase (Hegde *et al.* 1997). This novel mechanism for extending an intracellular signalling bears investigation in mammalian systems. Pharmacological inhibition of the proteosome in rat hippocampus can interfere with memory formation (Lopez-Salon *et al.* 2001), suggesting that this mechanism, too, may be preserved.

With the increased power and availability of gene profiling analyses and the sequencing of the mouse genome, our knowledge of the specific genes induced during long-lasting LTP and memory will doubtless increase dramatically in the next few years. It will be exciting to see to what extent the handful of genes known to be upregulated during the induction of long-term facilitation in *Aplysia* is recapitulated in mammals.

(c) Long-lasting synaptic depression

LTP is complemented by the capacity of hippocampal synapses to undergo synaptic depression; depression may be as important for information processing and storage as potentiation. Recently, several studies have demonstrated a long-term, protein synthesis-dependent form of synaptic depression in the hippocampus and elsewhere (e.g. Huber *et al.* 2000; Kauderer and Kandel 2000). This synaptic depression can be captured, at least in organotypic hippocampal cultures (Kauderer and Kandel 2000), indicating mechanisms of synaptic tagging and communication with the nucleus similar to those seen in synaptic potentiation. Long-term, transcription-dependent synaptic depression also occurs in *Aplysia* (Montarolo *et al.* 1988), once again making it an attractive model system for further mechanistic studies.

We have seen above that the induction of long-lasting synaptic plasticity leads to the transmittal of a signal to the nucleus, largely by p40/42 MAPK, and the induction of transcription of specific target genes, in both hippocampus and *Aplysia*. What are the parallel processes in long-lasting depression? In both rodents (Bolshakov *et al.* 2000) and *Aplysia* (Guan *et al.* 2003), p38 MAPK is an important carrier of this signal. In *Aplysia*, p38 MAPK targets and activates the transcription factors CREB2 and ATF2 in the nucleus (Guan *et al.* 2003). These data show that, in addition to being a repressor of CREB-mediated transcription (Bartsch *et al.* 1995), CREB2 has an important role as a transcriptional activator. This suggests that, in the nucleus as well as at the synapse, synaptic potentiation and synaptic depression are both mechanistically and functionally complementary.

(d) A new logic for long-term synaptic integration: interaction between synaptic events in the nucleus—the role of chromatin modulation

We have known for decades that different synapses on a single neuron interact non-linearly in the short term to determine whether and how that neuron responds. Only recently has it become clear that distant synapses on a single neuron also interact in their production of long-lasting, transcription-dependent changes (Kandel 2001). Heroic studies of this issue have been undertaken in mammalian cell culture, leading to some interesting phenomenology (Fitzsimonds *et al.* 1997). However, the power of

Aplysia as a cellular model of memory makes it an ideal system in which to study these interactions and their mechanisms.

The phenomenon of synaptic capture, described in Section 21.2d, was the first type of these long-term interactions to be described, in both *Aplysia* and mammals. A consequence of this phenomenon is that the effects of stimulation at one synapse on a neuron depend not only on the local environment and the recent history of that synapse, but also on the recent history of all other synapses on the neuron.

Do synaptic potentiation and depression at different synapses on the same neuron interact in a similar fashion? In the short term, these processes are independent. In the long term, however, when long-lasting potentiation is induced at one synapse and long-lasting depression at a distant synapse on the same neuron, depression dominates. The nuclear events accompanying long-lasting synaptic depression in *Aplysia* appear able to suppress those otherwise induced by the induction of potentiation, truncating the potentiation to the transcription-independent short term (Guan *et al.* 2002).

How does this competition in the nucleus occur? We have found a critical role for modulation of chromatin structure at induced genes. The induction of long-lasting facilitation leads to CREB1 activation, the recruitment of the transcription cofactor CBP, a histone acetylase, and acetylation of histones at the induced gene C/EBP. In this process, the basal level of CREB2, which normally competes with CREB1, is reduced at the C/EBP locus, presumably alleviating this competition. When long-lasting depression is induced, CREB2 at this locus increases and CREB1 decreases. CREB2 recruits the histone deacetylase HDAC5, which deacetylates histones and thereby makes the gene inaccessible for induction.

There is thus a competition, at least at the promoter of the C/EBP gene, between CREB1 and CREB2, between CBP and HDAC5, and between histone acetylation and histone deacetylation. When stimuli to induce long-lasting potentiation and long-lasting depression are presented simultaneously to widely separated synapses on the same neuron, the events related to depression outcompete those related to potentiation: CREB2 displaces CREB1, and deacetylation by HDAC5 dominates. As a result of this histone deacetylation, the C/EBP gene remains inaccessible to transcription (Guan *et al.* 2002).

It is much more difficult to study this level of integration in a complex mammalian structure such as the hippocampus. But it will be important to investigate whether chromatin modulation represents a mechanism of signal competition and integration in mammalian systems, too. If so, this mode of signal interaction in the nucleus may prove to be of broad importance. It may provide new insights into long-term integration—a process that appears to be fundamentally different from short-term synaptic integration.

(e) What is the molecular nature of the synaptic tag?

The products of induced genes need to be appropriately targeted to potentiated (or to depressed) synapses. As discussed in Section 21.2d, the phenomenon of synaptic capture suggests that this occurs through the creation of a synaptic 'tag', a marker at potentiated synapses. What is the nature of this synaptic tag? Experiments in *Aplysia* have provided us with some insight.

Using the bifurcated culture system, Martin *et al.* (1997*b*) showed local protein synthesis to be critical for the signal from the stimulated synapse back to the nucleus, but not for the initial phase of synaptic capture, producing facilitation lasting 24 hours. Continuing this analysis, Casadio *et al.* (1999) found that the synaptic tag for capture requires PKA. This second study revealed a role for local protein synthesis in the persistence of captured synaptic facilitation, and therefore in some aspect of the synaptic tag. Capture of long-term facilitation in the absence of local protein synthesis is not maintained; it can produce facilitation and synaptic growth lasting 24 hours but not 72 hours. The required local protein synthesis is sensitive to the drug rapamycin. As rapamycin blocks specific mechanisms of translational induction, this finding provides a first insight into the mechanisms of local protein synthesis in plasticity. Further experiments in our laboratory, as well as elsewhere, seek to further characterize the local synaptic tags involved in these temporally distinct capture phenomena (Martin and Kosik 2002; K. Si and E. R. Kandel, unpublished data).

Studies in mice and rats (Frey and Morris 1997; Barco *et al.* 2002) have found that synaptic capture also occurs in the hippocampus; the latter study suggests that protein synthesis is required for its full expression. Future experiments must address whether the two-phase nature of capture and the specific molecules involved in it recapitulate those found in *Aplysia*. These will be challenging experiments, as it is difficult to manipulate separate populations of synapses in the hippocampus. It is to be hoped that the more tractable *Aplysia* system will continue to provide mechanistic clues, telling us where to start looking in more complicated organisms.

21.4 Conclusion

The ability to ask an important scientific question in an answerable way often hinges on the choice of model system. As a central purpose of neurobiology is to cast light on the functions of the human brain, mammalian model systems are often preferable. However, the complexity of the mammalian brain encourages parallel work in simpler model systems.

The similarities in some mechanisms of lasting synaptic change in these two evolutionarily disparate contexts invite the suggestion that other synapses in the mammalian brain may use similar mechanisms for long-term plasticity. The amygdala, which is an important locus of the changes underlying learned fear (LeDoux 2000), is an attractive structure in which to study learning and memory, because its circuitry is simpler than that of the hippocampus, and the relationship between specific synaptic changes and specific changes in behaviour is perhaps more clear. The mechanisms of plasticity at synapses in the amygdala, especially long-lasting plasticity, are not yet as well understood as those in the hippocampus. However, similarities to some of the mechanisms outlined in Section 21.2 are already apparent. For example, PKA, MAPK and CREB are activated by synaptic stimuli that induce plasticity (Huang *et al.* 2000), and interference with CREB function can impair amygdala-dependent fear conditioning (Kida *et al.* 2002). Clearly, the mechanisms of lasting plasticity elucidated in *Aplysia* will bear investigation, not only at the Schaffer collateral synapse in the hippocampus, but at all synapses in which lasting potentiation is observed. While the mechanisms of plasticity at different synapses are unlikely to be identical, they appear to be variations on certain shared themes. This allows for a fruitful synergy between different model systems.

This synergistic approach has proven fruitful in the study of learning and memory, with *Aplysia* providing an important example of the relationship between learning and plasticity, as well as elucidation of various mechanisms of plasticity that are conserved across phylogeny. Ideally, different model systems complement each other and converge on conserved mechanisms. In a problem as complex as the nature of synaptic plasticity and its relationship to learning, we can be far more confident of the validity of our findings when they are reproduced in such disparate model systems. There have been a number of recent advances in our understanding of the details of long-lasting facilitation in *Aplysia*. We propose that some of the mechanisms we have reviewed are likely to be conserved, perhaps with variations or elaborations, at mammalian synapses important for various types of memory storage.

This work has been supported by the Mather foundation, HHMI, and the Columbia University Medical Scientist Training Programme.

References

Abel, T., Nguyen, P. V., Barad, M., Deuel, T. A., Kandel, E. R., and Bourtchouladze, R. (1997). Genetic demonstration of a role for PKA in the late phase of LTP and in hippocampus-based long-term memory. *Cell* **88**, 615–26.

Abel, T., Martin, K. C., Bartsch, D., and Kandel, E. R. (1998). Memory suppressor genes, inhibitory constraints on the storage of long-term memory. *Science* **279**, 338–41.

Agranoff, B. W. (1967). Memory and protein synthesis. *Sci. Am.* **216**, 115–22.

Alberini, C. M., Ghirardi, M., Metz, R., and Kandel, E. R. (1994). C/EBP is an immediate-early gene required for the consolidation of long-term facilitation in *Aplysia*. *Cell* **76**, 1099–114.

Antonov, I., Antonova, I., Kandel, E. R., and Hawkins, R. D. (2003). Activity-dependent presynaptic facilitation and Hebbian LTP are both required and interact during classical conditioning in *Aplysia*. *Neuron* **37**, 135–47.

Bacskai, B. J., Hochner, B., Mahaut-Smith, M., Adams, S. R., Kaang, B. K., Kandel, E. R., *et al.* (1993). Spatially resolved dynamics of cAMP and protein kinase A subunits in *Aplysia* sensory neurons. *Science* **260**, 222–6.

Barco, A., Alarcon, J. M., and Kandel, E. R. (2002). Expression of consitutively active CREB protein facilitates the late phase of long-term potentiation by enhancing synaptic capture. *Cell* **108**, 689–703.

Bartsch, D., Ghirardi, M., Skehel, P. A., Karl, K. A., Herder, S. P., Chen, M., *et al.* (1995). *Aplysia* CREB2 represses long-term facilitation, relief of repression converts transient facilitation into long-term functional and structural change. *Cell* **83**, 979–92.

Bartsch, D., Casadio, A., Karl, K. A., Serodio, P., and Kandel, E. R. (1998). CREB1 encodes a nuclear activator, a repressor, and a cytoplasmic modulator that form a regulatory unit critical for long-term facilitation. *Cell* **95**, 211–23.

Bartsch, D., Ghirardi, M., Casadio, A., Giustetto, M., Karl, K. A., Zhu, H., *et al.* (2000). Enhancement of memory-related long-term facilitation by ApAF, a novel transcription factor that acts downstream from both CREB1 and CREB2. *Cell* **103**, 595–608.

Bliss, T. V. and Lømo, T. (1973). Long-lasting potentiation of synaptic transmission in the dentate area of the anaesthetized rabbit following stimulation of the perforant path. *J. Physiol. (Lond.)* **232**, 331–56.

Blitzer, R. D., Wong, T., Nouranifar, R., Iyengar, R., and Landau, E. M. (1995). Postsynaptic cAMP pathway gates early LTP in hippocampal CA1 region. *Neuron* **15**, 1403–14.

Bolshakov, V. Y., Carboni, L., Cobb, M. H., Siegelbaum, S. A., and Belardetti, F. (2000). Dual MAP kinase pathways mediate opposing forms of long-term plasticity at CA3-CA1 synapses. *Nature Neurosci.* **3**, 1107–12.

Bourtchouladze, R., Frenguelli, B., Blendy, J., Cioffi, D., Schutz, G., and Silva, A. J. (1994). Deficient long-term memory in mice with a targeted mutation of the cAMP-responsive element binding protein. *Cell* **79**, 59–68.

Bourtchouladze, R., Abel, T., Berman, N., Gordon, R., Lapidus, K., and Kandel, E. R. (1998). Different training procedures recruit either one or two critical period for contextual memory consolidation, each of which requires protein synthesis and PKA. *Learn. Memory* **5**, 365–74.

Casadio, A., Martin, K. C., Giustetto, M., Zhu, H., Chen, M., Bartsch, D., *et al.* (1999). A transient, neuron-wide form of CREB-mediated long-term facilitation can be stabilized at specific synapses by local protein synthesis. *Cell* **99**, 221–37.

Castellucci, V., Frost, W. N., Goelet, P., Montarolo, P. G., Schacher, S., Morgan, J. A., *et al.* (1986). Cell and molecular analysis of long-term sensitization in *Aplysia. J. Physiol. (Lond.)* **81**, 349–57.

Chain, D. G., Hegde, A. N., Yamamoto, N., Liu-Marsh, B., and Schwartz, J. H. (1995). Persistent activation of cAMP-dependent protein kinase by regulated proteolysis suggests a neuron- specific function of the ubiquitin system in *Aplysia. J. Neurosci.* **15**, 7592–603.

Chen, A., Muzzio, I. A., Malleret, G., Bartsch, D., Verbitsky, M., Pavlidis P., *et al.* (2003). Inducible enhancement of memory storage and synaptic plasticity in transgenic mice expressing an inhibitor of ATF-4 (CREB-2) and C/EBP proteins. *Neuron.* **14**, 655–69.

Dash, P. K., Hochner, B., and Kandel, E. R. (1990). Injection of the cAMP-responsive element into the nucleus of *Aplysia* sensory neurons blocks long-term facilitation. *Nature* **345**, 718–21.

Dudek, S. M. and Fields, R. D. (2002). Somatic action potentials are sufficient for late-phase LTP-related cell signaling. *Proc. Natl Acad. Sci. USA* **99**, 3962–7.

English, J. D. and Sweatt, J. D. (1996). Activation of p42 mitogen-activated protein kinase in hippocampal long term potentiation. *J. Biol. Chem.* **271**, 24 329–32.

English, J. D. and Sweatt, J. D. (1997). A requirement for the mitogen-activated protein kinase cascade in hippocampal long term potentiation. *J. Biol. Chem.* **272**, 19 103–6.

Fitzsimonds, R. M., Song, H. J., and Poo, M. M. (1997). Propagation of activity-dependent synaptic depression in simple neural networks. *Nature* **388**, 439–48.

Flexner, L. B., Flexner, J. B., De La Haba, G., and Roberts, R. B. (1965). Loss of memory as related to cerebral protein synthesis. *J. Neurochem.* **12**, 535–41.

Freeman, F. M., Rose, S. P., and Scholey, A. B. (1995). Two time windows of anisomycin-induced amenesia for passive avoidance training in the day-old chick. *Neurobiol. Learn. Mem.* **63**, 291–5.

Frey, U. and Morris, R. G. (1997). Synaptic tagging and long-term potentiation. *Nature* **385**, 533–6.

Frey, U., Huang, Y. Y., and Kandel, E. R. (1993). Effects of cAMP simulate a late stage of LTP in hippocampal CA1 neurons. *Science* **260**, 1661–4.

Guan, Z., Giustetto, M., Lomvardas, S., Kim, J.-H., Miniaci, M. C., Schwartz, J. H., *et al.* (2002). Integration of long-term-memory-related synaptic plasticity involves bidirectional regulation of gene expression and chromatin structure. *Cell* **111**, 483–93.

Guan, Z., Kim, J.-H., Lomvardas, S., Holick, K., Xu, S., Kandel, E. R., *et al.* (2003). p38 MAP kinase mediates both short-term and long-term synaptic depression in *Aplysia. J. Neurosci.* (Submitted.)

Hegde, A. N., Inokuchi, K., Pei, W., Casadio, A., Ghirardi, M., Chain, D. G., *et al.* (1997). Ubiquitin C-terminal hydrolase is an immediate-early gene essential for long-term facilitation in *Aplysia. Cell* **89**, 115–26.

Huang, Y. Y., Nguyen, P. V., Abel, T., and Kandel, E. R. (1996). Long-lasting forms of synaptic potentiation in the mammalian hippocampus. *Learn. Mem.* **3**, 74–85.

Huang, Y. Y., Martin, K. C., and Kandel, E. R. (2000). Both protein kinase A and mitogen-activated protein kinase are required in the amygdala for the macromolecular synthesis-dependent late phase of long-term potentiation. *J. Neurosci.* **20**, 6317–25.

Huber, K. M., Kayser, M. S., and Bear, M. F. (2000). Role for rapid dendritic protein synthesis in hippocampal mGluR-dependent long-term depression. *Science* **288**, 1254–7.

Hummler, E., Cole, T. J., Blendy, J. A., Ganss, R., Aguzzi, A., Schmid, W., *et al.* (1994). Targeted mutation of the CREB gene, compensation within the CREB/ATF family of transcription factors. *Proc. Natl Acad. Sci. USA* **91**, 5647–51.

Impey, S., Obrietan, K., and Storm, D. R. (1999). Making new connections: role of ERK/MAP kinase signaling in neuronal plasticity. *Neuron* **23**, 11–14.

Kandel, E. R. (1979). *Behavioral biology of* Aplysia, *a contribution to the comparative study of opisthobranch mollusks.* San Francisco, CA: Freeman.

Kandel, E. R. (2001). The molecular biology of memory storage, a dialogue between genes and synapses. *Science* **294**, 1030–8.

Kauderer, B. S. and Kandel, E. R. (2000). Capture of a protein synthesis-dependent component of long-term depression. *Proc. Natl Acad. Sci. USA* **97**, 13 342–7.

Kida, S., Josselyn, S. A., de Ortiz, S. P., Kogan, J. H., Chevere, I., Masushige, S., *et al.* (2002). CREB required for the stability of new and reactivated fear memories. *Nature Neurosci.* **5**, 348–55.

LeDoux, J. E. (2000). Emotion circuits in the brain. *A. Rev. Neurosci.* **23**, 155–84.

Lopez-Salon, M., Alonso, M., Vianna, M. R., Viola, H., Mello e Souza, T., Izquierdo, I., *et al.* (2001). The ubiquitin-proteosome cascade is required for mammalian long-term memory formation. *Eur. J. Neurosci.* **14**, 1820–6.

Malleret, G., Haditsch, U., Genoux, D., Jones, M. W., Bliss, T. V., Vanhoose, A. M., *et al.* (2001). Inducible and reversible enhancement of learning, memory, and long-term potentiation by genetic inhibition of calcineurin. *Cell* **104**, 675–86.

Mansuy, I. M., Mayford, M., Jacob, B., Kandel, E. R., and Bach, M. E. (1998). Restricted and regulated overexpression reveals calcineurin as a key component in the transition from short-term to long-term memory. *Cell* **92**, 39–49.

Martin, K. C. and Kosik, K. S. (2002). Synaptic tagging—who's it? *Nature Rev. Neurosci.* **3**, 813–20.

Martin, K. C., Michael, D., Rose, J. C., Barad, M., Casadio, A., Zhu, H., *et al.* (1997a). MAP kinase translocates into the nucleus of the presynaptic cell and is required for long-term facilitation in *Aplysia. Neuron* **18**, 899–912.

Martin, K. C., Casadio, A., Zhu, H. E. Y., Rose, J. C., Chen, M., Bailey, C. H., *et al.* (1997b). Synapse-specific, long-term facilitation of *Aplysia* sensory to motor synapses, a function for local protein synthesis in memory storage. *Cell* **91**, 927–38.

Montarolo, P. G., Kandel, E. R., and Schacher, S. (1988). Long-term heterosynaptic inhibition in *Aplysia. Nature* **333**, 171–4.

Patterson, S. L., Pittenger, C., Morozov, A., Martin, K. C., Scanlin, H., Drake, C., *et al.* (2001). Some forms of cAMP-mediated long-lasting potentiation are associated with release of BDNF and nuclear translocation of phospho-MAP kinase. *Neuron* **32**, 123–40.

Pittenger, C., Huang, Y.-Y., Paletzki, R. F., Bourtchouladze, R., Scanlin, H., Vronskaya, S., *et al.* (2002). Reversible inhibition of CREB/ATF transcription factors in region CA1 of the dorsal hippocampus disrupts hippocampus-dependent spatial memory. *Neuron* **34**, 447–62.

Steward, O. and Schuman, E. M. (2001). Protein synthesis at synaptic sites on dendrites. *A. Rev. Neurosci.* **24**, 299–325.

Taubenfeld, S. M., Wiig, K. A., Monti, B., Dolan, B., Pollonini, G., and Alberini, C. M. (2001). Fornix-dependent induction of hippocampal CCAAT enhancer-binding protein β and δ co-localizes with phosphorylated cAMP response element-binding protein and accompanies long-term memory consolidation. *J. Neurosci.* **21**, 84–91.

Winder, D. G., Mansuy, I. M., Osman, M., Moallem, T. M., and Kandel, E. R. (1998). Genetic and pharmacological evidence for a novel, intermediate phase of long-term potentiation suppressed by calcineurin. *Cell* **92**, 25–37.

Glossary

C/EBP   CCAAT-enhancer-binding protein
CRE   cAMP-responsive element
CREB   cAMP-responsive element binding protein
L-LTP   late, transcription-dependent phase of long-term potentiation
LTP   long-term potentiation
MAPK   mitogen-activated protein kinase
PKA   protein kinase A

Function

22

Long-term potentiation and the ageing brain

C. A. Barnes

Ageing is associated with learning and memory impairments. Data are reviewed that suggest that age-related impairments of hippocampal-dependent forms of memory, may be caused, in part, by altered synaptic plasticity mechanisms in the hippocampus, including long-term potentiation (LTP). To the extent that the mechanisms responsible for LTP can be understood, it may be possible to develop therapeutic approaches to alleviate memory decline in normal ageing.

Keywords: ageing; long-term potentiation; hippocampus; learning; memory

A testimonial to the importance of a scientific observation is when many investigators 'remember when and where' they first heard about it. The discovery of LTP is among the shortlist of such empirical breakthroughs in neuroscience, and it is fitting that, at the thirtieth anniversary of the publication of the first full manuscript written about it, many will wish to reveal the impact this finding had on their individual scientific development. Several conceptual and empirical breakthroughs occurred during the early 1970s that gave rise to an optimistic feeling that understanding the neural mechanisms of memory might be a tractable problem. These included previews of a promising manuscript by O'Keefe and Nadel (1978), Marr's then recent papers on how memories could be stored in networks that resembled the architecture of the hippocampus (Marr 1970, 1971), and, of course, the landmark publications on LTP that were published in 1973 (Bliss and Lømo 1973). The *zeitgeist* was thereby primed for raising questions about how the ageing process might impact the way in which memories are laid down or retrieved.

I was at Carleton University in Ottawa, Canada, in 1973 when I first heard about LTP. Afterwards I shifted the direction of my dissertation to focus on the relationship between LTP and learning across the lifespan. If the process that Lømo, Bliss and Gardner-Medwin described *did* reflect a mechanism used by the hippocampus to store information, then the ability to modify synaptic weights should be correlated with how well hippocampal-dependent behavioural tasks are learned and remembered. Although there was a small literature on age-related memory impairments in humans in 1973, there were very few experiments that had addressed memory impairments in aged animals to investigate the underlying mechanisms. The review of the hippocampal lesion literature that O'Keefe and Nadel had outlined in an early version of their manuscript suggested that a comparison of spatial memory and hippocampal plasticity over the lifespan would be a productive experimental approach. To evaluate the persistence of memories in relation to synaptic change, it would be necessary to use relevant behavioural experiments and an electrophysiological preparation that could be monitored over days or weeks. The latter methods were in use by Graham Goddard's group in Halifax (Douglas and Goddard 1975). The issue of what behavioural task to use remained. The first experiments conducted on memory, LTP and ageing were performed in Goddard's laboratory.

22.1 Correlating electrophysiological changes with behaviour

The behavioural tasks that were in standard use at the time, and known to be hippocampal dependent, required the use of food restriction or shock. Because old rats were likely to be more frail than the young rats typically used in behavioural experiments, it was important to design any test of spatial memory, and specifically navigational accuracy, that stressed old animals minimally. A circular platform task was therefore developed, in which rats were required to learn which of 18 holes at the perimeter of a 1.2 m circular platform leads to a dark escape box. Rats naturally approach dark areas and avoid open, brightly illuminated spaces. Accordingly, when placed in the middle of the open platform, the rats would go to the edge to look for escape routes and eventually find the one hole under which the dark escape box was placed (Barnes 1979; Fig. 22.1). The apparatus was housed in a large open area (a television studio), and equipped for online manual video tracking, so that path-length could be monitored as the rats ran about the platform. Path-length is a measure independent of running speed, which changes over the lifespan. Latency and number of errors (nose pokes into holes not over the escape box) were also measured. Pilot studies with young rats showed that path-lengths, errors and latency measures all declined over trials and days, indicating an improvement in navigation to the correct location, despite the fact that olfactory cues were scrambled by randomly moving the surface of the platform from trial to trial. For the ageing experiment 32 young (around 14 months) and 32 old (around 32 months) male Long–Evans rats were given two trials per day for 6 days, and then a change in escape location was implemented for a further 5 days. The use of relatively many animals per group afforded the possibility of examining correlations between behaviour and electrophysiology with confidence.

After behavioural testing, all animals underwent surgery for the chronic bilateral implantation of electrodes used to record evoked extracellular field potentials. Recording electrodes were placed in the hilus of the fascia dentata and stimulating electrodes in the angular bundle, where the axons from the entorhinal cortex (the perforant pathway) converge. After behavioural testing, LTP was induced bilaterally using the robust stimulation parameters that had been developed by Douglas and Goddard (1975) to induce reliable enhancement of synaptic efficacy (20 ms bursts of 400 Hz stimuli, supra-threshold for population spikes, delivered at an overall rate of 0.2 Hz, repeated 15 times). First, one such high-frequency session was given (120 total stimulus pulses), and the resulting enhancement was monitored for 7 days. After this, high-frequency stimulation was delivered once every 24 h for 3 consecutive days, after which the synaptic responses were tested for two additional weeks. The slope of the average synaptic response was measured, and the fractional change of the evoked response, was calculated. Although other electrophysiological and behavioural measures were collected in this experiment, the main findings of interest for this review include observations of spatial acquisition on the circular platform, the induction of LTP of the synaptic potentials and decay of this LTP over time.

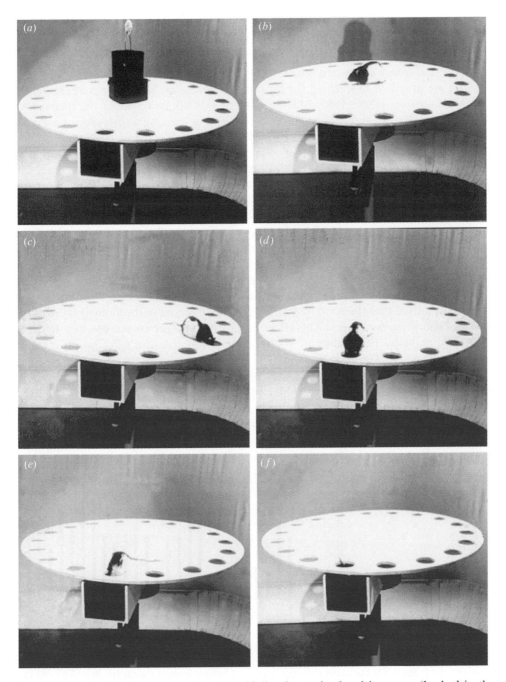

Fig. 22.1 Circular platform apparatus. (*a*) Initially, the rat is placed in a start 'bucket' in the centre of the platform. (*b*) When the start bucket is raised, the rat is free to move and the trial begins. (*c*) The rats explore the surface of the platform searching for the escape box, and make errors, as illustrated here. (*d*) When the rat finds the escape box (*e*) he descends into it (*f*) and is allowed to remain there for 30–60 s.

The data over the first 6 days of acquisition (two trials per day) are shown in Fig. 22.2*a*. Old rats exhibited longer path-lengths to the escape box (and more total errors and longer latencies) than did the young rats. From this first experiment with the circular platform, and others conducted later in ageing rats, the consistent finding has been that old rats are impaired in learning the location of the escape box (Barnes 1979; Barnes and McNaughton 1980*a*, 1985; Markowska *et al*. 1989), in retaining the memory of that location (Barnes and McNaughton 1980*a*) and in learning a reversal or change of location of the escape box (Barnes 1979). More recently, Bach *et al*. (1999) have found a similar pattern of spatial learning impairment in aged mice by using a modified version of the circular platform. In Bach's experiment, a visual discrimination problem was also administered, and revealed no impairment in the acquisition of a cued version of the task in the old, spatial memory-impaired, mice.

With the stimulation protocol used, there was no difference in the magnitude of LTP induced either after a single high-frequency session as a function of the age of the animals, nor after the first or second of the three consecutive daily high-frequency treatments. There was also no difference in LTP decay following a single LTP-inducing session, as measured over a one week period (Fig. 22.2*b*). The striking difference between age groups emerged in the persistence of LTP after three LTP-inducing sessions. It appeared that the good 'retention' of LTP observed in the young rats required repeated high-frequency input. This effect of repetition on persistence was not observed in the old animals. The finding in young animals was reminiscent of an observation made by Bliss and Gardner-Medwin (1973). The one rabbit that received repeated LTP-inducing sessions in their study showed more enduring LTP than did other rabbits with single sessions. In the present study, repeated stimulation extended the decay time-constant of LTP for the young adult, but not for the old rats. Finally, there was a statistically significant correlation between accuracy of performance on the circular

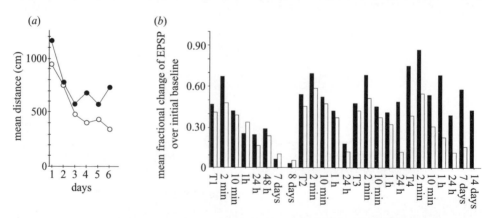

Fig. 22.2 (*a*) Behavioural performance on the circular platform task over 6 days of training (two trials per day). Shown is the mean distance traversed before finding the escape box. The old rats (filled circles) showed poorer acquisition scores than did young rats (open circles). (*b*) LTP-inducing stimulation was given four times during this experiment (T1, T2, T3 and T4). Shown is the mean fractional change of the field EPSP for the young (filled bars) and old rats (open bars). Although the old rats did not show LTP induction or decay differences following a single high-frequency stimulation session (T1), after three consecutive daily high-frequency sessions (T4), the old rats showed significantly less LTP than did the young rats (adapted from Barnes 1979).

platform task on the final day of acquisition and the amount of LTP after the third induction session. This correlation was statistically reliable in each age group alone, as well as across groups. The relationship indicated that the rats with the most durable LTP in a given age group tended to show the best spatial learning. These data provided the first support for the hypothesis that LTP at hippocampal synapses and spatial learning may depend on similar mechanistic processes.

Several questions remained outstanding: do the old rats simply require more repetition than do young rats to reach the same levels of LTP? With more repetitions, could the LTP decay time constant be extended equivalently? An additional study was designed specifically to examine these issues (Barnes and McNaughton 1980a). In this experiment, LTP-inducing stimuli were administered at 24 h intervals for 12 consecutive days to attempt to 'saturate' the LTP-induction process in both groups and perhaps allow sufficient repetitions for the old rats to show more durable LTP. The result of 12 daily LTP-inducing stimulation sessions was monitored for several weeks thereafter. Figure 22.3a shows the fractional change in the slope of the field EPSP at 24 h intervals following each daily LTP treatment (left of dotted line), and the magnitude of LTP after the cessation of high-frequency stimulation over several weeks (right of dotted line). The rate of growth of the decay time-constant for LTP was a decreasing function of the number of LTP-inducing sessions given (Fig. 22.3b). The young rats reached the maximum value on trial 5, whereas the old rats reached their maximum on trial 10. Even though the same absolute magnitude of LTP was reached in both age groups by the end of the 12 high-frequency sessions, the LTP decay time-constant was only 17 days for the old rats compared with 37 days in their young counterparts.

The faster decay of LTP in the older rats suggested that behavioural forgetting in young and old animals might share similar kinetics. Specifically, if the decay of

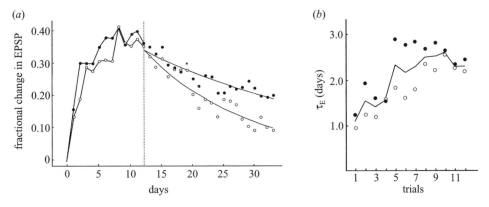

Fig. 22.3 (a) Mean fractional change in the field EPSP in the young (filled circles) and old (open circles) groups of rats. To the left of the dashed line are the data 24 h after high-frequency stimulation (12 in total), and to the right of the dashed line are the data that follow the end of LTP-inducing sessions, also obtained at 24 h intervals. Note that by the end of the high-frequency stimulation sessions, LTP in the young and old rats was equivalent; however, the old rats showed faster decay of LTP over the ensuing days. (b) Mean time-constant of LTP for each 24 h period after the 12 daily LTP-inducing sessions for the young (filled circles) and old (open circles) rats shown in (a). The solid line is the mean for both groups combined. The young group reached their maximum value earlier than did the old group (adapted from Barnes and McNaughton 1980a).

hippocampal LTP and behavioural forgetting of a spatial problem shared common mechanisms, the old rats should show similarly accelerated rates of decline in both processes. By using 90 rats, with separate groups of rats for each retention time-point measured (10, 20, 30, 45 and 60 days), the animals were first trained on the circular platform, one trial per day for 16 days. The old rats, indeed, forgot the location of the escape box on the circular platform about twice as fast as did the young rats (Barnes and McNaughton 1985). In fact, when the ratios of behavioural forgetting were compared with the ratios of decay of LTP between groups, there was only a 1% difference—in other words, old rats show rates of forgetting and LTP decay that are about twice as fast as those of young rats. This lent additional support to the idea that the maintenance of LTP may play an important role in sustaining a robust memory. At approximately the same time, de Toledo-Morrell and Morrell (1985) found a significant relationship between the durability of LTP over days at the perforant path— granule cell synapse and behavioural performance on the radial 8-arm maze (another task that had been shown to be dependent on an intact hippocampus). More recent experiments have examined the relationship between LTP at the Schaffer collateral– CA1 synapse, and spatial performance on the circular platform. Bach *et al.* (1999) uncovered aged-related LTP maintenance deficits in CA1 of old mice after 3 h using the *in vitro* slice preparation. These decay rates were correlated, across age groups, with spatial performance on the circular platform task.

22.2 Mechanisms underlying age-related changes in memory

LTP is often divided into phases—induction, expression and maintenance. It is appropriate to ask whether ageing affects any of the processes separately. The first reports indicated intact hippocampal LTP induction at the Schaffer collateral–CA1 synapse (Landfield and Lynch 1977; Landfield *et al.* 1978) and at the perforant path– granule cell synapse (Barnes 1979) in old rats. With few exceptions, this lack of an age-related LTP induction deficit has been repeatedly observed in CA1 and in the fascia dentata, when robust, high-intensity stimulation protocols are used. Experiments from two groups, however, in the early 1990s, helped to place the findings of experiments using robust stimulation parameters into the proper perspective. When fewer stimulus pulses and lower amplitude stimulus currents are used to induce LTP ('peri-threshold protocols'), old rats do show LTP induction deficits in the Schaffer collateral–CA1 synapse compared with their younger counterparts (Deupree *et al.* 1993; Moore *et al.* 1993). Furthermore, at the perforant path–granule cell synapse, Barnes *et al.* (2000*a*) have shown that a larger amplitude current injection is necessary for LTP to be induced in old rats when weak presynaptic stimulation is paired with direct depolarization of the postsynaptic granule cell. This points to a change in the induction threshold at this synapse as well. Taken together, these results show that LTP *can* be more difficult to induce in old rats.

What contributes to these changes in LTP characteristics in old rats relative to what is observed in younger animals? First, several anatomical and electrophysiological properties can be eliminated. There is no loss of hippocampal granule or CA1 pyramidal cells in old rats (Rapp and Gallagher 1996; Rasmussen *et al.* 1996), most biophysical properties of old pyramidal or granule cells do not differ from those in young cells (review in Barnes 1994), and there is no change in spontaneous firing rates of single cells in the hippocampus of freely behaving old rats compared with young rats (e.g. Shen *et al.* 1997). Second, there are certain changes observed during ageing that may contribute to the LTP deficits. For example, there is a reduction in the actual number of perforant-path synaptic contacts on granule cells (Geinisman *et al.* 1992) and a corresponding reduced amplitude of the presynaptic fibre potential and field EPSP elicited by perforant path stimulation (Barnes and McNaughton 1980*b*; Foster *et al.* 1991). In CA1, the field EPSP elicited by Schaffer collateral stimulation is also reduced, but the presynaptic-fibre-potential response is not (Kerr *et al.* 1991; Barnes *et al.* 1992; Potier *et al.* 2000). These two observations have also been confirmed *in vivo* (Barnes *et al.* 2000*b*), consistent with the hypothesis that there is a loss of functional synaptic contacts in CA1, although not of afferents *per se*. Such decreases in network connectivity certainly could contribute to plasticity changes during advanced age.

Third, Landfield and his colleagues have found deficits in several aspects of calcium regulation during ageing, including frequency potentiation (Landfield and Lynch 1977), an increased calcium-mediated inward potassium current in old rats (Landfield and Pitler 1984), and an increased density of L-type calcium channels in old rats (Thibault and Landfield 1996). These changes may also contribute to the altered plasticity characteristics of the ageing hippocampus. Consistent with this idea, a form of LTP that is NMDA-independent has been described (Grover and Teyler 1990), and can be induced if very high intensity stimuli are applied. This form of LTP appears to be mediated by calcium influx through vdcc. Shankar *et al.* (1998) observed that, if measured in isolation, vdccLTP in CA1 is increased in old rats. On the other hand, if NMDA-LTP was measured in isolation (vdccLTP blocked), an age-related LTP deficit was unmasked. These authors suggest that, in CA1, the observation of no age-related changes in LTP induction with robust stimulation parameters has arisen because of a shift in the balance between these two types of LTP in old rats. Furthermore, LTD and depotentiation are easier to induce in hippocampal slices from old rats than from adult rats (Norris *et al.* 1996). This may also be a result of alterations in calcium-mediated cascades in older animals, and certainly could contribute to the observed changes in decay rates of LTP in old rats.

22.3 Synaptic plasticity and the stabilization of hippocampal maps

If it is more difficult to induce LTP but easier to induce LTD, what impact might this have on the overall network properties of the ageing hippocampus? Although the correlations between artificially induced LTP and behaviour are consistent with the hypothesis that LTP-like processes may underlie learning, stronger support for this idea would be provided if LTP could be directly measured during some behavioural experience. Single-cell activity in the hippocampus of freely behaving rats shows striking modulation of firing rates of complex-spike cells, dependent on the location of an animal in a given environment. John O'Keefe first called these hippocampal cells 'place cells' because of this correlate (O'Keefe and Dostrovsky 1971). The region of the environment over which the cell responds is called its 'place field', and the distribution of these fields in a given environment is referred to as a hippocampal place field 'map'. With recent advances in multiple single-cell recording methods, it has become possible to record many hippocampal cells simultaneously (e.g. Wilson and McNaughton 1993). Because cell firing occurs in response to the animal's behaviour and sensory input, rather than because of artificial stimulation, the activity of hippocampal ensembles potentially provides a complementary window for viewing experience-dependent changes in brain function. In fact, Wilson and McNaughton (1993) demonstrated that it is possible to reconstruct a rat's location in an environment, simply from monitoring the activity of a large group of hippocampal cells. With repeated exposure to an environment, it has been suggested that hippocampal maps become stabilized as a consequence of LTP at the synapses carrying external and internal information to the hippocampus. Because LTP is compromised in old rats, this stabilization process may also be affected by the ageing process.

Can synaptic modification be inferred from the network dynamics of groups of hippocampal cells? Going back to Hebb's ideas on phase sequences or linked cell assemblies, several modern theoretical considerations of route learning predict that the pattern of place cell discharge should change as a consequence of repeated traversals of a route. Because of the temporal asymmetry of LTP (Levy and Steward 1983), repeated traversals of a route should eventually cause cells at a given location to activate subsequent cells in the sequence, before the rat actually reaches the original firing location. Just as predicted by theories of sequence learning (Levy 1989; Blum and Abbott 1996; Fig. 22.4a), when young rats traverse linear tracks, place fields do expand in the direction opposite to the direction of motion of the rat, and firing rates increase over the first few traversals of the track on a given day (Mehta et al. 1997). In addition to possibly encoding the sequences in which places have been visited, this experience-dependent place field expansion might cause an increase in the spatial information contained in the

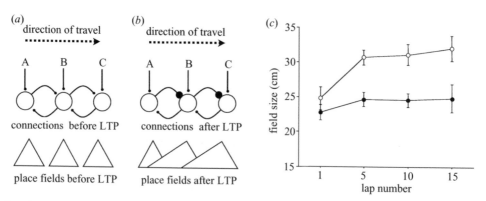

Fig. 22.4 (a) Diagram of the theoretical basis for sequence learning and the experience-dependent place field expansion effect. (b) Repeated activation of a sequence (ABC) of cells causes an LTP-like asymmetric strengthening of the forward connections. This causes a given cell to begin to fire in response to the activity of cells earlier in the sequence with repetitions of that sequence. Hence, the place fields expand in a direction opposite to the motion of the rat. (c) The effect of age on experience-dependent place field expansion as young rats (open circles) and old (filled circles) rats traverse a rectangular track. Shown here are mean, and standard error of the mean, place field sizes for laps 1, 5, 10, and 15. The place field sizes expanded significantly from lap 1 to lap 5 for the young rats, but the old rats did not exhibit this expansion. The lack of place field expansion in the old rats provides indirect evidence for a failure of asymmetric LTP-like processes in the hippocampus during ageing (adapted from Shen et al. 1997).

hippocampal map, producing more overlap in cell firing activity in an environment, potentially leading to greater map stabilization.

Although place field expansion was a theoretical prediction of route learning models, what other evidence suggests that it may be a behaviourally driven LTP-like process? Ekstrom *et al.* (2001) compared place field expansion characteristics in young rats given saline or the NMDA antagonist CPP while repeatedly traversing a rectangular track. If experience-dependent expansion of place fields shared common mechanisms with LTP, then a manipulation of the glutamate receptor that affects LTP, should correspondingly affect expansion of the place fields in these behavioural conditions. Experience-dependent place field expansion was, in fact, blocked by the NMDA receptor antagonist CPP, in similar doses to those that block LTP induction (Ekstrom *et al.* 2001). Because LTP mechanisms are disrupted in old rats, it was also reasoned that there should be a difference in place field expansion characteristics in old, spatial memory-deficient rats. Consistent with the hypothesis that LTP and the place field expansion effect share common mechanisms, Shen *et al.* (1997) confirmed that the expansion effect is much less robust in old, memory-impaired rats, than in young rats (Fig. 22.4b).

Recent studies have indicated that hippocampal cell-firing patterns during periods of quiet rest or sleep ('off-line' periods), reflect the patterns that were expressed during the immediately preceding behavioural experience (Wilson and McNaughton 1994). Moreover, the sequential order of neuronal firing, as reflected by asymmetry in neuronal cross-correlations, is significantly preserved (Skaggs and McNaughton 1996), suggesting that event sequences are reactivated during such periods. The deficit in experience-dependent place field expansion in old animals suggests that sequence encoding may be compromised, and this would be expected to affect the degree to which the sequential order of experiences is preserved during off-line reactivation in old animals. This expectation was recently confirmed by Gerrard *et al.* (2002). Moreover, preservation of sequence reactivation was positively correlated with spatial accuracy on the Morris swim task, in both age groups. This provides a further, albeit indirect, link between behaviourally observed memory performance and LTP-like processes in the hippocampus.

Another prediction of the hypothesis that LTP-like mechanisms may play a role in stabilizing hippocampal maps is that old rats should show less effective map retrieval. It has been shown that NMDA receptor blockade does not prevent the formation of coherent place fields in a novel environment, but this treatment does prevent hippocampal map stabilization and retrieval in young rats (Kentros *et al.* 1998). Barnes *et al.* (1997) found that when old rats are brought into a familiar environment, they occasionally retrieve a completely different hippocampal map than was retrieved in the same environment earlier in the day. On these occasions some fields changed location, some cells no longer fired in the environment and some previously silent cells began to fire. However, once a map had been retrieved by an old animal, it was stable throughout the entire session (as long as the rat was not taken out of the room), just as animals with NMDA receptor blockade show well-formed hippocampal maps when introduced into an environment. Again, analogous to young animals with reduced LTP mechanisms (NMDA receptor antagonism), old rats can show instability of the map retrieval process.

Another change in place-field dynamics observed in old rats is a delayed realignment in the hippocampal map when visual cues and self-motion information are mismatched (Rosenzweig *et al.* 2002). When rats are trained to run back and forth along a track with a journey origin that changes from trial to trial, in the journeys from the start box toward the end of the track, self-motion cues tend to provide information about the rat's position relative to the start box, while external visual cues provide independent information about the rat's position relative to the end of the track (Gothard *et al.* 1996; Redish *et al.* 2000). The start box in this task was moved from trial to trial, forcing a mismatch in the position estimates from the two forms of information. Under these conditions, place fields near the start box tend to be aligned to the start box, and place fields near the end of the track tend to be aligned to the room, indicating that the hippocampal map realigns during the course of each journey. In old rats, the map realignment from motion to room coordinates is delayed (Rosenzweig *et al.* 2002). That is, aged rats are closer to the end of the track when the hippocampal map changes from a self-motion-based alignment to a visual-cue-based alignment. Some models of hippocampal function (e.g. Samsonovich and McNaughton 1997; Redish 1999) suggest that cues and landmarks are bound to the map secondarily through an LTP-like process. The observed delay in map realignment in old rats is consistent with the idea that old rats possess a naturally occurring LTP deficit, and that weaker cue binding forces the hippocampal representation to depend more on self-motion information in old rats. Another hypothesis, tested in this same experiment, was that spatial localization accuracy should require a hippocampal map that is room aligned to facilitate finding a spatial goal. In fact, the position at which a given rat's map alignment switched from start-box coordinates (variable) to room coordinates (fixed), was significantly correlated with how well a given rat learned the location of a hidden reward zone at a fixed location in room coordinates (Rosenzweig *et al.* 2002), regardless of age group. That is, the further along the track map alignment occurred in individual rats, the less accurate was that rat's spatial performance.

As mentioned above, old rats can show map retrieval errors ('re-map') when the environment is unchanged (Barnes *et al.* 1997). Other observations, however, suggest that under different circumstances, old rats fail to re-map when the local cues in the environment are intentionally changed (Tanila *et al.* 1997; Oler and Markus 2000). These seemingly incompatible results can be conceptualized as indicative of age-related impairments in two opposing functions of the hippocampal network. Redish *et al.* (1998) have suggested that inappropriate re-mapping may reflect defects in pattern completion in the CA3 component of the hippocampal network, whereas the failure to re-map appropriately may reflect defects in pattern separation or the orthogonalization process, attributed to the fascia dentata (Marr 1971; McNaughton and Morris 1987; Redish 1999). That is, impaired pattern completion in aged rats might cause the occasional retrieval of an incorrect map upon entry to a familiar environment, whereas impaired pattern separation in aged rats might prevent the formation of a new map in response to environmental changes. Either way, if an inappropriate map is retrieved, or if an inappropriate map is maintained, the final result will be profound changes in spatial cognition.

22.4 Conclusion

It is plausible to propose that, at the core of most of the age-related changes discussed above, there is a fundamental defect in the basic mechanisms by which the hippocampus stores and retrieves information. It is more difficult to store and stabilize memory traces as we age, easier for these traces to decay, and consequentially harder for them to be retrieved. Changes in the plasticity characteristics of hippocampal circuits contribute to major alterations in network dynamics observed in older rats, and may explain the more general observation that older organisms have a greater tendency to become lost.

This leaves us with the fascinating issue of whether, having secured this basic understanding of what happens within the hippocampus over the lifespan, it will be possible to develop therapeutic treatments to alleviate memory decline in normal ageing. Some of the most promising approaches to this problem include alterations of glutamatergic receptors at hippocampal synapses (e.g. 'ampakines'; Staubli *et al.* (1994)), positioned strategically to affect LTP; however, many other avenues are being pursued to modify transmission through the synapses that are involved in memory formation and retrieval. Fortunately, most of us will not succumb to dementing illnesses that tend to occur at older ages. Nevertheless, memory decline does, indeed, appear to be a natural consequence of the ageing process. Ensuring the fidelity of memories from the past, as well as the laying down of future memories, would certainly contribute to life quality for those in their sixth decade and beyond. It is not unreasonable to suppose that, largely because of the past 30 years of work on LTP, a 'fountain of youth', at least where memory is concerned, may well be discovered.

The work from my laboratory described here was supported by grants from the US National Institute on Aging, AG03376 and AG12609.

References

Bach, M. E., Barad, M., Son, H., Zhuo, M., Lu, Y. F., Shih, R., *et al.* (1999). Age-related defects in spatial memory are correlated with defects in the late phase of hippocampal long-term potentiation *in vitro* and are attenuated by drugs that enhance the cAMP signaling pathway. *Proc. Natl Acad. Sci. USA* **96**, 5280–5.

Barnes, C. A. (1979). Memory deficits associated with senescence: a neurophysiological and behavioral study in the rat. *J. Comp. Physiol. Psychol.* **93**, 74–104.

Barnes, C. A. (1994). Normal aging: regionally specific changes in hippocampal synaptic transmission. *Trends Neurosci.* **17**, 13–18.

Barnes, C. A. and McNaughton, B. L. (1980*a*). Spatial memory and hippocampal synaptic plasticity in middle-aged and senescent rats. In *Psychobiology of aging: problems and perspectives* (ed. D. Stein), pp. 253–272. New York: Elsevier.

Barnes, C. A. and McNaughton, B. L. (1980*b*). Physiological compensation for loss of afferent synapses in rat hippocampal granule cells during senescence. *J. Physiol.* **309**, 473–85.

Barnes, C. A. and McNaughton, B. L. (1985). An age comparison of the rates of acquisition and forgetting of spatial information in relation to long-term enhancement of hippocampal synapses. *Behav. Neurosci.* **99**, 1040–8.

Barnes, C. A., Rao, G., Foster, T. C., and McNaughton, B. L. (1992). Region-specific age effects on AMPA sensitivity: electrophysiological evidence for loss of synaptic contacts in hippocampal field CA1. *Hippocampus* **2**, 457–68.

Barnes, C. A., Rao, G., and Houston, F. P. (2000*a*). LTP induction threshold change in old rats at the perforant path-granule cell synapse. *Neurobiol. Aging* **21**, 613–20.

Barnes, C. A., Rao, G., and Orr, G. 2000*b* Age-related decrease in the Schaffer collateral-evoked EPSP in awake, freely behaving rats. *Neural Plasticity* **7**, 167–78.

Barnes, C. A., Suster, M. S., Shen, J., and McNaughton, B. L. (1997). Multistability of cognitive maps in the hippocampus of old rats. *Nature* **388**, 272–5.

Bliss, T. V. P. and Gardner-Medwin, A. R. (1973). Long-lasting potentiation of synaptic transmission in the dentate area of the unanaesthetised rabbit following stimulation of the perforant path. *J. Physiol.* **232**, 357–74.

Bliss, T. V. P. and Lømo, T. (1973). Long-lasting potentiation of synaptic transmission in the dentate area of the anesthetized rabbit following stimulus of perforant path. *J. Physiol.* **232**, 331–56.

Blum, K. I. and Abbott, L. F. (1996). A model of spatial map formation in the hippocampus of the rat. *Neural Comp.* **8**, 85–93.

de Toledo-Morrell, L. and Morrell, F. (1985). Electrophysiological markers of aging and memory loss in rats. *Ann. NY Acad. Sci.* **444**, 296–311.

Deupree, D. L., Bradley, J., and Turner, D. A. (1993). Age-related alterations in potentiation in the CA1 region in F344 rats. *Neurobiol. Aging* **14**, 249–58.

Douglas, R. M. and Goddard, G. V. (1975). Long-term potentiation of the perforant path-granule cell synapse in the rat hippocampus. *Brain Res.* **86**, 205–15.

Ekstrom, A. D., Meltzer, J., McNaughton, B. L., and Barnes, C. A. (2001). NMDA receptor antagonism blocks experience-dependent expansion of hippocampal 'place fields'. *Neuron* **31**, 631–8.

Foster, T. C., Barnes, C. A., Rao, G., and McNaughton, B. L. (1991). Increase in perforant path quantal size in aged F-344 rats. *Neurobiol. Aging* **12**, 441–8.

Geinisman, Y., de Toledo-Morrell, L., Morrell, F., Persina, I. S., and Rossi, M. (1992). Age-related loss of axospinous synapses formed by two afferent systems in the rat dentate gyrus as revealed by the unbiased stereological dissector technique. *Hippocampus* **2**, 437–44.

Gerrard, J. L., Kudrimoti, H. K., Cowen, S. L., Redish, A. D., Rosenzweig, E. S., Barnes, C. A., et al. (2002). Dissociation of pattern and sequence reactivation efficiency in the aged rat hippocampus. Program no. 678.7. *Abstract Viewer/Itinerary Planner*. Washington, DC: Society for Neuroscience, Online.

Gothard, K. M., Skaggs, W. E., and McNaughton, B. L. (1996). Dynamics of mismatch correction in the hippocampal ensemble code for space: interaction between path integration and environmental cues. *J. Neurosci.* **16**, 8027–40.

Grover, L. M. and Teyler, T. J. (1990). Two components of long-term potentiation induced by different patterns of afferent activation. *Nature* **347**, 477–9.

Kentros, C., Hargreaves, E., Hawkins, R. D., Kandel, E. R., Shapiro, M., and Muller, R. V. (1998). Abolition of long-term stability of new hippocampal place cell maps by NMDA receptor blockade. *Science* **280**, 2121–6.

Kerr, D. S., Campbell, L. W., Applegate, M. D., Brodish, A., and Landfield, P. W. (1991). Chronic stress-induced acceleration of electrophysiologic and morphometric biomarkers of hippocampal aging. *J. Neurosci.* **11**, 1316–26.

Landfield, P. W. and Lynch, G. (1977). Impaired monosynaptic potentiation in *in vitro* hippocampal slices from aged, memory-deficient rats. *J. Gerontol.* **32**, 523–33.

Landfield, P. W. and Pitler, T. A. (1984). Prolonged Ca^{2+}-dependent after hyperpolarizations in hippocampal neurons of aged rats. *Science* **226**, 1089–92.

Landfield, P. W., McGaugh, J. L., and Lynch, G. (1978). Impaired synaptic potentiation process in the hippocampus of aged, memory deficient rats. *Brain Res.* **150**, 85–101.

Levy, W. B. (1989). A computation approach to hippocampal function. In *Computational models of learning in simple neural systems* (ed. R. D. Hawkins and G. H. Bower), pp. 243–305. New York: Academic Press.

Levy, W. B. and Steward, O. (1983). Temporal contiguity requirements for long-term associative potentiation/depression in the hippocampus. *Neuroscience* **8**, 791–7.

McNaughton, B. L. and Morris, R. G. M. (1987). Hippocampal synaptic enhancement and information storage within a distributed memory system. *Trends Neurosci.* **10**, 408–15.

Markowska, A. L., Stone, W. S., Ingram, D. K., Reynolds, J., Gold, P. E., Conti, L. H., *et al.* (1989). Individual differences in aging: behavioral and neurobiological correlates. *Neurobiol. Aging* **10**, 31–43.

Marr, D. (1970). A theory of cerebral neocortex. *Proc. R. Soc. Lond.* B **176**, 161–234.

Marr, D. (1971). Simple memory: a theory for archicortex. *Phil. Trans. R. Soc. Lond.* B **262**, 23–81.

Mehta, M. R., Barnes, C. A., and McNaughton, B. L. (1997). Experience-dependent, asymmetric expansion of hippocampal place fields. *Proc. Natl Acad. Sci. USA* **94**, 8918–21.

Moore, C. I., Browning, M. D., and Rose, G. M. (1993). Hippocampal plasticity induced by primed burst, but not long-term potentiation, stimulation is impaired in area CA1 of aged Fischer 344 rats. *Hippocampus* **3**, 57–66.

Norris, C. M., Korol, D. L., and Foster, T. C. (1996). Increased susceptibility to induction of long-term depression and long-term potentiation reversal during aging. *J. Neurosci.* **16**, 5382–92.

O'Keefe, J. and Dostrovsky, J. (1971). The hippocampus as a spatial map. Preliminary evidence from unit activity in the freely-moving rat. *Brain Res.* **34**, 171–5.

O'Keefe, J. and Nadel, L. (1978). *The hippocampus as a cognitive map.* Oxford: Clarendon Press.

Oler, J. A. and Markus, E. J. (2000). Age-related deficits in the ability to encode contextual change: a place cell analysis. *Hippocampus* **10**, 338–50.

Potier, B., Poindessous-Jazat, F., Dutar, P., and Billard, J. M. (2000). NMDA receptor activation in the aged rat hippocampus. *Exp. Gerontol.* **35**, 1185–99.

Rapp, P. R. and Gallagher, M. (1996). Preserved neuron number in the hippocampus of aged rats with spatial learning deficits. *Proc. Natl Acad. Sci. USA* **93**, 9926–30.

Rasmussen, T., Schliemann, T., Sorensen, J. C., Zimmer, J., and West, M. J. (1996). Memory impaired aged rats: no loss of principal hippocampal and subicular neurons. *Neurobiol. Aging* **17**, 143–7.

Redish, A. D. (1999). *Beyond the cognitive map from place cells to episodic memory.* Cambridge, MA: MIT Press.

Redish, A. D., McNaughton, B. L., and Barnes, C. A. (1998). Reconciling Barnes *et al.* (1997) and Tanila *et al.* (1997a,b). *Hippocampus* **8**, 438–43.

Redish, A. D., Rosenzweig, E. S., Bohanick, J. D., McNaughton, B. L., and Barnes, C. A. (2000). Dynamics of hippocampal ensemble activity realignment: time versus space. *J. Neurosci.* **20**, 9298–309.

Rosenzweig, E. S., Redish, A. D., McNaughton, B. L., and Barnes, C. A. (2002). Age-related changes in hippocampal map realignment. Program no. 678.6. *Abstract Viewer/ Itinerary Planner.* Washington, DC: Society for Neuroscience, Online.

Samsonovich, A. and McNaughton, B. L. (1997). Path integration and cognitive mapping in a continuous attractor neural network model. *J. Neurosci.* **17**, 5900–20.

Shankar, S., Teyler, T. J., and Robbins, N. (1998). Aging differentially alters forms of long-term potentiation in rat hippocampal area CA1. *J. Neurophysiol.* **79**, 334–41.

Shen, J., Barnes, C. A., McNaughton, B. L., Skaggs, W. E., and Weaver, K. L. (1997). The effect of aging on experience-dependent plasticity of hippocampal place cells. *J. Neurosci.* **17**, 6769–82.

Skaggs, W. E. and McNaughton, B. L. (1996). Replay of neuronal firing sequences in rat hippocampus during sleep following spatial experience. *Science* **271**, 1870–3.

Staubli, U., Perez, Y., Xu, F., Rogers, G., Ingvar, M., Stone-Elander, S., *et al.* (1994). Centrally active modulators of glutamate receptors facilitate the induction of long-term potentiation *in vivo. Proc. Natl Acad. Sci USA* **91**, 11 158–62.

Tanila, H., Shapiro, M., Gallagher, M., and Eichenbaum, H. (1997). Brain aging: changes in the nature of information coding by the hippocampus. *J. Neurosci.* **17**, 5155–66.

Thibault, O. and Landfield, P. W. (1996). Increase in single L-type calcium channels in hippocampal neurons during aging. *Science* **272**, 1017–20.

Wilson, M. A. and McNaughton, B. L. (1993). Dynamics of the hippocampal ensemble code for space. *Science* **261**, 1055–8.
Wilson, M. A. and McNaughton, B. L. (1994). Reactivation of hippocampal ensemble memories during sleep. *Science* **265**, 676–9.

Glossary

CPP   3-((I)-2-carboxypiperazin-4-yl)-propyl-1-phosphonic acid
EPSP   excitatory postsynaptic potential
LTD   long-term depression
LTP   long-term potentiation
NMDA   *N*-methyl-D-aspartate
vdcc   voltage-dependent L-type calcium channels

23

Elements of a neurobiological theory of the hippocampus: the role of activity-dependent synaptic plasticity in memory

R. G. M. Morris, E. I. Moser, G. Riedel, S. J. Martin, J. Sandin, M. Day, and C. O'Carroll

The hypothesis that synaptic plasticity is a critical component of the neural mechanisms underlying learning and memory is now widely accepted. In this article, we begin by outlining four criteria for evaluating the 'synaptic plasticity and memory (SPM)' hypothesis. We then attempt to lay the foundations for a specific neurobiological theory of hippocampal (HPC) function in which activity-dependent synaptic plasticity, such as long-term potentiation (LTP), plays a key part in the forms of memory mediated by this brain structure. HPC memory can, like other forms of memory, be divided into four processes: encoding, storage, consolidation and retrieval. We argue that synaptic plasticity is critical for the encoding and intermediate storage of memory traces that are automatically recorded in the hippocampus. These traces decay, but are sometimes retained by a process of cellular consolidation. However, we also argue that HPC synaptic plasticity is not involved in memory retrieval, and is unlikely to be involved in systems-level consolidation that depends on HPC–neocortical interactions, although neocortical synaptic plasticity does play a part. The information that has emerged from the worldwide focus on the mechanisms of induction and expression of plasticity at individual synapses has been very valuable in functional studies. Progress towards a comprehensive understanding of memory processing will also depend on the analysis of these synaptic changes within the context of a wider range of systems-level and cellular mechanisms of neuronal transmission and plasticity.

Keywords: synaptic plasticity; event memory; early long-term potentiation; late long-term potentiation; synaptic tagging; memory consolidation

23.1 The synaptic plasticity and memory hypothesis

During learning, spatio-temporal patterns of neural activity that represent events cause long-lasting changes in the strength of synaptic connections within the brain. Later reactivation of these altered connections causes patterns of cell firing that collectively constitute the experience of memory for these events or the expression of learned changes in behaviour triggered by them. These statements are the essence of the SPM hypothesis. The discovery of LTP, whereby brief high-frequency stimulation can induce long-lasting increases in synaptic efficacy (Bliss and Lømo 1973), provided the first experimental analogue of these postulated learning-induced changes in synaptic connectivity in the mammalian brain. Thirty years later, evidence consistent with the hypothesis has accumulated to the point where few doubt the general principle to be correct.

In a series of review articles, we have outlined criteria by which this hypothesis might be judged, the experimental strategies that have been used to address it, and the evidence that supports or conflicts with it (Martin *et al.* 2000; Grimwood *et al.* 2001; Martin and Morris 2002). A key aspect of our approach is the need to think about both synaptic plasticity on the one hand and memory on the other. Recognition that there are different forms of each makes the claim that 'LTP equals memory' too general to be useful, even if a million dollars may be on offer (Stevens 1998). It is a hypothesis that has to be specified more precisely—what forms of synaptic plasticity, what brain structures and circuits, and what forms of learning and memory are being considered? Partly because of this, numerous variants of the SPM hypothesis have been advanced over the years pertaining to the study of memory in different species, networks and brain regions (e.g. Marr 1971; Kandel and Schwartz 1982; Lynch and Baudry 1984; Teyler and Discenna 1984; McNaughton and Morris 1987; Bliss and Collingridge 1993; Izquierdo and Medina 1995; Maren and Baudry 1995; Jeffery 1997; Morris and Frey 1997). Notwithstanding important differences, the underlying core hypothesis is as follows.

Activity-dependent synaptic plasticity is induced at appropriate synapses during memory formation, and is both necessary and sufficient for the information storage underlying the type of memory mediated by the brain area in which that plasticity is observed.

In our reviews, we argued that this hypothesis should be tested in relation to four criteria: detectability, mimicry, anterograde alteration and retrograde alteration. The first and most intuitive of these criteria, detectability, states that the formation of memory must be associated with detectable changes in synaptic efficacy in relevant circuits of the nervous system. The main difficulty is deciding where to look. The second criterion, mimicry, is a critical test of whether changes in synaptic strength are sufficient for memory formation—sufficient, that is, within the context of a normally functioning nervous system. Our third and fourth criteria, anterograde and retrograde alteration, relate to whether synaptic plasticity is necessary for memory formation and expression respectively. We argued that, across a range of different types of learning and memory, including the experience-dependent reorganization of neural circuits, three of these criteria have largely been met. Work from our laboratories and those of many others provides relevant supporting evidence as summarized in our reviews. This evidence includes experiments documenting physiological, biochemical and structural changes during learning that are very likely to have been caused by activity-dependent synaptic plasticity (detectability criterion (e.g. Rioult-Pedotti *et al.* 2000)). Such experiments include physiological, pharmacological and gene-targeting interventions that alter or occlude the capacity to induce or express synaptic plasticity and simultaneously cause changes in learning anterograde alteration criterion (e.g. Morris *et al.* 1986; Silva *et al.* 1992; Moser *et al.* 1998). We recognize that the dependent consequences of a single independent treatment are not necessarily causally related, a logical issue we have discussed at length, but the weight of evidence is very suggestive. Meeting the criteria also includes experiments in which memory retrieval is affected after learning by similar experimental manipulations (retrograde alteration criterion (e.g. Brun *et al.* 2001)).

The outstanding problem is mimicry. This is the sufficiency or 'engineering' criterion. The supposition is that, if it were possible artificially to engineer a particular spatial distribution of synaptic weight changes across a network of neurons, an experimental subject would genuinely behave as if it remembered something that had not in fact happened. Unfortunately, however logically desirable the sufficiency criterion may be, it is unclear that such an experiment would be feasible in many mammalian brain structures owing to the distributed nature of memory storage. Nevertheless, simpler mammalian brain structures, or the nervous systems of lower vertebrates or invertebrates, may offer a more promising substrate for a meaningful test of this criterion (Pittenger and Kandel 2003).

23.2 Elements of a neurobiological theory of the hippocampus and the role of NMDA receptor-dependent synaptic plasticity

A difficulty with this way of assessing the generic SPM hypothesis is that it is somewhat formal and abstract. Although attractive logically, it lacks specifics. It needs to be complemented by the examination of specific neurobiological theories of particular brain regions in which activity-dependent synaptic-plasticity serves an identifiable role. Accordingly, in this paper, we pursue a different approach by outlining some elements of what might eventually become a neurobiological theory of HPC function. We stress that our proposals fall short of a comprehensive theory at this stage, but they represent a synthesis of the published ideas of others and our own thinking about the specific role of activity-dependent synaptic plasticity in HPC memory function.

The mammalian HPC formation is a set of brain structures that, following neuropsychological research on patients with selective brain damage, functional imaging studies, and work using experimental lesions in animals, is widely held to serve an important function in certain types of memory. Its specific contribution to memory remains a matter of dispute. Rival theories include proposals for a role in spatial and cognitive mapping (O'Keefe and Nadel 1978; Gaffan 2001), declarative and relational memory (Squire 1992; Eichenbaum and Cohen 2001), episodic memory (Tulving 1983; Mishkin *et al.* 1997; Morris and Frey 1997; Vargha-Khadem *et al.* 1997; Aggleton and Brown 1999) and the rapid acquisition of configural or conjunctive associations (Sutherland and Rudy 1989; O'Reilly and Rudy 2001). Neural network modelling studies indicate that its intrinsic anatomy and synaptic physiology could mediate the rapid encoding and distributed storage of many arbitrary associations (Marr 1971; McNaughton and Morris 1987; McClelland *et al.* 1995; Rolls and Treves 1998). In all mammals—man, monkey and mouse—the HPC formation seems to be a particular kind of associative memory network. It does not operate in isolation; inputs from midbrain and other forebrain nuclei modulate its activity, and several excitatory inputs and outputs reflect important functional interactions with the neocortex (Amaral and Witter 1989).

A focus of our thinking has been that HPC memory includes the ability to remember events. Events happen in particular places at particular times, and their later recall generally includes the memory of where and when an event happened (Gaffan 1994). Thus, event encoding is necessarily associative in character. Many events cannot be anticipated, occur only once, and may contain distinct features that, in sequence, form short episodes. It is vital that traces representing information about such episodes are encoded and stored in real time—as they happen—a process that we have previously described as the 'automatic recording of attended experience' (Morris and Frey 1997; Morris 2001). Not all events are remembered for any length of time; indeed to do so is not only unnecessary but might also saturate the storage capacity of the brain. In addition, although paradoxical to some, it is far from clear that the hippocampus need receive via its extrinsic afferents the detailed sensory/perceptual information pertaining to individual objects or events. Rather, all it needs to remember events and the sequence in which they happen are cartoons or 'indices' of the locations in the neo-cortex where this detail is processed and at least temporarily encoded. Our first pro-position is as follows.

Proposition 1. *Some animals have episodic-like memory and the HPC is one group of brain structures mediating it.*

A prominent candidate for the neural substrate of event memory is HPC NMDA receptor-dependent synaptic plasticity. Such plasticity, assessed by the experimental phenomenon of LTP, exhibits many properties that are suitable for a role in memory formation (Bliss and Collingridge 1993; Martin *et al.* 2000), and a growing body of evidence offers support for this view (Riedel *et al.* 2003). Accordingly, our second proposition is as follows.

Proposition 2. *A form of activity-dependent, NMDA receptor-dependent synaptic plas-ticity in the hippocampus is the primary neural mechanism responsible for inducing the temporary storage of HPC 'indices' of event memory.*

If most automatically encoded event memories are temporary, there must be psy-chological processes and neural mechanisms for selecting the subset of traces that are to be rendered longer lasting or even permanent. These include the emotional sig-nificance of the event to be remembered itself (or of other events happening close together in time or space), and the relevance of the event to the existing knowledge structures of the organism witnessing it (Bartlett 1932; Bransford 1979). Underlying these psychological processes are two separate neuronal mechanisms of memory con-solidation: cellular consolidation mechanisms that include the synthesis and synaptic capture of plasticity-proteins that stabilize memory traces within individual cells and at the level of the individual synapse; and systems-level consolidation mechanisms that reflect a dynamic interaction between populations of neurons within HPC and neo-cortex (Dudai and Morris 2001). These forms of consolidation are distinct but inter-dependent. This inter-dependence derives from the cellular consolidation mechanism enabling memory indices to last long enough in the HPC for the slower systems-level consolidation process to work. Reflecting new ideas about cellular consolidation, our third proposition is as follows.

Proposition 3. *An essential feature of cellular consolidation processes is the interaction between local 'synaptic tags' (set by glutamatergic activation), and diffusely targeted 'plasticity proteins' (that can be triggered by heterosynaptic activation of neuromodulat-ory inputs) (Frey and Morris 1997, 1998a; Dudai and Morris 2001).*

In contrast to cellular consolidation, systems-level consolidation refers to a process through which initially labile memory traces in the neocortex become gradually stronger through the strengthening of connections between cortical modules. Some theories hold that this requires a dynamic interaction between the HPC and neocortex that eventually enables the cortex to act as an associative memory, linking arbitrary items of information (Squire 1992). Other theories assert that long-lasting HPC traces may exist for certain kinds of memory (e.g. Nadel and Moscovitch 1997).

The defining functional characteristics of associative networks such as the HPC are believed by several theorists to include distributed representations, interleaved storage across multiple synapses and associative retrieval. These enable stored patterns of activity to be 'completed' from partial fragments of the original input (Marr 1971; McNaughton and Morris 1987; Paulsen and Moser 1998; Tonegawa et al. 2003). Several factors determine the operating characteristics and storage capacity of such networks. One, connectivity density (i.e. the number of connections per cell), provides an anatomical basis for understanding an important feature of the relationship between HPC and neocortex (McNaughton et al. 2003). Specifically, the average connectivity within the cortex is too low to support the encoding of arbitrary associations (Rolls and Treves 1998). The cortical mantle contains in the order of 10^{10} neurons, but each cortical principal neuron receives only about 10^4 connections. Thus, the average connection probability in the cortex is only $1 : 10^6$. To overcome this apparent biological limitation, mammals seem to have evolved an arrangement whereby distributed associative memory between items represented in different sensory modalities can be accomplished through indirect associations mediated by a hierarchical organization (McNaughton et al. 2003). In such a scheme, neocortical modules at the base of the hierarchy are reciprocally connected via modifiable synapses with one or more HPC modules at the apex. The HPC modules include CA3 as well as the dentate hilus, both characterized by high internal connectivity as well as modifiable synapses. In CA3, each pyramidal cell is contacted by around 4% of the pyramidal cells of the same subfield (Amaral 1990), implying that most CA3 pyramidal cells are connected via 2–3 synaptic steps (Rolls and Treves 1998). This high degree of internal recurrent connectivity is probably sufficient to allow autoassociation, or association among individual elements of a patterned input (Marr 1971). Activity patterns reflecting sensory detail in neocortical modules may generate a unique identifying pattern, a so-called 'index', in such a network (Teyler and DiScenna 1987). This higher-level index is no longer 'sensory' in any strict sense, but is stored associatively with other indices and the output fed back to lower level neocortical modules via modifiable synapses. Activation of a cortical pattern (e.g. a specific flavour of food) could then result in activation of its index in the hippocampus. In turn, this enables retrieval of associated indices and thence the complementary pattern in the other cortical modules (e.g. where the food is found). Indirect associations enable memory retrieval between cortical modules that are too sparsely connected to do this directly.

This principle of indirect association in memory places high demands on the synaptic storage capacity of the HPC that is otherwise in danger of becoming saturated. Once saturated, learning can no longer proceed effectively (McNaughton and Barnes 1986; Moser et al. 1998). One of several ways to limit this burden could, as already noted, be via the rapid decay of a high proportion of the traces that are automatically encoded online. Heterosynaptic depression may also serve a normalizing function and increase effective storage capacity (Willshaw and Dayan 1990). Another way, also an element of the ideas being described, would be to ensure that what is stored in the HPC is merely an index of the neocortical sites of trace storage where the full sensory/perceptual details are encoded. A fourth way would be to enable HPC associations that are repeatedly recalled, often representing environmental regularities, to trigger the gradual development of low-level intermodular connections within the neocortex, a process that is likely to require cortical, but not HPC, synaptic plasticity. These connections would enable cortical retrieval in the absence of activity in the hippocampus. This is the process of systems-level memory consolidation. Identified originally through experiments on retrograde amnesia revealing that damage to the HPC and related structures can impair new memory encoding while leaving old memories relatively intact (Squire and Zola-Morgan 1991; Kapur 1999), it is unlikely that insensitivity to brain damage is the adaptive pressure that led to its evolution. Our theoretical framework implies that, in part, its function is to avoid the distracting 'recovery to consciousness' of irrelevant associations that could otherwise interfere with ongoing mental activities (Moscovitch 1995). To work, it is vital that the inter-modular connections that develop are appropriate to the associations represented. This requires the gradual interleaving of appropriate connections (McClelland et al. 1995), perhaps during sleep (McNaughton et al. 2003). Interestingly, the rate of consolidation may not be strictly time-dependent. The process may be 'cladistic', with the rate of consolidation affected by the frequency with which HPC indices are reactivated. Thus, a further set of propositions to investigate is as follows.

Proposition 4. *Systems-level consolidation requires both HPC and neocortical neural activity, and may therefore not be strictly time-dependent.*

Proposition 5. *Systems-level consolidation does not require HPC plasticity, but does engage neocortical plasticity.*

23.3 Experimental observations

(a) Propositions 1 and 2

There has been considerable recent interest in the idea that the HPC is essential for episodic rather than all forms of declarative memory in humans (Vargha-Khadem et al. 1997, 2001; Duzel et al. 2001; Maguire et al. 2001). An immediate difficulty for neurobiological studies is that episodic memory is defined in a way that renders it difficult to study in animals, in particular, Tulving's (1983) insistence on concomitant 'autonoetic consciousness' (the sense of self). Notwithstanding this difficulty, there have been claims that vertebrates may possess an episodic-like memory system analogous to subcomponents of true human episodic memory. One-trial spatial working-memory tasks are of this character (Steele and Morris 1999; Aggleton and Pearce 2001; Brown and Aggleton 2001), but the argument is not watertight as these might be, and sometimes are, solved using familiarity (Griffiths et al. 1999; Brown and Aggleton 2001). A valuable breakthrough has been Clayton and Dickinson's (1998) food-caching paradigm with scrub-jays. They observed that jays can recall 'what, where and when' in appropriately securing, during cache retrieval, either a favoured foodstuff (mealworms) or, after several days, one that lasts better over time (peanuts).

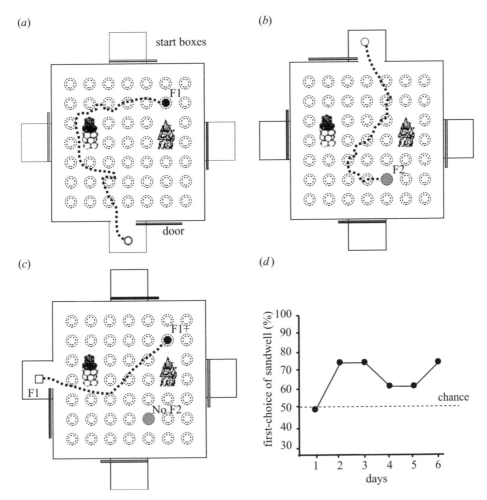

Fig. 23.1 The event arena. The 1.6 m² arena made of Perspex consisted of 49 sand wells (open circles), the two intramaze landmarks, and the four start boxes. (*a*) On sample trial one, the door to a start box is drawn back and the rat runs out into the arena (dotted line) where it displays occasional lateral head-movements to find food (F1) at the single open well. (*b*) Sample trial two to a different food (F2) at a different location. Double-sample presentation rats had sample trials one and two repeated at this point. (*c*) The cued-recall choice trial begins with presentation of either of the two sample trial foods (food F1 is shown) followed by the rat being rewarded selectively for digging at the sand well containing this same food. (*d*) Proportion of choice trials in which the first chosen sand well had been cued in the start box. Single sample presentation rats ($n = 8$) were above chance over days 2–6 of training.

Inspired by this experiment, Day *et al.* (2003) have developed a one-trial paired-associate task (Fig. 23.1) in which rats recall (rather than merely recognize) in which of two locations a particular flavour of rat food is to be found within a large 1.6 m × 1.6 m event arena. In each of two sample trials on each day, a few minutes apart, rats exit a start box to find a single open sand well where they can dig for a flavoured food. On the daily choice trial, 5 to 20 min later, the rat is given one of the two flavours to eat in the start box (its recall cue) and, 30 s later, exits to choose between the two sand wells now available. A win–stay rule applies whereby going to the location recalled by the flavour cue is usually rewarded by more of that same flavour (non-rewarded probes are also run). Up to 30 different locations and flavours are paired in novel combinations at the rate of two pairs per day. Video clips showing a rat performing two successive sample trials (where it encodes flavour–location associations) followed by a choice trial are available at: http://neuroweb-2.cfn.ed.ac.uk/ video/. This what–where paradigm, with one-trial encoding and recall as the expression of memory, constitutes evidence that rats are capable of episodic-like memory as proposed in Proposition 1, and in a species more amenable to neurobiological study than jays. In keeping with Proposition 2 above, we have also established that the encoding of one-trial memory of such paired-associates lasts more than 60 min before recall performance drops to chance. Encoding is sensitive to the acute intrahippocampal infusion of an NMDA receptor antagonist (D-AP5) without any effect on retrieval, whereas encoding and retrieval are sensitive to the AMPA receptor antagonist CNQX (Fig. 23.2).

These findings complement earlier work using the repeated one-trial learning paradigm in the water maze called DMP (Steele and Morris 1999). However, whereas DMP examines only spatial memory, this new training procedure looks at what–where associations and reveals that one-trial learning of such associations is possible and that they decay quite quickly (within a day). The training protocol does not (yet) incorporate the temporal 'when' component, as in Clayton and Dickinson (1998). However, from a neuropharmacological perspective, having even a what–where association is sufficient to point to a partial dissociation between the role of NMDA and AMPA receptors in the hippocampus with respect to memory encoding and memory retrieval respectively. A weakness of the experiment—as it stands—is that the deficit in choice behaviour observed when CNQX is infused before recall could be a strictly spatial deficit, rather than a deficit in the ability to recall a place given the cue of an appropriate flavour (the 'what–where' association). This ambiguity has been addressed in new work using overtrained flavour–place associations, but this weakness does not affect the interpretation of the AP5 experiments. Blocking HPC NMDA receptors *after* the daily sample trials but *before* a choice trial had no effect on choice accuracy relative to aCSF infusions. It follows that NMDA receptors are not critical for the recall of spatial information or place–flavour associations. In turn, this implies that the deficit in choice trials seen when AP5 is infused *before* sample trials also cannot be due to impaired spatial recall. Thus, the memory deficit in choice trials following pre-sample AP5 infusions must result from a failure of encoding and storage. As the representation of the environment has already been well learned at the time of the drug infusions, this must be a deficit in associating new information about flavours with information retrieved from the neocortex about locations within the familiar testing environment.

What, then, is the function of the hippocampus in the earlier stages of spatial memory and how might the spatial and non-spatial features of an event be put together? An important milestone in the understanding of spatial cognition was the discovery that most pyramidal cells in the hippocampus exhibit location-specific activity and that the activity of such place cells is influenced by the training history of the animal (O'Keefe and Dostrovsky 1971). The predominantly spatial nature of HPC neuronal activity led to the proposal that place cells form a distributed maplike

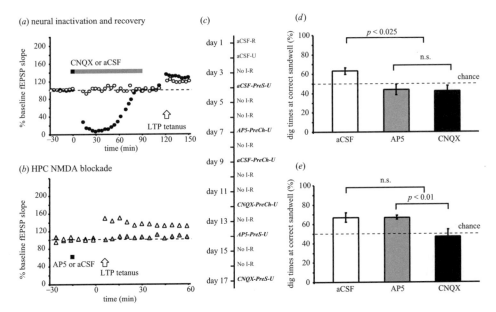

Fig. 23.2 Role of HPC NMDA and AMPA receptors in encoding and retrieval of memory. (*a*) CNQX and electrophysiology. Maximal neural inactivation in the hippocampus occurs within 10–15 min of CNQX infusion and lasts for around 60 min. Open circles, aCSF; closed circles, CNQX. (*b*) AP5 and electrophysiology. AP5 infusions do not affect fast synaptic transmission but block LTP induction 15 min post-infusion. Open triangles, aCSF; closed triangles, AP5. (*c*) Representative sequence of the treatments given to an individual rat across 17 days. Different sequences were used to achieve counterbalancing of treatment order. AP5, CNQX, aCSF: bilaterally infused with respective treatment; R,U: choice trial rewarded or unrewarded (dig time data only available for unrewarded trials); Pre-S and PreCh: infusions before the sample or choice trials. Dig time data secured from days assigned in bold italic. (*d,e*) Drug-infusions before sample trials (*d*) and before choice trials (*e*). Separate analyses of days when the drugs (aCSF, AP5 and CNQX) were infused before sample trials revealed a significant drug effect. There was no difference between days with AP5 and CNQX treatment, but both better and above-chance performance on aCSF days than drug days. Analyses of days when the drugs were infused before choice trials revealed no difference between days with aCSF and AP5 treatment, but better and above-chance performance on these days compared with those with CNQX infusions.

representation of the spatial environment that an animal uses for efficient navigation (O'Keefe and Nadel 1978). When a rat is exposed to a new environment, pyramidal cells develop distinct firing fields within few minutes (Hill 1978; Wilson and McNaughton 1993). The place fields then remain stable for weeks or more if the environment is constant (Thompson and Best 1990; Lever *et al.* 2002), as predicted if these cells contribute to a particular spatial memory.

It is commonly believed that the development of HPC firing patterns, like HPC memory, might depend on LTP at HPC excitatory synapses. Studies have primarily investigated the contribution of LTP to spatial firing in HPC pyramidal cells. Surprisingly, interventions that abolish HPC LTP have only weak effects on the development of place fields. For example, blockade of NMDA receptors does not prevent the formation of new place fields in rats that explore a novel environment. Place fields recorded in CA1 in mice with mutations of NMDA receptors either in CA3 or CA1 are somewhat less distinct than in control mice under certain conditions, but the fields remain stable across repeated tests on the same day (McHugh *et al.* 1996; Nakazawa *et al.* 2002). Place fields also develop normally in rats treated systemically with an NMDA receptor antagonist at a dose that prevents new LTP in the hippocampus (Kentros *et al.* 1998). Despite blockade of the NMDA receptor, place fields were maintained between consecutive test sessions in the same environment for at least 1.5 h. Similar results were obtained when LTP was blocked by interference with $Ca^{2+}/$ calmodulin-dependent protein kinase II (Rotenberg *et al.* 1996) or protein kinase A (Rotenberg *et al.* 2000). However, these interventions did decrease the long-term stability of the place fields, as measured 24 h after the initial exposure to the environment. Together, these studies suggest that NMDA receptor activation may not be necessary for the development or initial maintenance of place-related activity in HPC neurons, although it may contribute to the fine-tuning of place fields and aspects of the long-term stabilization of spatial representations. The latter function could involve the neocortex as well as the hippocampus.

The development of place fields during NMDA receptor blockade or other forms of disruption of LTP is consistent with several lines of work suggesting that spatial information can be generated and stored upstream of the hippocampus. First, location-specific firing is already expressed in the superficial layers of the entorhinal cortex (Quirk *et al.* 1992; Frank *et al.* 2000). The signal : noise ratio of these spatial signals is lower than in the hippocampus, but the fact that most principal cells in entorhinal cortex exhibit view-independent spatial modulation suggests that, by this stage, the fundamental computation may already have been made. It is possible, though, that spatial firing in superficial entorhinal neurons depends on spatial input from cells in deep layers, which in turn may rely on associative computations in afferent HPC structures. However, several studies suggest that place fields develop without the intrahippocampal trisynaptic circuitry. Pyramidal cells in CA1 exhibit spatial firing both after selective lesions of the dentate gyrus (McNaughton *et al.* 1989) and after disconnection of CA1 from CA3 (Brun *et al.* 2002; Fig. 23.3). In CA3-lesioned animals, CA1 pyramidal neurons receive cortical input only by the direct connections from the entorhinal cortex. The presence of place fields in these preparations suggests that direct entorhinal–HPC circuitry has significant capacity for transforming weak location-modulated signals from superficial layers of the entorhinal cortex into accurate spatial firing in CA1. Several simple filter mechanisms could accomplish such a transformation. For example, firing rates of perforant path fibres to CA1 could be thresholded by feed-forward inhibition, such that only the highest afferent firing rates, i.e. those in the centre of the entorhinal place field, are able to drive postsynaptic neurons in the hippocampus. Alternatively, single EPSPs in distal pyramidal-cell dendrites of CA1 may often not be sufficient to trigger somatic actional potentials in these cells; reliable discharge may require summation of EPSPs, i.e. high afferent firing rates (Golding and Spruston 1998; Golding *et al.* 2002).

It is important to note that the computation and storage of positional information outside the hippocampus does not preclude the processing, storage and use of spatial information (or indices of such information) within the hippocampus. Indeed, the internal recurrent connectivity of HPC area CA3 makes the region highly suitable for storage of just this type of patterned information, at least for an intermediate period of time. Recent results suggest that plasticity in associative synapses of CA3 is necessary

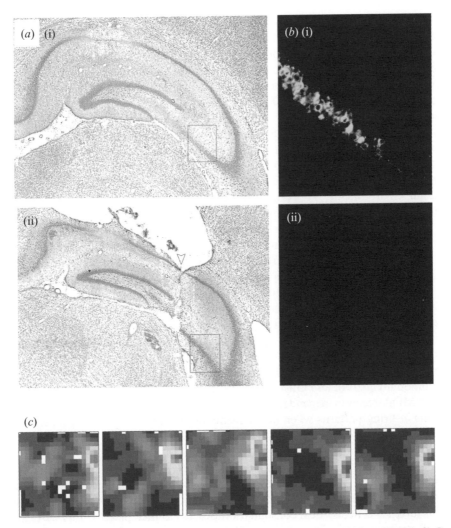

Fig. 23.3 Intact place fields in area CA1 after transection of fibres from CA3 to CA1. (*a,b*) Cresyl violet and fluorescence images from an unlesioned control rat (*a*(i) and *b*(i)) and a rat with CA1 isolated from CA3 by a longitudinal cut (arrowhead) at the border between these subfields (*a*(ii) and *b*(ii)). A retrograde tracer (aminostilbamidine) was infused at the recording position in dorsal CA1 (green). Fluorescence images in (*b*) correspond to red boxes in adjacent left sections in (*a*). (*c*) Colour-coded firing rate map for a cell from the lesioned rat in ((*a*) and (*b*)). The cell was recorded for 5 consecutive days (left to right). Dark red indicates maximum rate (left to right: 8, 12, 12, 17 and 11 Hz). (See Plate 8 of the Plate Section, at the centre of this book.)

for the successful encoding of spatial information in a manner that later allows recall with partial cues (Nakazawa *et al.* 2002; Tonegawa *et al.* 2003). Mice with targeted deletions of NMDA receptors in CA3 were trained in a reference memory task in the water maze. These mice were unable to localize the hidden platform on a recall trial with only a limited set of the landmarks used during training. When the full set of cues was available, retention was indistinguishable from that of control animals. Place fields in CA1 were more dispersed than in control mice in the limited-cue condition but not in the full-cue test. These findings suggest that the CA3 performs pattern completion during recall of spatial information. Longitudinal axon collaterals in CA3 may be important for successful retrieval of such information, as memory retention may be impaired by a single transversely-oriented cut through the dorsal CA3 region of each hippocampus (Steffenach *et al.* 2002).

The key novel feature of our argument and data is that the network of the hippocampus has the circuitry and the plasticity to store associations between locations and events. The location information that is encoded within these associations may be derived online from HPC spatial processing (e.g. that occurring during exploration of a novel environment) or retrieved via the direct entorhinal pathway (e.g. that concerning a familiar environment). To examine how HPC neurons respond to an unpredicted event in a well-consolidated environment, we trained rats to find a hidden platform at a fixed location in an annular water maze and then moved the platform to a new place (Fyhn *et al.* 2002). This movement of the platform constituted transferring a critical event (escaping from the water) from one location to another. Several cells fired vigorously at the new platform location, despite previously having been silent. Others that fired in different locations around the maze continued to do so after the platform relocation, arguing against spatial remapping. The new activity was paralleled by reduced discharge in a subset of simultaneously recorded interneurons. The pattern of activity largely returned towards its original configuration as the rat learned the new location. However, a few of the newly recruited neurons remained active. This persistent firing may reflect facilitated synaptic plasticity during the temporary reduction in inhibition (Wigstrom and Gustafsson 1983; Paulsen and Moser 1998; see also Lynch 2003). NMDA-receptor-dependent LTP may be necessary for these permanent modifications in firing patterns when novel events occur in a familiar environment.

(b) Proposition 3

The idea that HPC memory indices are encoded as distributed patterns of synaptic weights requires that changes in synaptic weight last long enough for the slower systems level HPC/neocortical consolidation process to take place. E-LTP lasts at most 3–4 h. Protein-synthesis-dependent L-LTP lasts longer but perhaps not indefinitely (c.f. Abraham 2003). The difference between these two forms of synaptic potentiation reflects a long-recognized difference between STM and LTM: that *de novo* protein synthesis is required for a short-lasting trace to be converted into a long-lasting one. It draws upon experimental work in *Drosophila* (Belvin and Yin 1997), *Aplysia* (Montarolo *et al.* 1986), early learning in birds (Rose 1995), mammalian memory (Davis and Squire 1984), neural models of memory formation such as LTP (Krug *et al.* 1984) and theories about the relationship between STM and LTM (Goelet *et al.* 1986).

A new perspective on these ideas is the synaptic tagging hypothesis of memory trace formation (Frey and Morris 1997, 1998*a,b*; Morris and Frey 1997; Dudai and Morris 2001). This hypothesis accepts that plasticity proteins are critical for the persistence of synaptic memory traces, but argues against obligatory *de novo* synthesis of these proteins in response to the events that are to be remembered. Our idea is that LTM trace formation is at least a two-stage process (the systems–neuroscience framework above actually implies a three-stage process). In one step, the potential for a LTM is established locally at synapses in the form of rapidly decaying E-LTP accompanied by the setting of a synaptic tag. In the other, a series of biochemical interactions, including protein–protein interactions, are triggered to convert this synaptic potentiality into a longer lasting trace at those synapses at which tags have been set. The somatic events that lead to these interactions can be set in motion shortly before the event to be remembered, at the same time (as in most behavioural and *in vitro* brain slice experiments so far), or shortly afterwards. Critically, the persistence of memory does not have to be determined at the time of initial memory trace formation. Frey and Morris (1998*b*) proposed that patterns of afferent glutamatergic activation and postsynaptic spiking, which together induce LTP, set synaptic tags and induce short-lasting changes in synaptic weights. Heterosynaptic activation, which we proposed in 1998 occurs through neuromodulatory inputs (particularly DA afferent to areas CA1 and CA3 of the hippocampus, and the noradrenergic inputs to the dentate gyrus), is responsible for *de novo* protein synthesis. These proteins travel diffusely in dendritic compartments until sequestered locally by the synaptic tags whereupon they help induce synaptic stabilization.

At present, we still do not know whether synaptic tagging occurs *in vivo* and whether the principle also extends to behavioural memory as implied by Proposition 3. That is, would it be possible to induce a long-lasting memory during the inhibition of protein synthesis if the synthesis and distribution of the relevant plasticity proteins had occurred earlier? Unlike brain slice or intracellular experiments, it would be necessary, *in vivo*, to ensure that the upregulation of protein synthesis occurred in a common population of neurons to those used by the animal later during learning. One way in which it may be possible to work towards this is to take advantage of the idea that heterosynaptic activation of neuromodulatory afferents, such as dopamine D1 and D5 receptors, is involved in the persistence of LTP (Swanson-Park *et al.* 1999) and, in particular, L-LTP (Frey *et al.* 1991). In new work, we have recently replicated the observation that the D1/D5 antagonist SCH23390 blocks L-LTP in HPC slices (Fig. 23.4*a*) and then explored the impact of this drug on STM and LTM.

The behavioural experiments used the DMP paradigm in the water maze. This is a repetitive one-trial learning protocol in which the hidden platform moves location each day, but remains in that day's location for each of four trials. The animals therefore have the opportunity to encode the new location on trial one of each day and so escape much more rapidly on trials two to four. The delay between trials one and two was varied between 20 min and 6 h. This study revealed that bilateral intrahippocampal infusion of the D1/D5 receptor antagonist SCH23390 causes a delay-dependent impairment of memory (Fig. 23.4*b*).

This study represents the first step of a systematic series of experiments in which we hope to test the implications of the synaptic tagging idea in behaving animals. As the critical predictions of the theory require protein synthesis to be triggered at one point in the sequence of events but not at another shortly thereafter (or shortly before), it is unclear whether gene-targeting techniques will be very useful. They will, as in the work of Barco *et al.* (2002) and Hédou and Mansuy (2003), help us identify many of the mechanisms of persistence of LTP and LTD at a genetic level. However, addressing the heterosynaptic issue will be more difficult as even inducible constructs require several days to work. By using physiological and pharmacological techniques, however, it may be possible to activate dopaminergic afferents to the hippocampus before a learning

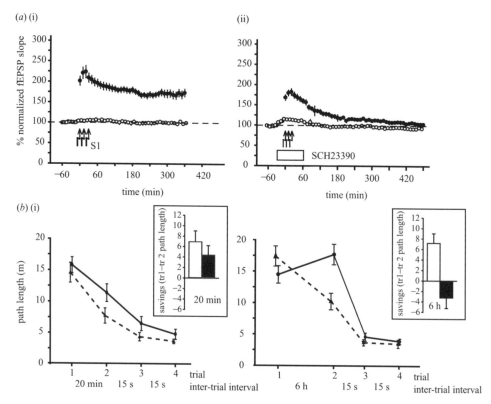

Fig. 23.4 The D1/D5 receptor antagonist blocks L-LTP and LTM for a single event. (*a*) Electrophysiological brain slice experiments confirmed earlier studies showing that SCH23390 blocks L-LTP but not E-LTP. Note stability of simultaneously monitored control pathway (S2, open circles). LTP was induced by three bursts of tetanic stimulation at 100 Hz spaced 10 min apart in HPC slices maintained at 32 °C (S1, closed circles). (*b*) Behavioural studies used rats (*n* = 36) prepared for acute bilateral infusion of drugs into the dorsal hippocampus. After recovery, they were given 8 days of drug-free training (four trials per day, 30 s on the platform after each trial). The inter-trial interval was 15 s between most trials. However, between trials one and two, it was 20 min on half the days and 6 h on the other half (in an ABBA design). The DMP protocol was then continued with bilateral intrahippocampal infusions of aCSF or SCH23390 in aCSF on different days (30 min before trial one of each day). Averaged across the 8 days of training, rats infused with the D1/D5 antagonist showed good memory of the new platform location on trial two each day at the 20 min interval between trials one and two, but substantial forgetting at the 6 h interval. Path-length on trial two was lower on the drug-treatment days for 20 min than for 6 h. The savings between trials one and two are shown in the inserts.

experience and then train in the presence of an antagonist. This and other related tests of the synaptic tagging hypothesis of the persistence of HPC indices are underway.

(c) Propositions 4 and 5

Our theoretical framework identifies the HPC as encoding indices linking disparate neocortical modules whose connectivity is too sparse to support the encoding of arbitrary associations. According to some, the HPC subsequently plays a time-limited role in memory by enabling the gradual development of intracortical connections that render the cortical memory traces enduring and self-sufficient, the process we have referred to as systems-level consolidation (Squire 1992; McClelland *et al.* 1995). Others argue that the HPC has a permanent role in memory storage for certain kinds of information and, thus, its retrieval (Nadel and Moscovitch 1997). Much of the conflicting evidence is derived from studies on patients with permanent brain damage (Kapur 1999) or animals with irreversible lesions. Such studies cannot easily dissociate the distinctive memory processes of storage, consolidation and retrieval.

Reversible pharmacological manipulations offer an alternative approach (Izquierdo and Medina 1998; McGaugh 2000). They have three advantages. (i) The experimental manipulation can be made after training during the consolidation period, but withdrawn during the next phase (e.g. retrieval). Any effects they then have cannot be on sensorimotor processes, or on memory encoding. (ii) They offer the opportunity of asking what aspects of neural activity are required because, in addition to studying the effects of regionally specific neural inactivation (induced by AMPA antagonists), one of our Propositions (5) implies that HPC plasticity should play no role in guiding neocortical consolidation. There is a clear controversy on this issue, particularly between genetic (Shimizu *et al.* 2000) and pharmacological data (Day and Morris 2001; Villarreal *et al.* 2002). Finally, (iii) if the HPC guides consolidation by establishing relevant intracortical connectivity, reversible pharmacological manipulations might be applied to the neocortex as well as to the HPC during the putative consolidation period.

We have previously shown that 7 days' infusion of a GLUR1-5 antagonist to inactivate the HPC, starting 1 to 5 days after training, disrupts spatial memory in the water maze when tested 16 days after training (Riedel *et al.* 1999; Fig. 23.5). This finding is consistent with systems-level consolidation requiring HPC neural activity post-training, but raises two questions relevant to Propositions 4 and 5. First, would a similar finding pertain if an NMDA antagonist were chronically infused into the hippocampus over the same time-period? This is a relevant follow-up of the work with the GLUR1-5 antagonist as this would, as a secondary effect, have also inhibited NMDA receptor mechanisms by preventing sufficient postsynaptic depolarization. Second, is interference with systems-level consolidation the only interpretation of the findings of Riedel *et al.* (1999)? We consider these two issues in turn.

New work using rats and mice indicates that chronic *post-training* infusion of D-AP5 into the dorsal hippocampus bilaterally has no effect on later memory (Fig. 23.5*b*). We put emphasis on both the location in the brain where the AP5 is infused (the hippocampus) and the time of administration of the drug (post-training) for our propositions do include that AP5 *during* learning disrupts memory encoding. In the rat studies, retrieval was tested 16 days after the end of training exactly as in Riedel *et al.* (1999), long after the 7 day minipumps implanted after training were exhausted. The concentration of D-AP5 used was sufficient to block dentate and CA1 LTP *in vivo* when this was tested during the period of drug infusion.

However, second, it is possible that the chronic blockade of AMPA receptors actually disrupts trace storage within the HPC itself rather than the HPC/neocortical consolidation process. This may happen by a breakdown in the quantitative scaling of homeostatic plasticity (Turrigiano *et al.* 1998). One way of distinguishing these possibilities would be to contrast HPC inactivation starting soon after training ('recent

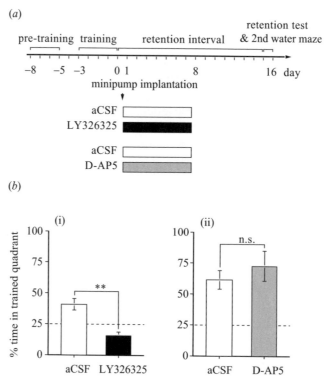

Fig. 23.5 HPC neural activity but not NMDA receptor activity is involved in systems-level memory consolidation. (*a*) Experimental design shows training phases and periods when aCSF (n.s. = 17 and 5, respectively), the GLUR1-5 antagonist LY326325 ($n = 8$), and D-AP5 ($n = 7$) were chronically infused after spatial reference memory training using an Atlantis platform. Retention tests consisting of a 60 s swim with the platform absent were conducted 16 days after the end of training. (*b*) Selective impairment of spatial memory following AMPA receptor (i) but not NMDA receptor blockade (ii). The variation in performance of the two aCSF groups was unexpected and reflects variability in performance of rats tested at different times.

memory' group as in Riedel *et al.* (1999)) with inactivation starting several weeks later ('remote memory' group). If the recent memory group were to display amnesia while the remote memory group did not, the most parsimonious explanation would be in terms of a systems-level consolidation process. However, if an equivalent memory impairment is observed in both groups, suggesting that memory traces do not survive a prolonged period of AMPA receptor blockade, an HPC site of storage has likely been disrupted. These traces may be the 'indices' that are persistently required to link information in disparate neocortical modules, in the manner of Nadel and Moscovitch's (1997) theory. An experiment to test this prediction of our hypothesis is currently underway. Overall, the experimental philosophy is that use of reversible inactivation rather than conventional lesions should enable us to distinguish theoretically between a putative consolidation process and any contributions that HPC activity may be making to storage and retrieval processes. The data at hand point to a clear difference between post-training neural inactivation and post-training inhibition of NMDA receptor-dependent plasticity, and are inconsistent with recent gene-targeting experiments.

We find no support for the notion that HPC NMDA receptor-dependent synaptic plasticity is involved in long-term consolidation.

However, the persistence of spatial memory after post-training blockade of HPC NMDA receptors leaves several questions unresolved. One is that other forms of activity-dependent plasticity may be engaged—our experiment is silent on this issue. Another relates to the role of synaptic plasticity during offline reactivation in neuronal ensembles that were active during the preceding behavioural experience. In the context of place cells, reactivation refers to the striking observation that cells with overlapping place fields continue to exhibit correlated firing during slow-wave and rapid-eye-movement sleep episodes subsequent to the behavioural session (Wilson and McNaughton 1994; Louie and Wilson 2001). Reactivation occurs throughout large areas of the posterior cortex (Hoffman and McNaughton 2002) and is seen particularly during sharp waves. Sharp waves are bursts of synchronous activity in HPC pyramidal cells that may be necessary for the induction of plasticity in downstream areas in behaving animals (Buszaki 1989; King *et al.* 1999). The poor long-term stability of place fields after blockade of HPC LTP suggests that HPC or neocortical plasticity during offline states may play a role in the modification of spatial representations. This modification may take place in the cortex, in the hippocampus, or both. Our proposition states only that HPC plasticity is unlikely to be involved in circumstances in which information that has been encoded online in the HPC network is to be protected from change during the course of systems consolidation. However, it remains to be determined whether there is a direct link between sharp-wave related reactivation and NMDA receptor-dependent synaptic modifications in efferent synapses within the HPC formation (e.g. subiculum) or in neocortical target areas. Reactivation is strongest immediately after the behavioural session, during a time-period much shorter than that thought to underlie systems consolidation. This shorter time-course includes the very time-periods over which place field instability has been observed. Examining whether reactivation gives rise to NMDA receptor-dependent plasticity within the hippocampus would therefore require an experimental design in which the receptors were blocked almost instantly after termination of the training experience (Packard and Teather 1997).

23.4 Conclusion

Bliss and Lømo (1973, p. 355) ended their article on long-lasting potentiation with a somewhat embedded conundrum: 'whether or not the intact animal makes use in real life of a property which has been revealed by synchronous, repetitive volleys to a population of fibres the normal rate and pattern of activity along which are unknown, is another matter.' Thirty years later, our appraisal of the literature indicates that there is now overwhelming evidence that activity-dependent synaptic plasticity is engaged during learning, is required for learning and, if induced physiologically after learning, alters an animal's memory of past experience. Accordingly, three of the four formal criteria by which the SPM hypothesis can be assessed have been satisfied in one or more brain systems of learning and memory, although not always within a single brain system.

Beyond this abstract assessment of this hypothesis, we have also outlined some elements of an emerging neurobiological theory of the HPC formation together with

new data pertaining to a series of specific propositions. Both behavioural and electrophysiological data are consistent with the idea that activity-dependent HPC synaptic
potentiation is critical for the automatic recording of unique event–place associations.
This involves both encoding and intermediate storage of memory traces that constitute
indices of the locations in the neocortex where more detailed sensory/perceptual detail
may be found. Many automatically encoded traces decay rapidly. However, if encoding
happens around the time of the synthesis and dendritic distribution of plasticity-related
proteins to activated synapses, the traces may persist long enough to enable, through a
process of indirect association, the much slower HPC/neocortical consolidation process
to build direct connections between relevant cortical modules. Retrieval of remote
memories is a process through which this passive storehouse of cortically located traces
can then be reactivated. With recent memories, HPC neural activity is likely to be
involved; with more remote memories, it need not be. HPC LTP engages mechanisms
used in some but not all of these processes that collectively enable the seamless
execution of what we understand as memory.

We are grateful to the Medical Research Council (grant number G9200370/2), the Norwegian
Research Council (G 139398/300; and CBM 145993), and the European Union (QLG3-CT-1999-
00192) for their support of this research.

References

Abraham, W. C. (2003). How long will long-term potentiation last? *Phil. Trans. R. Soc. Lond.* B
    358, 735–44. (DOI 10.1098/rstb.2002.1222.)
Aggleton, J. P. and Brown, M. W. (1999). Episodic memory, amnesia, and the hippocampal-
    anterior thalamic axis. *Behav. Brain Sci.* **22**, 425–89.
Aggleton, J. P. and Pearce, J. M. (2001). Neural systems underlying episodic memory: insights from
    animal research. *Phil. Trans. R. Soc. Lond.* B **356**, 1467–82. (DOI 10.1098/rstb. 2001.0946.)
Amaral, D. G. (1990). Neurons, numbers and the hippocampal network. In *Progress in brain
    research* (ed. J. Storm-Mathisen, J. Zimmer and O. P. Ottersen), pp. 1–11. Amsterdam, The
    Netherlands: Elsevier.
Amaral, D. G. and Witter, M. P. (1989). The three dimensional organization of the hippocampal
    formation: a review of anatomical data. *Neuroscience* **31**, 571–91.
Barco, A., Alarcon, J. M., and Kandel, E. R. (2002). Expression of a constitutively active CREB protein
    facilitates the late phase of long-term potentiation by enhancing synaptic capture. *Cell* **108**, 689–703.
Bartlett, F. C. (1932). *Remembering*. Cambridge University Press.
Belvin, M. P. and Yin, J. C. (1997). *Drosophila* learning and memory: recent progress and new
    approaches. *Bioessays* **19**, 1083–9.
Bliss, T. V. P. and Collingridge, G. L. (1993). A synaptic model of memory: long-term poten-
    tiation in the hippocampus. *Nature* **361**, 31–9.
Bliss, T. V. P. and Lømo, T. (1973). Long-lasting potentiation of synaptic transmission in
    the dentate area of the anaesthetized rabbit following stimulation of the perforant path.
    J. Physiol. (*Lond.*) **232**, 331–56.
Bransford, J. D. (1979). *Human cognition: learning, understanding and remembering*. Belmont,
    CA: Wadsworth.
Brown, M. W. and Aggleton, J. P. (2001). Recognition memory: what are the roles of the
    perirhinal cortex and hippocampus? *Trends Cogn. Sci.* **2**, 51–61.
Brun, V. H., Ytterbo, K., Morris, R. G., Moser, M. B., and Moser, E. I. (2001). Retrograde
    amnesia for spatial memory induced by NMDA receptor-mediated long-term potentiation.
    J. Neurosci. **21**, 356–62.

Brun, V. H., Otnass, M. K., Molden, S., Steffenach, H. A., Witter, M. P., Moser, M.-B., et al. (2002). Place cells and place recognition maintained by direct entorhinal–hippocampal circuitry. *Science* **296**, 2243–6.

Buszaki, G. (1989). Two-stage model of memory-trace formation: a role for 'noisy' brain states. *Neuroscience* **31**, 551–70.

Clayton, N. S. and Dickinson, A. (1998). What, where and when: episodic-like memory during cache recovery by scrub jays. *Nature* **395**, 272–4.

Davis, H. P. and Squire, L. R. (1984). Protein synthesis and memory: a review. *Psychol. Bull.* **96**, 518–59.

Day, M. and Morris, R. G. M. (2001). Memory consolidation and NMDA receptors: discrepancy between genetic and pharmacological approaches. *Science* **293**, 755.

Day, M., Langston, R. F., and Morris, R. S. M. (2003). Glutamate recepter mediated encoding and retrival of paired associate learning. *Nature* **424**, 205–9.

Dudai, Y. and Morris, R. G. M. (2001). To consolidate or not to consolidate: what are the questions? In *Brain, perception and memory: advances in cognitive sciences* (ed. J. Bolhuis), pp. 147–62. Oxford University Press, Oxford.

Duzel, E., Vargha-Khadem, F., Heinze, H. J., and Mishkin, M. (2001). Brain activity evidence for recognition without recollection after early hippocampal damage. *Proc. Natl. Acad. Sci. USA* **98**, 8101–6.

Eichenbaum, H. and Cohen, N. J. (2001). *From conditioning to conscious recollection*. New York: Oxford University Press.

Frank, L. M., Brown, E. N., and Wilson, M. (2000). Trajectory encoding in the hippocampus and entorhinal cortex. *Neuron* **27**, 169–78.

Frey, U. and Morris, R. G. M. (1997). Synaptic tagging and longterm potentiation. *Nature* **385**, 533–6.

Frey, U. and Morris, R. G. M. (1998a). Weak before strong: dissociating synaptic-tagging and plasticity-factor accounts of late-LTP. *Neuropharmacology* **37**, 545–52.

Frey, U. and Morris, R. G. M. (1998b). Synaptic tagging: implications for late maintenance of hippocampal long-term potentiation. *Trends Neurosci.* **21**, 181–8.

Frey, U., Matthies, H., Reymann, K. G., and Matthies, H. (1991). The effect of dopaminergic d1-receptor blockade during tetanization on the expression of long-term potentiation in the rat CA1 region *in vitro*. *Neurosci. Lett.* **129**, 111–14.

Fyhn, M., Molden, S., Hollup, S. A., Moser, M.-B., and Moser, E. I. (2002). Hippocampal neurons responding to first-time dislocation of a target object. *Neuron* **35**, 555–66.

Gaffan, D. (1994). Scene-specific memory for objects: a model of episodic memory impairment in monkeys with fornix transection. *J. Cogn. Neurosci.* **6**, 305–20.

Gaffan, D. (2001). What is a memory system? Horel's critique revisited *Behav. Brain Res.* **127**, 5–11.

Goelet, P., Castellucci, V. F., Schacher, S., and Kandel, E. R. (1986). The long and the short of long-term memory—a molecular framework. *Nature* **322**, 419–22.

Golding, N. L. and Spruston, N. (1998). Dendritic sodium spikes are variable triggers of axonal action potentials in hippocampal CA1 pyramidal neurons. *Neuron* **21**, 1189–200.

Golding, N. L., Staff, N. P., and Spruston, N. (2002). Dendritic spikes as a mechanism for cooperative long-term potentiation. *Nature* **418**, 326–31.

Griffiths, D., Dickinson, A., and Clayton, N. (1999). Episodic memory: what can animals remember about their past? *Trends Cogn. Sci.* **3**, 74–80.

Grimwood, P. D., Martin, S. J., and Morris, R. G. M. (2001). Synaptic plasticity and memory. In *Synapses* (ed. W. M. Cowan, T. C. Sudhof and C. F. Stevens), pp. 519–70. Baltimore, MD: Johns Hopkins University Press.

Hédou, G. and Mansuy, I. M. (2003). Inducible molecular switches for the study of long-term potentiation. *Phil. Trans. R. Soc. Lond.* B **358**, 797–804. (DOI 10.1098/rstb.2002.1245.)

Hill, A. J. (1978). First occurrence of hippocampal spatial firing in a new environment. *Exp. Neurol.* **62**, 282–97.

Hoffman, K. L. and McNaughton, B. L. (2002). Sleep on it: cortical reorganization after-the-fact. *Trends Neurosci.* **25**, 1–2.

Izquierdo, I. and Medina, J. H. (1995). Correlation between the pharmacology of long-term potentiation and the pharmacology of memory. *Neurobiol. Learning Memory* **63**, 19–32.

Izquierdo, I. and Medina, J. H. (1998). On brain lesions, the milkman and Sigmunda. *Trends Neurosci.* **21**, 423–6.

Jeffery, K. J. (1997). LTP and spatial learning: where to next? *Hippocampus* **7**, 95–110.

Kandel, E. R. and Schwartz, J. H. (1982). Molecular biology of learning: modulation of transmitter release. *Science* **218**, 433–43.

Kapur, N. (1999). Syndromes of retrograde amnesia: a conceptual and empirical synthesis. *Psychol. Bull.* **125**, 800–25.

Kentros, C., Hargreaves, E., Hawkins, R. D., Kandel, E. R., Shapiro, M., and Muller, R. V. (1998). Abolition of long-term stability of new hippocampal place cell maps by NMDA receptor blockade. *Science* **280**, 2121–6.

King, C., Henze, D. A., Leinekugel, X., and Buzsaki, G. (1999). Hebbian modification of a hippocampal population pattern in the rat. *J. Physiol.* **521**, 159–67.

Krug, M., Lossner, B., and Ott, T. (1984). Anisomycin blocks the late phase of long-term potentiation in the dentate gyrus of freely moving rats. *Brain Res. Bull.* **13**, 39–42.

Lever, C., Wills, T., Cacucci, F., Burgess, N., and O'Keefe, J. (2002). Long-term plasticity in hippocampal place-cell representation of environmental geometry. *Nature* **416**, 90–4.

Louie, K. and Wilson, M. A. (2001). Temporally structured REM sleep replay of awake hippocampal ensemble activity. *Neuron* **29**, 145–56.

Lynch, G. (2003). Long-term potentiation in the Eocene. *Phil. Trans. R. Soc. Lond.* B **358**, 625–8. (DOI 10.1098/rstb.2002.1253.)

Lynch, G. and Baudry, M. (1984). The biochemistry of memory: a new and specific hypothesis. *Science* **224**, 1057–63.

McClelland, J. L., McNaughton, B. L., and O'Reilly, R. C. (1995). Why there are complementary learning systems in the hippocampus and neocortex: insights from the successes and failures of connectionist models of learning and memory. *Psychol. Rev.* **102**, 419–57.

McGaugh, J. L. (2000). Memory: a century of consolidation. *Science* **287**, 248–51.

McHugh, T. J., Blum, K. I., Tsien, J. Z., Tonegawa, S., and Wilson, M. A. (1996). Impaired hippocampal representation of space in CA1-specific NMDAR1 knockout mice. *Cell* **87**, 1339–49.

McNaughton, B. L. and Barnes, C. A. (1986). Long-term enhancement of hippocampal synaptic transmission and the acquisition of spatial information. *J. Neurosci.* **6**, 563–571.

McNaughton, B. L. and Morris, R. G. M. (1987). Hippocampal synaptic enhancement and information storage within a distributed memory system. *Trends Neurosci.* **10**, 408–15.

McNaughton, B. L., Barnes, C. A., Meltzer, J., and Sutherland, R. J. (1989). Hippocampal granule cells are necessary for normal spatial learning but not for spatially-selective pyramidal cell discharge. *Exp. Brain Res.* **76**, 485–96.

McNaughton, B. L., Barnes, C. A., Battaglia, F. A., Bower, M. R., Cowen, S. L., Ekstrom, A. D., *et al.* (2003). Off-line reprocessing of recent memory and its role in memory consolidation: a progress report. In *Sleep and brain plasticity* (ed. P. Maquet, C. Smith, and R. Stickgold), pp. 225–46. Oxford University Press, Oxford.

Maguire, E. A., Vargha-Khadem, F., and Mishkin, M. (2001). The effects of bilateral hippocampal damage on fMRI regional activations and interactions during memory retrieval. *Brain* **124**, 1156–70.

Maren, S. and Baudry, M. (1995). Properties and mechanisms of long-term synaptic plasticity in the mammalian brain: relationships to learning and memory. *Neurobiol. Learning Memory* **63**, 1–18.

Marr, D. (1971). Simple memory: a theory for archicortex. *Phil. Trans. R. Soc. Lond.* B **262**, 23–81.

Martin, S. J. and Morris, R. G. M. (2002). New life in an old idea: the synaptic plasticity and memory hypothesis revisited. *Hippocampus* **12**, 609–36.

Martin, S. J., Grimwood, P. D., and Morris, R. G. (2000). Synaptic plasticity and memory: an evaluation of the hypothesis. *A. Rev. Neurosci.* **23**, 649–711.

Mishkin, M., Suzuki, W. A., Gadian, D. G., and Vargha-Khadem, F. (1997). Hierarchical organization of cognitive memory. *Phil. Trans. R. Soc. Lond.* B **352**, 1461–7. (DOI 10.1098/rstb.1997.0132.)

Montarolo, P. G., Goelet, P., Castellucci, V. F., Morgan, J., Kandel, E. R., and Schacher, S. (1986). A critical period for macromolecular synthesis in long-term heterosynaptic facilitation in *Aplysia. Science* **234**, 1249–54.

Morris, R. G. M. (2001). Episodic-like memory in animals: psychological criteria, neural mechanisms and the value of episodic-like tasks to investigate animal models of neurode-generative disease. *Phil. Trans. R. Soc. Lond.* B **356**, 1453–65. (DOI 10.1098/rstb.2001.0945.)

Morris, R. G. M. and Frey, U. (1997). Hippocampal synaptic plasticity: role in spatial learning or the automatic recording of attended experience? *Phil. Trans. R. Soc. Lond.* B **352**, 1489–503. (DOI 10.1098/rstb.1997.0136.)

Morris, R. G. M., Anderson, E., Lynch, G. S., and Baudry, M. (1986). Selective impairment of learning and blockade of longterm potentiation by an N-methyl-D-aspartate receptor antagonist, AP5. *Nature* **319**, 774–6.

Moscovitch, M. (1995). Recovered consciousness: a hypothesis concerning modularity and episodic memory. *J. Clin. Exp. Neuropsychol.* **17**, 276–90.

Moser, E. I., Krobert, K. A., Moser, M. B., and Morris, R. G. M. (1998). Impaired spatial learning after saturation of long-term potentiation. *Science* **281**, 2038–42.

Nadel, L. and Moscovitch, M. (1997). Memory consolidation, retrograde amnesia and the hippocampal complex. *Curr. Opin. Neurobiol.* **7**, 217–27.

Nakazawa, K., Quirk, M. C., Chitwood, R. A., Watanabe, M., Yechel, M. F., Sun, L. D., *et al.* (2002). Requirement for hippocampal CA3 NMDA receptors in associative memory recall. *Science* **297**, 211–18.

O'Keefe, J. and Dostrovsky, J. (1971). The hippocampus as a spatial map. Preliminary evidence from unit activity in the freely-moving rat. *Brain Res.* **34**, 171–5.

O'Keefe, J. and Nadel, L. (1978). *The hippocampus as a cognitive map.* Oxford: Clarendon.

O'Reilly, R. C. and Rudy, J. W. (2001). Conjunctive representations in learning and memory: principles of cortical and hippocampal function. *Psychol. Rev.* **108**, 311–45.

Packard, M. G. and Teather, L. A. (1997). Double-dissociation of hippocampal and dorsal-striatal memory systems by posttraining intracerebral injections of 2-amino-5-phosphono-pentanoic acid. *Behav. Neurosci.* **111**, 543–51.

Paulsen, O. and Moser, E. I. (1998). A model of hippocampal memory encoding and retrieval: GABAergic control of synaptic plasticity. *Trends Neurosci.* **21**, 273–8.

Pittenger, C. and Kandel, E. R. (2003). In search of general mechanisms for long-lasting plasticity: *Aplysia* and the hippocampus. *Phil. Trans. R. Soc. Lond.* B **358**, 757–63. (DOI 10. 1098/rstb.2002.1247.)

Quirk, G. J., Muller, R. U., Kubie, J. L., and Ranck, J. B. (1992). The positional firing properties of medial entorhinal neurons: description and comparison with hippocampal place cells. *J. Neurosci.* **12**, 1945–63.

Riedel, G., Micheau, J., Lam, A. G. M., Roloff, E. V. L., Martin, S. J., Bridge, H., *et al.* (1999). Reversible neural inactivation reveals hippocampal participation in several memory processes. *Nature Neurosci.* **2**, 898–905.

Riedel, G., Platt, B., and Micheau, J. (2003). Glutamate receptor function in learning and memory. *Behav. Brain Res.* **140**, 1–47.

Rioult-Pedotti, M.-S., Friedman, D., and Donoghue, J. P. (2000). Learning-induced LTP in neocortex. *Science* **290**, 533–6.

Rolls, E. T. and Treves, A. (1998). *Neural networks and brain function.* Oxford University Press.

Rose, S. P. R. (1995). Glycoproteins and memory formation. *Behav. Brain Formation* **66**, 73–8.

Rotenberg, A., Mayford, M., Hawkins, R. D., Kandel, E. R., and Muller, R. U. (1996). Mice expressing activated CaMKII lack low frequency LTP and do not form stable place cells in the CA1 region of the hippocampus. *Cell* **87**, 1351–61.

Rotenberg, A., Abel, T., Hawkins, R. D., Kandel, E. R., and Muller, R. U. (2000). Parallel instabilities of long-term potentiation, place cells, and learning caused by decreased protein kinase A activity. *J. Neurosci.* **20**, 8096–102.

Shimizu, E., Tang, Y. P., Rampon, C., and Tsien, J. Z. (2000). NMDA receptor-dependent synaptic reinforcement as a crucial process for memory consolidation. *Science* **290**, 1170–4.

Silva, A. J., Stevens, C. F., Tonegawa, S., and Wang, Y. (1992). Deficient hippocampal long-term potentiation in α-calciumcalmodulin kinase II mutant mice. *Science* **257**, 201–6.

Squire, L. R. (1992). Memory and the hippocampus: a synthesis from findings with rats, monkeys, and humans. *Psychol. Rev.* **99**, 195–231.

Squire, L. R. and Zola-Morgan, S. (1991). The primate hippocampal formation: evidence for a time-limited role in memory storage. *Science* **253**, 1380–6.

Steele, R. J. and Morris, R. G. M. (1999). Delay-dependent impairment of a matching-to-place task with chronic and intrahippocampal infusion of the NMDA-antagonist D-AP5. *Hippocampus* **9**, 118–36.

Steffenach, H. A., Sloviter, R. S., Moser, E. I., and Moser, M. B. (2002). Impaired retention of spatial memory after transection of longitudinally oriented axons of hippocampal CA3 pyramidal cells. *Proc. Natl. Acad. Sci. USA* **99**, 3194–8.

Stevens, C. F. (1998). A million dollar question: does LTP = memory? *Neuron* **20**, 1–2.

Sutherland, R. J. and Rudy, J. W. (1989). Configural association theory: the role of the hippocampal formation in learning, memory, and amnesia. *Psychobiol.* **17**, 129–44.

Swanson-Park, J. L., Coussens, C. M., Mason-Parker, S. E., Raymond, C. R., Hargreaves, E. L., Dragunow, M., *et al.* (1999). A double dissociation within the hippocampus of dopamine D1/D5 receptor and beta-adrenergic receptor contributions to the persistence of long-term potentiation. *Neuroscience* **92**, 485–97.

Teyler, T. J. and Discenna, P. (1984). Long-term potentiation as a candidate mnemonic device. *Brain Res. Rev.* **7**, 15–28.

Teyler, T. J. and Discenna, P. (1987). Long-term potentiation. *A. Rev. Neurosci.* **10**, 131–61.

Thompson, L. T. and Best, P. J. (1990). Long-term stability of the place-field activity of single units recorded from the dorsal hippocampus of freely behaving rats. *Brain Res.* **509**, 299–308.

Tonegawa, S., Nakazawa, K., and Wilson, M. A. (2003). Genetic neuroscience of mammalian learning and memory. *Phil. Trans. R. Soc. Lond.* B **358**, 787–95. (DOI 10.1098/rstb.2002.1243.)

Tulving, E. (1983). *Elements of episodic memory*. Oxford: Clarendon.

Turrigiano, G., Leslie, K. R., Desai, N., Rutherford, L. C., and Nelson, S. (1998). Activity-dependent scaling of quantal amplitude in neocortical neurons. *Nature* **391**, 892–5.

Vargha-Khadem, F., Gadian, D. G., Watkins, K. E., Connely, A., Van Paesschen, W., and Mishkin, M. (1997). Differential effects of early hippocampal pathology on episodic and semantic memory. *Science* **277**, 376–80.

Vargha-Khadem, F., Gadian, D. G., and Mishkin, M. (2001). Dissociations in cognitive memory: the syndrome of developmental amnesia. *Phil. Trans. R. Soc. Lond.* B **356**, 1435–40.

Villarreal, D. M., Do, V., Haddad, E., and Derrick, B. E. (2002). NMDA receptor antagonists sustain LTP and spatial memory: active processes mediate LTP decay. *Nature Neurosci.* **5**, 48–52.

Wigstrom, H. and Gustafsson, B. (1983). Facilitated induction of hippocampal long-lasting potentiation during blockade of inhibition. *Nature* **301**, 603–4.

Willshaw, D. and Dayan, P. (1990). Optimal plasticity from matrix memories: what goes up must come down. *Neural Commun.* **2**, 85–93.

Wilson, M. A. and McNaughton, B. L. (1993). Dynamics of the hippocampal ensemble code for space. *Science* **261**, 1055–8.

Wilson, M. A. and McNaughton, B. L. (1994). Reactivation of hippocampal ensemble memories during sleep. *Science* **265**, 676–82.

Glossary

aCSF	artificial cerebrospinal fluid
AMPA	α-amino-3-hydroxy-5-methylisoxazole-4-propionic acid
CA1–3	Cornu Ammonis areas 1–3
DMP	delayed matching-to-place
E-LTP	early long-term potentiation
EPSP	excitatory postsynaptic potential
HPC	hippocampal
L-LTP	late long-term potentiation
LTD	long-term depression
LTM	long-term memory
LTP	long-term potentiation
NMDA	*N*-methyl-D-aspartate
SPM	synaptic plasticity and memory
STM	short-term memory

24

Genetic neuroscience of mammalian learning and memory

Susumu Tonegawa, Kazu Nakazawa, and Matthew A. Wilson

Our primary research interest is to understand the molecular and cellular mechanisms on neuronal circuitry underlying the acquisition, consolidation and retrieval of hippocampus-dependent memory in rodents. We study these problems by producing genetically engineered (i.e. spatially targeted and/or temporally restricted) mice and analysing these mice by multifaceted methods including molecular and cellular biology, *in vitro* and *in vivo* physiology and behavioural studies. We attempt to identify deficits at each of the multiple levels of complexity in specific brain areas or cell types and deduce those deficits that underlie specific learning or memory. We will review our recent studies on the acquisition, consolidation and recall of memories that have been conducted with mouse strains in which genetic manipulations were targeted to specific types of cells in the hippocampus or forebrain of young adult mice.

Keywords: memory; hippocampus; N-methyl-D-aspartate receptors

24.1 The general strategy

An understanding of the brain mechanisms of cognition, such as learning and memory, requires the identification of the underlying events and processes occurring at multiple levels of complexity; from molecular, synaptic and cellular levels to neuronal ensemble and brain systems level. One would then have to deduce cause–consequence relationships among these multilevel events and processes. This is an enormous challenge because cognitive phenomena manifest themselves as behaviours of live animals, while many of the analytical methods for the study of underlying mechanisms rely on *in vitro* preparations. Among *in vivo* analytical methods, non-invasive imaging such as functional magnetic resonance imaging and positron emission tomography are powerful in correlating cognitive phenomena to the activities of neuronal ensembles or brain systems, but the current technology of this type cannot reach down to cellular or molecular levels (reviewed in Schacter and Wagner 1999). Single-unit and multi-unit recording techniques have been powerful in monitoring activities of individual neurons and neuronal ensembles as an animal undergoes a specific type of cognition (Wilson and McNaughton 1993; Wessberg *et al.* 2000). The recent advent of invasive imaging techniques is filling in the gaps between the levels of complexity addressed by the non-invasive imaging approach and the *in vivo* electrophysiology (reviewed in Helmchen and Denk 2002). However, all of these approaches are primarily designed to identify events or processes that *can* occur while the subjects or animals go through a specific cognitive behaviour but are, in principle, mute in identifying lower-level events or processes that are *necessary* for the higher-level phenomenon. For this latter purpose, lesion and pharmacological intervention techniques have been widely used.

Lesion studies address whether a certain brain region or a global neuronal circuitry is necessary for a given cognitive function but are not designed to identify a specific type of molecule or cell necessary for a specific cognition. Traditionally, for an intervention at the molecular level, pharmacological administration has been used because of the availability of a range of receptor antagonists and enzyme inhibitors. Examples are AP5 for NRs and CNQX for AMPA receptors (Morris *et al.* 1986; Izquierdo and Medina 1997; Steele and Morris 1999). The advantages of a pharmacological intervention are: (i) not only can it block a physiological process at the molecular level, but (ii) it can also block a specific physiological process acutely and reversibly. However, it is difficult to target a drug to a specific brain area, for example, area CA1 of the hippocampus and it is even more difficult to do so reproducibly from one animal to another. This last point is particularly relevant in rodent memory research because most memory tasks require averaging of at least a dozen individual animals. In addition, many of the drugs used are not entirely specific to a single receptor or enzyme. As the question posed becomes increasingly sophisticated, the intrinsic limitation associated with a pharmacological blockade is emerging, namely the lack of cell type specificity—for instance, even if one manages to target the delivery of AP5 to area CA1, it will block NRs expressed on both excitatory pyramidal cells and inhibitory interneurons.

Given this background, it was desirable to develop an alternative intervention technique aimed at the molecular level. For relatively simple invertebrate systems such as fruit flies or worms, molecular genetics has been used for this purpose with substantial success (Benzer 1967; Brenner 1974). With the advent of the transgenic and 'knockout' techniques, it became possible in the early 1990s to apply genetics or 'reverse genetics' to neuroscience of a mammalian (mouse) system for the study of cognitive mechanisms (Silva *et al.* 1992*a*, *b*). However, because of the inherent complexity of mammalian central nervous systems, it was necessary to add a spatial and/or temporal restriction to the genetic manipulations for them to be a truly effective approach. Thus, our experimental strategy was to create new mouse strains in which a gene of interest is deleted or overexpressed or the activity of its protein product is inhibited, in a limited brain area or, preferably, in a specific cell type of a restricted brain area of adult inbred mice (Tsien *et al.* 1996*a*; Nakazawa *et al.* 2002). We will then subject these genetically engineered mice, together with normal littermates, to a variety of analytical methods each designed to detect a defect or impairment at a particular level of complexity (Fig. 24.1). The

approach:	molecular genetic	slice and culture electrophysiology	multielectrode physiology of freely moving animals	behavioural studies
		cell biology biochemistry	imaging	
level of complexity:	molecule	individual neurons and synapses	neuronal ensembles	cognition and behaviour
			neuronal circuitries	

Fig. 24.1 The general strategy based on cell type-restricted knockout mice. Approaches and techniques designed to identify a deficit or impairment at a particular level of complexity in the organization of the brain are listed. Analysis of targeted gene knockout mice can potentially allow the identification of causal relationships among events occurring at different levels of complexity.

advantages of this approach are that the blockade can be highly specific with respect to the gene and its protein product, the brain area and the type of cells. Furthermore, animal to animal reproducibility of the blockade is guaranteed. However, this type of genetic blockade is generally inferior to the pharmacological blockade with respect to temporal control. Nevertheless, there have been cases in the literature in which a reversible temporal control was combined with a certain degree of spatial restriction by genetic manipulations (Mayford *et al.* 1996; Mansuy *et al.* 1998).

24.2 Memory acquisition

Using the Cre/loxP system (Sauer and Henderson 1988) we previously targeted a knockout of the obligatory NR subunit, NR1, to the CA1 pyramidal cells of young adult mice (Tsien *et al.* 1996*a, b*). These mice displayed impairments in the SC CA1 LTP and in spatial learning tested in the hidden platform version of the Morris watermaze. The mutant's inability to form normal memory representations as CA1 place cells (McHugh *et al.* 1996) suggested that this mutant mouse is defective in the acquisition rather than the retrieval of the memory. During recent years, we have demonstrated that the mutants are also impaired in non-spatial hippocampus-dependent learning; trace-fear conditioning (Huerta *et al.* 2000) and olfaction-based transverse patterning (Rondi-Reig *et al.* 2001). These findings provide the most cogent evidence for Hebb's hypothesis (Hebb 1949).

The standard Morris watermaze task tests animals' ability for 'reference memory', which is acquired incrementally over multiple trials and involves information constant across trials. Another type of memory supported by the hippocampus is 'episodic memory' (for humans) (Tulving 1972) or 'episodic-like memory' (for rodents) (Griffiths *et al.* 1999) which is acquired rapidly with one trial or one-time experience and involves trial- or event-specific information (Marr 1971; Tulving 1995). It is probable that different mechanisms underlie these two types of declarative memory (Squire 1994; Eichenbaum 1997; Vargha-Khadem *et al.* 1997). However, little is known about underlying differential mechanisms. We investigated two theories, both of which are based on mathematical modelling of memory systems. First, it has been suggested that the learning rate and the number of unambiguous patters are greater in a network with bidirectional modifiability of synaptic strength than in a network with unidirectional modifiability (Willshaw and Dayan 1990). For instance, the information storage efficiency of a network with only LTP capability would be lower than that of a network with both LTP and LTD capability. We generated a mouse strain (CN-KO) in which the gene encoding the sole regulatory subunit of calcineurin in the brain (CNB1) is only deleted in the postnatal forebrain (Zeng *et al.* 2001). At the SC-CA1 synapses, LTD was significantly diminished while the LTP elicited by saturating stimulation (100 Hz, 1 s) was normal (a collaboration with Mark Bear). The mutant mice were normal in the acquisition and retrieval of spatial reference memory but were specifically impaired in two tasks for spatial episodic-like memory, namely a DMP version of the Morris water-maze (Steele and Morris 1999) and the working memory version of Olton's eight-arm radial maze (Olton and Papas 1979). These results support the notion that a network with bi-directional modifiability of synaptic strength plays a crucial role in the acquisition of episodic-like memory, while it is dispensable for reference memory.

In rodents, infusion of an NR antagonist into the hippocampus has been shown to result in a deficit in 'episodic-like' memory (Morris and Frey 1997; Steele and Morris 1999). However, to date, there has been no study, to our knowledge, that directly implicates a specific sub-field of the hippocampus or a specific protein therein in this mnemonic process. It has been suggested that recurrent networks with modifiable synaptic strength could support the rapid acquisition of memories of a one-time experience (Marr 1971). The CA3 sub-field of the hippocampus is known to have a robust recurrent network with pyramidal cells receiving synaptic contacts from around 2% of other CA3 pyramidal cells (MacVicar and Dudek 1980; Miles and Traub 1986). Hebbian-type synaptic plasticity in the form of LTP has also been demonstrated at the synapses of recurrent collaterals in CA3 (Harris and Cotman 1986; Williams and Johnston 1988; Zalutsky and Nicoll 1990; Berger and Yeckel 1991). In conjunction with a set of inhibitory feed-back inputs to CA3 pyramidal cells, such a CA3 recurrent network has been suggested to provide a mechanism for maintaining coherent information for short-term duration and to serve as a temporary storage site for short-term, episodic or working memories by reverberating activity in the recurrent collateral connections (Rawlins 1985; Wiebe *et al.* 1997; Kesner and Rolls 2001).

To test this proposal, we generated a knockout mouse (CA3-NR1 KO) in which the deletion of the NR1 gene is restricted to the CA3 pyramidal cells of an adult mouse (Fig. 24.2; Nakazawa *et al.* 2003). These mice were impaired in the spatial DMP task when the platform was placed in a novel location, but were normal when the platform location employed a few days earlier was reused. This behavioural deficit was highly specific in that the mutants were normal in the acquisition of spatial reference memory as tested by the standard hidden platform version of the Morris watermaze task (see below). In order to investigate the cellular mechanism underlying this specific behavioural impairment observed in the mutant mice, we monitored the activities of the pyramidal cells in CA1, the area downstream of CA3 and the site for the hippocampal output, before and after the animals entered a novel space from a familiar space.

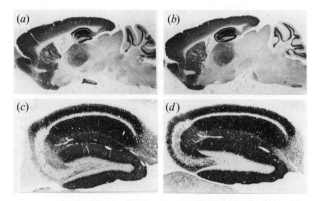

Fig. 24.2 Immunoperoxidase staining of medial parasagittal sections of brains (*a,b*) or transverse sections (*c,d*) of the hippocampus derived from 18-week-old CA3-NR1 KO mice (*a,c*) and their control littermates (*b,d*) visualized with 3,3′-diaminobenzidine. The primary antibody used was specific for NR1. The immunoreactivity was specifically deficient in the apical and basal dendrite areas of mutant CA3.

We found that the specificity of spatial tuning in the mutants was reduced during the first 15 min of exploration in the novel space compared with the same period in the familiar space. By contrast, no space shift-associated change of spatial tuning was observed when the mutant mice were returned 1 day later to the pair of spaces experienced on the previous day. The spatial tuning of CA1 place cells of control animals did not exhibit any space shift-associated changes. These results suggest that CA3 NRs, most probably those in the recurrent network, play a crucial role in rapid hippocampal encoding of a novel encounter and in one trial- or one experience-based rapid learning.

How does the lack of CA3 NRs lead to the decreased spatial specificity of CA1 pyramidal cells in the novel space? CA1 receives inputs from both the layer III stellate cells of the EC via the temporo-ammonic pathway, and from CA3 pyramidal cells via the SCs. During spatial exploration, cells in the superficial layer of the EC show spatially related responses with significantly lower specificity than that observed in CA3 (Barnes et al. 1990; Quirk et al. 1992; Frank et al. 2000), and it has been suggested that they provide a major source of input to CA1 (Vinogradova 1975; McNaughton et al. 1989; Brun et al. 2002), particularly during tasks that require encoding of novel information (Sybirska et al. 2000). The activity of the temporo-ammonic pathway has been shown to regulate the gating of CA1 spikes in EC-hippocampal slices (Remondes and Schuman 2002). Our result, demonstrating that CA1 place fields are less spatially tuned in the mutant animals when a new spatial representation is required, is consistent with the notion that a new spatial context is conveyed via the temporo-ammonic pathway. Moreover, our finding supports a long-standing hypothesis that the CA1 network acts as a comparator: detecting novelty or mismatches between actual sensory information from the EC and the expectation from memory in CA3 (Vinogradova 1970; Gray 1982; McNaughton et al. 1989; Moser and Paulsen 2001; Fyhn et al. 2002).

We propose that during exposure to a novel context, CA1 response is initially driven by the spatially broadly tuned, direct EC input. In control animals, NR function in CA3, perhaps via recurrent connections, allows the rapid formation of more spatially specific responses that can then drive correspondingly specific response in CA1 as the input through the SCs comes to dominate that from the EC. In CA3-NR KO mice, CA3 NR ablation leading to the lack of dominant CA3 input (Nakazawa et al. 2002, 2003) may result in the more gradual spatial refinement of CA1 place fields implemented by other hippocampal circuit plasticity. CA1 place field enlargement may be due to the prolonged influence of direct EC input to CA1 during this slow refinement process. Our results indicate that the reduced spatial tuning in mutants' CA1 lasts for at least 15 min (duration of place cell recording sessions). Thus, at some time between 15 min after the onset of exploration of a novel environment and the return to it 24 h later, normal place cell activity seems to be restored in the mutants. This reduced spatial tuning may, in turn, affect the accuracy of spatial learning during this period. The time-course of these physiological effects was roughly consistent with those of the behavioural deficits observed in the DMP tasks in which the mutants exhibited memory impairment for at least 20 min (four trials each taking around 2 min plus three inter-trial intervals of 5 min) in a test session with a novel platform location while they behaved normally for the platform locations experienced 4 days earlier.

24.3 Memory consolidation

A critical feature of both memory consolidation and the formation of long-lasting synaptic plasticity is a requirement for new mRNA and protein synthesis (Frey *et al.* 1988; Milner *et al.* 1998). Previous studies of memory consolidation have largely focused on the regulation of gene expression, establishing an important role for the transcription factor CREB in this process (Bourtchuladze *et al.* 1994; Bartsch *et al.* 1995). We have studied the roles of two kinases, CaMKIV and ERK, in memory consolidation and long-lasting synaptic plasticity using conditional gene engineering techniques.

Among several Ca^{2+}-dependent protein kinases that phosphorylate CREB at Ser-133 for its activation, CaMKIV is the only one detected predominantly in the nuclei of neurons (Jensen *et al.* 1991). However, global CaMKIV knockout mice exhibited developmental impairments and conflicting data regarding the role of this kinase in LTP and memory (Ho *et al.* 2000; Wu *et al.* 2000). We generated and analysed transgenic mice in which a dominant-negative form of CaMKIV (dnCaMKIV) inhibits Ca^{2+}-stimulated CaMKIV activity only in the postnatal forebrain (a collaboration with Tom Soderling) (Kang *et al.* 2001). In these transgenic mice, activity-induced CREB phosphorylation and *c*-Fos expression were significantly attenuated. Hippocampal L-LTP was also impaired whereas basic synaptic function and E-LTP were unaffected. Further, these deficits correlated with impairments in long-term memory, specifically in its consolidation–retention phase but not in the acquisition phase. These results indicate that neural activity-dependent CaMKIV signalling in the neuronal nucleus plays an important role in the consolidation–retention of hippocampus- dependent long-term memory.

In another study in my laboratory (currently unpublished), Ray Kelleher and Arvind Govindarajan focused on the ERK signalling cascade which is known to play a central role in the response to mitogenic signals in many cell types by regulating the phosphorylation of key transcription factors. In neurons, the ERK pathway is activated in response to calcium influx and neurotrophin stimulation. Although previous studies relying on the use of pharmacological inhibitors have implicated ERK activation in LTP and memory (Impey *et al.* 1999; Orban *et al.* 1999), the underlying cellular and molecular mechanisms remain unclear. We generated transgenic mice in which ERK activation is inhibited by a dominant-negative ERK kinase (dnMEK1) transgene only in the postnatal forebrain. The protein synthesis-dependent portion of L-LTP was impaired at SC-CA1 synapses, whereas E-LTP, paired pulse facilitation, and basal synaptic transmission were normal. Consistent with this selective impairment in hippocampal L-LTP, the mutant mice exhibited a selective impairment in long-term memory in contextual fear conditioning. We further investigated the role of the ERK signalling pathway in activity-dependent protein synthesis by applying transfection techniques to cultured hippocampal neurons. We propose that the ERK signalling pathway governs memory consolidation and long-lasting synaptic plasticity, at least in part, through a novel role in the regulation of protein synthesis in neurons.

24.4 Memory recall

In the past, the neuroscience of associative memory has largely focused on the mechanisms underlying its acquisition and consolidation, while the mechanism of memory recall has been relatively ignored. In day-to-day life, recall of associative memory almost always occurs under the constraints of limited cues. For instance, recalling the rich content of interesting conversations with someone can be triggered merely by the subsequent sighting of that person. In the past, a study of the mechanism underlying this fundamental feature of memory recall, referred to as 'pattern completion,' has been limited to computational modelling. These theoretical studies proposed that a recurrent network with modifiable synaptic strength, such as that in hippocampal area CA3, could provide this pattern completion capability (Marr 1971; Gardner-Medwin 1976; Hopfield 1982; McNaughton and Morris 1987; Rolls 1989; Hasselmo *et al.* 1995). However, because of technical difficulties, at least 30 years have passed with virtually no experimental evidence for or against the hypothesis since David Marr's first publication on this subject (Marr 1971). We addressed this issue with CA3-NR1 KO mice (Nakazawa *et al.* 2002). A set of immunocytochemical and cytochemical experiments demonstrated the integrity of the cytoarchitecture of the mutant hippocampus (a collaboration with Masahiko Watanabe's laboratory). Wholecell patch-clamp recordings performed on visually identified cells in acute hippocampal slices showed the normal intrinsic properties of CA3 pyramidal cells. The evoked N-methyl-D-aspartate currents were entirely missing at C/A-CA3 synapses while those at the MF-CA3 synapses as well as the medial perforant path–dentate gyrus synapses and SC-CA1 synapses were normal. LTP was deficient at C/A-CA3 synapses, whereas it was intact at MF-CA3 and SC-CA1 synapses (a collaboration with Dan Johnston's laboratory). The mutant mice were normal in the acquisition and retrieval of spatial memory tested in the hidden platform version of the Morris watermaze. However, when the memory of the location of the hidden platform was tested following removal of three of the four major extramaze cues (partial cue conditions), the mutants exhibited a clear deficit of memory retrieval compared with the control animals (Fig. 24.3). That this specific recall deficit was not due to faster loss of the memory was confirmed by demonstrating that the mutants reached the platform as fast as the control mice in a trial carried out 1 h after the partial cue probe test following the restoration of the platform and the complete set of cues (full-cue conditions).

To investigate the neural mechanisms that might underlie the specific recall deficit we examined the neurophysiological consequences of CA3-NR1 deletion by analysing CA1 place cell activity. While the complex spike bursting was significantly reduced, the basic cellular properties of CA1 pyramidal cells, such as mean firing rate and spike width, were normal in the mutants. No significant differences were observed between the mutant and control mice in either place field size or average firing rate within a cell's place field (integrated firing rate). Furthermore, the ability of cells with overlapping place fields to fire in a coordinated manner did not differ between control and mutant mice (note that this is in contrast to CA1-NR1 KO mice). Thus, spatial information within CA1 is relatively preserved despite the loss of CA3 NRs providing a physiological correlate of the intact spatial performance of the CA3-NR1 KO mice in the Morris watermaze under full-cue conditions. We examined the effect of partial cue removal on CA1 output as follows. Mice were allowed to explore a familiar arena for 20–30 min under full-cue conditions, and then removed to their home cage. Following a 2 h delay, mice were returned to the open field with either the same four major extramaze cues present (full-cue conditions) or with three of the four cues removed (partialcue conditions). In the control mice, there were no significant changes in place

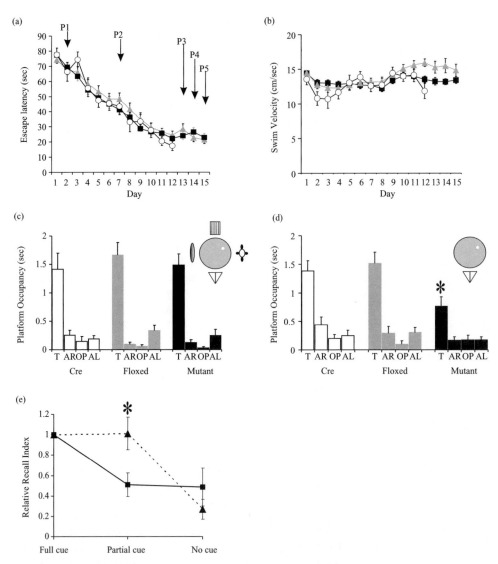

Fig. 24.3 Performance of CA3-NR1 KO mice in the standard Morris watermaze task and recall capability under various cue conditions. (*a,b*) 18–24-week-old male CA3-NR1 KO mice (mutant, filled squares, $n = 44$), *fNR1* (grey triangles, $n = 37$), Cre ($n = 14$, not shown), and their wild-type littermates (open circles, $n = 11$) were subjected to training trials under full-cue conditions. The four types of mouse did not differ significantly in (*a*) escape latency or (*b*) swimming velocity (genotype effect for each measure, $F_{3,102} < 2.5$, $p > 0.05$; genotype × trial interaction for each measure, $p > 0.05$). (*c*) Day 13 probe trial (*P3*) of randomly selected subsets of Cre ($n = 14$), *fNR1* ($n = 20$) and mutant ($n = 23$) mice by absolute platform occupancy (time (s) the mice spent in the area which corresponded exactly to the area occupied by the platform during the training session) (Cre, $F_{3,52} = 15.8$, $p < 0.0001$; *fNR1*, $F_{3,76} = 37.4$, $p < 0.0001$; mutant, $F_{3,88} = 35.5$, $p < 0.0001$; Newman–Keuls *post hoc* comparison (the target platform position compared with all the other platform positions); $p < 0.01$ for all genotypes). (*d*) The same sets of mice as in (*c*) were subjected to partial-cue probe trials on day 14 (*P4*) and absolute platform occupancy was assessed. Cre and *fNR1* mice exhibited similar recall under partial-cue conditions as under full-cue conditions

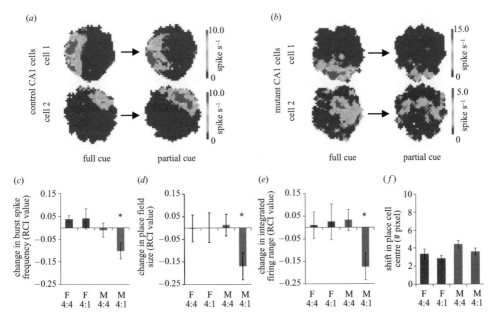

Fig. 24.4 CA1 place cell activity in CA3-NR1 KO mice. (*a,b*) Examples of place fields that are representative of cells that showed no reduction (*fNR1*; (*a*)) and a reduction of field size (mutant; (*b*)) before and after partial cue removal. (*c–e*) Relative change in the place field properties for each cell recorded across two conditions quantified with a relative change index (RCI, defined as the difference between the cell's firing between two conditions divided by the sum of the cell's firing across the two conditions). Among the cells that were identified as the same cells throughout the two recording sessions, the average burst spike frequency ((*c*) $F_{3,140} = 4.16$, $p < 0.007$; Fisher's *post hoc* comparison (mutant 4 : 1 versus all the other three paradigms), *$p < 0.05$), place field size over 1 Hz ((*d*) $F_{3,140} = 2.68$, $p < 0.049$; Fisher's *post hoc* comparison (mutant 4 : 1 versus all the other three paradigms), *$p < 0.05$) and the integrated firing rate ((*e*) $F_{3,140} = 3.20$, $p < 0.025$; Fisher's *post hoc* comparison (mutant 4 : 1 versus all the other three paradigms), *$p < 0.05$) were significantly reduced in the mutant animals (red bars) only after partial cue removal (4 : 1). By contrast, partial cue removal did not affect the CA1 place cell activity in the control mice (blue bars). (*f*) Location of the CA1 place field centre between the two recording sessions was not shifted regardless of genotype and cue manipulation ($F_{3,140} = 2.15$, $p = 0.097$). F, *fNR1* control mice; M, mutant mice. (See Plate 9 of the Plate Section, at the centre of this book.)

field properties associated with the change in the cue conditions; burst frequency, place field size or integrated firing rate was maintained upon partial cue removal. By contrast, mutant CA1 cells showed significant reduction in all of these properties (Fig. 24.4).

(paired *t*-test, $p > 0.9$ for each genotype), while recall by the mutant mice was impaired (paired *t*-test, *$p < 0.01$). (*e*) Relative recall index (RRI, averaged ratio of the target platform occupancy of the partial-cue (*P4*) or no-cue (*P5*) probe trial to that of the full-cue (*P3*) probe trial for each animal) of *fNR1* mice ($n = 18$, dotted line) and mutant mice ($n = 22$, solid line). The RRI value difference between the *fNR1* and the mutant mice under the partial-cue conditions was significant (*$p < 0.009$, Mann–Whitney *U*-test), while that under no-cue conditions was not ($p = 0.9$, Mann–Whitney *U*-test). T, target quadrant; AR, adjacent right quadrant; OP, opposite quadrant; AL, adjacent left quadrant.

Interestingly, however, the centre of individual place fields did not shift across conditions, suggesting that some reflection of past experience is maintained in the firing of mutant CA1 place cells even under conditions of partial cue removal. These physiological results are compatible with the behavioural results, suggesting that reductions in CA1 output as a consequence of reduced CA3 drive resulting from cue removal may make it more difficult for mutants to retrieve spatial memories. This impairment may underlie the inability of mutants to solve spatial memory tasks such as the watermaze when only partial distal cues are available.

A substantial portion of aged individuals exhibit deficits of memory recall (Gallagher and Rapp 1997). In early Alzheimer patients, retrieval is the first type of memory function to decline; such retrieval deficits may serve as an early predictor of Alzheimer's disease (Tuokko et al. 1991; Backman et al. 1999). Normal ageing produces a CA3-selective pattern of neurochemical alterations (Le Jeune et al. 1996; Kadar et al. 1998; Adams et al. 2001). Exposure to chronic stress, which can lead to memory deficits, also selectively causes atrophy in the apical dendrites of CA3 pyramidal cells (McEwen 1999). These results are consistent with our findings in mice that the CA3 region is critical for cognitive functions related to memory recall through pattern completion.

24.5 Conclusions

The multifaceted analyses of the CA1-NR1 KO mice and CA3-NR1 KO mice dramatically illustrated the power of cell type-restricted, adult-onset gene manipulations in the study of molecular, cellular, neuronal ensemble and neural circuitry mechanisms underlying learning and memory. These studies provide evidence that the same neurotransmitter receptors, NRs, can play quite distinct roles in the mnemonic process— memory acquisition versus memory recall—depending on where in the brain, and in which hippocampal circuitries, they are expressed. The desired level of temporal control of blockade has yet to be attained (i.e. reversibly regulated control of gene expression), but the exquisite cell-type specificity and developmentally late onset of the gene knockout attained in the mutant mice allowed us to dissect the mnemonic mechanisms at a level of resolution that could not be reached by other methods. In the future, it is expected that a number of genetically engineered mouse strains will be generated that harbour spatially restricted and/or temporally regulated expression of genes. Multifaceted analyses of these mice will help dissect mechanisms, not only for memory but also other cognitive functions.

The authors thank their collaborators, Daniel Johnston, Raymond A. Chitwood, Mark F. Yeckel, Michael C. Quirk, Linus D. Sun, Masahiko Watanabe, Akira Kato, Candice A. Carr, Laure Rondi-Reig, Sumantra Chattarji, Michaela Barbarosie, Benjamin D. Philpot, Tsuyoshi Miyakawa, Raymond Kelleher, Arvind Govindarajan, Hyejin Kang, and Mark Bear, for their invaluable contributions. They also thank Frank Bushard, Lorene Leiter and Chanel Lovett for their excellent technical assistance. This work was supported by the Howard Hughes Medical Institute (S.T.), RIKEN (S.T., K.N., and M.W.), and NIH grants RO1-NS32925 (S.T.) and P50-MH58880 (S.T. and M.W.), and Human Frontier Science Program (K.N.).

References

Adams, M. M., Smith, T. D., Moga, D., Gallagher, M., Wang, Y., Wolfe, B. B., *et al.* (2001). Hippocampal dependent learning ability correlates with N-methyl-D-aspartate (NMDA) receptor levels in CA3 neurons of young and aged rats. *J. Comp. Neurol.* **432**, 230–43.

Backman, L., Andersson, J. L., Nyberg, L., Winblad, B., Nordberg, A., and Almkvist, O. (1999). Brain regions associated with episodic retrieval in normal aging and Alzheimer's disease. *Neurology* **52**, 1861–70.

Barnes, C. A., McNaughton, B. L., Mizumori, S. J., Leonard, B. W., and Lin, L. H. (1990). Comparison of spatial and temporal characteristics of neuronal activity in sequential stages of hippocampal processing. *Prog. Brain Res.* **83**, 287–300.

Bartsch, D., Ghirardi, M., Skelhel, P. A., Karl, K. A., Herder, S. P., Chen, M., *et al.* (1995). *Aplysia* CREB2 represses long-term facilitation: relief of repression converts transient facilitation into long-term functional and structural change. *Cell* **83**, 979–92.

Benzer, S. (1967). Behavioral mutants of *Drosophila* isolated by countercurrent distribution. *Proc. Natl Acad. Sci. USA* **58**, 1112–19.

Berger, T. W. and Yeckel, M. F. (1991). Long-term potentiation of entorhinal afferents to the hippocampus enhanced propagation of activity through the trisynaptic pathway. In *Long-term potentiation: a debate of current issues* (ed. M. Baudry and J. L. Davis), pp. 327–56. Cambridge, MA: MIT Press.

Bourtchuladze, R., Frengulli, B., Blendy, J., Cioffi, D., Schultz, G., and Silva, A. J. (1994). Deficient long-term memory in mice with a targeted mutation of the cAMP-responsive element-binding protein. *Cell* **79**, 59–68.

Brenner, S. (1974). The genetics of *Caenorhabditis elegans. Genetics* **77**, 71–94.

Brun, V. H., Otnaess, M. K., Molden, S., Steffenach, H.-A., Witter, M. P., Moser, M.-B., *et al.* (2002). Place cells and place recognition maintained by direct entorhinal–hippocampal circuitry. *Science* **296**, 2243–6.

Eichenbaum, H. (1997). Declarative memory: insights from cognitive neurobiology. *A. Rev. Psychol.* **48**, 547–72.

Frank, L. M., Brown, E. N., and Wilson, M. A. (2000). Trajectory encoding in the hippocampus and entorhinal cortex. *Neuron* **27**, 169–78.

Frey, U., Krug, M., Reymann, K. G., and Matthies, H. (1988). Anisomycin, an inhibitor of protein synthesis, blocks late phases of LTP phenomena in the hippocampal CA region *in vitro. Brain Res.* **452**, 57–65.

Fyhn, M., Molden, S., Hollup, S., Moser, M.-B., and Moser, E. I. (2002). Hippocampal neurons responding to first-time dislocation of a target object. *Neuron* **35**, 555–66.

Gallagher, M. and Rapp, P. R. (1997). The use of animal models to study the effects of aging on cognition. *A. Rev. Psychol.* **48**, 339–70.

Gardner-Medwin, A. R. (1976). The recall of events through the learning of associations between their parts. *Proc. R. Soc. Lond.* B **194**, 375–402.

Gray, J. A. (1982). *The neuropsychology of anxiety: an enquiry into functions of the septo-hippocampal system.* Oxford: Oxford Unversity Press.

Griffiths, D., Dickinson, A., and Clayton, N. (1999). Episodic memory: what can animals remember about their past? *Trends Cogn. Sci.* **3**, 74–80.

Harris, E. W. and Cotman, C. W. (1986). Long-term potentiation of guinea pig mossy fiber response is not blocked by N-methyl D-aspartate antagonist. *Neurosci. Lett.* **70**, 132–7.

Hasselmo, M. E., Schnell, E., and Barkai, E. (1995). Dynamics of learning and recall at excitatory recurrent synapses and cholinergic modulation in rat hippocampal region CA3. *J. Neurosci.* **15**, 5249–62.

Hebb, D. O. (1949). *The organization of behavior.* New York: Wiley.

Helmchen, F. and Denk, W. (2002). New developments in multiphoton microscopy. *Curr. Opin. Neurobiol.* **12**, 593.

Ho, N., Liauw, J. A., Blaeser, F., Wei, F., Hanissian, S., Muglia, L. M., *et al.* (2000). Impaired synaptic plasticity and cAMP response element-binding protein activation in Ca^{2+}/calmodulin-dependent protein kinase type IV/Gr-deficient mice. *J. Neurosci.* **20**, 6459–72.

Hopfield, J. J. (1982). Neural networks and physical systems with emergent collective computational abilities. *Proc. Natl Acad. Sci. USA* **79**, 2554–8.

Huerta, P. T., Sun, L. D., Wilson, M. A., and Tonegawa, S. (2000). Formation of temporal memory requires NMDA receptors within CA1 pyramidal neurons. *Neuron* **25**, 473–80.

Impey, S., Obrietan, K., and Storm, D. R. (1999). Making new connections: role of ERK/MAP kinase signaling in neuronal plasticy. *Neuron* **23**, 11–14.

Izquierdo, I. and Medina, J. H. (1997). Memory formation: the sequence of biochemical events in the hippocampus and its connection to activity in other brain structures. *Neurobiol. Learn. Mem.* **68**, 285–316.

Jensen, K. F., Ohmstede, C.-A., Fisher, A. S., and Sahyoun, N. (1991). Nuclear and axonal localization of Ca^{2+}/calmodulin-dependent protein kinase type Gr in rat cerebellar cortex. *Proc. Natl Acad. Sci. USA* **88**, 2850–3.

Kadar, T., Dachir, S., Shukitt-Hale, B., and Levy, A. (1998). Sub-regional hippocampal vulnerability in various animal models leading to cognitive dysfunction. *J. Neural Transm.* **105**, 987–1004.

Kang, H., Sun, L. D., Atkins, C. M., Soderling, T. R., Wilson, M. A., and Tonegawa, S. (2001). An important role of neural activity-dependent CaMKIV signaling in the consolidation of long-term memory. *Cell* **106**, 771–83.

Kesner, R. P. and Rolls, E. T. (2001). Role of long-term synaptic modification in short-term memory. *Hippocampus* **11**, 240–50.

Le Jeune, H., Cecyre, D., Rowe, W., Meaney, M. J., and Quirion, R. (1996). Ionotropic glutamate receptor subtypes in the aged memory-impaired and unimpaired Long–Evans rat. *Neuroscience* **74**, 349–63.

McEwen, B. S. (1999). Stress and hippocampal plasticity. *A. Rev. Neurosci.* **22**, 105–22.

McHugh, T. J., Blum, K. I., Tsien, J. Z., Tonegawa, S., and Wilson, M. A. (1996). Impaired hippocampal representation of space in CA1-specific NMDAR1 knockout mice. *Cell* **87**, 1339–49.

McNaughton, B. L. and Morris, R. G. M. (1987). Hippocampal synaptic enhancement and information storage within a distributed memory system. *Trends Neurosci.* **10**, 408–15.

McNaughton, B. L., Barnes, C. A., Meltzer, J., and Sutherland, R. J. (1989). Hippocampal granule cells are necessary for normal spatial learning but not for spatially-selective pyramidal cell discharge. *Exp. Brain Res.* **76**, 489–96.

MacVicar, B. and Dudek, F. (1980). Local synaptic circuits in rat hippocampus: interaction between pyramidal cells. *Brain Res.* **184**, 220–3.

Mansuy, I. M., Mayford, M., Jacob, B., Kandel, E. R., and Bach, M. E. (1998). Restricted and regulated overexpression reveals calcineurin as a key component in the transition from short-term to long-term memory. *Cell* **92**, 39–49.

Marr, D. (1971). Simple memory: a theory for archicortex. *Phil. Trans. R. Soc. Lond.* B **262**, 23–81.

Mayford, M., Bach, M. E., Huang, Y. Y., Hawkins, R. D., and Kandel, E. R. (1996). Control of memory formation through regulated expression of a CaMKII transgene. *Science* **274**, 1678–83.

Miles, R. and Traub, R. (1986). Excitatory synaptic interactions between CA3 neurons in the guinea-pig hippocampus. *J. Physiol. (Lond.)* **373**, 397–418.

Milner, B., Squire, L. R., and Kandel, E. R. (1998). Cognitive neuroscience and the study of memory. *Neuron* **20**, 445–68.

Morris, R. G. and Frey, U. (1997). Hippocampal synaptic plasticity: role in spatial learning or the automatic recording of attended experience? *Phil. Trans. R. Soc. Lond.* B **352**, 1489–503. (DOI 10.1098/rstb.1997.0136.)

Morris, R. G. M., Anderson, E., Lynch, G. S., and Baudry, M. (1986). Selective impairment of learning and blockade of long-term potentiation by an N-methyl-D-aspartate receptor antagonist, AP5. *Nature* **319**, 774–6.

Moser, E. I. and Paulsen, O. (2001). New excitement in cognitive space: between place cells and spatial memory. *Curr. Opin. Neurobiol.* **11**, 745–51.

Nakazawa, K., Quirk, M. C., Chitwood, R. A., Watanabe, M., Yeckel, M. F., Sun, L. D., *et al.* (2002). Requirement for hippocampal CA3 NMDA receptors in acquisition and recall of associative memory. *Science* **297**, 211–18.

Nakazawa, K., Wilson, M. A., and Tonegawa, S. (2003). On crucial roles of hippocampal NMDA receptors in acquisiton and recall of associative memory. In *Neurobiology of perception and communication* (ed. L. Squire). Cambridge: Cambridge University Press. (In press.)

Olton, D. S. and Papas, B. C. (1979). Spatial memory and hippocampal function. *Neuropsychologia* **17**, 669–82.

Orban, P. C., Chapman, P. F., and Brambilla, R. (1999). Is the Ras-MAPK signalling pathway necessary for long-term memory formation? *Trends Neurosci.* **22**, 38–44.

Quirk, G. J., Muller, R. U., Kubie, J. L., and Ranck Jr, J. B. (1992). The positional firing properties of medial entorhinal neurons: description and comparison with hippocampal place cells. *J. Neurosci.* **12**, 1945–63.

Rawlins, J. N. P. (1985). Associations across time: the hippocampus as a temporary memory store. *Behav. Brain Res.* **8**, 479–96.

Remondes, M. and Schuman, E. M. (2002). Direct cortical input modulates plasticity and spiking in CA1 pyramidal neurons. *Nature* **416**, 736–40.

Rolls, E. T. (1989). The representation and storage of information in neural networks in the primate cerebral cortex and hippocampus. In *The computing neuron* (ed. R. Durbin, C. Miall and G. Mitchison), pp. 125–59. Wokingham, UK: Addison-Wesley.

Rondi-Reig, L., Libbey, M., Eichenbaum, H., and Tonegawa, S. (2001). CA1-specific N-methyl-D-aspartate receptor knockout mice are deficient in solving a nonspaital transverse patterning task. *Proc. Natl Acad. Sci. USA* **98**, 3543–8.

Sauer, B. and Henderson, N. (1988). Site-specific DNA recombination in mammalian cells by the Cre recombinase of bacteriophage P1. *Proc. Natl Acad. Sci. USA* **85**, 5166–70.

Schacter, D. L. and Wagner, A. D. (1999). Medial temporal lobe activations in fMRI and PET studies of episodic encoding and retrieval. *Hippocampus* **9**, 7–24.

Silva, A. J., Stevens, C. F., Tonegawa, S., and Wang, Y. (1992a). Deficient hippocampal long-term potentiation in α-calcium-calmodulin kinase II mutant mice. *Science* **257**, 201–6.

Silva, A. J., Paylor, R., Wehner, J. M., and Tonegawa, S. (1992b). Impaired spatial learning in alpha-calcium-calmodulin kinase II mutant mice. *Science* **257**, 206–11.

Squire, L. R. (1994). Declarative and nondeclarative memory: multiple brain systems supporting learning and memory. In *Memory systems* (ed. D. L. Schacter and E. Tulving), pp. 203–31. Cambridge, MA: MIT Press.

Steele, R. J. and Morris, R. G. (1999). Delay-dependent impairment of a matching-to-place task with chronic and intrahippocampal infusion of the NMDA-antagonist D-AP5. *Hippocampus* **9**, 118–36.

Sybirska, E., Davachi, L., and Goldman-Rakic, P. S. (2000). Prominence of direct entorhinal-CA1 pathway activation in sensorimotor and cognitive tasks revealed by 2-DG functional mapping in nonhuman primate. *J. Neurosci.* **20**, 5827–34.

Tsien, J. Z., Chen, D. F., Gerber, D., Tom, C., Mercer, E. H., Anderson, D. J., *et al.* (1996a). Subregion- and cell type-restricted gene knockout in mouse brain. *Cell* **87**, 1317–26.

Tsien, J. Z., Huerta, P. T., and Tonegawa, S. (1996b). The essential role of hippocampal CA1 NMDA receptor-dependent synaptic plasticity in spatial memory. *Cell* **87**, 1327–38.

Tulving, E. (1972). Episodic and semantic memory. In *Organization of memory* (ed. E. Tulving and W. Donaldson), pp. 381–403. New York: Academic Press.

Tulving, E. (1995). Organization of memory: quo vadis? In *The cognitive neurosciences* (ed. M. S. Gazzaniga), pp. 839–47. Cambridge, MA: MIT Press.

Tuokko, H., Vernon-Wilkinson, R., Weir, J., and Beattie, B. L. (1991). Cued recall and early identification of dementia. *J. Clin. Exp. Neuropsychol.* **13**, 871–9.

Vargha-Khadem, F., Gadian, D. G., Watkins, K. E., Connelly, A., Van Paesschen, W., and Mishkin, M. (1997). Differential effects of early hippocampal pathology on episodic and semantic memory. *Science* **277**, 376–80.

Vinogradova, O. (1970). Registration of information and the limbic system. In *Short-term changes in neural activity and behavior* (ed. G. Horn and R. A. Hinde), pp. 99–140. Cambridge University Press.

Vinogradova, O. S. (1975). Functional organization of the limbic system in the process of registration of information: facts and hypothesis. In *The hippocampus*, vol. 2 (ed. R. L. Isaacson and K. H. Pribram), pp. 3–69. New York: Plenum Press.

Wessberg, J., Stambaugh, C. R., Kralik, J. D., Beck, P. D., Laubach, M., and Chapin, J. K. (2000). Real-time prediction of hand trajectory by ensembles of cortical neurons in primates. *Nature* **408**, 361–5.

Wiebe, S. P., Staubli, U. V., and Ambros-Ingerson, J. (1997). Short-term reverberant memory model of hippocampal field CA3. *Hippocampus* **7**, 656–65.

Williams, S. and Johnston, D. (1988). Muscarinic depression of long-term potentiation in CA3 hippocampal neurons. *Science* **242**, 84–7.

Willshaw, D. and Dayan, P. (1990). Optimal plasticity from matrix memories: what goes up must come down. *Neural Comput.* **2**, 85–93.

Wilson, M. A. and McNaughton, B. L. (1993). Dynamics of the hippocampal ensemble code for space. *Science* **261**, 1055–8.

Wu, J. Y., Ribar, T. J., Cummings, D. E., Burton, K. A., McKnight, G. S., and Means, A. R. (2000). Spermiogenesis and exchange of basic nuclear proteins are impaired in male germ cells lacking Camk4. *Nature Genet.* **25**, 448–52.

Zalutsky, R. A. and Nicoll, R. A. (1990). Comparison of two forms of long-term potentiation in single hippocampal neurons. *Science* **248**, 1619–24.

Zeng, H., Chattarji, S., Barbarosie, M., Rondi-Reig, L., Philpot, B. D., Miyakawa, T., *et al.* (2001). Forebrain-specific calcineurin knockout selectively impairs bidirectional synaptic plasticity and working/episodic-like memory. *Cell* **107**, 617–29.

Glossary

C/A	commissural/associational
CaMKIV	Ca^{2+}/calmodulin-dependent protein kinase IV
CNQX	6-cyano-7-nitroquinoxaline-2,3-dione
CREB	cAMP response element binding protein
DMP	delayed-matching-to-place
EC	entorhinal cortex
E-LTP	early phase long-term potentiation
ERK	extracellular signal-regulated protein kinase
LTD	long-term depression
L-LTP	late phase long-term potentiation
LTP	long-term potentiation
MF	mossy fibre
NR	*N*-methyl-D-aspartate receptor
SC	Schaffer collateral

25

Inducible molecular switches for the study of long-term potentiation

Gaël Hédou and Isabelle M. Mansuy

This article reviews technical and conceptual advances in unravelling the molecular bases of long-term potentiation (LTP), learning and memory using genetic approaches. We focus on studies aimed at testing a model suggesting that protein kinases and protein phosphatases balance each other to control synaptic strength and plasticity. We describe how gene 'knock-out' technology was initially exploited to disrupt the Ca^{2+}/calmodulin-dependent protein kinase IIα (CaMKIIα) gene and how refined knock-in techniques later allowed an analysis of the role of distinct phosphorylation sites in CaMKII. Further to gene recombination, regulated gene expression using the tetracycline-controlled transactivator and reverse tetracycline-controlled transactivator systems, a powerful new means for modulating the activity of specific molecules, has been applied to CaMKIIα and the opposing protein phosphatase calcineurin. Together with electro-physiological and behavioural evaluation of the engineered mutant animals, these genetic methodologies have helped gain insight into the molecular mechanisms of plasticity and memory. Further technical developments are, however, awaited for an even higher level of finesse.

Keywords: gene targeting; inducible gene expression; protein kinase; protein phosphatases; long-term potentiation; learning and memory

25.1 Introduction

Learning about learning is a great challenge for neuroscientists because it deals with one of our most essential and intimate skills. Not only the pursuit of knowledge *per se*, but also its potential application to the therapeutic benefit of memory dysfunctions after stroke or post-traumatic disorder, and the improvement of skills in children with learning disabilities and of ageing-related memory decline, justify the urge to elucidate the fundamental bases of learning and memory. The phenomenon of LTP (Bliss and Collingridge 1993) and, by extension, of other kinds of plasticity including LTD (Lynch *et al.* 1977) and depotentiation (Staubli and Lynch 1990) are experimental models of choice to study these processes. Although a direct parallel between plasticity and memory formation has not been firmly established, multiple evidence suggests that they do share common features (Martin *et al.* 2000).

The groundbreaking character of the discovery of LTP in the early 1970s (Bliss and Gardner-Medwin 1973; Bliss and Lømo 1973) and the recognition that the discovery has brought about a new dimension to memory research are now important milestones of neuroscience history. The celebration of the 30th birthday of LTP acknowledges the extent to which it has yielded a mass of new, sometimes unexpected, knowledge about the basic physiological rules of brain plasticity and the fundamental functioning of neurons (Malenka and Nicoll 1999). It also stresses, to a large extent, the intellectual stimulation it prompted and the resulting new concepts about learning and memory.

25.2 A calcium–calmodulin switch

One of the concepts that addressed the potential molecular mechanisms of LTP was first formulated by John Lisman in the 1980s, and has largely been adjusted and perfected since then (see Lisman 2003). This model suggests that synaptic weight is bi-directionally controlled by protein kinases and protein phosphatases in a Ca^{2+}-dependent fashion (Lisman 1985, 1989) and that the balance between protein phosphorylation and dephosphorylation dynamically sets physiological synaptic strength (Wang and Kelly 1996). CaMKII is believed to play a central role in this model and has a number of properties that make it a strong candidate for being a memory molecule (Lisman et al. 2002). CaMKII is extremely abundant in the brain and is particularly enriched in postsynaptic terminals of neurons in hippocampus, neocortex, amygdala and basal ganglia. These brain structures are known to experience plastic changes upon stimulation (LTP, LTD) and to support some aspects of learning and memory. Further, after initial stimulation by calcium, CaMKII has the ability to maintain itself in an active state for long periods of time by autophosphorylation on threonine 286 (Hanson and Schulman 1992; Ouyang et al. 1997), a process thought to leave a molecular trace of previous Ca^{2+}-induced activity. A counterpart to CaMKII is the protein phosphatase CN, the only known Ca^{2+}/calmodulin-dependent protein phosphatase in the brain. CN would oppose CaMKII by activating PP1, a downstream phosphatase belonging to the same Ser/Thr protein phosphatase family. PP1 is able to dephosphorylate CaMKII presumably through CN-dependent dephosphorylation of inhibitor-1, an inhibitor of PP1 that is activated by phosphorylation by the cAMP-dependent PKA (Fig. 25.1).

Numerous pharmacological, electrophysiological, biochemical and genetic studies have been carried out to challenge this model and determine the functions of CaMKII and CN in plasticity, learning and memory. We discuss studies that have exploited gene targeting and transgenic technologies, and we try to describe how the use of inducible approaches or systems have helped gain insight into the role of these molecules in LTP.

25.3 Initial strategy and recent elaborations on the gene targeting approach to study the role of CAMKII in LTP

The development of refined genetic techniques such as knockout and transgenesis significantly advanced the understanding of the mechanisms of plasticity, learning and memory. Analyses of in vitro LTP and cross-comparison with behaviour in genetically modified animals has been a useful means to investigate the molecular pathways underlying these processes and their potential commonalities.

The first important experiments in the field were carried out by the laboratory of Susumu Tonegawa who developed a line of mutant mice in which gene coding for the alpha subunit of CaMKII (CaMKIIα), a predominant CaMKII isoform in the brain, was inactivated by homologous recombination. Disruption of the CaMKIIα gene resulted in a defect in the induction of LTP in area CA1 of the hippocampus (Silva et al. 1992a; Hinds et al. 1998) and in impaired experience-dependent plasticity in sensory cortex in vivo (Glazewski et al. 1996; Gordon et al. 1996). These deficits in plasticity were accompanied by an impairment of spatial and associative learning and memory

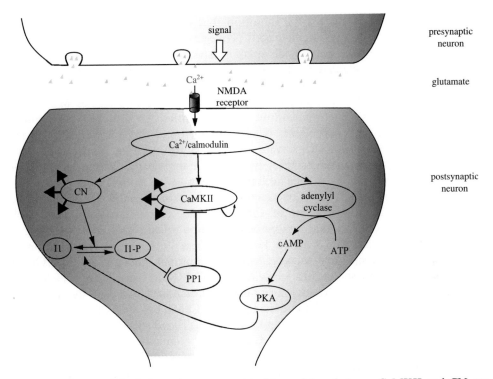

Fig. 25.1 Scheme of the balance between protein kinases/phosphatases. CaMKII and CN are activated by Ca^{2+} and act on multiple targets (represented by small arrows) including CaMKII itself. CN dephosphorylates inhibitor-1 (I1), an inhibitor of PP1 that is phosphorylated by PKA, a cAMP-dependent protein kinase. When relieved from inhibition, PP1 dephosphorylates CaMKII. Although not represented, a similar balance may also be operating presynaptically.

(Silva *et al.* 1992*b*). Interestingly, later on, the extent of these deficits was found to depend on the degree of elimination of CaMKIIα expression. When only one of the mutated alleles was introduced in heterozygous mice, sufficient CaMKIIα was still present in hippocampal neurons to sustain the induction of LTP (although LTP magnitude was attenuated). By contrast, in the neocortex, this partial reduction in CaMKIIα was substantial enough to prevent the induction of LTP. This selective defect in neocortical plasticity was associated with impaired long-term memory but short-term hippocampal-dependent memory was intact in heterozygous animals (Frankland *et al.* 2001). These results highlighted the critical role of CaMKIIα in both hippocampal and neocortical LTP and corroborated the hypothesis that normal plasticity is required in the hippocampus for the initial encoding of memory while plasticity in the neocortex is needed for the establishment of permanent memory traces. These data indicated, in turn, that LTP, depending on the brain structure that sustains it, appears to accompany distinct forms and phases of cognitive functions, possibly by using different mechanisms that share the recruitment of CaMKIIα.

The gene targeting approach as used in these studies, however, suffers from a number of pitfalls that limit the interpretation of the results. These include the lack of spatial restriction, the all-or-none nature of the mutation, and the irreversibility and the early occurrence of the genetic mutation that is associated with the likelihood that compensatory pathways are activated (Tonegawa *et al.* 1995; Gerlai 1996, 2000; Gingrich and Hen 2000). To provide spatial restriction to gene recombination, the Cre-loxP system was adapted to the brain and has allowed the disruption of genes in specific brain areas, for instance, in hippocampal sub-fields (Tsien *et al.* 1996a,b; Nakazawa *et al.* 2002; see Tonegawa *et al.* 2003). These approaches are a considerable improvement, but not without new difficulties, for example, the regional restriction may be age dependent, being present up to a certain age but not thereafter. Additional refinements were introduced by inserting point mutation(s) in the coding sequence of target genes by knock-in specifically altering the function of the encoded protein. With this technique, the role of distinct phosphorylation sites on CaMKIIα was examined by placing inhibitory or activating point mutations in selected residues. Replacement of threonine 286 with a non-phosphorylatable alanine (T286A) revealed that autophosphorylation of CaMKIIα at this site is required for hippocampal LTP and learning (Giese *et al.* 1998). In addition to Thr286, Thr305/306, sites that undergo inhibitory autophosphorylation after Thr286 is activated, were also shown to be essential for CaMKIIα function, specifically for its translocation to PSDs. Blockade of phosphorylation at Thr305/306 by valine and alanine substitutions increased the association of CaMKIIα with PSDs resulting in a reduction of the threshold for hippocampal LTP induction and a diminished flexibility of learning and memory. Conversely, simulating phosphorylation by replacing Thr305 with Asp decreased the level of CaMKIIα in terminals and impaired LTP and learning (Elgersma *et al.* 2002). Although not inducible, nor yet regionally specific, these genetic manipulations provided a high level of sophistication in the dissection of the mechanisms of CaMKIIα function and demonstrated the distinct role of independent residues in LTP and memory.

Another technical advance was recently achieved by combining this approach with pharmacology to spatially circumscribe the genetic manipulation and, additionally, confer inducibility. This method is based on the use of a drug that, when administered at a sub-threshold dose to animals or derived tissue slices carrying a recessive null mutation, leads to full or partial inactivation (depending on the dose) of a gene (Ohno *et al.* 2001). With this method, the effect of the loss of a gene product or function similar to that provoked by a homozygous mutation can be induced in heterozygous animals. Thus, in CaMKIIα T286A hippocampal slices from heterozygous mice, blockade of CaMKII activation by pretetanic application of a low dose of the NMDA-receptor antagonist (CPP) induced a deficit in LTP similar to that observed in slices from homozygous mice. The dose of CPP necessary to reveal this defect had no effect in wild-type slices. Further, in heterozygous slices, the drug did not affect LTP once induced, confirming that CaMKIIα is involved in induction rather than expression or maintenance mechanisms. Finally, because LTP was normal before CPP treatment, it can be concluded that its impairment resulted from the drug-induced blockade of CaMKII activation and not from a developmental anomaly (Ohno *et al.* 2001, 2002). This combined approach therefore constitutes a valuable and flexible tool to gain temporal and spatial control over recessive genetic mutations. Its rapidity, dose dependence and reversibility may allow analyses of distinct phases of LTP *in vitro* and *in vivo*.

25.4 Transgenesis from the test-tube to the behaving animal

In parallel to the knockout and knock-in approach, a number of molecular switches have been developed to provide alternative strategies to modulate gene expression and activity in a spatially and temporally controlled fashion in the brain. The emergence of tissue-specific, inducible promoters for restricting genetic manipulations to specific brain structures during selected temporal windows in higher organisms have allowed these developments. Inducible systems for gene expression benefited from the expertise of the group of Hermann Bujard, who developed an inducible promoter—based on the regulatory elements of the tetracycline resistance operon of *E. coli* (Furth *et al.* 1994; Gossen *et al.* 1994, 1995). In this operon, the tetracycline-controlled repressor (*tetR*) binds to its operator to repress the expression of resistance genes conferring survival in the presence of the antibiotic. This system was made functional in eukaryotic cells by fusion to the virion protein 16 (VP16) of the herpes simplex virus. The resulting hybrid tTA after binding to the tetracycline operator (tetO), induces the expression of a gene fused to tetO in a tetracycline- or doxycycline (dox)-dependent manner. A rtTA factor was later engineered by chemical mutation of tTA. The rtTA factor has the exclusive property of requiring dox for binding to tetO and therefore constitutes a truly inducible system for gene expression.

The tTA system was first applied to the mouse brain by Mark Mayford to temporally restrict the expression of a Ca^{2+}-independent active mutant of CaMKIIα mutated on Asp286 (Mayford *et al.* 1996*a*). For spatial restriction, Mayford combined the tTA factor with a fragment of the CaMKIIα promoter known to be active in forebrain neurons postnatally (Mayford *et al.* 1996*b*). The increase in CaMKII activity in hippocampus provided by tTA-controlled expression of CaMKII-Asp286 was found to alter the induction of LTP in response to a 10 Hz stimulation and to impair spatial and associative memory. The power of the tTA system in this study was to demonstrate that the transgene itself mediated these defects and not a developmental anomaly resulting from CaMKII-Asp286 transgene expression early in life. Thus, by suppressing CaMKII-Asp286 transgene expression with dox, normal LTP and memory could be fully restored in adult mutant animals, confirming the specificity of the effect (Mayford *et al.* 1996*a*). Although consistent with previous findings that the constitutive expression of CaMKII-Asp286 shifts the threshold for LTP in favour of LTD (Mayford *et al.* 1995) and impairs memory (Bach *et al.* 1995), these results did not corroborate the model suggesting that autophosphorylation of CaMKII is an essential trigger for LTP and contradicted the previous knockout data (Silva *et al.* 1992*a,b*).

It is only recently that an explanation for this discrepancy was proposed after re-analysis of the CaMKII-Asp286 animals based on a feature of the combined CaMKIIα promoter/tTA system (Bejar *et al.* 2002).

Bejar *et al.* (2002) used the original line of transgenic mice that expressed high levels of CaMKII-Asp286 to produce a group of low-expressor animals. For this, transgene expression was suppressed during gestation and postnatal development and then restored in adulthood. This manipulation was taking advantage of a previous observation that long-term transgene suppression often reduces the level of expression when reactivated in adult animals. The difference in CaMKII-Asp286 levels achieved that way in the same line of mice helped to reveal a dose-dependent effect of CaMKII-Asp286 on LTP. While high levels were again found to impair low-frequency LTP, low levels enhanced LTP such as expected by the model and in accordance with the results obtained in the CaMKII T286A mice (Giese *et al.* 1998). Since compensatory mechanisms were suspected to be responsible for the LTP impairment in the high expressors, gene chip analyses were carried out to identify the affected genes. These analyses revealed that several genes were upregulated in response to high CaMKII activity, some of which were already known to be activated by LTP-inducing stimuli. Thus, CaMKIIα over-activation during development appeared to prompt compensatory changes that altered LTP. These changes may also possibly have led to an enhanced potentiation that occluded further tetanic LTP. Regardless of the mechanisms involved, this evidence stresses the potentially deleterious effect of excessive overexpression or overactivation of a protein which, in the case of CaMKII, is consistent with the fact that physiologically, only a small increase (15%) in CaMKII levels is triggered by LTP (Ouyang *et al.* 1997). By extension, this confirms that complete or even partial downregulation of a gene may impose non-physiological conditions and engage non-specific responses obscuring the expected effect. Finally, it also underscores the confounding effect of the early occurrence of a genetic mutation, implying that systematic genetic analyses should be considered in plain knockout animals for verification, and that tight and temporally controlled systems should be more widely used to regulate genetic manipulations.

25.5 Inducible transgenesis for the study of protein phosphatases in LTP

We have adopted an inducible approach based on the rtTA system to investigate the protein phosphatase side of the kinase/phosphatase balance thought to regulate LTP. The idea was to shift the balance either in favour of protein phosphatases by increasing CN activity, or in favour of protein kinases by decreasing CN activity. For this, the rtTA system was combined with the CaMKIIα promoter (Fig. 25.2*a*) to express either a truncated active form of the Aα catalytic subunit of CN, or the autoinhibitory domain of CNAα in forebrain neurons (Mansuy *et al.* 1998*a*; Malleret *et al.* 2001). In both cases, the shift was induced only in adulthood just a few days before experimentation to avoid any possible detrimental effect of transgene expression during development, and it could be fully reversed by suppressing transgene expression. Further, in both cases the achieved increase or reduction in CN activity was moderate, 77% and 35–45%, respectively, which more closely mimicked physiological conditions. CN overactivity was found to reversibly impair a PKA-dependent intermediate phase of LTP (I-LTP) (Fig. 25.3*a*) without affecting early-phase LTP, a phase distinguished from I-LTP by its PKA independency (Mansuy *et al.* 1998*a*; Winder *et al.* 1998). Conversely, inhibiting CN facilitated early LTP both *in vitro* in area CA1 of the hippocampus (Fig. 25.3*b*), and in anaesthetized mice in area CA1, and the dentate gyrus and made it PKA dependent (Fig. 25.3*c*; Malleret *et al.* 2001). In addition to increasing the overall magnitude of LTP, CN inhibition also significantly prolonged LTP in freely moving animals. Thus while in control mice, *in vivo* LTP started to decay soon after induction and was gone 3 days later, it remained high and persisted over 3–4 days in the mutant mice (Fig. 25.3*d*). Mechanistically, the facilitation of early LTP appeared to result from the intervention of PKA since it was blocked by a PKA inhibitor KT5720 (Fig. 25.3*b*), suggesting a failure of CN to oppose PKA. Overall, the

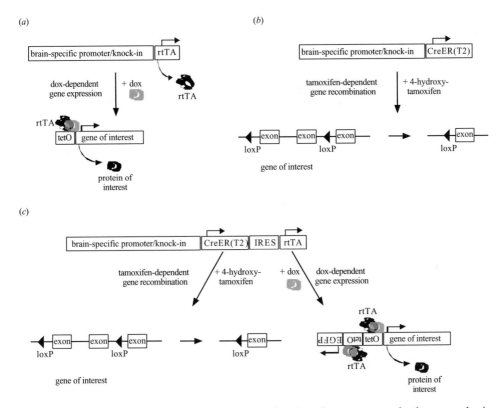

Fig. 25.2 Strategy to achieve inducible gene expression, knockout or rescue in the mouse brain. (*a*) Inducible gene expression with the rtTA system based on the combination of a transgene expressing rtTA under the control of a brain-specific promoter or of an endogenous promoter by knock-in, with a transgene carrying a rtTA-specific tetO promoter fused to the gene of interest. Expression of the gene of interest is induced by dox and is suppressed by dox removal. (*b*) Inducible gene knockout. The inducible CreER(T2) (ER: oestrogen receptor) recombinase is expressed under the control of a brain-specific promoter or of an endogenous promoter by knock-in. It excises a DNA fragment between loxP sites in the gene of interest only in the presence of 4-hydroxy-tamoxifen. (*c*) Inducible gene knockout and rescue. CreER(T2) and rtTA expressed simultaneously under the control of a brain-specific promoter or of an endogenous promoter by knock-in through an internal ribosomal entry site (IRES) induce gene recombination and/or gene expression (gene of interest + marker such as EGFP) in the presence of 4-hydroxy-tamoxifen and/or dox.

apparent PKA dependency of both the impairment and enhancement of LTP confirmed that CN acts by interfering with PKA-controlled pathway(s) as predicted by the kinase/phosphatase balance model.

Further to its modulatory effect on LTP, CN was found to influence learning and memory. While an excess of CN perturbed spatial learning and a temporal phase of memory between short- and long-term memory (Mansuy *et al.* 1998*b*), CN inhibition facilitated learning and prolonged memory (Malleret *et al.* 2001). Recently, the downstream protein phosphatase PP1 was similarly demonstrated to improve learning efficacy and the persistence of memory (Genoux *et al.* 2002). Strikingly, with CN, comparable temporal phases of LTP and memory were affected by the genetic modulation of its

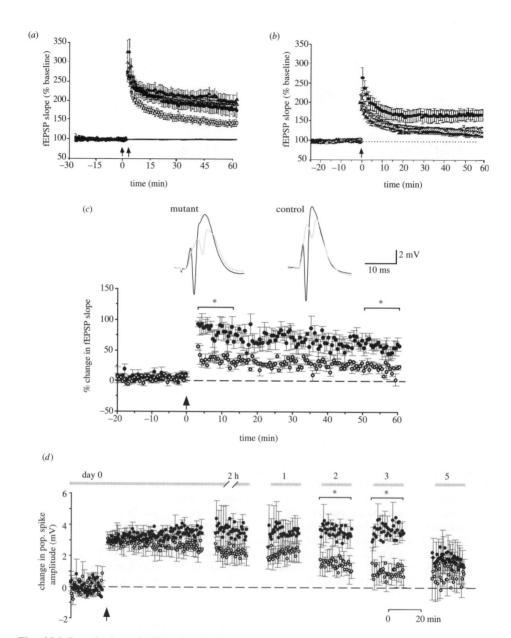

Fig. 25.3 Impaired or facilitated LTP by overexpression or inhibition of CN. (*a*) A PKA-dependent intermediate phase of CA1 LTP induced by 2-train of high-frequency stimulation is impaired in slices from mutant mice expressing an active CN upon dox treatment. Filled triangles, control; open triangles, mutant; filled circles, control dox; open circles, mutant dox. (*b*) A PKA-independent early phase of CA1 LTP induced by 1-train of high-frequency stimulation is facilitated in slices from mutant mice expressing a CN inhibitor upon dox treatment. The PKA inhibitor KT5720 reverses this facilitation. Open circles, control dox; filled circles, mutant dox; open triangles, control dox + KT5720; filled triangles, mutant dox + KT5720. (*c,d*) Enhanced 1-train dentate gyrus LTP in (*c*) anaesthetized and (*d*) freely moving mutant mice expressing a CN inhibitor. Open circles, control dox; filled circles, mutant dox.

activity, suggesting a temporally correlated effect of CN on plasticity and behaviour. Interestingly, the transient overexpression of CN after learning was found to reversibly impair retrieval, a specific phase of memory that allows the recovery of previously learned information (Mansuy *et al.* 1998*a*). Although the mechanisms of retrieval remain unclear, initial evidence has recently suggested that LTP in area CA3 of the hippocampus might sustain memory recall (Nakazawa *et al.* 2002).

Taken together, these data demonstrated that the level of CN activity is critical for determining synaptic strength and, in turn, the degree of LTP. Notably, and even more convincing than impairment, a correlated improvement of similar temporal phases of LTP and memory provides strong evidence in support of LTP being a cellular substrate of memory. In these studies, the rtTA system was instrumental in that it allowed the subtle perturbation of fine-tuning mechanisms required by the balance between kinases and phosphatases to regulate synaptic processes over only short time-windows and to only a limited extent. In contrast to such moderate change, the complete elimination of CN activity by CA1-restricted knockout of the major regulatory subunit of CN, CNB, appeared to have no effect on LTP but diminished LTD. It also impaired working memory, an immediate phase of memory, without affecting long-term memory (Zeng *et al.* 2001). These results conflict with the kinase/phosphatase balance model and with our data, and may be explained by compensatory mechanisms that would gain by being identified by genetic analyses.

25.6 Technical improvements and future directions

As illustrated by the studies reviewed above, the mechanisms that regulate LTP, learning and memory are extremely complex and are subjected to discrete regulatory mechanisms. To fully understand these mechanisms, it is thus essential that refined methodological approaches are employed. Recent developments in the use of tTA and rtTA inducible expression systems and their combination with gene recombination techniques such as the Cre-loxP system now make these approaches suitable. In a recent study for instance, an inducible genetic rescue of the NR1 gene deletion was achieved in knockout animals by expressing a NR1 transgene in a dox-dependent and brain-specific fashion with the tTA system and the CaMKIIα promoter (Shimizu *et al.* 2000). This study showed that defects in LTP and memory resulting from NR1 gene disruption (Tsien *et al.* 1996*b*) could be reversed by dox-induced expression of the NR1 transgene while reproduced by its suppression. This approach provided proof of the principle that inducible gene expression and recombination can be achieved together. However, this strategy requires a considerable labour-intensive investment for generating and breeding the multiple transgenic lines needed (floxed NR1 × Cre transgenic × tTA transgenic × NR1 transgenic). Further, it does not provide true inducibility since only the transgenic rescue and not the knockout itself can be turned on or off. Finally, the degree of rescue is contingent upon the spatial restriction and the level of transgene expression driven by the tTA system and does not optimally mimic endogenous gene expression.

An alternative strategy to achieve inducible gene inactivation would be to express the Cre protein itself under the control of an inducible expression system. In that respect, the second generation of rtTA factors, rtTA2(s)-M2 and -S2, with increased sensitivity to dox and higher transactivation activity, may help improve the efficiency and rapidity of such genetic manipulations (Urlinger *et al.* 2000; Lamartina *et al.* 2002; Salucci *et al.* 2002). Another powerful approach would be to use inducible versions of Cre like, for instance, CreER(T2) (Indra *et al.* 1999; Fig. 25.2*b*) or CrePR (Wunderlich *et al.* 2001). These recombinases contain the ligand-binding domain of the oestrogen or progesterone receptors, which renders their activity dependent on the synthetic ligand 4-hydroxy-tamoxifen. In combination with the rtTA system, they should allow inducible gene knockout and rescue via tamoxifen-induced gene recombination and dox-dependent reversible transgene expression (Fig. 25.2*c*). The association of various inducible recombination–expression systems is a promising means for targeting–expressing several genes and fluorescent markers simultaneously (Baron *et al.* 1999; Moser *et al.* 2001) to further advance research on LTP.

References

Bach, M. E., Hawkins, R. D., Osman, M., Kandel, E. R., and Mayford, M. (1995). Impairment of spatial but not contextual memory in CaMKII mutant mice with a selective loss of hippocampal LTP in the range of the theta frequency. *Cell* **81**, 905–15.

Baron, U., Schnappinger, D., Helbl, V., Gossen, M., Hillen, W., and Bujard, H. (1999). Generation of conditional mutants in higher eukaryotes by switching between the expression of two genes. *Proc. Natl Acad. Sci. USA* **96**, 1013–18.

Bejar, R., Yasuda, R., Krugers, H., Hood, K., and Mayford, M. (2002). Transgenic calmodulin-dependent protein kinase II activation: dose-dependent effects on synaptic plasticity, learning, and memory. *J. Neurosci.* **22**, 5719–26.

Bliss, T. V. and Collingridge, G. L. (1993). A synaptic model of memory: long-term potentiation in the hippocampus. *Nature* **361**, 31–9.

Bliss, T. V. and Gardner-Medwin, A. R. (1973). Long-lasting potentiation of synaptic transmission in the dentate area of the unanaesthetized rabbit following stimulation of the perforant path. *J. Physiol.* (*Lond.*) **232**, 357–74.

Bliss, T. V. and Lømo, T. (1973). Long-lasting potentiation of synaptic transmission in the dentate area of the anaesthetized rabbit following stimulation of the perforant path. *J. Physiol.* (*Lond.*) **232**, 331–56.

Elgersma, Y., Fedorov, N. B., Ikonen, S., Choi, E. S., Elgersma, M., Carvalho, O.M., *et al.* (2002). Inhibitory autophosphorylation of CaMKII controls PSD association, plasticity, and learning. *Neuron* **36**, 493–505.

Frankland, P. W., O'Brien, C., Ohno, M., Kirkwood, A., and Silva, A. J. (2001). Alpha-CaMKII-dependent plasticity in the cortex is required for permanent memory. *Nature* **411**, 309–13.

Furth, P. A., St Onge, L., Boger, H., Gruss, P., Gossen, M., Kistner, A., *et al.* (1994). Temporal control of gene expression in transgenic mice by a tetracycline-responsive promoter. *Proc. Natl Acad. Sci. USA* **91**, 9302–6.

Genoux, D., Haditsch, U., Knobloch, M., Michalon, A., Storm, D., and Mansuy, I. M. (2002). The protein phosphatase 1 is a molecular constraint on learning and memory. *Nature* **418**, 970–5.

Gerlai, R. (1996). Gene-targeting studies of mammalian behavior: is it the mutation or the background genotype? *Trends Neurosci.* **19**, 177–81.

Gerlai, R. (2000). Targeting genes and proteins in the analysis of learning and memory: caveats and future directions. *Rev. Neurosci.* **11**, 15–26.

Giese, K. P., Fedorov, N. B., Filipkowski, R. K., and Silva, A. J. (1998). Autophosphorylation at Thr286 of the alpha calcium-calmodulin kinase II in LTP and learning. *Science* **279**, 870–3.

Gingrich, J. A. and Hen, R. (2000). The broken mouse: the role of development, plasticity and environment in the interpretation of phenotypic changes in knockout mice. *Curr. Opin. Neurobiol.* **10**, 146–52.

Glazewski, S., Chen, C. M., Silva, A., and Fox, K. (1996). Requirement for alpha-CaMKII in experience-dependent plasticity of the barrel cortex. *Science* **272**, 421–3.

Gordon, J. A., Cioffi, D., Silva, A. J., and Stryker, M. P. (1996). Deficient plasticity in the primary visual cortex of alpha-calcium/calmodulin-dependent protein kinase II mutant mice. *Neuron* **17**, 491–9.

Gossen, M., Bonin, A. L., Freundlieb, S., and Bujard, H. (1994). Inducible gene expression systems for higher eukaryotic cells. *Curr. Opin. Biotechnol.* **5**, 516–20.

Gossen, M., Freundlieb, S., Bender, G., Muller, G., Hillen, W., and Bujard, H. (1995). Transcriptional activation by tetracyclines in mammalian cells. *Science* **268**, 1766–9.

Hanson, P. I. and Schulman, H. (1992). Neuronal Ca^{2+}/calmodulin-dependent protein kinases. *A. Rev. Biochem.* **61**, 559–601.

Hinds, H. L., Tonegawa, S., and Malinow, R. (1998). CA1 long-term potentiation is diminished but present in hippocampal slices from alpha-CaMKII mutant mice. *Learn. Mem.* **5**, 344–54.

Indra, A. K., Warot, X., Brocard, J., Bornert, J. M., Xiao, J. H., Chambon, P., *et al.* (1999). Temporally-controlled site-specific mutagenesis in the basal layer of the epidermis: comparison of the recombinase activity of the tamoxifen-inducible Cre-ER(T) and Cre-ER(T2) recombinases. *Nucleic Acids Res.* **27**, 4324–7.

Lamartina, S., Roscilli, G., Rinaudo, C. D., Sporeno, E., Silvi, L., Hillen, W., *et al.* (2002). Stringent control of gene expression *in vivo* by using novel doxycycline-dependent transactivators. *Hum. Gene Ther.* **13**, 199–210.

Lisman, J. E. (1985). A mechanism for memory storage insensitive to molecular turnover: a bistable autophosphorylating kinase. *Proc. Natl Acad. Sci. USA* **82**, 3055–7.

Lisman, J. (1989). A mechanism for the Hebb and the anti-Hebb processes underlying learning and memory. *Proc. Natl Acad. Sci. USA* **86**, 9574–8.

Lisman, J. (2003). Long-term potentiation: outstanding questions and attempted synthesis. *Phil. Trans. R. Soc. Lond.* B **358**, 829–42. (DOI 10.1098/rstb.2002.1242.)

Lisman, J., Schulman, H., and Cline, H. (2002). The molecular basis of CaMKII function in synaptic and behavioural memory. *Nature Rev. Neurosci.* **3**, 175–90.

Lynch, G. S., Dunwiddie, T., and Gribkoff, V. (1977). Heterosynaptic depression: a postsynaptic correlate of long-term potentiation. *Nature* **266**, 737–9.

Malenka, R. C. and Nicoll, R. A. (1999). Long-term potentiation—a decade of progress? *Science* **285**, 1870–4.

Malleret, G., Haditsch, U., Genoux, D., Jones, M. W., Bliss, T. V., Vanhoose, A. M., *et al.* (2001). Inducible and reversible enhancement of learning, memory, and long-term potentiation by genetic inhibition of calcineurin. *Cell* **104**, 675–86.

Mansuy, I. M., Winder, D. G., Moallem, T. M., Osman, M., Mayford, M., Hawkins, R. D., *et al.* (1998*a*). Inducible and reversible gene expression with the rtTA system for the study of memory. *Neuron* **21**, 257–65.

Mansuy, I. M., Mayford, M., Jacob, B., Kandel, E. R., and Bach, M. E. (1998*b*). Restricted and regulated overexpression reveals calcineurin as a key component in the transition from short-term to long-term memory. *Cell* **92**, 39–49.

Martin, S. J., Grimwood, P. D., and Morris, R. G. M. (2000). Synaptic plasticity and memory: an evaluation of the hypothesis. *A. Rev. Neurosci.* **23**, 649–711.

Mayford, M., Wang, J., Kandel, E. R., and O'Dell, T. J. (1995). CaMKII regulates the frequency-response function of hippocampal synapses for the production of both LTD and LTP. *Cell* **81**, 891–904.

Mayford, M., Bach, M. E., Huang, Y. Y., Wang, L., Hawkins, R. D., and Kandel, E. R. (1996*a*). Control of memory formation through regulated expression of a CaMKII transgene. *Science* **274**, 1678–83.

Mayford, M., Baranes, D., Podsypanina, K., and Kandel, E. R. (1996b). The 3′-untranslated region of CaMKII alpha is a cis-acting signal for the localization and translation of mRNA in dendrites. *Proc. Natl Acad. Sci. USA* **93**, 13 250–5.

Moser, S., Rimann, M., Fux, C., Schlatter, S., Bailey, J. E., and Fussenegger, M. (2001). Dual-regulated expression technology: a new era in the adjustment of heterologous gene expression in mammalian cells. *J. Gene Med.* **3**, 529–49.

Nakazawa, K., Quirk, M. C., Chitwood, R. A., Watanabe, M., Yeckel, M. F., Sun, L. D., *et al.* (2002). Requirement for hippocampal CA3 NMDA receptors in associative memory recall. *Science* **297**, 211–18.

Ohno, M., Frankland, P. W., Chen, A. P., Costa, R. M., and Silva, A. J. (2001). Inducible, pharmacogenetic approaches to the study of learning and memory. *Nature Neurosci.* **4**, 1238–43.

Ohno, M., Frankland, P. W., and Silva, A. J. (2002). A pharmacogenetic inducible approach to the study of NMDA/alphaCaMKII signaling in synaptic plasticity. *Curr. Biol.* **12**, 654–6.

Ouyang, Y., Kantor, D., Harris, K. M., Schuman, E. M., and Kennedy, M. B. (1997). Visualization of the distribution of autophosphorylated calcium/calmodulin-dependent protein kinase II after tetanic stimulation in the CA1 area of the hippocampus. *J. Neurosci.* **17**, 5416–27.

Salucci, V., Scarito, A., Aurisicchio, L., Lamartina, S., Nicolaus, G., Giampaoli, S., *et al.* (2002). Tight control of gene expression by a helper-dependent adenovirus vector carrying the rtTA2(s)-M2 tetracycline transactivator and repressor system. *Gene Ther.* **9**, 1415–21.

Shimizu, E., Tang, Y. P., Rampon, C., and Tsien, J. Z. (2000). NMDA receptor-dependent synaptic reinforcement as a crucial process for memory consolidation. *Science* **290**, 1170–4.

Silva, A. J., Stevens, C. F., Tonegawa, S., and Wang, Y. (1992a). Deficient hippocampal long-term potentiation in alpha-calcium-calmodulin kinase II mutant mice. *Science* **257**, 201–6.

Silva, A. J., Paylor, R., Wehner, J. M., and Tonegawa, S. (1992b). Impaired spatial learning in alpha-calcium-calmodulin kinase II mutant mice. *Science* **257**, 206–11.

Staubli, U. and Lynch, G. (1990). Stable depression of potentiated synaptic responses in the hippocampus with 1–5 Hz stimulation. *Brain Res.* **513**, 113–18.

Tonegawa, S., Li, Y., Erzurumlu, R. S., Jhaveri, S., Chen, C., Goda, Y., *et al.* (1995). The gene knockout technology for the analysis of learning and memory, and neural development. *Prog. Brain Res.* **105**, 3–14.

Tonegawa, S., Nakazawa, K., and Wilson, M. A. (2003). Genetic neuroscience of mammalian learning and memory. *Phil. Trans. R. Soc. Lond.* B **358**, 787–95. (DOI 10.1098/rstb. 2002. 1243.)

Tsien, J. Z., Chen, D. F., Gerber, D., Tom, C., Mercer, E. H., Anderson, D. J., *et al.* (1996a). Subregion- and cell type-restricted gene knockout in mouse brain. *Cell* **87**, 1317–26.

Tsien, J. Z., Huerta, P. T., and Tonegawa, S. (1996b). The essential role of hippocampal CA1 NMDA receptor-dependent synaptic plasticity in spatial memory. *Cell* **87**, 1327–38.

Urlinger, S., Baron, U., Thellmann, M., Hasan, M. T., Bujard, H., and Hillen, W. (2000). Exploring the sequence space for tetracycline-dependent transcriptional activators: novel mutations yield expanded range and sensitivity. *Proc. Natl Acad. Sci. USA* **97**, 7963–8.

Wang, J. H. and Kelly, P. T. (1996). The balance between postsynaptic Ca^{2+}-dependent protein kinase and phosphatase activities controlling synaptic strength. *Learn. Mem.* **3**, 170–81.

Winder, D. G., Mansuy, I. M., Osman, M., Moallem, T. M., and Kandel, E. R. (1998). Genetic and pharmacological evidence for a novel, intermediate phase of long-term potentiation suppressed by calcineurin. *Cell* **92**, 25–37.

Wunderlich, F. T., Wildner, H., Rajewsky, K., and Edenhofer, F. (2001). New variants of inducible Cre recombinase: a novel mutant of Cre-PR fusion protein exhibits enhanced sensitivity and an expanded range of inducibility. *Nucleic Acids Res.* **29**, 47.

Zeng, H., Chattarji, S., Barbarosie, M., Rondi-Reig, L., Philpot, B. D., Miyakawa, T., *et al.* (2001). Forebrain-specific calcineurin knockout selectively impairs bidirectional synaptic plasticity and working/episodic-like memory. *Cell* **107**, 617–29.

Glossary

CaMKII	Ca^{2+}/calmodulin-dependent protein kinase II
CN	calcineurin
CPP	3-(2-carboxypiperazin-4-yl)propyl-1-phosphonic acid
fEPSP	field excitatory postsynaptic potential
LTD	long-term depression
LTP	long-term potentiation
NMDA	N-methyl-D-aspartate
NR1	N-methyl-D-aspartate receptor 1
PKA	protein kinase A
PP1	protein phosphatase 1
PSD	postsynaptic density
rtTA	reverse tetracycline-controlled transactivator
tTA	tetracycline-controlled transactivator

26

MAPK, CREB and *zif268* are all required for the consolidation of recognition memory

Bruno Bozon, Áine Kelly, Sheena A. Josselyn, Alcino J. Silva,
Sabrina Davis, and Serge Laroche

There has been nearly a century of interest in the idea that encoding and storage of information in the brain requires changes in the efficacy of synaptic connections between neurons that are activated during learning. Recent research into the molecular mechanisms of long-term potentiation (LTP) has brought about new knowledge that has provided valuable insights into the neural mechanisms of memory storage. The evidence indicates that rapid activation of the genetic machinery can be a key mechanism underlying the enduring modification of neural networks required for the stability of memories. In recent years, a wealth of experimental data has highlighted the importance of mitogen-activated protein kinase/extracellular signal-regulated kinase (MAPK/ERK) signalling in the regulation of gene transcription in neurons. Here, we briefly review experiments that have shown MAPK/ERK, cAMP response element-binding protein (CREB) and the immediate early gene (IEG) *zif268* are essential components of a signalling cascade required for the expression of late phase LTP and of certain forms of long-term memory. We also present experiments in which we have assessed the role of these three molecules in recognition memory. We show that pharmacological blockade of MAPK/ERK phosphorylation, functional inactivation of CREB in an inducible transgenic mouse and inactivation of *zif268* in a mutant mouse result in a similar deficit in long-term recognition memory. In the continuing debate about the role of LTP mechanisms in memory, these findings provide an important complement to the suggestion that synaptic changes brought about by LTP and memory consolidation and storage share, at least in part, common underlying molecular mechanisms.

Keywords: learning; long-term potentiation; synaptic plasticity; hippocampus; gene expression; transgenic mice

26.1 Introduction

In 1973, when Tim Bliss and Terje Lømo published their research and discovery of LTP (Bliss and Lømo 1973), they warned that 'whether or not the intact animal makes use in real life of a property which has been revealed by synchronous, repetitive volley to a population of fibres the normal rate and pattern of activity along which are unknown, is another matter'; the central, simple question being: does LTP have a role to play in the laying down and/or readout of memories? Since then, as some of the key molecular biological mechanisms underlying the induction and expression of LTP were being elucidated, many groups were striving to characterize the function of this particular property of brain synapses in the intact behaving animal. The results of the past 30 years of research have firmly established that the type of synaptic change that is brought about by LTP is a key player in memory function and dysfunction, even if there are still issues and questions about the role of LTP that are the subject of intensive debate. All along, a more profound, paradigmatic shift has been set in motion; no sooner was LTP discovered and a wealth of molecular information on its underlying mechanisms made available, than the beginnings of a new era in the cellular and molecular exploration of memory under both normal conditions and in disease states were framed. This has been driven by the increasing knowledge about LTP mechanisms, and also by the development of novel technologies specifically designed to exploit these molecular data. The net result has been a closer interaction between the fields of molecular, cellular, system and cognitive neuroscience that culminated in the past decade in the birth of the field of molecular and cellular cognition.

Among the many important advances that have been made in uncovering some of the mechanisms of LTP, one of the most intriguing is the realization that the mechanisms underlying the longer-lasting phases of LTP engage the genetic programme of neurons and result in the synthesis of new proteins. The evidence came from two main sources: the fact that inhibitors of either protein synthesis (Krug et al. 1984; Otani and Abraham 1989; Frey and Morris 1997) or transcription (Nguyen et al. 1994) affect the duration of LTP; and the finding that LTP itself induces transcriptional regulation of a variety of genes, including inducible transcription factors (Cole et al. 1989; Wisden et al. 1990; Abraham et al. 1993; Worley et al. 1993; French et al. 2001) and genes encoding synaptic proteins (e.g. Smirnova et al. 1993; Thomas et al. 1994, 1996; Link et al. 1995; Lyford et al. 1995; Bramham et al. 1996; Hicks et al. 1997; Génin et al. 2001). Remarkably, experimental evidence also indicates that the expression of long-term memories shares many characteristics with LTP, including similar molecular mechanisms, a requirement for protein synthesis (Davis and Squire 1984; Meiri and Rosenblum 1998) and, in specific areas of the brain, the regulated transcription of a variety of genes (Nikolaev et al. 1992; Davis et al. 1996, 1998; Okuno and Miyashita 1996; Guzowski et al. 1999, 2001; Tischmeyer and Grimm 1999; Hall et al. 2000; Zhao et al. 2000; Cavallaro et al. 2001). Many genes have been shown to be up- and downregulated in a finely tuned and coordinated manner and the full genomic response of neurons associated with specific aspects of LTP and memory processes is currently the subject of intensive investigation using newly available large-scale screening methods.

An important issue in this context is to understand how synaptic events signal gene regulation. Again, studies of synapse-to-nuclear signalling in LTP have provided important inroads for exploring memory mechanisms and in the past 10 years several important operating molecules have been identified. In LTP, as in many other aspects of cell function involving regulated gene transcription, two important steps appear to be critical: the activation of protein kinases and of constitutively expressed transcription factors and shortly after, the expression of a class of IEGs encoding regulatory transcription factors which interact with promoter regulatory elements of a host of downstream effector genes. To illustrate this process, and although not intended as a comprehensive overview of the topic, this article focuses on three key molecules, the ERK family of MAPK, the transcription factor CREB and the IEG *zif268*.We begin with a brief review of recent findings suggesting these three molecules are components of a signalling system from the synapse to the nucleus that is crucial for the long-term stabilization of neural plasticity and for the consolidation of certain forms of memories. We also report experiments evaluating their role in recognition memory, a form of memory based on the ability to discriminate between novel and familiar objects which in humans, monkeys and rodents is affected by damage to structures of the medial temporal lobe, including the hippocampus and adjacent entorhinal and para-hippocampal cortices (reviewed in Clark *et al.* 2000; Zola *et al.* 2000). We have assessed the role of these three molecules in trial-unique recognition memory by using three different strategies: pharmacological blockade of MAPK/ERK activation in rats, functional inactivation of CREB in inducible transgenic mice and inactivation of the *zif268* gene in a null mutant mouse. Our results indicate that the MAPK/ERK-CREB-*zif268* signalling pathway is essential for long-term recognition memory.

26.2 The IEG *zif268*, LTP and memory consolidation

Zif268, also known as *Egr-1*, *Krox-24*, *NGFI*-A or *Zenk*, is an IEG encoding a zinc finger transcription factor originally identified as a nerve growth factor response gene product in PC12 cells and an immediate–early serum response gene product in fibroblasts (Milbrandt 1987; Christy *et al.* 1988; Lemaire *et al.* 1988; Sukhatme *et al.* 1988). The gene encodes a three zinc finger protein which binds to cognate GC-rich response elements in the DNA to regulate downstream expression of late-response genes (Christy and Nathans 1989; Swirnoff and Milbrandt 1995). The mRNA and protein are expressed in several areas of the neocortex, hippocampus, entorhinal cortex, amygdala, striatum and cerebellum (Christy *et al.* 1988; Mack *et al.* 1990; Worley *et al.* 1991). In the hippocampus, its expression gradually increases in the second week after birth and remains elevated in the CA1/CA3 regions, but it is only transient in the dentate gyrus where its constitutive expression fades after three weeks (Watson and Milbrandt 1990; Herms *et al.* 1994). *Zif268* was found to be rapidly and transiently turned on by a variety of pharmacological and physiological stimuli including neurotransmitters, growth factors, peptides, depolarization, seizures, ischemia and brain injury or cellular stress (reveiwed in Gashler and Sukhatme 1995; Beckmann and Wilce 1997; O'Donovan *et al.* 1999). Further emphasizing the role of *zif268* in cellular physiology, two independent groups showed rapid and robust activation of *zif268* in the dentate gyrus after the induction of LTP (Cole *et al.* 1989; Wisden *et al.* 1990). Even though tens of distinct IEGs, including other members of the *Egr* family, can be induced by synaptic activity in an *N*-methyl-D-aspartate receptor-dependent manner, *zif268* has attracted much attention because its regulated transcription in the dentate gyrus is both reliably associated with the expression of the protein synthesis-dependent late phase of LTP and appears to correlate with the persistence of LTP (Abraham *et al.* 1991, 1993; Richardson *et al.* 1992; Worley *et al.* 1993). Recently, the analysis of *Zif268* DNA binding activity using gel-shift assays revealed that the increase in zif268 protein following induction of LTP is associated with increased binding of the protein to its response element (Williams *et al.* 2000), indicating functional activation of downstream genes containing zif268 response elements.

Behavioural studies also provided evidence that the expression of *zif268* is sensitive to natural environmental stimuli following exposure of rats to novel environments (Hall *et al.* 2000) or in a learning context (Tischmeyer and Grimm 1999). The induction occurs rapidly and is transient, indicating a role in the transition from short- to long-term memory. For example, Okuno and Miyashita (1996) found that zif268, but not c-Fos or JunD, is activated in the infero-temporal cortex of macaque monkeys trained in a form of explicit memory task, visual paired associate learning. Learning-related increases in *zif268* expression have also been observed in the hippocampus after active avoidance learning (Nikolaev *et al.* 1992), brightness discrimination (Grimm and Tischmeyer 1997), recall of contextual fear memory (Hall *et al.* 2001) or spatial learning (Guzowski *et al.* 2001), and in the amygdala after acquisition (Malkani and Rosen 2000) or recall (Hall *et al.* 2001) of contextual fear conditioning.

In recent experiments in collaboration with Tim Bliss and colleagues, we were able to investigate the role of *zif268* in LTP and learning using mutant mice (Jones *et al.* 2001). In these experiments, we found that basal synaptic transmission, cell excitability, forms of short-term plasticity such as paired-pulse facilitation and paired-pulse depression were normal in the dentate gyrus of *zif268* mutant mice; however, LTP, which was normal for the first hour, was not maintained over 24 h in awake animals, showing that the *zif268* gene is necessary for the expression of the later phases of LTP. The construct used to inactivate *zif268* in the mutant mice (Topilko *et al.* 1998) involved the insertion of a *LacZ* cassette downstream of the *zif268* promoter; we found that in the mutant mice the constitutive and LTP-inducible expression of the *LacZ* gene was comparable to that of *zif268* in wild-type (WT) mice, indicating that signalling events upstream of *zif268* transcription were not affected by the mutation. We examine short-term and long-term memory in these mice, by using a variety of behavioural tasks that make use of single or repeated training, different types of reinforcement, and the processing of spatial or non-spatial information. The results showed that short-term memory is intact in *zif268* mutant mice. Analysis of the mutants revealed normal levels of spontaneous alternation in a T-maze, a readily observed pattern of behaviour that relies upon spatial working memory, normal short-term retention for odours as tested in a social transmission of food preference task, and normal short-term memory for object recognition. In contrast, we found that long-term memory in *zif268* mutant mice was severely impaired in several tasks including social transmission of food preference, object recognition, conditioned taste aversion and a spatial navigation task in the water-maze (Jones *et al.* 2001). Thus, these experiments establish that *zif268* is essential for the expression of late LTP in the dentate gyrus and for the expression of long-term memories.

26.3 The MAPK/ERK signalling pathway, *zif268* transcription and LTP

What are the intracellular signalling mechanisms that are responsible for the induction and regulation of *zif268* in synaptic plasticity and learning? A crucial event in signal transduction leading to gene regulation in neurons is the activation of protein kinases. Although several kinases, including PKC, PKA, αCaMKII are known to play an important role in LTP (see Soderling and Derkach (2000) for a review), recent work has highlighted the potential role of the MAPK/ERK cascade as a critical trigger to initiate gene transcription after synaptic activation (see Sweatt (2001) for a review). Moreover, cross-talk between kinase pathways indicates that MAPK/ERK may be a point of convergence integrating PKC, PKA and CaMK signals (Impey *et al.* 1998*a*; Roberson *et al.* 1999; Vanhoutte *et al.* 1999), in addition to the activation of other kinase-selective target substrates. In cell lines, experimental evidence indicates that MAPK/ERK, once activated, translocates from the cytosol to the nucleus where it can regulate transcriptional activity of many IEGs (reviewed in Treisman 1996). This is likely to be accomplished via two prime nuclear targets of activated MAPK/ERK, the transcription factors CREB and Elk-1. CREB is transactivated by MAPK/ERK via the CREB kinase ribosomal protein S6 kinase (Rsk2), and homo or heterodimers of the CREB/ATF family that can bind to CRE sites in the upstream regulatory region of several IEGs (see Lonze and Ginty (2002) for a review). Elk-1 is directly activated by MAPK/ERK and plays a pivotal role in IEG induction by various extracellular signals (Marais *et al.* 1993; Hipskind *et al.* 1994) via a ternary complex assembled on the SRE, another DNA sequence motif also present within the upstream regulatory region of many IEGs (Wasylyk *et al.* 1998). The upstream promoter region of the *zif268* gene contains two putative CRE sites and a series of six SREs in the 5′-flanking region (reviewed in Beckmann and Wilce 1997). The expression of *zif268* is therefore likely to be strongly controlled by the MAPK/ERK–CREB pathway targeting CRE and the MAPK/ERK–Elk pathway targeting SRE.

Several studies have shown that MAPK/ERK is rapidly phosphorylated after LTP and that this activation is essential for the expression of LTP in CA1 *in vitro* (English and Sweatt 1996, 1997; Patterson *et al.* 2001) and in the dentate gyrus *in vivo* (Davis *et al.* 2000; Rosenblum *et al.* 2000). CREB is also critical for hippocampal LTP (Bourtchuladze *et al.* 1994) and studies in CRE-*LacZ* transgenic mice indicate activation of CRE-mediated transcription in CA1 by the induction of LTP (Impey *et al.* 1996). Furthermore, LTP is enhanced in transgenic mice expressing a constitutively active form of CREB (Barco *et al.* 2002). In a recent study, we examined whether MAPK/ERK, CREB and Elk-1 were activated and required for LTP-induced transcriptional regulation of *zif268 in vivo* (Davis *et al.* 2000). We found that LTP in the dentate gyrus leads to rapid phosphorylation and nuclear translocation of MAPK/ERK and a subsequent coordinated phosphorylation of both CREB and Elk-1. Inhibition of MAPK/ERK phosphorylation by an MEK inhibitor was shown to block phosphorylation of both CREB and Elk-1, and also to block LTP-dependent transcriptional activation of *zif268* in dentate granule cells, resulting in a rapidly decaying LTP. Thus, these results show that MAPK/ERK controls *zif268* expression in LTP and that this is mediated by two parallel and possibly cooperating signalling pathways, one targeting CRE-mediated transcription via CREB and the second targeting SRE-mediated transcription via Elk-1 (Davis *et al.* 2000). This cascade is likely to control the transcriptional activation of many other IEGs under the control of CRE and SRE elements, as has been shown for example for *c-fos* (Sgambato *et al.* 1998) or *arg3.1/arc* (Waltereit *et al.* 2001).

The identification of the crucial role of the MAPK/ERK signalling pathway in LTP precipitated an intensive search for its role in learning and memory. Within a few years, several groups had shown that MAPK/ERK is activated in the hippocampus and is required for a variety of hippocampal-dependent forms of learning (reviewed in Impey *et al.* 1999; Sweatt 2001). For example, inhibition of the upstream kinase MEK produces deficits in memory for cued and contextual fear associations (Atkins *et al.* 1998) and in spatial memory (Blum *et al.* 1999; Selcher *et al.* 1999). Similar results have been obtained in the lateral nucleus of the amygdala in the consolidation of fear memory (Schafe *et al.* 2000) where *zif268* is also activated (Malkani and Rosen 2000; Hall *et al.* 2001). Moreover, coordinated activation of MAPK/ERK, CREB and Elk-1 has also been reported in the hippocampus after one-trial avoidance learning (Cammarota *et al.* 2000) and in the insular cortex. LTP in the insular cortex is associated with *zif268* expression and blocked by inhibition of MAPK/ERK (Jones *et al.* 1999). The insular cortex is also associated with long-term storage of taste memory (Berman *et al.* 1998).

Several studies have shown that CREB is also strongly implicated in memory formation in different paradigms. Deficits in long-term, but not short-term, memory have been observed in fear conditioning and spatial learning in mice with a targeted disruption of the $\alpha\Delta$CREB isoforms (Bourtchuladze *et al.* 1994). More recent experiments have shown deficits in spatial long-term memory after functional inactivation of CREB in the hippocampus using antisense oligodeoxynucleotides (Guzowski and McGaugh 1997), in memory for taste aversion after functional inactivation of CREB in the amygdala (Lamprecht *et al.* 1997), or in the memory for fear associations after induction of an inducible CREB repressor in transgenic mice (Kida *et al.* 2002). Conversely, a gain-of-function study by Josselyn *et al.* (2001) showed that over-expression of CREB in the amygdala via viral vector-mediated gene transfer enhances fear memory. Finally, Impey *et al.* (1998*b*), using CRE-*LacZ* transgenic mice, provided support for the recruitment of CRE-mediated transcription in CA1 during contextual fear conditioning. A more recent report suggests this is associated with MAPK/ERK activation and essential for long-term contextual memory (Athos *et al.* 2002). Thus, together with the functional implication of *zif268* as we have seen above, these findings indicate that the MAPK/ERK–CREB/Elk-1–*zif268* signalling pathway is one important route for inducing molecular changes underlying the type of synaptic plasticity required for formation of long-term memories.

26.4 Requirement of MAPK/ERK activation for recognition memory

To assess the role of MAPK/ERK in recognition memory, we used an object recognition task; this is a task based on the natural preference of rodents for novelty and their ability to discriminate the familiarity of previously encountered objects. In the standard task, rodents are placed in a small arena and briefly exposed to two objects that they can explore freely. Then, after a variable delay interval, one object is replaced by a new one. Normal animals prefer to explore the novel rather than the familiar object, thus demonstrating they remember the two objects they had previously had experience with. If the memory of the familiar objects has faded, however, they would spend equal time exploring the two objects.

In the present experiment, adult male Sprague–Dawley rats were allowed to explore and become familiarized to an empty circular open-field arena (five sessions of 20 min) before training. A single training session was then given where in the arena were placed two different complex-shaped three-dimensional objects constructed with Lego pieces that rats were allowed to explore freely (three 5 min periods separated by a 5 min interval). Retention was tested 24 h later in a single session (5 min) in which one of the two objects was replaced by a novel-shaped object and the time spent exploring each object was recorded. Objects were cleaned thoroughly between trials to ensure the absence of olfactory cues. We tested in this protocol normal rats ($n = 8$) and rats implanted with a cannula in the lateral ventricle with which we injected an inhibitor of the upstream MAPK/ERK kinase MEK. The MEK inhibitor, UO126 (4 µl, 1 µg µl^{-1}, injected at a rate of 1 µl min^{-1}; $n = 6$) or the vehicle, DMSO ($n = 7$) were injected 40 min before the training session. We found that both normal rats and rats injected

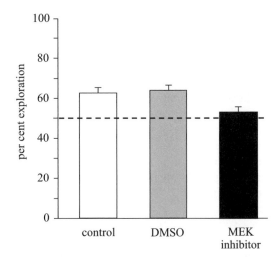

Fig. 26.1 Long-term recognition memory is impaired by injection of the MEK inhibitor. Control rats (white bar) and rats with an implanted cannula receiving either the MEK inhibitor U0126 (black bar) or the vehicle DMSO (grey bar) were exposed to two objects (sample phase) and memory was tested 24 h later with one of the previously encountered objects replaced by a novel object. DMSO or U0126 were injected 40 min before the sample phase. The histograms represent the time spent exploring the novel object during the test session at a 24 h delay, expressed as a per cent of the total time of exploration of objects. Control rats and DMSO-injected rats spent significantly more time exploring the novel object, indicating good recognition memory. Rats injected with the MEK inhibitor showed no preference for the novel object.

with DMSO explored the novel object more than the familiar object (Fig. 26.1). Exploration of the novel object was significantly above chance ($p < 0.01$ in each case). In contrast, rats injected with the MEK inhibitor just before the training session did not show preference for the novel object ($p > 0.05$) during the retention test 24 h later and explored the novel and familiar objects equally (Fig. 26.1). The performance of these rats was significantly different from both the noninjected and DMSO-injected rats ($p < 0.05$ in each case). Inhibition of MAPK/ERK did not affect exploration during the training phase, and short-term memory tested 10 min after the initial exposure. By contrast, 24 h after training, memory was impaired by the MEK inhibitor (Fig. 26.1), indicating that blocking MAPK/ERK function does not impair behavioural exploration of novel objects, the encoding of a new experience or short-term memory for objects, but impairs the consolidation or expression of long-term recognition memory.

26.5 Requirement of CREB for recognition memory

To test the role of CREB in recognition memory, we used a transgenic mouse line with a brain-specific and inducible CREB repressor (Kida *et al.* 2002). In these mice, the CREB repressor, a Ser[133] mutated αCREB isoform, is fused to a LBD of a human oestrogen receptor with a G521R mutation, allowing induction of the CREB repressor by the drug 4-hydroxytamoxifen (tamoxifen). Injection of tamoxifen disrupts

CRE-mediated transcription in transgenic mice expressing this inducible CREB repressor (LBD–CREB^{IR}) under the control of the αCaMKII promoter (Kida *et al.* 2002). With this inducible, spatially restricted CREB transgenic mouse, it is possible to switch CREB function off. Inducing the activation of the transgenic CREB repressor with tamoxifen 6 h before training in a cued or a contextual fear conditioning paradigm had no effect on short-term memory, but resulted in impaired long-term memory for both cued and contextual fear associations (Kida *et al.* 2002). Injection of tamoxifen 6 h before training produced the largest deficit in fear memory.

To test the impact of CREB inactivation in recognition memory in these mice, we opted for a more complex recognition task in which we could distinguish between spatial and non-spatial recognition memory in the same paradigm. To this end, we modified the object recognition task to assess separately memory for objects and memory for the spatial configuration of objects, based on the discrimination between novel and familiar objects (Fig. 26.2*a*) or between a novel and a familiar spatial location of an object (Fig. 26.2*b*). In this protocol, three distinct objects were used instead of two during the training phase, and a cue card was placed above one of the side walls of the open field (58 cm in length and 35 cm in height) to aid the mapping of the location of each object in space. The mice were habituated to the empty open field (two sessions of 20 min) before training. On the first day of the experiment, mice were exposed to three novel objects that they were allowed to explore for two 10 min sessions with a 10 min interval. On the second day, one object was displaced to a new

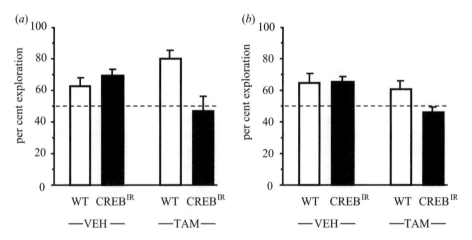

Fig. 26.2 Long-term recognition memory is impaired after activation of the CREB repressor in transgenic mice. WT and CREB^{IR} mice were exposed to three objects (sample phase) and memory was tested 24 h later with either (*a*) one familiar object replaced by a novel object or (*b*) one familiar object moved to a new location in the arena. The histograms represent the time spent exploring the novel object or the displaced object during the test phase at a 24 h delay, expressed as a per cent of the total time of exploration of objects (mean time for the two familiar/undisplaced objects plus time for novel or displaced objects). When the vehicle was injected (VEH), both WT mice (white bars) and CREB^{IR} mice (black bars) spent significantly more time exploring the novel object or the displaced object. Activating CREB^{IR} with an injection of tamoxifen (TAM) 6 h before the sample phase disrupted recognition memory in both the novel object task and the spatial change task, whereas it had no effect in WT mice.

position and mice were given a 10 min session of exploration, thus testing the spatial version of the recognition memory task. On the third day, mice were exposed to three new objects and given the same exploration protocol as that on day 1, and then tested 24 h later (day 4) during a 10 min session in which one of the three objects was replaced by a novel object, testing the nonspatial version of the task. The time spent exploring each object was recorded and preference for the novel object or the displaced object was expressed as a per cent exploration of these objects over the total exploration time of objects.

Groups of CREB^{IR} mice and WT litter-mate mice were tested twice in this protocol, with new sets of objects each time and a few days rest between sets. In one condition, CREB^{IR} and WT mice were injected with tamoxifen (16 mg kg^{-1}, i.p.) 6 h before the training phase, whereas in the other condition they were injected with the peanut oil vehicle solution. No difference in basic locomotor activity or in the time spent exploring objects during the training phase was observed, indicating tamoxifen injection or inducing the CREB repressor does not impair motor activity or the spontaneous tendency of mice to explore novelty. In the absence of tamoxifen, all mice, CREB^{IR} ($n = 8$) and WT ($n = 10$), displayed strong preference for the novel object 24 h after training (Fig. 26.2a). There was no difference between groups ($p > 0.05$) and exploration of the novel object was significantly greater than chance (50%) for both groups ($p < 0.05$). When one of the familiar objects was moved to a new position, again both CREB^{IR} ($n = 8$) and WT ($n = 6$) mice injected with the vehicle solution showed significantly greater exploration of the displaced object (Fig. 26.2b; $p < 0.05$) with no significant difference between groups ($p > 0.05$). Similarly, when tamoxifen was injected in the WT mice, these mice displayed a strong preference for the novel (Fig. 26.2a) or the displaced (Fig. 26.2b) object. By contrast, when the CREB repressor was turned on by injecting tamoxifen 6 h before training in CREB^{IR} mice, retention performance fell to chance levels in both the non-spatial (Fig. 26.2a) and spatial (Fig. 26.2b) version of the task. There was no preferential exploration of the novel object or of the object placed in a new position ($p > 0.05$ in each case) and performance of the tamoxifen-injected CREB^{IR} mice was significantly different from that of the tamoxifen-injected WT mice ($p < 0.05$). Thus, these results indicate that disruption of CREB function impairs both memory for objects and memory for spatial location of objects at the 24 h delay.

26.6 Requirement of the IEG *zif268* for recognition memory

To test the role of the IEG *zif268* in recognition memory, we used mice with a null mutation in the *zif268* gene generated by Patrick Charnay's group (Topilko *et al.* 1998). The targeted inactivation of the *zif268* gene was obtained by insertion of a *LacZ-neo* cassette between the promoter and coding region, and the addition of a frame-shift mutation upstream of the DNA-binding domain, resulting in a complete absence of constitutive and regulated *zif268* expression. In our first study we found these mice have profound deficits in several types of long-term memory (Jones *et al.* 2001). We tested recognition memory in *zif268* mutant mice in this study by using a standard two-object task and found that *zif268* inactivation spares short-term, but impairs long-term, object recognition memory. We next examined performance of the

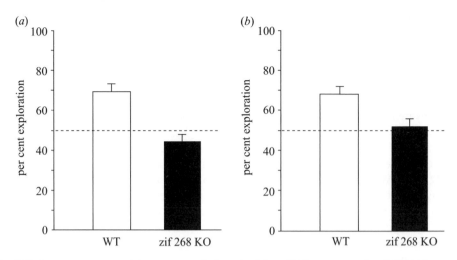

Fig. 26.3 Long-term recognition memory is impaired in *zif268* mutant mice. WT and mutant mice (zif268 KO) were exposed to three objects (sample phase) and memory was tested 24 hours later with either (*a*) one familiar object replaced by a novel object or (*b*) one familiar object moved to a new location in the arena. The histograms represent the time spent exploring the novel object or displaced object (see legend to Fig. 26.2). WT mice (white bars) spent significantly more time exploring the novel or the displaced object, showing long-term recognition memory for objects and for location of objects, whereas *zif268* mutant mice (black bars), showed no preference for the novel or the displaced object.

zif268 mutant mice in the more complex three-object task and tested their ability to remember objects and the spatial location of objects using an identical protocol to that used with the CREB[IR] mutant mice (Bozon *et al.* 2002). As shown in Fig. 26.3, we found that *zif268* mutant mice were severely impaired in the novel object recognition task 24 h after the initial exposure to the objects (Fig. 26.3*a*). *Zif268* mutant mice ($n = 11$) explored all three objects equally ($p > 0.05$), compared with their WT littermates ($n = 11$) that explored the novel object significantly more than the two familiar objects ($p < 0.05$). When we tested the same mice in the spatial version of the task, a similar impairment was found: WT mice displayed significantly greater exploration of the displaced object ($p < 0.05$), whereas *zif268* mutant mice spent an equal amount of time exploring each of the objects ($p > 0.05$; Fig. 26.3*b*). Thus, in complement to the previous findings that inactivation of *zif268* results in long-term memory deficits in several types of task, these results show that *zif268* mutant mice are unable to consolidate or recall information about the characteristics of objects or the spatial location of the objects in these tasks.

In all, these data indicate that MAPK/ERK, CREB and the transcription factor *zif268* are essential components of a signalling cascade required for the expression of long-term recognition memory. Furthermore, our data are also consistent with recent findings showing, in another transgenic mouse, a deficit in long-term object recognition memory in a two-object task when an inhibitor of CREB, cAMP-responsive element modulator and ATF1 isoforms is expressed in the CA1 area of the hippocampus (Pittenger *et al.* 2002). Interestingly, genetic inhibition of calcineurin phosphatase activity (Malleret *et al.* 2001) or of protein phosphatase 1 improves object recognition memory and in the latter case, the mutation also increased training-induced activation of CRE-mediated gene transcription (Genoux *et al.* 2002).

26.7 Conclusion

The laying-down of a stable memory trace is thought to require a molecular consolidation cascade. A central concept in most neurobiological models of memory is that this process involves activity-dependent changes in gene and protein expression, which result in long-lasting alterations in the strength of synaptic connectivity and remodelling of neural networks activated during the encoding of experience. Over the last few decades, research into the mechanisms underlying LTP has helped exploring the mechanisms of memory consolidation and storage, based on the idea that LTP and the formation of memories share, at least in part, common mechanistic properties at the neuronal level. Molecular accounts of consolidation have identified the requirement of regulated gene expression and synthesis of new proteins and insights have been gained into some of the signal transduction mechanisms that convey the signal from cell surface receptors to the nucleus to control the genomic response of synaptically activated neurons.

One critical mediator in this process is the activation of a class of inducible IEGs encoding nuclear transcription factors that can regulate the expression of downstream late-response genes. Here, as an example of this approach, we have focused on one such IEG, *zif268*, and on two molecules, the MAPK/ERK and CREB, known to be implicated in activity-dependent activation of *zif268* in a variety of cell processes. We have examined the role of these molecules in a fundamental memory ability: recognition memory. Using three different approaches, our results show that blocking MAPK/ERK activation, turning CREB function off or inactivating *zif268* all resulted in the same deficit in long-term recognition memory. In the continuing debate about the role of LTP mechanisms in memory, these findings provide an important complement to the suggestion that synaptic changes brought about by LTP and during memory consolidation and storage share, at least in part, common underlying molecular mechanisms. Together with a wealth of experimental data showing that each of these molecules plays important roles in mediating long-term changes in neuronal function, our results are consistent with the view that a MAPK/ERK– CREB pathway targeting CRE, and possibly a MAPK/ERK–Elk pathway targeting SRE and the subsequent transcriptional regulation of *zif268* and other IEGs, is an important molecular mechanism recruited in neurons during the establishment of long-term recognition memory.

Apart from the MAPK/ERK/CRE–Elk/*zif268* pathway, it is probable that there are many other interacting molecules and pathways mediating the full genomic response of neurons required for memory formation. Unravelling these is a great challenge for future research. It will be important to define precisely how a selective set of kinases, phosphatases, transcriptional activators and regulators are put into motion in a coordinated manner to provide neurons with an orchestrated gene response underlying the expression of selective types of plasticity; in what manner any specific type of genomic response corresponds to certain conditions, phases or processes of memory; how it translates into changes in neurons and network properties;

and which structures and pathways express these mechanisms in relation to the laying down and/or recall of distinct categories of memories. Armed with ever more specific and powerful technologies, such as those used here, the field of molecular and cellular cognition is starting to make inroads into the core of mechanisms underlying learning and memory.

We are grateful to Patrick Charnay and his colleagues for the generous gift of *zif268* mutant mice. The work presented in this article was supported by grants from the Centre National de la Recherche Scientifique, programme PICS no. 756 to S.L., the Health Research Board, Ireland, to A.K., an SNRPNIH to A.J.S., and by a doctorate fellowship to B.B. from the Fondation pour la Recherche Médicale.

References

Abraham, W. C., Dragunow, M., and Tate, W. P. (1991). The role of immediate early genes in the stabilization of long-term potentiation. *Mol. Neurobiol.* **5**, 297–314.

Abraham, W. C., Mason, S. E., Demmer, J., Williams, J. M., Richardson, C. L., Tate, W. P., *et al.* (1993). Correlations between immediate early gene induction and the persistence of long-term potentiation. *Neuroscience* **56**, 717–27.

Athos, J., Impey, S., Pineda, V. V., Chen, X., and Storm, D. R. (2002). Hippocampal CRE-mediated gene expression is required for contextual memory formation. *Nature Neurosci.* **5**, 1119–20.

Atkins, C. M., Selcher, J. C., Petraitis, J. J., Tzaskos, J. M., and Sweatt, J. D. (1998). The MAPK cascade is required for mammalian associative learning. *Nature Neurosci.* **1**, 602–9.

Barco, A., Alarcon, J. M., and Kandel, E. R. (2002). Expression of constitutively active CREB protein facilitates the late phase of long-term potentiation by enhancing synaptic capture. *Cell* **108**, 689–703.

Beckmann, A. M. and Wilce, P. A. (1997). Egr transcription factors in the nervous system. *Neurochem. Int.* **31**, 477–510.

Berman, D. E., Hazvi, S., Rosenblum, K., Seger, R., and Dudai, Y. (1998). Specific and differential activation of mitogen-activated protein kinase cascades by unfamiliar taste in the insular cortex of the behaving rat. *J. Neurosci.* **18**, 10 037–44.

Bliss, T. V. P. and Lømo, T. (1973). Long-lasting potentiation of synaptic transmission in the dentate area of the anaesthetized rabbit following stimulation of the perforant path. *J. Physiol. Lond.* **232**, 331–56.

Blum, S., Moore, A. N., Adams, F., and Dash, P. K. (1999). A mitogen-activated protein kinase cascade in the CA1/CA2 subfield of the dorsal hippocampus is essential for long-term spatial learning. *J. Neurosci.* **19**, 3535–44.

Bourtchuladze, R., Frenguelli, B., Blendy, J., Cioffi, D., Schutz, G., and Silva, A. J. (1994). Deficient long-term memory in mice with a targeted mutation of the cAMP-responsive element-binding protein. *Cell* **79**, 59–68.

Bozon, B., Davis, S., and Laroche, S. (2002). Regulated transcription of the immediate early gene Zif268: mechanisms and gene dosage-dependent function in synaptic plasticity and memory formation. *Hippocampus* **12**, 570–7.

Bramham, C. R., Southard, T., Sarvey, J. M., Herkenham, M., and Brady, L. S. (1996). Unilateral LTP triggers bilateral increases in hippocampal neurotrophin and trk receptor mRNA expression in behaving rats: evidence for interhemispheric communication. *J. Comp. Neurol.* **368**, 371–82.

Cammarota, M., Bevilaqua, L. R., Ardenghi, P., Paratcha, G., Levi de Stein, M., Izquierdo, I., *et al.* (2000). Learning-associated activation of nuclear MAPK, CREB and Elk-1, along with Fos production, in the rat hippocampus after a one-trial avoidance learning: abolition by NMDA receptor blockade. *Mol. Brain Res.* **76**, 36–46.

Cavallaro, S., Schreurs, B. G., Zhao, W., D'Agata, V., and Alkon, D. L. (2001). Gene expression profiles during long-term memory consolidation. *Eur. J. Neurosci.* **13**, 1809–15.

Christy, B. A. and Nathans, D. (1989). DNA binding site of the growth factor-inducible protein Zif268. *Proc. Natl Acad. Sci. USA* **86**, 8737–41.

Christy, B. A., Lau, L. F., and Nathans, D. (1988). A gene activated in mouse 3T3 cells by serum growth factors encodes a protein with 'zinc finger' sequences. *Proc. Natl Acad. Sci. USA* **85**, 7857–61.

Clark, R. E., Zola, S. M., and Squire, L. R. (2000). Impaired recognition memory in rats after damage to the hippocampus. *J. Neurosci.* **20**, 8853–60.

Cole, A. J., Saffen, D. W., Baraban, J. M., and Worley, P. F. (1989). Rapid increase of an immediate early gene messenger RNA in hippocampal neurons by synaptic NMDA receptor activation. *Nature* **340**, 474–6.

Davis, H. P. and Squire, L. R. (1984). Protein synthesis and memory: a review. *Psychol. Bull.* **96**, 518–9.

Davis, S., Rodger, J., Hicks, A., Mallet, J., and Laroche, S. (1996). Brain structure and task-specific increase in the expression of the gene encoding syntaxin 1B during learning in the rat: a potential molecular marker for learning-induced synaptic plasticity in neural networks. *Eur. J. Neurosci.* **8**, 2068–74.

Davis, S., Rodger, J., Stéphan, A., Hicks, A., Mallet, J., and Laroche, S. (1998). Increase in syntaxin 1B mRNA in hippocampal and cortical circuits during spatial learning reflects a mechanism of transsynaptic plasticity involved in establishing a memory trace. *Learn. Mem.* **5**, 375–90.

Davis, S., Vanhoutte, P., Pages, C., Caboche, J., and Laroche, S. (2000). The MAPK/ERK cascade targets both Elk-1 and cAMP response element-binding protein to control longterm potentiation-dependent gene expression in the dentate gyrus *in vivo*. *J. Neurosci.* **20**, 4563–72.

English, J. D. and Sweatt, J. D. (1996). Activation of p42 mitogen-activated protein kinase in hippocampal long-term potentiation. *J. Biol. Chem.* **271**, 24 329–32.

English, J. D. and Sweatt, J. D. (1997). Requirement for the mitogen-activated protein kinase cascade in hippocampal long-term potentiation. *J. Biol. Chem.* **272**, 19 103–6.

French, P. J., O'Connor, V., Jones, M. W., Davis, S., Errington, M. L., Voss, K., *et al.* (2001). Subfield-specific immediate early gene expression associated with hippocampal longterm potentiation *in vivo*. *Eur. J. Neurosci.* **13**, 968–76.

Frey, U. and Morris, R. G. M. (1997). Synaptic tagging and longterm potentiation. *Nature* **385**, 533–6.

Gashler, A. and Sukhatme, V. P. (1995). Early growth response protein 1 (Egr-1): prototype of a zinc-finger family of transcription factors. *Progr. Nucleic Acid Res. Mol. Biol.* **50**, 191–224.

Génin, A., Davis, S., Meziane, H., Doyère, V., Jeromin, A., Roder, J., *et al.* (2001). Regulated expression of the neuronal calcium sensor-1 gene during long-term potentiation in the dentate gyrus *in vivo*. *Neuroscience* **106**, 571–7.

Genoux, D., Haditsch, U., Knobloch, M., Michalon, A., Storm, D., and Mansuy, I. M. (2002). Protein phosphatase 1 is a molecular constraint on learning and memory. *Nature* **418**, 970–5.

Grimm, R. and Tischmeyer, W. (1997). Complex patterns of immediate early gene induction in rat brain following brightness discrimination training and pseudotraining. *Behav. Brain Res.* **84**, 109–16.

Guzowski, J. F. and McGaugh, J. L. (1997). Antisense oligodeoxy-nucleotide-mediated disruption of hippocampal cAMP response element binding protein levels impairs consolidation of memory for water maze training. *Proc. Natl Acad. Sci. USA* **94**, 2693–8.

Guzowski, J. F., McNaughton, B. L., Barnes, C. A., and Worley, P. (1999). Environment-specific expression of the immediateearly gene Arc in hippocampal neuronal ensembles. *Nature Neurosci.* **2**, 1120–4.

Guzowski, J. F., Setlow, B., Wagner, E. K., and McGaugh, L. (2001). Experience-dependent gene expression in the rat hippocampus after spatial learning: a comparison of the immediate-early genes *Arc, c-fos*, and *zif268*. *J. Neurosci.* **21**, 5089–98.

Hall, J., Thomas, K. L., and Everitt, B. J. (2000). Rapid and selective induction of BDNF expression in the hippocampus during contextual learning. *Nature Neurosci.* **3**, 533–5.

Hall, J., Thomas, K. L., and Everitt, B. J. (2001). Cellular imaging of *zif268* expression in the hippocampus and amygdala during contextual and cued fear memory retrieval: selective activation of hippocampal CA1 neurons during recall of contextual memories. *J. Neurosci.* **21**, 2186–93.

Herms, J., Zurmohle, U., Schlingensiepen, R., Brysch, W., and Schlingensiepen, K. H. (1994). Developmental expression of the transcription factor zif268 in rat brain. *Neurosci. Lett.* **165**, 171–4.

Hicks, A., Davis, S., Rodger, J., Helme-Guizon, A., Laroche, S., and Mallet, J. (1997). Synapsin I and syntaxin 1B: key elements in the control of neurotransmitter release are regulated by neuronal activation and long-term potentiation *in vivo. Neuroscience* **79**, 329–40.

Hipskind, R. A., Baccarini, M., and Nordheim, A. (1994). Transient activation of RAF-1, MEK and ERK2 coinsides kinetically with ternary complex factor phosphorylation and immediate-early gene promoter activity *in vivo. Mol. Cell Biol.* **14**, 6219–31.

Impey, S., Mark, M., Villacres, E. C., Chavkin, C., and Storm, D. R. (1996). Induction of CRE-mediated gene expression by stimuli that generate long-lasting LTP in area CA1 of the hippocampus. *Neuron* **16**, 973–82.

Impey, S., Obrietan, K., Wong, S. T., Poser, S., Yano, S., Wayman, G., *et al.* (1998*a*). Cross talk between ERK and PKA is required for Ca^{2+} stimulation of CREB-dependent transcription and ERK nuclear translocation. *Neuron* **21**, 869–83.

Impey, S., Smith, D. M., Obrietan, K., Donahue, R., Wade, C., and Storm, D. R. (1998*b*). Stimulation of cAMP response element (CRE)-mediated transcription during contextual learning. *Nature Neurosci.* **1**, 595–601.

Impey, S., Obrietan, K., and Storm, D. R. (1999). Making new connections: role of ERK /MAP kinase signaling in neuronal plasticity. *Neuron* **23**, 11–14.

Jones, M. W., French, P. J., Bliss, T. V. P., and Rosenblum, K. (1999). Molecular mechanisms of LTP in the insular cortex *in vivo. J. Neurosci.* **19**, 1–8.

Jones, M. W., Errington, M. L., French, P. J., Fine, A., Bliss, T. V. P., Garel, S., *et al.* (2001). A requirement for the immediate early gene Zif268 in the expression of late LTP and the consolidation of long-term memories. *Nature Neurosci.* **4**, 289–96.

Josselyn, S. A., Shi, C., Carlezon Jr, W. A., Neve, R. L., Nestler, E. J., and Davis, M. (2001). Long-term memory is facilitated by cAMP response element-binding protein overexpression in the amygdala. *J. Neurosci.* **21**, 2404–12.

Kida, S., Josselyn, S. A., de Ortiz, S. P., Kogan, J. H., Chevere, I., Masushige, S., *et al.* (2002). CREB required for the stability of new and reactivated fear memories. *Nature Neurosci.* **5**, 348–55.

Krug, M., Lossner, B., and Ott, T. (1984). Anisomycin blocks the late phase of long-term potentiation in the dentate gyrus of freely moving rats. *Brain Res. Bull.* **13**, 39–42.

Lamprecht, R., Hazvi, S., and Dudai, Y. (1997). cAMP response element-binding protein in the amygdala is required for long- but not short-term conditioned taste aversion memory. *J. Neurosci.* **17**, 8443–50.

Lemaire, P., Revelant, O., Bravo, R., and Charnay, P. (1988). Two mouse genes encoding potential transcription factors with identical DNA-binding domains are activated by growth factors in cultured cells. *Proc. Natl Acad. Sci. USA* **85**, 4691–5.

Link, W., Konietzko, U., Kauselmann, G., Krug, M., Schwanke, B., Frey, U., *et al.* (1995). Somatodendritic expression of an immediate early gene is regulated by synaptic activity. *Proc. Natl Acad. Sci. USA* **92**, 5734–8.

Lonze, B. E. and Ginty, D. D. (2002). Function and regulation of CREB family transcription factors in the nervous system. *Neuron* **35**, 605–23.

Lyford, G. L., Yamagata, K., Kaufmann, W. E., Barnes, C. A., Sanders, L. K., Copeland, N. G., *et al.* (1995). Arc, a growth factor and activity-regulated gene, encodes a novel cytoskeleton-associated protein that is enriched in neuronal dendrites. *Neuron* **14**, 433–45.

Mack, K., Day, M., Milbrandt, J., and Gottlieb, D. I. (1990). Localization of the NGFI-A protein in the rat brain. *Mol. Brain Res.* **8**, 177–80.

Malkani, S. and Rosen, J. B. (2000). Specific induction of early growth response gene 1 in the lateral nucleus of the amygdala following contextual fear conditioning in rats. *Neuroscience* **97**, 693–702.

Malleret, G., Haditsch, U., Genoux, D., Jones, M. W., Bliss, T. V., Vanhoose, A. M., *et al.* (2001). Inducible and reversible enhancement of learning, memory, and long-term potentiation by genetic inhibition of calcineurin. *Cell* **104**, 675–86.

Marais, R., Wynne, J., and Treisman, R. (1993). The SRF accessory protein ELK-1 contains a growth factor-regulated transcriptional activation domain. *Cell* **73**, 381–93.

Meiri, N. and Rosenblum, K. (1998). Lateral ventricle injection of the protein synthesis inhibitor anisomycin impairs longterm memory in a spatial memory task. *Brain Res.* **789**, 48–55.

Milbrandt, J. (1987). A nerve growth factor-induced gene encodes a possible transcriptional regulatory factor. *Science* **238**, 797–9.

Nguyen, P. V., Abel, T., and Kandel, E. R. (1994). Requirements of a critical period of transcription for induction of a late phase of LTP. *Science* **265**, 1104–7.

Nikolaev, E., Werka, T., and Kaczmarek, L. (1992). C-fos protooncogene expression in rat brain after long-term training of two-way avoidance reaction. *Behav. Brain Res.* **48**, 91–4.

O'Donovan, K. J., Tourtellotte, W. G., Milbrandt, J., and Baraban, J. M. (1999). The EGR family of transcription-regulatory factors: progress at the interface of molecular and systems neuroscience. *Trends Neurosci.* **22**, 167–73.

Okuno, H. and Miyashita, Y. (1996). Expression of the transcription factor Zif268 in the temporal cortex of monkeys during visual paired associate learning. *Eur. J. Neurosci.* **8**, 2118–28.

Otani, S. and Abraham, W. C. (1989). Inhibition of protein synthesis in the dentate gyrus, but not the entorhinal cortex, blocks the maintenance of long-term potentiation in rats. *Neurosci. Lett.* **106**, 175–80.

Patterson, S. L., Pittenger, C., Morozov, A., Martin, K. C., Scanlin, H., Drake, C., *et al.* (2001). Some forms of cAMP-mediated long-lasting potentiation are associated with release of BDNF and nuclear translocation of phospho-MAP kinase. *Neuron* **32**, 123–40.

Pittenger, C., Huang, Y. Y., Paletzki, R. F., Bourtchouladze, R., Scanlin, H., Vronskaya, S., *et al.* (2002). Reversible inhibition of CREB/ATF transcription factors in region CA1 of the dorsal hippocampus disrupts hippocampusdependent spatial memory. *Neuron* **34**, 447–62.

Richardson, C. L., Tate, W. P., Mason, S. E., Lawlor, P. A., Dragunow, M., and Abraham, W. C. (1992). Correlation between the induction of an immediate early gene, zif268, and long-term potentiation in the dentate gyrus. *Brain Res.* **580**, 147–54.

Roberson, E. D., English, J. D., Adams, J. P., Selcher, J. C., Kondratick, C., and Sweatt, J. D. (1999). The mitogen-activated protein kinase cascade couples PKA and PKC to cAMP response element binding protein phosphorylation in area CA1 of the hippocampus. *J. Neurosci.* **19**, 4337–48.

Rosenblum, K., Futter, M., Jones, M., Hulme, E. C., and Bliss, T. V. P. (2000). ERKI/II regulation by the muscarinic acetylcholine receptors in neurons. *J. Neurosci.* **20**, 977–85.

Schafe, G. E., Atkins, C. M., Swank, M. W., Bauer, E. P., Sweatt, J. D., and LeDoux, J. E. (2000). Activation of ERK /MAP kinase in the amygdala is required for memory consolidation of pavlovian fear conditioning. *J. Neurosci.* **20**, 8177–87.

Selcher, J. C., Atkins, C. M., Trzaskos, J. M., Paylor, R., and Sweatt, J. D. (1999). A necessity for MAP kinase activation in mammalian spatial learning. *Learn. Mem.* **6**, 478–90.

Sgambato, V., Pagès, C., Rogard, M., Besson, M. J., and Caboche, J. (1998). Extracellular signal-regulated kinase (ERK) controls immediate early gene induction on corticostriatal stimulation. *J. Neurosci.* **18**, 8814–25.

Smirnova, T., Laroche, S., Errington, M. L., Hicks, A. A., Bliss, T. V. P., and Mallet, J. (1993). Transsynaptic expression of a presynaptic glutamate receptor during hippocampal long-term potentiation. *Science* **262**, 433–6.

Soderling, T. R. and Derkach, V. A. (2000). Postsynaptic protein phopshorylation and LTP. *Trends Neurosci.* **23**, 75–80.

Sukhatme, V. P., Cao, X. M., Chang, L. C., Tsai–Morris, C. H., Stamenkovich, D., Ferreira, P. C., *et al.* (1988). A zinc finger-encoding gene coregulated with c-fos during growth and differentiation, and after cellular depolarization. *Cell* **53**, 37–43.

Sweatt, J. D. (2001). The neuronal MAP kinase cascade: a biochemical signal integration system subserving synaptic plasticity and memory. *J. Neurochem.* **76**, 1–10.

Swirnoff, A. H. and Milbrandt, J. (1995). DNA-binding specificity of NGFI-A and related zinc finger transcription factors. *Mol. Cell Biol.* **15**, 2275–87.

Thomas, K. L., Laroche, S., Errington, M. L., Bliss, T. V. P., and Hunt, S. P. (1994). Spatial and temporal changes in signal transduction pathways during LTP. *Neuron* **13**, 737–45.

Thomas, K. L., Davis, S., Hunt, S. P., and Laroche, S. (1996). Alterations in the expression of specific glutamate receptor subunits following hippocampal LTP *in vivo*. *Learn. Mem.* **3**, 197–208.

Tischmeyer, W. and Grimm, R. (1999). Activation of immediate early genes and memory formation. *Cell. Mol. Life Sci.* **55**, 564–74.

Topilko, P., Schneider-Maunoury, S., Levi, G., Trembleau, A., Gourdji, D., Driancourt, M. A., *et al.* (1998). Multiple pituitary and ovarian defects in Krox-24 (NGFI-A, Egr-1)-targeted mice. *Mol. Endocrinol.* **12**, 107–22.

Treisman, R. (1996). Regulation of transcription by MAP kinase cascade. *Curr. Opin. Cell Biol.* **8**, 205–15.

Vanhoutte, P., Barnier, J. V., Guibert, B., Pagès, C., Besson, M. J., Hipskind, R. A., *et al.* (1999). Glutamate induces phosphorylation of Elk-1 and CREB, along with c-fos activation via an extracellular signal-regulated kinasedependent pathway in brain slices. *Mol. Cell Biol.* **19**, 136–46.

Waltereit, R., Dammermann, B., Wulff, P., Scafidi, J., Staubli, U., Kauselmann, G., Bundman, M., and Kuhl, D. (2001). Arg3.1/Arc mRNA induction by Ca^{2+} and cAMP requires protein kinase A and mitogen-activated protein kinase/extracellular regulated kinase activation. *J. Neurosci.* **21**, 5484–93.

Wasylyk, B., Hagman, J., and Gutierrez-Hartmann, A. (1998). Ets transcription factors/nuclear effectors of the Ras-MAP-kinase signaling pathway. *Trends Biol. Sci.* **23**, 213–16.

Watson, M. A. and Milbrandt, J. (1990). Expression of the nerve growth factor-regulated NGFI-A and NGFI-B genes in the developing rat. *Development* **110**, 173–83.

Williams, J. M., Beckmann, A. M., Mason-Parker, S. E., Abraham, W. C., Wilce, P. A., and Tate, W. P. (2000). Sequential increase in Egr-1 and AP-1 DNA binding activity in the dentate gyrus following the induction of long-term potentiation. *Mol. Brain Res.* **77**, 258–66.

Wisden, W., Errington, M. L., Williams, S., Dunnett, S. B., Waters, C., Hitchcock, D., *et al.* (1990). Differential expression of immediate early gene in the hippocampus and spinal cord. *Neuron* **4**, 603–14.

Worley, P. F., Christy, B. A., Nakabeppu, Y., Bhat, R. V., Cole, A. J., and Baraban, J. M. (1991). Constitutive expression of *zif268* in neocortex is regulated by synaptic activity. *Proc. Natl Acad. Sci. USA* **88**, 5106–10.

Worley, P. F., Bhat, R. V., Baraban, J. M., Erickson, C. A., McNaughton, B. L., and Barnes, C. A. (1993). Threshold for synaptic activation of transcription factors in hippocampus: correlation with long-term enhancement. *J. Neurosci.* **13**, 4776–86.

Zhao, W., Meiri, N., Xu, H., Cavallaro, S., Quattrone, A., Zhang, L., *et al.* (2000). Spatial learning induced changes in expression of the ryanodine type II receptor in the rat hippocampus. *FASEB J.* **14**, 290–300.

Zola, S. M., Squire, L. R., Teng, E., Stefanacci, L., Buffalo, E. A., and Clark, R. E. (2000). Impaired recognition memory in monkeys after damage limited to the hippocampal region. *J. Neurosci.* **20**, 451–63.

Glossary

CaMK	calcium–calmodulin kinase
CRE	cAMP response element
CREB	cAMP response element-binding protein
CREB/ATF	cAMP response element-binding protein/activating transcription factor
DMSO	dimethylsulphoxide
Elk	Ets-like protein
ERK	extracellular signal-regulated kinase
IEG	immediate early gene
LBD	ligand-binding domain
LTP	long-term potentiation
MAPK	mitogen-activated protein kinase
MEK	MAPK/ERK kinase
PKA	cAMP-dependent protein kinase A
PKC	protein kinase C
SRE	serum response element
WT	wild-type

New directions

27

Synaptic plasticity in the mesolimbic dopamine system

Mark J. Thomas and Robert C. Malenka

Long-term potentiation (LTP) and long-term depression (LTD) are thought to be critical mechanisms that contribute to the neural circuit modifications that mediate all forms of experience-dependent plasticity. It has, however, been difficult to demonstrate directly that experience causes long-lasting changes in synaptic strength and that these mediate changes in behaviour. To address these potential functional roles of LTP and LTD, we have taken advantage of the powerful *in vivo* effects of drugs of abuse that exert their behavioural effects in large part by acting in the nucleus accumbens (NAc) and ventral tegmental area (VTA); the two major components of the mesolimbic dopamine system. Our studies suggest that *in vivo* drugs of abuse such as cocaine cause long-lasting changes at excitatory synapses in the NAc and VTA owing to activation of the mechanisms that underlie LTP and LTD in these structures. Thus, administration of drugs of abuse provides a distinctive model for further investigating the mechanisms and functions of synaptic plasticity in brain regions that play important roles in the control of motivated behaviour, and one with considerable practical implications.

Keywords: addiction; dopamine; drugs of abuse; nucleus accumbens; ventral tegmental area

27.1 Introduction

A fundamental issue in neuroscience is how experience modifies synaptic circuitry in the mammalian brain to mediate long-lasting changes in cognition and behaviour. To address this issue experimentally, two basic questions have been posed. First, what are the molecular mechanisms by which patterns of neural activity can stably modify synaptic efficacy? Progress in answering this question has come chiefly through the study of LTP and LTD using *in vitro* slice preparation of the hippocampus. Indeed, such work has greatly expanded our understanding of the molecular mechanisms underlying synaptic function. The second, no less challenging question is—what are the functional consequences of these modifications on neural circuits and behaviour? A very attractive and, we believe, underused model for the study of these sorts of functional questions is the experience-dependent plasticity elicited by *in vivo* exposure to drugs of abuse.

Repeated exposure to drugs of abuse, most notably psychostimulants such as cocaine, leads to a persistent increase in their rewarding and locomotor effects (Robinson and Berridge 1993; Kalivas 1995; Wolf 1998; Carlezon and Nestler 2002; Everitt and Wolf 2002). This enhanced response is thought to be a model for the intensification of drug craving in human addicts. Pharmacological, biochemical and lesion experiments indicate that these enhanced behavioural responses are mediated, at least in part, by long-lasting drug-induced adaptations in the mesolimbic dopamine system—the chief components of which are the VTA, the NAc and their afferent and efferent connections. In particular, modifications in the VTA appear to mediate the induction of behavioural sensitization, whereas adaptations in the NAc are involved in its long-term maintenance (Robinson and Berridge 1993; Kalivas 1995; Wolf 1998; Carlezon and Nestler 2002; Everitt and Wolf 2002). For example, repeated injection of psychostimulants into the VTA induces behavioural sensitization, whereas in sensitized animals, the injection of psychostimulants into the NAc is sufficient to elicit sensitized responses. Although the detailed modifications in neural circuitry that mediate this drug-induced behavioural plasticity remain unknown, attention is beginning to be focused on the idea that mechanisms of synaptic plasticity in operation in other regions of the brain, such as the hippocampus, may also be at work in the mesolimbic dopamine system where they play critically important roles in both adaptive forms of learning and memory (Hernandez *et al.* 2002) as well as the pathological behaviours that underlie addiction.

27.2 Mechanisms of synaptic plasticity

(a) LTP and LTD in the NAc

Before determining whether drugs of abuse elicit synaptic plasticity in the mesolimbic dopamine system, it was necessary to address the more straightforward question of whether synaptic plasticity can in fact be induced at excitatory synapses in the NAc and VTA? Studies primarily from our laboratory have shown that both LTP and LTD can be elicited at excitatory synapses on medium spiny neurons in the NAc (Kombian and Malenka 1994; Bonci and Malenka 1999; Thomas *et al.* 2000). Experiments thus far have focused primarily on the synapses made by prelimbic cortical afferents and it remains to be determined whether other glutamatergic afferents to the NAc, such as those from the hippocampus, express similar forms of plasticity. There are several similarities between the plasticity at prelimbic afferent-medium spiny neuron synapses and those commonly studied in the CA1 region of the hippocampus. For example, high-frequency tetani of presynaptic fibres induces LTP whereas low-frequency stimulation during modest depolarization of the postsynaptic cell induces LTD. Also as in the hippocampus, activation of NMDA receptors and elevation of postsynaptic calcium levels are required for both LTP and LTD. Alternatively, LTP in the NAc has the unique feature that the enhancement of the AMPA receptor-mediated component of the synaptic response is accompanied by a decrement in the NMDA receptor-mediated component (Kombian and Malenka 1994). Although the significance of this feature is not yet clear, it may be some kind of a negative feedback mechanism to limit further potentiation at synapses having undergone LTP. Although it seems likely that the signalling processes downstream of NMDA receptor activation would be shared between NMDA receptor-dependent forms of plasticity in different brain regions, very little is known about the signalling cascades that regulate either LTP or LTD in the NAc. However, a recent study reports that strong enhancement of ERK2 signalling in the absence of ERK1 can facilitate LTP induction in the NAc while having little influence on LTP in the hippocampus or amygdala (Mazzucchelli *et al.* 2002). This may indicate that different signalling pathways act downstream of NMDA receptor activation to trigger LTP in NAc cells than in other forms of plasticity elsewhere in the brain.

Surprisingly, there are several key differences in the mechanisms of LTD induced in medium spiny neurons by cortical afferent stimulation in the dorsal striatum compared with the NAc (which is also known as the ventral striatum). For example, although activation of mGluRs is reported to be necessary for the induction of LTD in the dorsal striatum (Calabresi *et al.* 2000) it is not required for NAc LTD (Thomas *et al.* 2000). In addition, in contrast to findings in the dorsal striatum, the activation of dopamine receptors is not required for the generation of LTD or for that matter LTP in the NAc. However, in both the dorsal striatum and the NAc a form of LTD dependent on the release of endocannabinoids has been reported (Gerdeman *et al.* 2002; Robbe *et al.* 2002).

(b) LTP and LTD in midbrain dopamine cells

Excitatory synapses on dopamine neurons in the midbrain dopamine regions (the VTA and substantia nigra pars compacta) can also undergo both LTP and LTD. LTP at these synapses is NMDA receptor dependent but for reasons that remain unclear, it is difficult to generate in that it requires perforated patch recording and is often small in magnitude (Bonci and Malenka 1999). Nothing is currently known about its underlying mechanisms. LTD, however, is triggered through the activation of postsynaptic voltage-gated calcium channels (Jones *et al.* 2000; Thomas *et al.* 2000). In fact, activation of these channels with depolarizing voltage steps induces LTD even in the absence of synaptic stimulation, indicating that this form of LTD does not necessarily occur specifically at activated synapses. This property would, in theory, enable a subset of activated synapses to effectively decrease excitatory synaptic strength throughout a significant proportion of the dendritic tree.

LTD in the VTA is strongly inhibited by dopamine and amphetamine through the activation of D2-like receptors (Jones *et al.* 2000; Thomas *et al.* 2000)—a modulation with potentially important functional implications. Recent studies have begun to investigate the signalling pathways that mediate LTD in the VTA. Thus, far, the pathways are quite different than those that underlie LTD in other brain regions. For example, although both VTA and hippocampal LTD appear to be mediated by the loss of surface AMPA receptors (Carroll *et al.* 2001), in VTA LTD this appears to involve increases in cAMP and the activation of PKA (Gutlerner *et al.* 2002), whereas at hippocampal synapses PKA activation inhibits AMPA receptor endocytosis. Future studies will be required to determine how the same signalling pathway can subserve seemingly opposite functions in these different brain regions.

27.3 Drug-induced synaptic plasticity

(a) Midbrain dopamine cells

In addition to the demonstration of synaptic plasticity at excitatory synapses in mesolimbic dopamine structures, there is abundant correlative evidence that supports the idea that synaptic plasticity may play a role in mediating the behavioural consequences of *in vivo* exposure to drugs of abuse and thus the development of addiction (Robinson and Berridge 1993; Kalivas 1995; Wolf 1998; Hyman and Malenka 2001; Nestler 2001; Carlezon and Nestler 2002; Everitt and Wolf 2002). This includes drug-induced changes in the levels of glutamate receptor expression and single-unit responses to glutamate as well as the behavioural effects of glutamate receptor antagonists injected into specific brain loci. A key question that had not been addressed, however, was whether drugs of abuse actually elicit changes in synaptic strength *in vivo*.

To address this issue, Ungless *et al.* (2001) prepared midbrain slices from animals that had received a single injection of cocaine one day earlier, and measured synaptic strength using whole-cell recording techniques. The single *in vivo* exposure to cocaine caused a large and robust potentiation of synaptic strength that appeared to be due, in large part, to an upregulation of the number and/or function of AMPA receptors (Fig. 27.1). This potentiation was specific in that it did not occur at excitatory synapses on hippocampal CA1 pyramidal neurons nor on GABA neurons in the VTA. Importantly, this cocaine-induced potentiation occluded LTP induction *in vitro*, indicating that the two processes share some underlying mechanisms. Two additional features of the cocaine-induced potentiation suggest a relationship between this phenomenon and the induction of behavioural sensitization. The first is that cocaine-induced potentiation is detectable 5 but not 10 days after exposure to cocaine. This is analogous to the essential but transient role that the VTA is thought to play in the induction of sensitization (Robinson and Berridge 1993; Kalivas 1995; Wolf 1998; Carlezon and Nestler 2002; Everitt and Wolf 2002). The second feature is that like

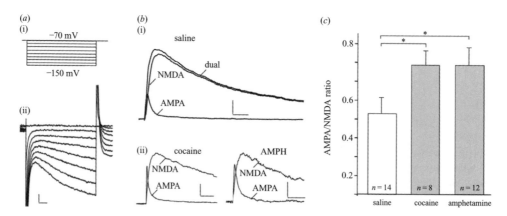

Fig. 27.1 Synaptic strength at excitatory synapses on midbrain DA neurons, as measured by measuring the ratio of AMPA-receptor to NMDA-receptor-mediated synaptic currents, is increased by *in vivo* administration of cocaine or amphetamine. (*a*) An example of I_h currents that are used to identify midbrain DA cells (calibration bars: 20 pA/50 ms). (*b*) (i) An example from a control cell of how AMPA/NMDA ratios were obtained. EPSCs were recorded at $+40$ mV (dual trace) then D-APV (50 μM) was applied to obtain the AMPA EPSC. The NMDA EPSC was obtained by digital subtraction of the AMPA EPSC from the dual EPSC. (ii) Examples of AMPA and NMDA EPSCs obtained from cocaine- and amphetamine-treated animals (calibration bars: 20 pA/15 ms). (*c*) Summary of AMPA/NMDA ratios obtained from animals that were administered saline, cocaine or amphetamine (*$p < 0.02$). Numbers within the bars indicate the number of cells examined. (Reprinted with permission from Saal *et al.* (2003).)

sensitization, cocaine-induced potentiation is blocked *in vivo* by the co-administration of cocaine with an NMDA receptor antagonist. Although the critical site of action of the NMDA receptor antagonist is unknown, a tantalizing observation (A. Bonci *et al.*, personal communication) is that cocaine appears to transiently enhance NMDA receptor-mediated responses in VTA dopamine neurons. This effect appears to be mediated through dopamine receptor activation and may be the first step towards LTP induction by cocaine exposure *in vivo*.

The existence of cocaine-induced potentiation at excitatory synapses on VTA dopamine neurons raises the question of the relationship between this cellular phenomenon and core features of addiction? That this synaptic modification may indeed be functionally important is suggested by recent findings that *in vivo* administration of a wide variety of drugs of abuse with very different molecular mechanisms of action (i.e. amphetamine, morphine, nicotine, ethanol) all cause an enhancement of strength at excitatory synapses on midbrain dopamine cells (Saal *et al.* 2003) (Figs. 27.1 and 27.2). Importantly, non-abused psychoactive drugs such as fluoxetine and carbamazepine did not cause a change. As stress has a profound facilitatory effect on the initiation and reinstatement of drug self-administration (Piazza and Le Moal 1998) the effect of an acute stress was also examined and, like drugs of abuse, was found to cause a robust increase in synaptic strength in midbrain dopamine cells (Saal *et al.* 2003). These results indicate that plasticity at excitatory synapses on dopamine cells may be a key neural adaptation contributing to addiction and its interactions with stress. Specifically, as external stimuli that are associated with the firing of midbrain dopamine cells are granted high appetitive or motivational significance, we suggest that by increasing synaptic drive onto these cells, drugs of abuse or stress enhance the motivational significance of drugs themselves as well as stimuli closely associated with drug seeking and self-administration.

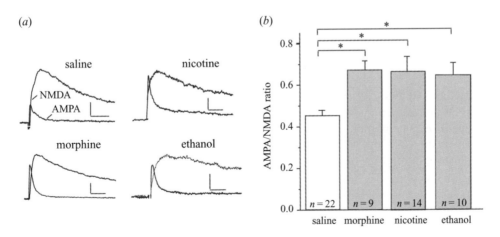

Fig. 27.2 Commonly abused drugs other than psychostimulants also increase the AMPA/NMDA ratio. (*a*) Examples of AMPA and NMDA EPSCs obtained from animals given the indicated substance (calibration bars: 20 pA/15 ms). (*b*) Summary of AMPA/NMDA ratios obtained from animals administered saline, morphine, nicotine or ethanol (*$p < 0.03$). (Reprinted with permission from Saal *et al.* (2003).)

(b) NAc

While neural adaptations in the VTA are involved in the induction of behavioural sensitization, long-lasting changes in the NAc are thought to mediate its expression. Thus, Thomas *et al.* (2001) sought to examine synaptic strength at excitatory synapses in NAc slices prepared 10–14 days after repeated (5 day) *in vivo* administration of cocaine—a treatment that caused robust behavioural sensitization. Neurons in the shell, but not the core region of NAc slices prepared from the cocaine-treated animals showed a decrease in strength at excitatory synapses made by prelimbic cortical afferents. LTD was also diminished; an occlusion that suggests that the decrease was due to mechanisms shared with LTD. As is the case for changes in the VTA, the mechanisms responsible for this drug-induced synaptic plasticity in the NAc are unclear. One intriguing hypothesis is suggested by the finding that persistent upregulation of the ΔFosB transcription factor, which is known to occur following repeated cocaine treatment, induces NAc expression of the AMPA receptor subunit GluR2 (Kelz *et al.* 1999). Owing to conductance differences in GluR2-containing versus non-GluR2-containing AMPA receptors, increases in GluR2 expression could potentially reduce AMPA receptor-mediated responses. This hypothesis, however, depends on the existence of a significant population of non-GluR2-containing synaptic AMPA receptors before cocaine exposure. If such a population existed, it should be identifiable because of the strong inward rectification of non-GluR2-containing receptors. Although this hypothesis remains intriguing, preliminary studies have failed to detect inward-rectifying AMPA receptor-mediated responses in NAc medium spiny neurons, suggesting that GluR2 incorporation does not explain the cocaine-induced depression. Another possibility is suggested by the fact that the acute administration of amphetamine to slices blocks LTP in the NAc (Li and Kauer 2000). This effect disappears in slices prepared from animals that have been repeatedly exposed to amphetamine. If this also occurs after *in vivo* cocaine exposure, such an action could initially enhance the likelihood of generating LTD.

27.4 Conclusion

Behavioural studies over the past two decades have provided compelling evidence that drugs of abuse exert powerful control over behaviour in large part because of their actions in the mesolimbic dopamine system. We have found that synaptic plasticity occurs in the NAc and VTA, two main components of this system, and that *in vivo* administration of drugs of abuse causes changes in synaptic strength probably because of the activation of the mechanisms that underlie LTP and LTD in these structures. Although the work reviewed here is still in its infancy, it hopefully illustrates that the powerful *in vivo* effects of drugs of abuse may be a valuable model for studying the role of synaptic plasticity in mediating experience-dependent plasticity. Indeed, it is already apparent that, like other forms of experience-dependent plasticity such as learning and memory (Martin *et al.* 2000), persistent drug-induced behavioural changes probably occur because of their ability to elicit long-lasting changes in synaptic weights in crucial brain circuits. Furthermore, it is important to note that the mesolimbic dopamine system did not evolve to respond to drugs of abuse but rather plays very important roles in adaptive behaviours including various types of learning and memory. Thus, examining the neural adaptations elicited by drugs of abuse will not only inform us about the pathophysiology of addiction but will also provide important information about how neural circuit modifications in the NAc and VTA contribute to normal, motivated behaviour.

References

Bonci, A. and Malenka, R. C. (1999). Properties and plasticity of excitatory synapses on dopaminergic and GABAergic cells in the ventral tegmental area. *J. Neurosci.* **19**, 3723–30.

Calabresi, P., Centonze, D., and Bernardi, G. (2000). Electrophysiology of dopamine in normal and denervated striatal neurons. *Trends Neurosci.* **23**, S57–63.

Carlezon, W. A. and Nestler, E. J. (2002). Elevated levels of GluR1 in the midbrain: a trigger for sensitization to drugs of abuse? *Trends Neurosci.* **25**, 610–15.

Carroll, R. C., Beattie, E. C., Von Zastrow, M., and Malenka, R. C. (2001). Role of AMPA receptor endocytosis in synaptic plasticity. *Nature Rev. Neurosci.* **2**, 315–24.

Everitt, B. J. and Wolf, M. E. (2002). Psychomotor stimulant addiction: a neural systems perspective. *J. Neurosci.* **22**, 3312–20.

Gerdeman, G. L., Ronesi, J., and Lovinger, D. M. (2002). Postsynaptic endocannabinoid release is critical to long-term depression in the striatum. *Nature Neurosci.* **5**, 446–51.

Gutlerner, J. L., Penick, E. C., Snyder, E. M., and Kauer, J. A. (2002). Novel protein kinase A-dependent long-term depression of excitatory synapses. *Neuron* **36**, 921–31.

Hernandez, P. J., Sadeghian, K., and Kelley, A. E. (2002). Early consolidation of instrumental learning requires protein synthesis in the nucleus accumbens. *Nature Neurosci.* **5**, 1327–31.

Hyman, S. E. and Malenka, R. C. (2001). Addiction and the brain: the neurobiology of compulsion and its persistence. *Nature Rev. Neurosci.* **2**, 695–703.

Jones, S., Kornblum, J. L., and Kauer, J. A. (2000). Amphetamine blocks long-term synaptic depression in the ventral tegmental area. *J. Neurosci.* **20**, 5575–80.

Kalivas, P. W. (1995). Interactions between dopamine and excitatory amino acids in behavioral sensitization to psychostimulants. *Drug Alcohol Depend.* **37**, 95–100.

Kelz, M. B., Chen, J., Carlezon Jr, W. A., Whisler, K., Gilden, L., Beckmann, A. M., et al. (1999). Expression of the transcription factor deltaFosB in the brain controls sensitivity to cocaine. *Nature* **401**, 272–6.

Kombian, S. B. and Malenka, R. C. (1994). Simultaneous LTP of non-NMDA- and LTD of NMDA-receptor-mediated responses in the nucleus accumbens. *Nature* **368**, 242–6.

Li, Y. and Kauer, J. A. (2000). Amphetamine interferes with longterm potentiation in the nucleus accumbens. *Soc. Neurosci. Abstr.* **26**, 1398.

Martin, S. J., Grimwood, P. D., and Morris, R. G. M. (2000). Synaptic plasticity and memory: an evaluation of the hypothesis. *A. Rev. Neurosci.* **23**, 649–711.

Mazzucchelli, C., Vantaggiato, C., Ciamei, A., Fasano, S., Pakhotin, P., Krezel, W., et al. (2002). Knockout of ERK1 MAP kinase enhances synaptic plasticity in the striatum and facilitates striatal-mediated learning and memory. *Neuron* **34**, 807–20.

Nestler, E. J. (2001). Molecular basis of long-term plasticity underlying addiction. *Nature Rev. Neurosci.* **2**, 119–28.

Piazza, P. V. and Le Moal, M. (1998). The role of stress in drug self-administration. *Trends Pharmacol. Sci.* **19**, 67–74.

Robbe, D., Kopf, M., Remaury, A., Bockaert, J., and Manzoni, O. J. (2002). Endogenous cannabinoids mediate long-term synaptic depression in the nucleus accumbens. *Proc. Natl Acad. Sci. USA* **99**, 8384–8.

Robinson, T. E. and Berridge, K. C. (1993). The neural basis of drug craving: an incentive-sensitization theory of addiction. *Brain Res. Brain Res. Rev.* **18**, 247–91.

Saal, D., Dong, Y., Bonci, A., and Malenka, R. C. (2003). Drugs of abuse and stress trigger a common synaptic adaptation in dopamine neurons. *Neuron* **37**, 577–82.

Thomas, M. J., Malenka, R. C., and Bonci, A. (2000). Modulation of long-term depression by dopamine in the mesolimbic system. *J. Neurosci.* **20**, 5581–6.

Thomas, M. J., Beurrier, C., Bonci, A., and Malenka, R. C. (2001). Long-term depression in the nucleus accumbens: a neural correlate of behavioural sensitization to cocaine. *Nature Neurosci.* **4**, 1217–23.

Ungless, M. A., Whistler, J. L., Malenka, R. C., and Bonci, A. (2001). Single cocaine exposure in vivo induces long-term potentiation in dopamine neurons. *Nature* **411**, 583–7.

Wolf, M. E. (1998). The role of excitatory amino acids in behavioral sensitization to psychomotor stimulants. *Prog. Neurobiol.* **54**, 679–720.

Glossary

AMPA	α-amino-3-hydroxy-5-methyl-4-isoxazolepropionic acid
EPSC	excitatory postsynaptic current
LTD	long-term depression
LTP	long-term potentiation
mGluR	metabotropic glutamate receptor
NAc	nucleus accumbens
NMDA	*N*-methyl-D-aspartate
VTA	ventral tegmental area

28

Synaptic plasticity in animal models of early Alzheimer's disease

Michael J. Rowan, Igor Klyubin, William K. Cullen, and Roger Anwyl

Amyloid β-protein (Aβ) is believed to be a primary cause of Alzheimer's disease (AD). Recent research has examined the potential importance of soluble species of Aβ in synaptic dysfunction, long before fibrillary Aβ is deposited and neurodegenerative changes occur. Hippocampal excitatory synaptic transmission and plasticity are disrupted in transgenic mice overexpressing human amyloid precursor protein with early onset familial AD mutations, and in rats after exogenous application of synthetic Aβ both *in vitro* and *in vivo*. Recently, naturally produced soluble Aβ was shown to block the persistence of long-term potentiation (LTP) in the intact hippocampus. Sub-nanomolar concentrations of oligomeric Aβ were sufficient to inhibit late LTP, pointing to a possible reason for the sensitivity of hippocampus-dependent memory to impairment in the early preclinical stages of AD. Having identified the active species of Aβ that can play havoc with synaptic plasticity, it is hoped that new ways of targeting early AD can be developed.

Keywords: long-term potentiation; β-amyloid; excitatory synaptic transmission; glutamate; NMDA receptors; acetylcholine

28.1 Introduction

A major goal of current research on AD is to determine the causes of the mild cognitive impairment that usually presages the insidious onset of clinical dementia. Mild cognitive impairment of preclinical AD is characterized by deficits in the forms of memory that are known to be dependent on the function of the medial temporal lobe, including the hippocampus and related structures (Laakso 2002). It is argued here that potentially reversible impairments of synaptic memory mechanisms in these brain regions are likely to precede neurodegenerative changes that are characteristic of clinical AD.

Other contributors to this volume see Chapters 7, 8, 21, 24, 25, 26, and 27) give cogent reasons why studies of synaptic plasticity, in particular LTP of fast excitatory synaptic transmission, are particularly suited to the elucidation of mechanisms of memory function. Our hope is that investigations of how putative causes of AD affect excitatory synaptic transmission and plasticity in the hippocampus will aid the discovery of the processes underlying the early memory deficits of preclinical AD. Such an approach should help to provide a fertile basis, for probing not only the causes of the synaptic dysfunction underlying memory impairment, but also possible targets for therapeutic intervention very early in the disease process.

28.2 Synaptic plasticity and the Aβ hypothesis of Alzheimer's disease

AD has been suggested to be a form of neuroplasticity failure (Mesulam 1999; Selkoe 2002). Consistent with this, the potential for neuroplasticity in the adult brain occurs unevenly in different regions, with synaptic plasticity, axonal and dendritic remo-delling and synaptogenesis being particularly high in areas affected early in AD (Arendt 2001). For example, plasticity-related increases in the length and branching of the dendritic tree during adulthood (Arendt et al. 1998), expression of the growth associated protein GAP 43 (a marker for axonal sprouting; Lin et al. 1992) and the expression levels of mRNAs for brain-derived neurotrophic factor and TrkB receptors (Okuno et al. 1999) are all relatively high in the hippocampus and entorhinal cortex. This indicates that the processes underlying experience-dependent remodelling and synaptic turnover in the adult are particularly vulnerable to the primary causes of AD.

The Aβ hypothesis of AD proposes that Aβ is a primary cause (Hardy and Selkoe 2002). The APP is axonally transported to presynaptic axon terminals where it is a transmembrane protein with a large extracellular amino terminus and a short cyto-plasmic carboxy terminus. Aβ is a 4 kDa peptide of 39–43 amino acids located at the part of APP that spans the transmembrane domain, lying partly outside and partly within the membrane (Glenner and Wong 1984; Kang et al. 1987). APP is cleaved in the middle of the Aβ between sites 16 and 17 by α-secretase to yield a secreted form of APP, sAPPα (a large 90 kDa N-terminal portion; Esch et al. 1990), which is secreted into the extracellular space and can act as a neuronal survival-promoting factor. Cleavage at the N-terminal site by β-secretase (Seubert et al. 1993) results in an approximately 99-amino-acid transmembrane fragment, C-99. This is further cleaved inside the membrane by α-secretase (which includes PS1) to yield APP intracellular domain, a fragment with a putative nuclear signalling role, and Aβ (predominantly Aβ1–40 and Aβ1–42). The latter species of Aβ is highly hydrophobic and has been particularly implicated in causing AD (Pike et al. 1995).

28.3 Transgenic animal models

(a) Familial Alzheimer's disease APP mutations

Strong support for the Aβ hypothesis came from a small proportion of familial AD clusters that are caused by mutations of APP, which lead to increased Aβ levels and the relatively early onset of dementia. Many groups have developed transgenic mice that overexpress these mutant forms of human APP. Most currently studied models show cognitive deficits and age-related disruption of synaptic markers and amyloid plaque deposition, but few strains show evidence of significant cell death (Janus et al. 2000; Ashe 2001; Chapman et al. 2001; Richardson and Burns 2002).

The neurophysiological consequences of such mutations have been examined in the hippocampus of these mutant mice. This has allowed the investigation of the role of age-related factors such as plaque deposition and synaptic loss in functional deficits. Most studies have reported, principally, either inhibition of LTP or reduction in baseline fast excitatory transmission prior to plaque deposition. The relative importance of these changes and apparent discrepancies still need to be resolved (see also Section 28.5b). For example, transgenic mice (called PDAPP mice) overexpressing hAPP mutated at valine to phenylalanine at amino acid 717 (V717F, Indiana mutation) were studied initially at age 4–5 months, prior to the deposition of Aβ. These mice had a small (less than 20%) reduction in basal synaptic transmission in the CA1 area *in vitro*. LTP induced by theta-burst conditioning stimulation was inhibited, and was associated with a change in the synaptic response during burst stimulation. In aged mice (27 months), which had Aβ plaque formation, baseline transmission was reduced by 70%, but LTP was normal (Larson *et al.* 1999). Complete inhibition of LTP of the population spike with no significant effect on baseline amplitude was detected in the CA1 area *in vivo* in PDAPP mice both at ages 3–4.5 and 24–27 months. No changes were detected in the dentate gyrus (Giacchino *et al.* 2000). In a further study on a separate line with the same mutation, greatly reduced (around 40%) basal synaptic transmission was observed *in vitro* at 1–4 months, probably owing to a decrease in the number of functional synapses even though no amyloid plaques were present at this age. LTP induction in response to strong HFS was unchanged in these animals or at a later stage (8–10 months) when amyloid plaques had been deposited (Hsia *et al.* 1999).

Transgenic mice overexpressing hAPP 695 mutated with both K670N and M671L (Swedish mutation, called Tg2576 mice) also show age-dependent plaque deposition but no major disruption of synaptic markers or cell viability. At 15–17 months, such mice had normal excitatory synaptic transmission in CA1 and dentate gyrus, but were severely impaired in LTP induction in these areas when assessed both *in vitro* and *in vivo*. Young mice of 2–8 months had no such deficits (Chapman *et al.* 1999). However, further *in vitro* studies by other researchers failed to observe a reduction in LTP in the same transgenic line at 12 or 18 months despite compromised baseline transmission (Fitzjohn *et al.* 2001). A further transgenic mouse line, with both the Swedish and Indiana mutations present, had a major loss of basal transmission *in vitro* at 2–4 months. Aβ in these animals was expressed at a high level, whereas hAPP levels remained relatively low, strongly suggesting that the loss in synapses and in synaptic transmission is caused by Aβ (Hsia *et al.* 1999).

Another mutant hAPP line (V642I, London mutation, termed TgAPP/Ld/2 mice) had a deficit in the persistence of LTP of the EPSP induced by strong HFS in CA1 at age 5–7 months, even though amyloid plaque formation was only detected in animals older than 12 months (Moechars *et al.* 1999). Recently, the inhibition of LTP was confirmed in similar mice (V717I, London mutation) but was absent in double transgenic mice that also had a conditional knockout of PS1. Since Aβ production was blocked in the double transgenics, the inhibition of LTP in V717I mice was attributed to Aβ (Dewachter *et al.* 2002). Neither of these reports included detailed analysis of baseline transmission.

In summary, hippocampal transmission and plasticity at excitatory glutamatergic synapses have been found to be sensitive markers of early dysfunction, often being reduced in young animals long before Aβ is found deposited in neuropathological plaques. This indicates that soluble Aβ (i.e. Aβ that remains in aqueous solution after high-speed centrifugation, composed of monomeric, oligomeric and protofibrillary species) may be a critical player in producing functional synaptic deficits in the absence of fibrillar Aβ or cell death.

(b) Other APP and PS mutants

Several other related transgenic models have examined the effects of modifying APP and PS expression on synaptic transmission and plasticity and therefore may help to elucidate their normal and/or pathological roles. Overall, mice with loss of APP had reduced LTP in response only to certain conditioning protocols. Generally, transgenic mice expressing human familial AD PS mutations had facilitated LTP, possibly owing to alterations in Ca buffering, whereas transgenic mice underexpressing PSs had decreased LTP induction, possibly owing to increased GABAergic transmission. None of these mutations was reported to affect basal fast excitatory synaptic transmission.

Transgenic mice lacking the APP gene (APP null) at age 8–12 months or 20–24 months had normal LTP induced by a weak HFS (10 stimuli at 100 Hz) but had reduced LTP induced by a subsequent (30 min later) stronger theta-burst HFS (4×10 stimuli at 100 Hz), with the level of LTP being reduced immediately following the HFS (Seabrook et al. 1999; see also Dawson et al. 1999). By contrast, LTP induced by a strong HFS of 100 Hz for 1 s was not reduced, either in control media or in the presence of picrotoxin (Seabrook et al. 1999; Fitzjohn et al. 2000). GABAergic inhibition was also reduced in these mice, the inhibitory postsynaptic current amplitude being reduced (Seabrook et al. 1999).

Transgenic mice expressing human PS mutations (familial AD-linked mutants PS1[A246E] or PS2[N141I]) did not display any pathological deficiencies. They had normal LTP induction in CA1 in response to strong HFS, but LTP induction was enhanced in response to a weak HFS, with controls showing LTP declining to baseline over 2 h, but mutants having non-declining LTP. Glutamate application led to a higher than normal Ca^{2+} elevation in transgenic mice (Schneider et al. 2001). Further studies in mice with familial AD-linked mutations in PS1 (deletion of exon 9 variant, M146L and A246E mutations) also showed normal basal transmission and enhanced LTP (larger amplitude and more persistent) in response to theta burst and HFS (Parent et al. 1999; Barrow et al. 2000; Zaman et al. 2000) and also showed enhanced inhibitory transmission (Zaman et al. 2000).

In transgenic mice in which PS1 conditional knockout was restricted to the postnatal forebrain (PS1 expression was progressively eliminated from the third postnatal week), levels of $A\beta 1–40$ and $A\beta 1–42$ were reduced compared with controls, while APP C-terminal fragments increased. Basal transmission and LTP induction in response to theta burst or HFS was normal in such mice (Yu et al. 2001). Somewhat similarly, mutant mice underexpressing PS1 (PS1± mice) from birth had normal basal transmission in CA1. Although LTP induction in response to a single theta burst or a single tetanus was normal in these mice, LTP induction in response to multiple tetanus was reduced, with LTP declining more rapidly than in controls (Morton et al. 2002). In view of the role of PS in the metabolism of the APP C-terminal, it is interesting that transgenic mice expressing an amyloidogenic C-terminal fragment of APP (C104 mice) exhibited age-related amyloid deposition and decrease in CA1 cell number. Although basal synaptic transmission was not reported, 8–10-month-old transgenic mice showed deficient LTP induction, with significant inhibition at times greater than 10 min post-HFS (Nalbantoglu et al. 1997).

28.4 Exogenously applied Aβ

Overall, although transgenic animals offer many advantages in the study of possible causes of AD, it has not been possible to disentangle clearly the role of APP *per se* or its breakdown products, including the different soluble and fibrillar Aβ species. Direct exogenous application of Aβ provides an alternative approach to determine whether Aβ can cause deficits in hippocampal excitatory synaptic transmission/plasticity and the necessity for amyloid plaque formation and neurodegeneration.

(a) Effect of Aβ on LTP in vitro

Several studies have shown that synthetic Aβ inhibits LTP induction *in vitro*. Thus, in hippocampal slices prepared from 20–30-day-old rats, soluble Aβ1–42 (500 nM) was found to inhibit LTP induction by strong HFS of the medial perforant path in the dentate gyrus both of the population spike (Lambert *et al.* 1998) and EPSPs (Wang *et al.* 2002). Both early- and late-phase LTP were strongly inhibited in these studies, whereas basal AMPA receptormediated synaptic transmission was not altered, although there was a reduction in paired-pulse depression at a short (20 ms) inter-pulse interval (Wang *et al.* 2002). In these studies, Aβ1–42 was specially prepared to contain large metastable Aβ oligomeric assemblies (termed ADDLs), providing evidence that non-fibrillar Aβ can selectively disrupt both short-term and long-term synaptic plasticity.

Similarly, LTP of field EPSPs in rat CA1 and the medial perforant path of the dentate gyrus was inhibited by Aβ1–40, Aβ1–42 and the truncated Aβ fragment 25–35 at concentrations of 200 nM or 1 μM. The N-terminal sequence of Aβ25–35 was found to be necessary for inhibition of LTP induction (Chen *et al.* 2000). In contrast to these studies showing an inhibition of LTP induction, synthetic Aβ1–40 (200 nM) enhanced LTP induction in the associational–commissural pathway of the dentate gyrus of 30–50-day-old rats (Wu *et al.* 1995a). Basal AMPA receptor-mediated synaptic transmission was not affected in this study.

In summary, the inhibitory effects of Aβ on LTP *in vitro* occurred in the absence of changes in baseline transmission and thus do not appear to be caused by a toxic action of the Aβ resulting in rapid neurodegeneration. Moreover, truncated Aβ variants that were not lethal to cultured neurons also blocked LTP induction (Chen *et al.* 2000). Intriguingly, non-fibrillar Aβ 1–42 (Wang *et al.* 2002) and Aβ variants that did not form fibrils *in vitro* (Chen *et al.* 2000) inhibited LTP, pointing to a critical role for soluble peptide.

(b) Effect of Aβ on LTP in vivo

Consistent with most *in vitro* studies, synthetic Aβ also inhibits LTP in the intact hippocampus. Thus late-phase LTP of field EPSPs in the CA1 area was strongly inhibited at doses that had no acute effect on baseline excitatory transmission in adult rats by intracerebroventricular (i.c.v.) injection of Aβ1–40 (0.4 and 3.5 nmol, but not 0.1 nmol), Aβ 1–42 (0.01 nmol) and the Aβ-containing C-terminal fragment CT105 (0.05 nmol). In these studies, LTP was only significantly inhibited at a time greater than 2 h post-HFS, and the LTP was completely blocked by Aβ1–40 and Aβ 1–42 at

3 h post-HFS (Cullen *et al.* 1997*a*), implicating late LTP. Somewhat similarly, LTP of EPSPs in the CA1 area was inhibited by the truncated fragments Aβ25–35 (10 nmol, 100 nmol) and Aβ35–25, but not Aβ 15–25, at times greater than 30 min post HFS (Freir *et al.* 2001).

Other studies have examined the delayed neurophysiological effects of Aβ *in vivo*. In contrast to the acute effect of Aβ1–40 (3.5 nmol), there was a small reduction in baseline transmission in the CA1 area 24 h after a single i.c.v. injection. The reduction was present for at least 5 days, whereas LTP was not affected at this time (Cullen *et al.* 1996).

In another study, induction of LTP of field EPSPs in the dentate gyrus by strong HFS was inhibited after direct intrahippocampal injection of Aβ1–43 or a combination of Aβ1–40 and Aβ1–43 in adult rats. Late-phase LTP of the EPSP was most sensitive to disruption, whereas EPSP-spike LTP was largely intact. The effect of the Aβ was examined *ca.* 7–16 weeks after the injections, a time when focal amyloid deposits and cell atrophy were detected. A reduction in baseline synaptic transmission and deficits in working memory were also present (Stéphan *et al.* 2001).

Somewhat analogous to the *in vitro* studies on transgenic mice, two studies examined the effects of *in vivo* Aβ exposure on synaptic function in the hippocampal slice of adult rats. Whereas acute single i.c.v. injection of synthetic Aβ1–40 (0.4 or 3.5 but not 0.1 nmol) caused a reduction in baseline transmission and no change in LTP in the dentate gyrus 48 h later (Cullen *et al.* 1996), continuous i.c.v. infusion of Aβ1–40 (300 pmol day^{-1}) for 10–11 days inhibited LTP of the population spike in the CA1 area (Itoh *et al.* 1999). In the latter study, there was a tendency to require a greater current to evoke equivalent-sized spikes.

(c) Effects of naturally produced Aβ on synaptic plasticity

The brains of transgenic animals accumulate a variety of Aβ species, both soluble and insoluble, the relative importance of which in the disruption of synaptic transmission and plasticity is difficult if not impossible to separate. One of the problems with most published studies of exogenously applied Aβ is that the synthetic Aβ peptides are usually present in several different undefined states of association/aggregation. Some of these states may never occur naturally. We therefore believe that it is necessary to study the effects of naturally produced Aβ species as well as synthetic peptides.

By using medium collected from cells transfected with mutant hAPP (V717F) that secrete nanomolar concentrations of soluble Aβ, in the absence of fibrillar Aβ, we were able to examine the contribution of soluble monomers and oligomers of variable length (including Aβ1–42) to the effects of Aβ on synaptic function in the intact hippocampus (Walsh *et al.* 2002; Fig. 28.1). Although basal glutamatergic transmission was unaffected by such low amounts of Aβ, the persistence of LTP was reduced to less than 3 h when i.c.v. injected shortly before HFS. Remarkably, when all of the monomers were selectively cleared from the medium using the protease insulin-degrading enzyme, leaving only oligomers, the block was unaffected. This means that the oligomers are by far the most active species even though they were present only in sub-nanomolar concentrations. By contrast, medium from cells that were exposed to low doses of a γ-secretase inhibitor DAPM (N-[N-3,5-difluorophenacetyl)-L-alanyl]-S-phenylglycine methyl ester) to partially block the production of Aβ, thereby preferentially reducing oligomer formation but leaving monomers relatively unaffected, did not block LTP.

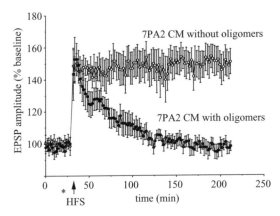

Fig. 28.1 Naturally secreted oligomers of Aβ inhibit LTP of excitatory synaptic transmission in the intact hippocampus of anaesthetized rats (adapted from Walsh *et al.* 2002). i.c.v. (asterisk) injection of conditioned medium from cells transfected with mutant APP that release soluble Aβ oligomers (7PA2 CM with oligomers, closed circles) completely blocked LTP measured at 3 h after HFS (arrow), whereas conditioned medium from cells pretreated with a γ-secretase inhibitor, at a concentration that reduced Aβ oligomer production relatively selectively, prevented the block (7PA2 CM without oligomers, open circles).

This finding thus confirms the role of soluble Aβ oligomers and also gives support to the use of relatively low doses of γ- and possibly β-secretase inhibitors as a viable pharmacological approach to the therapy of AD.

Recently we have confirmed that medium containing sub-nanomolar concentrations of naturally produced Aβ oligomers also inhibits LTP in the rat dentate gyrus *in vitro* (H.-W. Wang, D. M. Walsh, M. J. Rowan, D. J. Selkoe and R. Anwyl, unpublished observations).

In view of the apparently limited ability of exogenously applied Aβ to penetrate into cells (Bi *et al.* 2002), this approach does not directly address the potentially important role of raised intracellular Aβ. In this context, it will be interesting to examine the effect of viral application of Aβ.

28.5 Cellular mechanisms of Aβ action

Many cellular mechanisms have been proposed to explain the toxic effects of high concentrations of fibrillar Aβ. Relatively little is known about the mechanisms of action of low concentrations of soluble Aβ. We focus on possible cholinergic and NMDA receptor-mediated mechanisms given the current, albeit limited, pharmacotherapy of AD with cholinesterase inhibitors such as donepezil and the NMDA receptor antagonist memantine.

(a) Role of acetylcholine and related signalling

There is extensive support for the involvement of cholinergic mechanisms in the biochemical and behavioural effects of soluble Aβ (Auld *et al.* 2002). Recent studies have found that alterations in acetylcholine and related signalling can reverse the inhibitory effect of Aβ on LTP, thereby providing a mechanistic basis for this important therapeutic target. Thus co-administration of an acetycholinesterase inhibitor, huperzine A, at a concentration that did not by itself enhance LTP induction completely prevented the suppression of LTP of the population spike by acute application of truncated Aβ fragments 25–35 and 31–35 in the CA1 area of the rat (Ye and Qiao 1999). These authors suggested that the inhibitory effect of Aβ on LTP induction may be via inhibiting cholinergic transmission, perhaps suppressing synthesis and/or release of acetylcholine (Hoshi et al. 1997) or blocking acetylcholine receptors (Kelly et al. 1996). Similarly, the block of LTP persistence by Aβ1–40 (3.5 nmol, i.c.v.) in vivo was completely prevented by pretreatment with the cholinesterase inhibitor physostigmine (0.1 mg kg^{-1}, i.p.). This dose of physostigmine on its own did not have a significant effect on baseline transmission or on the magnitude of LTP induced by HFS (Cullen et al. 1997b). Recently, Sun and Alkon (2002) reported that the truncated Aβ 25–35 (but not Aβ 35–25) injected i.c.v. 4–6 days before recording in vitro greatly reduced a long-term synaptic modification of GABA$_A$ receptor-mediated synaptic potentials that depends on the associative activation of cholinergic and GABAergic inputs. Cholinergic (muscarinic)-induced theta in CA1 pyramidal cells was inhibited, but LTP was unaffected.

Much interest has been generated in the possible role of nicotinic receptors in the actions of Aβ. The α7 subunit-containing nicotinic receptor (α7nAChR) that has been suggested to be a high-affinity receptor for Aβ1–42. Aβ1–42, at very low concentration (0.1–100 nM), activates the ERK2 MAPK cascade acutely in hippocampal slices, an effect that is blocked by selective α7nAChR antagonists and prevents external Ca^{2+} influx (Dineley et al. 2001). It was suggested that Ca^{2+} influx via α7nAChR and α7nAChR-dependent depolarization led to MAPK activation. Subchronic exposure of organotypic hippocampal slice cultures for 6 days to Aβ1–42 upregulated α7nAChR. In addition, hAPP transgenic mice (Tg2576) had pronounced age-dependent upregulation of α7nAChR, which was accompanied by biphasic alterations in downstream ERK2 and CREB protein activation (Dineley et al. 2001). Whether or not these changes are related to the previously described disruption of synaptic function in these mice (Chapman et al. 1999; Fitzjohn et al. 2001) remains to be determined. Itoh et al. (1999) reported that nicotine failed to affect potentiation of the population spike in slices from animals treated with subchronic infusion of Aβ1–40 in vivo, and LTP was blocked. Since nicotine enhanced short-term potentiation in controls, this finding is consistent with a loss of nicotinic regulation of glutamatergic mechanisms. The involvement of GABAergic mechanisms needs to be addressed as α7nAChRs are located primarily on inhibitory interneurons (Frazier et al. 1998; Pettit et al. 2001). Clearly, any involvement of ERK/MAPK/CREB also potentially implicates many other transmitter pathways, including glutamatergic directly (see below).

(b) Role of NMDA receptor-mediated synaptic transmission

Since many forms of hippocampal synaptic plasticity and toxicity are NMDA receptor-dependent, alterations in NMDA receptor-mediated synaptic transmission and related mechanisms may contribute to the effects of Aβ. Overall, although there is some evidence of increased NMDA receptor-mediated function and excitotoxicity under defined in vivo and in vitro experimental conditions, it will be important to evaluate their general significance. Thus, Aβ1–40 (200 nM) can selectively elicit a rapid and persistent increase in NMDA receptor-mediated, but not AMPA receptor-mediated, transmission in the dentate gyrus *in vitro* (Wu *et al.* 1995*b*). Moreover, the delayed reduction in baseline synaptic transmission in the CA1 area *in vivo* caused by Aβ1–40 (3.5 nmol) can be prevented by treatment with the NMDA receptor antagonist CPP (7 mg kg^{-1} x2, i.p.) (Cullen *et al.* 1996).

Transgenic mice overexpressing hAPP (V717F) had a relative upregulation of NMDA receptor-mediated synaptic transmission at a time when AMPA receptor-mediated transmission was reduced (Hsia *et al.* 1999). Consistent with an age-related increased potential for NMDA receptor-dependent excitotoxicity, Fitzjohn *et al.* (2001) reported that the non-selective glutamate receptor antagonist kynurenic acid (1 mM), when present at the anoxic period of slice preparation, prevented the reduction in baseline transmission at 12 months in hAPP K670N/ M671L mice. However, this strategy was not effective at a later age (18 months) or at 8–9 months in V717F mice (Hsia *et al.* 1999; see also Chapman *et al.* 2001). In this context, it is interesting that glutamate can potentiate the inhibitory effect of Aβ1–42 on LTP (Nakagami and Oda 2002). In view of the putative involvement of the p38 MAPK pathway in excitotoxicity, it is of interest that the acute reduction in baseline synaptic transmission and block of LTP in the dentate gyrus of young rats by the truncated fragment Aβ25–35 (1 μM) was prevented by perfusion with the inhibitor SB203580 (1 μM) (Saleshando and O'Connor 2000).

By contrast, Aβ 1–42 (200 nM and 1 μM) has recently been reported to reduce NMDA receptor-mediated synaptic currents in the dentate gyrus (Chen *et al.* 2002). Aβ1–42 and ADDLs at the sublethal concentrations of 5 μM and 100 nM, respectively, also strongly suppressed a NMDA-evoked/depolarization-induced increase in CREB phosphorylation in cultured cortical neurons, whereas Aβ25–35 (10 μM) was inactive (Tong *et al.* 2001). CREB phosphorylation has been implicated in late LTP. Remarkably, in a recent study rolipram and forskolin, agents that enhance the cAMP-signalling pathway can reverse inhibition of LTP by Aβ1–42. This reversal was blocked by H89, an inhibitor of protein kinase A (Vitolo *et al.* 2002).

An intriguing corollary to the block of LTP by Aβ is the facilitation of LTD induction by low-frequency stimulation and time-dependent LTP reversal in the CA1 area by very low-dose Aβ1–42 (1 pmol i.c.v.) and CT105 (1– 2 pmol), respectively, in the adult rat. Both effects were blocked by the NMDA receptor antagonist D-AP5 (100 nmol), indicating their NMDA receptor dependence (Kim *et al.* 2001). Somewhat similarly, Aβ1–42 applied in the first hour after HFS inhibited LTP, and inhibition of calcineurin activity with FK506 or cyclosporin A completely prevented this effect (Chen *et al.* 2002). By contrast, ADDLs (500 nM) failed to affect a large, apparently NMDA receptor-independent form of LTD in the dentate gyrus of young (14–19-day-old) rats (Wang *et al.* 2002).

28.6 Conclusion

Extracellular deposition of fibrillar Aβ and cell death are not required for the development of functional deficits in AMPA receptor-mediated hippocampal synaptic transmission and plasticity in transgenic mutant hAPP mouse and acute Aβ rat models. Good evidence that the disruption of LTP is caused by highly mobile Aβ oligomers is

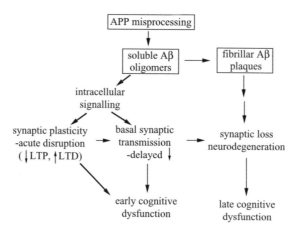

Fig. 28.2 Speculative overview of the actions of Aβ oligomers on hippocampal synaptic transmission and plasticity that may underlie the mild cognitive impairment of early AD. Soluble Aβ oligomers released into the extracellular space consequent to APP misprocessing may, in the absence of adequate clearance, diffuse to neighbouring cells. The presence of sub-nanomolar concentrations of Aβ oligomers would rapidly block LTP and promote LTD of fast excitatory transmission in a use-dependent manner, as a result of disruption of intracellular signalling, NMDA receptor-mediated transmission and cholinergic transmission. A delayed reduction in basal AMPA receptor-mediated transmission would be caused possibly by the shift from LTP-like to LTD-like synaptic plasticity and increased vulnerability to excitotoxicity. The rapid disruption of synaptic plasticity and delayed reduction in basal transmission may lead to the insidious but intermittent mild cognitive impairment of preclinical AD. In clinical AD, such mechanisms may be superimposed on the irreversible neurodegeneration and synaptic loss that may be caused primarily by (proto-) fibrillary Aβ and thereby contribute to progressive dementia.

provided by experiments using exogenously applied natural and synthetic Aβ. Further studies are required to determine the roles of recently discovered specific receptor/ signalling mechanisms and facilitated LTD/depotentiation in either the block of LTP or reductions in baseline transmission.

This research may provide insight into the likely causes and possible treatments of mild cognitive impairment in preclinical AD (see Fig. 28.2 for a schematic view of possible mechanisms and targets). Clearly, the mechanisms that are described here are probably more relevant to the very early rather than late symptoms of AD. Progressively higher concentrations of fibrillar Aβ associated with major neurodegenerative changes are found in clinical AD and are considered to be significant factors in the later course of the disease. However, it is possible that a disruption of synaptic plasticity-related mechanisms by soluble Aβ also contributes to clinical symptoms (Lue *et al.* 1999; McLean *et al.* 1999). Indeed, if the changes in synaptic function described here occur in the early preclinical stages they may provide the necessary trigger that interacts with age, oxidative status, energy supply and other major vulnerability factors to precipitate the onset of clinical disease.

The authors gratefully acknowledge the continued support of the Wellcome Trust, Irish Health Research Board, Irish Higher Education Authority (PRTLI), EU, and Science Foundation Ireland. They thank Professor Dennis Selkoe, Dr Dominic Walsh, Dr Joung-Hun Kim, and Dr Jianqun Wu for their major contribution to the work described.

References

Arendt, T. (2001). Disturbance of neuronal plasticity is a critical pathogenetic event in Alzheimer's disease. *Int. J. Dev. Neurosci.* **19**, 231–45.

Arendt, T., Brueckner, M. K., Gertz, H. J., and Marcova, L. (1998). Cortical distribution of neurofibrillary tangles in Alzheimer's disease matches the pattern of neurones that retain their capacity of plastic remodelling in the adult brain. *Neuroscience* **83**, 991–1002.

Ashe, K. H. (2001). Learning and memory in transgenic mice modeling Alzheimer's disease. *Learn. Mem.* **8**, 301–8.

Auld, D. S., Kornecook, T. J., Bastianetto, S., and Quirion, R. (2002). Alzheimer's disease and the basal forebrain cholinergic system: relations to beta-amyloid peptides, cognition, and treatment strategies. *Prog. Neurobiol.* **68**, 209–45.

Barrow, P. A., Empson, R. M., Gladwell, S. J., Anderson, C. M., Killick, R., Yu, X., *et al.* (2000). Functional phenotype in transgenic mice expressing mutant human presenilin-1. *Neurobiol. Dis.* **7**, 119–26.

Bear, M. F. (2003). Bidirectional synaptic plasticity: from reality to theory. *Phil. Trans. R. Soc. Lond.* B **358**, 649–55. (DOI 10.1098/rstb.2002.1255.)

Bi, X., Gall, C. M., Zhou, J., and Lynch, G. (2002). Uptake and pathogenic effects of amyloid beta peptide 1–42 are enhanced by integrin antagonists and blocked by NMDA receptor antagonists. *Neuroscience* **112**, 827–40.

Bozon, B., Kelly, Á., Josselyn, S. A., Silva, A. J., Davis, S., and Laroche, S. (2003). MAPK, CREB and *zif268* are all required for the consolidation of recognition memory. *Phil. Trans. R. Soc. Lond.* B **358**, 805–14. (DOI 10.1098/rstb.2002.1224.)

Chapman, P. F., Falinska, A. M., Knevett, S. G., and Ramsay, M. F. (2001). Genes, models and Alzheimer's disease. *Trends Genet.* **17**, 254–61.

Chapman, P. F. Seabrook, G. R., Zheng, H., Smith, D. W. Graham, S., O'Dowd, G., *et al.* (1999). Impaired synaptic plasticity and learning in aged amyloid precursor protein transgenic mice. *Nat. Neurosci.* **2**, 271–6.

Chen, Q., Kagan, B. L., Hirakura, Y., and Xie, C. (2000). Impairments of hippocampal long-term potentiation by Alzheimer amyloid-β peptide. *J. Neurosci. Res.* **60**, 65–72.

Chen, Q. S., Wei, W. Z., Shimahara, T., and Xie, C. W. (2002). Alzheimer amyloid β-peptide inhibits the late phase of long-term potentiation through calcineurin-dependent mechanisms in the hippocampal dentate gyrus. *Neurobiol. Learn. Mem.* **77**, 354–71.

Cullen, W. K., Wu, J., Anwyl, R., and Rowan, M. J. (1996). β-Amyloid produces a delayed NMDA receptor-dependent reduction in synaptic transmission in rat hippocampus. *NeuroReport* **8**, 87–92.

Cullen, W. K., Suh, Y. H., Anwyl, R., and Rowan, M. J. (1997*a*). Block of LTP in rat hippocampus *in vivo* by β-amyloid precursor protein fragments. *NeuroReport* **8**, 3213–17.

Cullen, W. K., Anwyl, R., and Rowan, M. J. (1997*b*). β-amyloid produces a selective block of late-phase long-term potentiation in rat hippocampus *in vivo*. *Br. J. Pharmacol.* **122**, 330P.

Dawson, G. R., White, G. L., Jones, M. W., Cooper-Blacketer, D., Marshall, V. J., Irizarry, M., *et al.* (1999). Age-related cognitive deficits, impaired long-term potentiation and reduction in synaptic marker density in mice lacking the beta-amyloid precursor protein. *Neuroscience* **90**, 1–13.

Dewachter, I., Reverse, D., Caluwaerts, N., Ris, L., Kuiperi, C., Van den Haute, C., *et al.* (2002). Neuronal deficiency of presenilin 1 inhibits amyloid plaque formation and corrects hippocampal long-term potentiation but not a cognitive defect of amyloid precursor protein [V717I] transgenic mice. *J. Neurosci.* **22**, 3445–53.

Dineley, K. T., Westerman, M., Bui, D., Bell, K., Ashe, K. H., and Sweatt, J. D. (2001). β-Amyloid activates the mitogen-activated protein kinase cascade via hippocampal α7 nicotinic acetylcholine receptors: *in vitro* and *in vivo* mechanisms related to Alzheimer's disease. *J. Neurosci.* **21**, 4125–33.

Esch, F. S., Keim, P. S., Beatie, E. C., Blacher, R. W., Culwell, A. R., Olterdorf, T., *et al.* (1990). Cleavage of amyloid beta peptide during constitutive processing of its precursor. *Science* **248**, 1122–4.

Fitzjohn, S. M., Morton, R. A., Davies, C. H., Seabrook, G. R., and Collingridge, G. L. (2000). Similar levels of long-term potentiation in amyloid precursor protein null and wild type mice in the CA1 region of picrotoxin treated slices. *Neurosci. Lett.* **288**, 9–12.

Fitzjohn, S. M., Morton, R. A., Kuenzi, F., Rosahl, T. W., Shearman, M., Lewis, H., *et al.* (2001). Age-related impairment of synaptic transmission but normal long-term potentiation in transgenic mice that overexpress the human APP695SWE mutant form of amyloid precursor protein. *J. Neurosci.* **21**, 4691–8.

Frazier, C. J., Rollins, Y. D., Breese, C. R., Leonard, S., Freedman, R., and Dunwiddie, T. V. (1998). Acetylcholine activates an α-bungarotoxin-sensitive nicotinic current in rat hippocampal interneurons, but not pyramidal cells. *J. Neurosci.* **18**, 1187–95.

Freir, D. B., Holscher, C., and Herron, C. E. (2001). Blockade of long-term potentiation by beta-amyloid peptides in the CA1 region of the rat hippocampus *in vivo*. *J. Neurophysiol.* **85**, 708–13.

Giacchino, J., Criado, J. R., Games, D., and Henriksen, S. (2000). *In vivo* synaptic transmission in young and aged amyloid precursor protein transgenic mice. *Brain Res.* **876**, 185–90.

Glenner, G. G. and Wong, C. W. (1984). Alzheimer's disease and Down's syndrome: sharing of a unique cardiovascular amyloid fibril protein. *Biochem. Biophys. Res. Commun.* **122**, 1131–5.

Hardy, J. and Selkoe, D. J. (2002). The amyloid hypothesis of Alzheimer's disease: progress and problems on the road to therapeutics.*Science* **297**, 353–6.

Hédou, G. and Mansuy, I. M. (2003). Inducible molecular switches for the study of long-term potentiation. *Phil. Trans. R. Soc. Lond.* B **358**, 797–804. (DOI 10.1098/rstb.2002. 1245.)

Hoshi, M., Takashima, A., Murayama, M., Yasutake, K., Yoshida, N., Ishiguro, K., *et al.* (1997). Non-toxic amyloid β-peptide 1–42 suppresses acetylcholine synthesis. *J. Biol. Chem.* **272**, 2038–41.

Hsia, A. Y., Masliah, E., McCologue, L., Nicoll, R. A., and Mucke, L. (1999). Plaque-independent disruption of neural circuits in Alzheimer's disease mouse models. *Proc. Natl Acad. Sci. USA* **96**, 3228–33.

Itoh, A., Akaike, T., Sokabe, M., Nitta, A., and Nabeshima, T. (1999). Impairment of long-term potentiation in hippocampal slices of β-amyloid-infused rats. *Eur. J. Pharmacol.* **3**, 167–75.

Janus, C., Chishti, M., and Westaway, D. (2000). Transgenic mouse models of Alzheimer's disease. *Biochim. Biophys. Acta* **1502**, 63–75.

Kang, J., Lemaire, H. G., Unterbeck, A., Salbaum, J. M., Masters, C., Grzchik, K. H., *et al.* (1987). The precursor of Alzheimer's disease amyloid A4 resembles a cell surface receptor. *Nature* **325**, 733–6.

Kelly, J. F., Furukawa, K., Barger, S. W., Rengen, M. R., Mark, R. J., Blanc, E. M., *et al.* (1996). Amyloid β-peptide disrupts muscaricic transmission. *Proc. Natl Acad. Sci. USA* **93**, 6753–8.

Kim, J.-H., Anwyl, R., Suh, Y.-H., Djamgoz, M. B., and Rowan, M. J. (2001). Use-dependent effects of amyloidogenic fragments of β-amyloid precursor protein on synaptic plasticity in rat hippocampus *in vivo*. *J. Neurosci.* **21**, 1327–33.

Laakso, M. P. (2002). Structural imaging in cognitive impairment and the dementias: an update. *Curr. Opin. Neurol.* **15**, 415–21.

Lambert, M. P., Barlow, A. K., Chromy, B. A., Kraaft, G. A., and Klein, W. L. (1998). Diffusible nonfibrillar ligands derived from Aβ1–42 are potent central nervous system neurotoxins. *Proc. Natl Acad. Sci. USA* **95**, 6448–53.

Larson, J., Lynch, G., Games, D., and Seubert, P. (1999). Alterations in synaptic transmission and long-term potentiation in hippocampal slices from young and aged PDAPP mice. *Brain Res.* **840**, 23–35.

Lin, L. H., Bock, S., Carpenter, K., Rose, M., and Norden, J. J. (1992). Synthesis and transport of GAP-43 in entorhinal cortex of neurons and perforant pathway during lesion-induced sprouting and reactive neurogenesis. *Mol. Brain Res.* **14**, 147–53.

Lisman, J. (2003). Long-term potentiation: outstanding questions/attempted synthesis. *Phil. Trans. R. Soc. Lond.* B **358**, 829–42. (DOI 10.1098/rstb.2002.1242.)

Lue, L. F., Kuo, Y. M., Roher, A. E., Brachova, L., Shen, Y., Sue, L., *et al.* (1999). Soluble amyloid beta peptide concentration as a predictor of synaptic change in Alzheimer's disease. *Am. J. Pathol.* **155**, 853–62.

McLean, C. A., Cherny, R. A., Fraser, F. W., Fuller, S. J., Smith, M. J., Beyreuther, K., *et al.* (1999). Soluble pool of A beta amyloid as a determinant of severity of neurodegeneration in Alzheimer's disease. *Ann. Neurol.* **46**, 860–6.

Mesulam, M. M. (1999). Neuroplasticity failure in Alzheimer's disease: bridging the gap between plaques and tangles. *Neuron* **24**, 521–29.

Moechars, D., Dewachter, I., Lorent, K., Reverse, D., Baekelandt, V., Naidu, A., *et al.* (1999). Early phenotypic changes in transgenic mice that overexpress different mutants of amyloid precursor protein in brain. *J. Biol. Chem.* **274**, 6483–92.

Morris, R. G. M. (2003). Long-term potentiation and memory. *Phil. Trans. R. Soc. Lond.* B **358**, 643–7. (DOI 10.1098/ rstb.2002.1230.)

Morton, R. A., Kuenzi, F. M., Fitzjohn, S. M., Rosahl, T. W., Smith, D., Zheng, H., *et al.* (2002). Impairment in hippocampal long-term potentiation in mice under-expressing the Alzheimer's disease related gene presenillin-1. *Neurosci. Lett.* **319**, 37–40.

Nakagami, Y. and Oda, T. (2002). Glutamate exacerbates amyloid β1–42-induced impairment of long-term potentiation in rat hippocampal slices. *Jpn J. Pharmacol.* **88**, 223–6.

Nalbantoglu, J. Tirado-Santiago, G., Lahsaini, A., Poirier, J., Goncalves, O., Verge, G., *et al.* (1997). Impaired learning and LTP in mice expressing the carboxy terminus of the Alzheimer amyloid precursor protein. *Nature* **387**, 500–5.

Okuno, H., Tokuyama, W., and Miyashita, Y. (1999). Quantitative evaluation of neurotrophin and trk mRNA expression in visual and limbic areas along the occipito-tempor-hippocampal pathway in adult macaque monkeys. *J. Comp. Neurol.* **408**, 378–98.

Parent, A., Linden, D. J., Sisodia, S. S., and Borchelt, D. R. (1999). Synaptic transmission and hippocampal long-term potentiation in transgenic mice expressing FAD-linked presenilin-1. *Neurobiol. Dis.* **6**, 56–62.

Pettit, D. L., Shao, Z., and Yakel, J. L. (2001). β-Amyloid 1–42 peptide directly modulates nicotinic receptors in the rat hippocampal slice. *J. Neurosci.* **21**, 1–5.

Pike, C. J., Walencewicz, A. J., Kosmoski, J., Cribbs, D. H., Glabe, C. G., and Cotman, C. W. (1995). Structure–activity analyses of β-amyloid peptides: contribution of the β25–35 region to aggregation and neurotoxicity. *J. Neurochem.* **64**, 253–65.

Pittenger, C. and Kandel, E. R. (2003). In search of general mechanisms for long-lasting plasticity: *Aplysia* and the hippocampus. *Phil. Trans. R. Soc. Lond.* B **358**, 757–63. (DOI 10. 1098/ rstb.2002.1247.)

Richardson, J. A. and Burns, D. K. (2002). Mouse models of Alzheimer's disease: a quest for plaques and tangles. *Inst. Lab. Anim. Resources J.* **43**, 89–99.

Saleshando, G. and O'Connor, J. J. (2000). SB203580, the p38 mitogen-activated protein kinase inhibitor blocks the inhibitory effect of β-amyloid on long-term potentiation in the rat hippocampus. *Neurosci. Lett.* **288**, 119–22.

Schneider, I. Reverse, D., Dewachter, I., Ris, L., Caluwaerts, N., Kuiperi, C., *et al.* (2001). Mutant presenilins disturb neuronal calcium homeostasis in the brain of transgenic mice, decreasing the threshold for excitotoxicity and facilitating long-term potentiation. *J. Biol. Chem.* **276**, 11 539–44.

Seabrook, G. R. (1999). Mechanisms contributing to the deficits in hippocampal synaptic plasticity in mice lacking amyloid precursor protein. *Neuropharmacology* **38**, 349–59.

Selkoe, D. J. (2002). Alzheimer's disease is a synaptic failure. *Science* **298**, 789–91.

Seubert, P., Oltersdorf, T., Lee, M. G., Barbow, R., Blomquist, C., Davis, D. L., *et al.* (1993). Secretion of β-amyloid precursor protein cleaved at the amino-terminus of the β-amyloid peptide. *Nature* **361**, 260–3.

Stéphan, A., Laroche, S., and Davis, S. (2001). Generation of aggregated β-amyloid in the rat hippocampus impairs synaptic transmission and plasticity and causes memory deficits. *J. Neurosci.* **21**, 5703–14.

Sun, M. K. and Alkon, D. L. (2002). Impairment of hippocampal CA1 heterosynaptic transformation and spatial memory by β-amyloid(25–35). *J. Neurophysiol.* **87**, 2441–9.

Tonegawa, S., Nakazawa, K., and Wilson, M. A. (2003). Genetic neuroscience of mammalian learning and memory. *Phil. Trans. R. Soc. Lond.* B **358**, 787–95. (DOI 10.1098/rstb.2002.1243.)

Tong, L., Thornton, P.L., Balazs, R., and Cotman, C.W. (2001). β-Amyloid-(1–42) impairs activity-dependent cAMP-response element-binding protein signaling in neurons at concentrations in which cell suvival is not compromised. *J. Biol. Chem.* **276**, 17 301–6.

Vitolo, O. V., Sant'Angelo, A., Costanzo, V., Battaglia, F., Arancio, O., and Shelanski, M. 2002 Amyloid β-peptide inhibition of the PKA/CREB pathway and long-term potentiation: reversibility by drugs that enhance cAMP signaling. *Proc. Natl Acad. Sci. USA* **99**, 13 217–21.

Walsh, D. M., Klyubuin, I., Fadeeva, J., Cullen, W. K., Anwyl, R., Wolfe, M. S., *et al.* (2002). Naturally secreted oligomers of the Alzheimer amyloid β-protein potently inhibit long-term potentiation *in vivo. Nature* **416**, 535–9.

Wang, H.-W., Pasternak, J. F., Kuo, H., Ristic, H., Lambert, M. P., Chromy, B., *et al.* (2002). Soluble oligomers of β-amyloid. 1–42 inhibit long-term potentiation but not longterm depression in rat dentate gyrus. *Brain Res.* **924**, 133–40.

Wu, J., Anwyl, R., and Rowan, M. J. (1995*a*). β-amyloid-(1–40) increases long-term potentiation in rat hippocampus *in vitro. Eur. J. Pharmacol.* **284**, R1–R3.

Wu, J., Anwyl, R., and Rowan, M. J. (1995*b*). β-Amyloid selectively augments NMDA receptor-mediated synaptic transmission in rat hippocampus. *NeuroReport* **6**, 2409–13.

Ye, L. and Qiao, J. T. (1999). Suppressive action produced by β-amyloid peptide fragment 31–35 on long-term potentiation in rat hippocampus is N-methyl-D-aspartate receptor-independent: it's offset by (-)huperzine A. *Neurosci. Lett* **275**, 187–90.

Yu, H., Saura, C. A., Choi, S. Y., Sun, L. D., Yang, X., Handler, M., *et al.* (2001). APP processing and synaptic plasticity in presenilin-1 knockout mice. *Neuron* **31**, 713–26.

Zaman, S. H., Parent, A., Laskey, A., Lee, M. K., Borchelt, D. R., Sisodia, S. S., *et al.* (2000). Enhanced synaptic potentiation in transgenic mice expressing presenilin 1 familial Alzheimer's disease mutation is normalised with a benzodiazapine. *Neurobiol. Dis.* **7**, 54–63.

Glossary

Aβ	amyloid β-protein
AD	Alzheimer's disease
ADDL	Aβ-derived diffusible ligand
APP	β-amyloid precursor protein
CREB	cAMP-regulatory element binding
EPSP	excitatory postsynaptic potential
ERK	extracellular signal-regulated kinase
hAPP	human β-amyloid precursor protein
HFS	high-frequency stimulation
LTD	long-term depression
LTP	long-term potentiation
MAPK	mitogen-activated protein kinase
NMDA	N-methyl-D-aspartate
PS	presenilin

29

Long-term potentiation: outstanding questions and attempted synthesis

John Lisman

This article attempts an overview of the mechanism of NMDAR-dependent long-term potentiation (LTP) and its role in hippocampal networks. Efforts are made to integrate information, often in speculative ways, and to identify unresolved issues about the induction, expression and molecular storage processes. The pre/post debate about LTP expression has been particularly difficult to resolve. The following hypothesis attempts to reconcile the available physiological evidence as well as anatomical evidence that LTP increases synapse size. It is proposed that synapses are composed of a variable number of trans-synaptic modules, each having presynaptic release sites and a postsynaptic structure that can be AMPAfied by the addition of a hyperslot assembly that anchors 10–20 AMPA channels. According to a newly developed view of transmission, the quantal response is generated by AMPA channels near the site of vesicle release and so will depend on whether the module(s) where release occurs has been AMPAfied. LTP expression may involve two structurally mediated processes: (i) the AMPAfication of existing modules by addition of hyperslot assemblies: this is a purely postsynaptic process and produces an increase in the probability of an AMPA response, with no change in the NMDA component; and (ii) the addition of new modules: this is a structurally coordinated pre/post process that leads to LTP-induced synapse enlargement and potentiation of the NMDA component owing to an increase in the number of release sites (the number of NMDA channels is assumed to be fixed). The protocol used for LTP induction appears to affect the proportion of these two processes; pairing protocols that involve low-frequency presynaptic stimulation induce only AMPAfication, making LTP purely postsynaptic, whereas high-frequency stimulation evokes both processes, giving rise to a presynaptic component. This model is capable of reconciling much of the seemingly contradictory evidence in the pre/post debate. The structural nature of the postulated changes is relevant to a second debate: whether a CaMKII switch or protein-dependent structural change is the molecular memory mechanism. A possible reconciliation is that a reversible CaMKII switch controls the construction of modules and hyperslot assemblies from newly synthesized proteins.

Keywords: long-term potentiation; long-term depression; protein synthesis; CaMKII; quantal analysis; memory

29.1 Introduction

In this article I will discuss some of the outstanding issues in the LTP field as we celebrate its 30th birthday. I will try to integrate the available information, often in speculative ways, and indicate the kind of experiments that may help to resolve important issues. For the sake of brevity, my discussion will focus on the best studied form of plasticity—the NMDAR-dependent form of LTP in the CA1 hippocampal region.

29.2 LTP/LTD/Silent synapses: what is the state diagram of the synapse?

As a field focused on the changes in the state of the synapse, it is crucial to know the number of states a synapse can have. In Fig. 29.1 I have summarized results from different publications that are relevant to this still unsolved issue. In the simplest case, the strength of synapses would be controlled by changes in a single process. It now appears, however, that LTP and LTD involve fundamentally different processes. The clearest evidence comes from the study of the GluR1 phosphorylation (Lee *et al.* 2000). Synapses start out in the 'naive' state (this is an operational definition meaning that the experimenter has not yet performed a manipulation). The induction of LTP then brings about an increase in the phosphorylation of the CaMKII site on GluR1, a process that can be reversed by 'depotentiation'. By contrast, if LTD is induced from the 'naive' state, there is dephosphorylation of the PKA site on GluR1, a process that is reversed by 'de-depression'. These findings suggest the state diagram shown in Fig. 29.1*a*. An important conclusion is that there must be two separate molecular memories at the synapse, one for LTD and one for LTP.

Note, however, that Fig. 29.1*a* contains no mention of 'silent' synapses (lacking AMPA, but not NMDA channels). Is this yet another state? Recent work (Montgomery and Madison 2002) studied the 'unitary responses' made by a single axon on a target cell and thus gives a clearer view than previous work utilizing large populations of synapses. This study showed that LTD induction could often drive the synapse to a silent state. Perhaps then, there are two fundamental reversible processes, as illustrated in Fig. 29.1*b*:

(i) The unsilencing of synapses produces an 'active state'; when LTD is then induced, synapses can be silenced.
(ii) Activated synapses can be further potentiated, a process that can be reversed by depotentiation (interestingly, this occurs by a process that differs pharmacologically from 'silencing').

According to this view, the reason that experimentalists working on large populations of synapses cannot drive transmission to zero with LTD induction protocols is that some of the synapses are already in the potentiated state and that these undergo depotentiation, not LTD. The further study of unitary connections is a promising way to resolve this issue and to reconcile the state diagrams in Figs 27.1*a* and 27.1*b*.

When a synapse undergoes LTP, does it undergo a gradual strengthening or is there a large discrete change? Petersen *et al.* (1998) used a repetitive induction protocol and found that the unitary response increased suddenly in an all-or-none manner (Fig. 29.1*c*). Importantly, the increase in synaptic current (as large as 15 pA) was much larger than could be carried by a single AMPA channel (around 1 pA), suggesting that a group of about 10–20 channels is involved. The term 'slot' has been used to denote the mechanism by which a channel is held in the synapse (Shi *et al.* 2001). I will use the term 'hyperslot' to describe an anchoring system capable of holding 10–20 AMPA channels. The average mushroom spine has 80 AMPA channels (Matsuzaki *et al.* 2001) and an area of 0.2 μm^2 (Harris *et al.* 1992). Based on these values, it can be estimated that a hyperslot diameter is around 0.2 μm, on the same order as the smallest CA1 synapses (Lisman and Harris 1993).

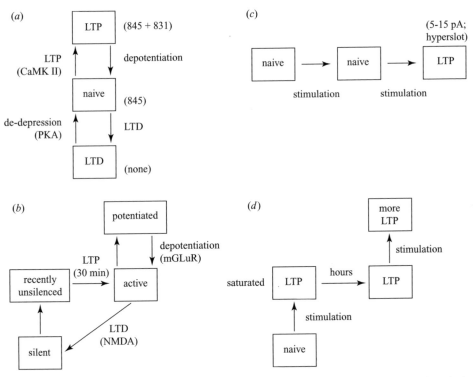

Fig. 29.1 State diagrams of the synapse. (*a*) Three states having different GluR1 phosphorylation (845/831): states based on the phosphorylation changes of GluR1 produced by various stimulation protocols (Lee *et al.* 2000). (*b*) States of unsilenced synapse: states based on the study of unitary silent and active connections in the CA3 region (Montgomery and Madison 2002). After unsilencing, there is a 30 minute period before the synapse can be weakened. Note that depotentiation is mGluR dependent whereas LTD is NMDA dependent. (*c*) Potentiation occurs by discrete addition of a multi-channel unit: a unitary connection is given repeated moderate stimulation. At some point an all-or-none increase in the synaptic response occurs. The increase in current is much larger than can be carried by a single channel as it is envisioned to involve the incorporation of a 'hyperslot' into the synapse (Petersen *et al.* 1998). (*d*) Further LTP can be induced after delay: after LTP saturation, the synapse can again undergo LTP, but only after several hours (Frey *et al.* 1995). An additional state-change not illustrated here is that mGluR receptors are initially required for LTP induction, but are then not further required for subsequent LTP induction (Bortolotto *et al.* 1994).

Having undergone LTP, is this the end of the road for a synapse or is further potentiation possible? Petersen *et al.* (1998) did not observe further potentiation, but they did not wait very long. In a different study (Frey *et al.* 1995) it was found that it was possible to induce further LTP if several hours progressed after LTP saturation (Fig. 29.1*d*; see also Dixon *et al.* (2002)). Taken together, these results suggest that with repeated LTP episodes, multiple hyperslots can be added to the synapse. This interpretation meshes well with the finding that at the largest CA1 synapses there are over 100 AMPA channels (Matsuzaki *et al.* 2001). Other ideas about states of the synapse are not dealt with in Fig. 29.1 (see Fig. 29.1 caption and other ideas about synaptic growth introduced later in this paper). It is not yet possible to integrate all of these ideas in a simple way. Thus, the specification of a state diagram of the synapse must be considered to be a future goal of the field.

29.3 LTP induction: Ca^{2+} sensors

One of the major accomplishments in the LTP field has been to elucidate the role of the NMDA channel in LTP. There is general agreement that Ca^{2+} entry through NMDA channels triggers LTP, but it remains unclear whether induction is caused by Ca^{2+} elevation in the spine cytoplasm or in a local domain close to the mouth of the NMDA channel. A recent study analysed the effect of buffer concentration on LTP induction and concluded that during some induction protocols, a local domain is involved (Hoffman et al. 2002). Interestingly, different induction protocols were not only differentially sensitive to Ca^{2+} buffers, but also differentially sensitive to the knockout of GluR1. The kinetics of onset and decay were also different. These results suggest that there are multiple Ca^{2+} sensors, each of which is coupled to a different potentiation mechanism. More generally, it seems difficult to escape the conclusion that LTP is complex, with even the early phase of LTP involving multiple mechanisms.

The primary Ca^{2+} sensor for LTP is CaMKII. Direct measurements show that CaMKII is activated and autophosphorylated by LTP induction (Fukunaga et al. 1993). This activation is required for LTP induction (Otmakhov et al. 1997; Giese et al. 1998), as indicated by genetic and pharmacological experiments. Importantly, the block of LTP in mature animals is nearly complete, suggesting that all components and phases of LTP require CaMKII activation. Other experiments show that the introduction of active CaMKII induces potentiation that closely mimics LTP and occludes with it (Lledo et al. 1995). A broad range of results support the idea that CaMKII activation is necessary and sufficient for LTP induction and is integral to the synaptic plasticity processes that occur during development and learning (Lisman et al. 2002).

The activation of CaMKII occurs in multiple steps and these may initiate different LTP expression mechanisms (Fig. 29.2). During synaptic activity, the kinase translocates from the cytoplasm to the PSD (Shen et al. 2000; Dosemeci et al. 2001). There, it binds to the NMDA channel where it becomes ideally positioned to sense the very high Ca^{2+} levels in the microdomain of the NMDA channel (Gardoni et al. 1998; Strack et al. 2000). The translocation requires the activation of CaMKII activity, but does not require autophosphorylation of the enzyme—the change that leads to persistent Ca^{2+}-independent activity. Such autophosphorylation is much more likely to occur once the kinase is bound to the NMDA channel, both because the Ca^{2+} levels are higher there and because the binding to the NMDA channel itself promotes autophosphorylation (Bayer et al. 2001). Theoretical work suggests that there may be another step in CaMKII activation that requires the crossing of an additional threshold: the nearly full autophosphorylation of multiple (n) nearby CaMKII holoenzymes in the PSD (Lisman and Zhabotinsky 2001). Only in this condition, can a CaMKII switch remain 'on' despite phosphatase activity (see Section 29.8), a necessary condition for a stable molecular memory. As suggested in Fig. 29.2, this form of CaMKII is likely to control the addition of hyperslots to the synapse.

A second Ca^{2+} sensor involved in LTP is the Ca/calmodulin-activated adenylate cyclase (Chetkovich and Sweatt 1993; Wong et al. 1999). The cAMP pathway apparently

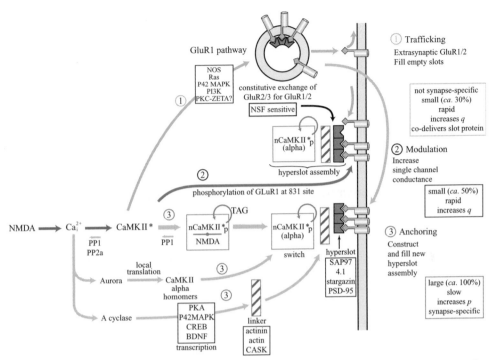

Fig. 29.2 Three postsynaptic pathways by which CaMKII produces LTP expression. Two Ca^{2+} sensors are shown, CaMKII and adenylate cyclase (how Aurora is activated remains unclear). CaMKII has sequential activation states, which may be differentially coupled to three different expression mechanisms. (1) Trafficking: GluR1 vesicular delivery pathway produces quasi-local delivery of microclusters of GluR1 and associated slot proteins to the plasma membrane. An existing synapse is strengthened by filling an unfilled slot with an AMPAR. (2) Neuromodulation: strengthening may also occur by CaMKIIdependent phosphorylation of GluR1, leading to enhanced single channel conductance. (3) Anchoring: a hyperslot assembly may be added to a silent synapse or, as shown, to a synapse that already has one assembly. The building blocks for the hyperslot assembly may come from several sources, including the GluR1 containing vesicle. In addition, transcription and translation may provide building blocks, one of which is CaMKII alpha homomers. A hyperslot assembly includes the CaMKII switch in its 'on' phosphorylated state, AMPA channels, the hyperslot that anchors the channels at the synapse and linker proteins that bind the switch to the hyperslot. A major goal is to determine the time course and magnitude of different expression mechanisms, as well as their effect on quantal analysis parameters. Tentative answers are given on the right-hand side.

does not directly trigger potentiation, but stimulates neural activity that triggers LTP by the normal NMDA-dependent process (Ma *et al.* 1999; Makhinson *et al.* 1999; Bozdagi *et al.* 2000). Elevation of cAMP can work synergistically with CaMKII-dependent process. In particular, elevation of cAMP leads to inhibition of PP1, thereby enhancing CaMKII autophosphorylation and CREB activation (Brown *et al.* 2000; Genoux *et al.* 2002). The CREB pathways then trigger the synthesis of proteins that may be important for the structural component of CaMKII-dependent potentiation (see Section 29.4). Other potential Ca^{2+} sensors include PKC, calpain and NOS.

Biophysical work is badly needed to measure the Ca^{2+} dynamics during LTP induction and to determine the properties of Ca^{2+} sensors. Although great progress has been made in Ca^{2+} imaging, there has not yet been a study of the Ca^{2+} dynamics during LTP or LTD induction at synapses that are demonstrably active during the process. It will also be important to understand more about calmodulin, the protein that couples Ca^{2+} to many enzymes. This adaptor molecule is not completely free in the cytoplasm, but can itself be 'buffered'. A recent study shows that synaptic plasticity undergoes major changes after knockout of the postsynaptic calmodulin buffer, RC3 (Krucker *et al.* 2002).

29.4 CaMKII potentiates by three different postsynaptic mechanisms: neuromodulation, trafficking and anchoring

It initially appeared as though LTP expression could be accounted for by a simple neuromodulatory process, the CaMKII-dependent phosphorylation of existing AMPA channels and the consequent increase in their single channel conductance (Barria *et al.* 1997a; Benke *et al.* 1998) (pathway 2 in Fig. 29.2). More recent work shows, however, that this component is relatively small (Poncer *et al.* 2002) and that LTP can still occur in its absence (Benke *et al.* 1998; Hayashi *et al.* 2000; Lee *et al.* 2003), indicating that other mechanisms are also involved.

There is now good evidence for a second mechanism (pathway 1 in Fig. 29.2): CaMKII drives a 'trafficking' process that involves vesicular delivery of GluR1 into the extrasynaptic membrane. This is followed by the diffusion of channels to synapses and their anchoring there (Chen *et al.* 2000; Hayashi *et al.* 2000; Passafaro *et al.* 2001). The extrasynaptic delivery of GluR1 is likely to occur in a large dendritic region near the active synapse. This would explain the finding that LTP induction enhances the response to the quasi-local application of glutamate (Montgomery *et al.* 2001), an increase that is hard to understand if the only change in AMPA channels occurs at the small fraction of synapses that undergo LTP. It would seem likely that some of the slots that anchor AMPA channels at synapses (see below) are empty; increasing the extrasynaptic concentration of channels could fill these slots. As this could happen at any synapse near the site of GluR1 delivery, one can understand why there should be a component of LTP that is not specific to stimulated synapses (Engert and Bonhoeffer 1999). Consistent with the somewhat diffuse character of the GluR1 delivery mechanism is its mediation by a cascade involving Ras and the soluble MAPK amplification system (Zhu *et al.* 2002). One of the most remarkable manipulations of GluR1 delivery involves the effect of PI3K inhibitors. These block the delivery of GluR1 to the extrasynaptic membrane (Passafaro *et al.* 2001) and selectively interfere with transmission at synapses that have undergone LTP (Sanna *et al.* 2002). The effect of PI3K inhibitors is reversible, indicating that the process is driven by some upstream synaptic memory. PKC also appears to be involved in this process (Daw *et al.* 2002; Ling *et al.* 2002). According to the ideas developed by Malinow and his associates (Shi *et al.* 2001) this persistent 'GluR1 pathway' will eventually subside, to be replaced by a constitutive 'GluR2 pathway' for AMPA channel delivery. It will be important to determine the timing of this transition. It will also be important to obtain direct evidence for the concept of an unfilled slot. So far there is only suggestive evidence: the gradual slide in the separation of quantal peaks observed during low-frequency depression (Larkman *et al.* 1997). A direct demonstration would be evidence for a change in the ratio of slot proteins to AMPA channels at the synapse.

The third CaMKII-dependent expression mechanism (pathway 3 in Fig. 29.2) involves the generation of new AMPA anchoring sites ('hyperslots') at synapses (Shi *et al.* 2001). AMPAfication of silent synapses has been widely discussed, but as argued previously, it is also likely that hyperslots can be added to synapses that already have AMPA-mediated transmission. There is still no consensus on the identity of slot proteins. The candidates are proteins known to interact with AMPA channels including SAP97, protein 4.1, GRIP and APB. Recent work suggests that PSD95 may be a critical slot protein (Schnell *et al.* 2002). AMPA channels are linked to PSD95 by the protein, stargazin. Overexpression of PSD-95 can enhance synaptic transmission (El-Husseini *et al.* 2000) whereas delocalizing the protein from the synapse by depalmitolaytion decreases transmission (El-Husseini *et al.* 2002).

It remains unclear how the phosphorylated state of CaMKII can control the addition of hyperslots. It is known that CaMKII bound in the PSD is less than 30 nm from the channels (Peterson *et al.* 2003) so the distances involved are not large. One possible linkage is CaMKII to actinin to actin to the protein 4.1/SAP97 complex that anchors AMPAR (Lisman and Zhabotinsky 2001). Each of these individual binding interactions has been demonstrated. Whatever the exact structural linkage, it seems likely that there is an entire assembly of proteins that produce AMPAfication; this includes the reversible CaMKII switch, the hyperslots that directly anchor AMPA channels and linker proteins that couple CaMKII to the hyperslots. I term this entire structure the hyperslot assembly (Fig. 29.2). In addition, there must be a trans-synaptic structure that ensures that the hyperslot assembly is added to the postsynaptic membrane in proper alignment with the presynaptic structures. Changes in the number of such transynaptic structures could give rise to a presynaptic component of LTP—a possibility that will be discussed in Section 29.6.

29.5 A structurally explicit theory of quantal analysis

The discovery that synapses can be 'silent' revolutionized the interpretation of quantal analysis by demonstrating the existence of a postsynaptic mechanism that could change the probability of transmission, a change that was previously interpreted to imply a presynaptic mechanism. Here, I will briefly describe further revisions of quantal analysis that we have developed in my laboratory. In essence what we are proposing is that AMPA-mediated transmission at large synapses is modular; multiple vesicles can be released, each acting preferentially on the local pool of AMPA receptors near the site of release. Some local regions of the synapse may lack AMPA receptors. Such synapses can be considered 'partially silent' since vesicles released at non-AMPAfied subregions will not generate a substantial AMPA response.

Central to this new view are five concepts.

(i) Quantal size can be estimated from the separation of quantal peaks in amplitude histograms (Foster and McNaughton 1991; Larkman *et al.* 1991; Malinow 1991; Kuhnt *et al.* 1992; Kullmann and Nicoll 1992; Liao *et al.* 1992; Stricker *et al.* 1996*a*; Magee and Cook 2000). The quantal size of 5–10 pA can be accounted for by the opening of about 10–20 AMPA channels (Magee and Cook 2000). Importantly, the narrowness of quantal peaks implies that the CV of the quantal response is small (< 0.2) (Stricker et al. 1996b).

(ii) Average mEPSCs (< 10 pA) activate only a small fraction of the total channels at a synapse (Liu et al. 1999; McAllister and Stevens 2000). Large mEPSCs are probably multiquantal (Bolshakov et al. 1997; Raghavachari and Lisman 2003).

(iii) EPSCs at large CA1 synapses are multiquantal, with the number of vesicles released being potentially greater than 10 (Oertner et al. 2002; Conti and Lisman 2003). Quanta summate nearly linearly; the variability of the number of effective release events accounts for the very high trial-to-trial variation of the AMPAR-mediated EPSC (4–40 pA) and NMDAR-mediated Ca^{2+} entry (Conti and Lisman 2003).

(iv) The rise time of small mEPSCs recorded with improved methodology is very fast (< 50 µs) (Magee and Cook 2000). In this brief period, glutamate remains highly concentrated near the site of vesicle release (100 nm). This 'spike' of glutamate is efficient at activating the AMPA channels in this region (Raghavachari and Lisman 2003). As glutamate spreads, its concentration falls and AMPA channels are no longer efficiently activated, particularly because low concentrations drive desensitization better than activation. The net result is that each vesicle release causes a hotspot of channel activation around 200 nm in diameter. This hotspot is of the same order as our estimate of the dimension of a hyperslot, which contains a sufficient number of AMPA channels to generate a quantal event. Thus, synapses may be modular, with AMPA transmission occurring relatively independently in each module.

(v) Some modules may be 'silent', whereas others are not; thus synapses can be 'partially silent'. Vesicles released in 'silent' modules generate an NMDA component (which does not depend on the location of vesicle release), but not a significant AMPA component. Other vesicles released over AMPAfied modules would generate both components. This could explain two remarkable recent findings. The first is that the AMPA/NMDA ratio of evoked responses at single synapses can vary dramatically from trial to trial (Renger et al. 2001). Lack of an AMPA response could be explained if release occurred at a silent module. The second result is that block of desensitization can dramatically increase the probability of response at low p synapses (Diamond and Jahr 1995; Choi et al. 2000; Gasparini et al. 2000). Our simulations (Raghavachari and Lisman 2003) indicate that that this can be explained because the glutamate released at silent modules can affect distant AMPA channels when desensitization is blocked (an alternative explanation (Choi et al. 2000) is that some vesicles release their content too slowly to activate AMPA channels).

In summary, many vesicles may be released at large synapses, with each activating an independent group of channels near the site of vesicle release.

This view of transmission has substantial impact on the way quantal analysis is interpreted. Importantly, the progressive addition of hyperslots and AMPA channels will *not* substantially affect quantal size, which is determined by other factors including the single channel conductance, the fraction of unfilled slots and the transmitter content of the vesicles. The probability of the response can be affected either by AMPAfication of modules or by changes in the probability of release. Thus, neither quantal size nor the probability of response can be used to unambiguously determine the locus of LTP expression. Several further implications should be noted. First, the shortcut method for monitoring synaptic strength by measuring mEPSP size is now dubious; there seems no alternative but to directly measure the average evoked responses, a technically demanding task at single synapses. Second, the concept of partially silent synapses makes it possible to understand how the pairing protocol for LTP induction can routinely produce massive potentiation (up to 400%) through a purely postsynaptic process (see Section 29.6) and do so under conditions (age 2–3 weeks) where there are relatively few (around 25%) silent synapses (Nusser *et al.* 1998; Petralia *et al.* 1999; Takumi *et al.* 1999).

29.6 LTP expression: a unifying pre/post hypothesis

Figure 29.3*a,b* shows a silent synapse and its AMPAfication by the addition of a hyperslot assembly. I have drawn a box through the pre- and postsynaptic region to emphasize that the entire structure must be a trans-synaptic module with a given number of release sites on the presynaptic side and the ability to bind a hyperslot assembly into the postsynaptic side. In addition, the synapse contains several NMDA channels, which are placed outside the modules.

Consider now how to draw this picture if LTP causes additional hyperslot assemblies to be added to the same synapse. One view would be that the number of modules is fixed; all that can occur is that more and more of the existing modules become AMPAfied. But according to this view, LTP will produce no change in synapse size, contrary to the available evidence. Recent work (Ostroff *et al.* 2002) provides the strongest indication so far that LTP induction produces an increase in the size of synapses measured 2 h after induction, consistent with previous work (Geinisman *et al.* 1995; Buchs and Muller 1996; Bozdagi *et al.* 2000; Weeks *et al.* 2003). If this is true, there must be a change in the size of the presynaptic active zone, an increase in the number of release sites and thus a presynaptic component of LTP.

A simple model that can account for both the structural changes and the evidence for silent synapses is as follows. The synapse consists of a variable number of trans-synaptic modules. The presynaptic side of the module contains a certain number of release sites; the postsynaptic side may or may not contain a hyperslot assembly and thus may be AMPAfied or silent. LTP expression involves two structural processes.

(i) Addition of 'silent' trans-synaptic modules: this produces a growth in the size of the synapse and an increase in the number of presynaptic release sites.
(ii) Postsynaptic AMPAfication of 'silent' modules by addition of a hyperslot assembly.

It is envisioned that these processes occur together or independently, depending on the induction conditions, and that the number of NMDA channels is not strongly affected by either process (Racca *et al.* 2000). If only AMPAfication occurs, LTP will appear postsynaptic; if module addition occurs, there will be enhanced presynaptic release owing to the increase in number of release sites. In essence what is being proposed is a hybrid of the silent synapse model and the model of Bolshakov *et al.* (1997). The proposal that synapses grow by the addition of transsynaptic modules provides a simple explanation for one of the most striking features of synapse

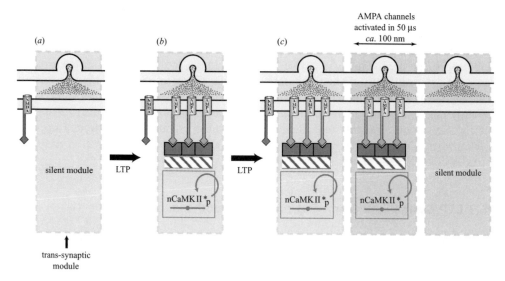

Fig. 29.3 Both presynaptic and postsynaptic processes can contribute to LTP at synapses composed of trans-synaptic modular elements. (*a*) A silent synapse containing a single 'silent' module. LTP induction leads to its AMPAfication (*b*). This is a structural process that occurs through the addition of a hyperslot assembly under the control of an 'on' CaMKII switch. The number of NMDA channels and the number of release sites is not changed; thus only AMPA-mediated transmission is enhanced. A second LTP induction (*c*) leads to the addition of two new modules, enlarging the synapse pre- and postsynaptically. Furthermore, one of these modules becomes AMPAfied whereas the other does not (it is unclear what determines the relative proportion of these two processes). Because vesicles primarily activate the AMPA channels in the module where they are released, the rightmost module, which lacks AMPA channels will be 'silent'. The synapse as a whole is therefore 'partly silent'. The enhancement of the number of release sites will produce LTP of the NMDA component of transmission. At large synapses, release is multiquantal. The details of the LTP induction procedure may determine the relative proportion of the two LTP processes (see Section 29.6).

architecture: the exact registration of the presynaptic active zone and the PSD despite wide variation in synapse size (Lisman and Harris 1993).

Of particular importance to resolving the pre/post debate is that different induction protocols may evoke process 1 and 2 in different proportions. When LTP is induced by standard pairing protocols (low-frequency presynaptic stimulation and strong post-synaptic depolarization), there is little or no change in the NMDA component (Kullmann 1994; Selig *et al.* 1995; Montgomery *et al.* 2001). This is what would be expected by process 2 alone and provides one of the strongest lines of support for the purely postsynaptic model of LTP. However, LTP of the NMDA component is large when LTP is induced by high-frequency stimulation (Bashir *et al.* 1991; Asztely *et al.* 1992; Xie *et al.* 1992). This would be consistent with the idea that high-frequency presynaptic activity is required for the addition of trans-synaptic modules and the consequent increase in presynaptic release. Thus, a potential resolution of the pre/post debate would be that under some induction conditions only a postsynaptic component of expression is involved, whereas under others condition both pre- and postsynaptic components are involved.

Before this resolution can be accepted, it will be necessary to strengthen the case that the LTP of the NMDA component is indeed caused by enhanced release rather than by a postsynaptic change in the number or conductance of NMDA channels. There has been surprisingly little work on this issue, but the available evidence points to a presynaptic mechanism. Kullmann *et al.* (1996) reported that LTP of the NMDA component is associated with a decrease in the CV, consistent with a presynaptic change. More directly, a recent report (Emptage *et al.* 2003) indicates that the probability of the NMDAR-mediated Ca^{2+} signals at single spines increases after LTP induction. If confirmed, these results would provide strong support for an increase in release.

29.7 LTP maintenance: synaptic memory versus attractors

One of the major goals of the study of LTP is to understand the molecular basis of synaptic memory. A key question is whether our ability to remember something for a lifetime requires that synaptic biochemical memory be stable for that duration. This may not be the case. One interesting alternative (Wittenberg and Tsien 2002) is that the molecular memory of a synapse is relatively short (perhaps only months) and that longer-term storage relies on the ability of autoassociative attractor networks to refresh this memory. What stores autoassociative information in an attractor network is the mutual enhancement of excitatory transmission between the subgroup of cells that represent a memory. It is exactly this kind of mutual enhancement that can be produced by the Hebbian form of LTP. Once synapses are strengthened in this way, the subgroup of cells that represent a memory form an ensemble that can be easily reactivated and fire persistently. Owing to the redundancy of the connections, such reactivation can occur even after partial decay of LTP. The reactivation could strengthen weakened synapses through additional LTP, restoring the strength of the original memory. There is increasing evidence that memories are in fact reactivated periodically, probably during sleep. Thus, the requirement at the synaptic level is that the average stability of LTP be long compared with the interval at which memories are reactivated. Unfortunately, no estimate is yet available for this interval.

29.8 Molecular memory mechanisms: CaMKII and protein-synthesis-dependent structural change

There have been two main proposals regarding the molecular basis of synaptic memory, the CaMKII hypothesis (Lisman and Zhabotinsky 2001) and protein synthesis hypothesis (Kandel 2001). I will first discuss these separately and then suggest ways in which they can be reconciled.

CaMKII is a potential memory molecule because it undergoes persistent activation after LTP induction (Fukunaga *et al.* 1993). Importantly, a single amino-acid substitution at Thr286 that blocks the generation of persistent activation, blocks LTP and interferes strongly with memory in behavioural tests (Giese *et al.* 1998). It has been argued that the kinase acts as a reversible memory switch localized at each synapse. Detailed models now exist showing how the biochemically established properties of the kinase could give rise to a stable memory switch (Lisman and Zhabotinsky 2001). The key properties are as follows.

(i) The ability of phosphorylation of Thr286 to make the subunit display Ca^{2+}-independent activity (Miller and Kennedy 1986).

(ii) The ability of such an active subunit to phosphorylate a neighbouring subunit, thereby providing a positive feedback autocatalytic reaction (Hanson *et al.* 1994).

(iii) The demonstration that the PP1 held in the PSD is the *only* phosphatase allowed access to PSD-associated CaMKII (Strack *et al.* 1997). This implies that the relevant chemistry is local and has the important consequence that PP1 will be saturated when CaMKII becomes hyperphosphorylated.

Simulations of these reactions show that a group of CaMKII holoenzymes in the PSD can have the stable 'on' and 'off' states required of a memory switch. Furthermore, the PP1 saturation provides a novel mechanism for interactions among holoenzymes that is important for longterm stability; during protein turnover a newly inserted holoenzyme will become phosphorylated if PP1 is saturated by neighbouring phosphorylated holoenzymes. Because of this process, a switch of this kind can be stable despite the protein turnover of its constituents. As noted earlier, there is growing evidence that CaMKII acts as a reversible memory switch; its phosphorylation is increased during LTP and decreased by depotentiation (Barria *et al.* 1997b; Huang *et al.* 2001). An important outstanding question is whether inhibition of PSD CaMKII can reverse LTP or memory maintenance, as would be expected if CaMKII is a memory molecule.

According to the protein synthesis model, LTP induction activates transcription and translation. The newly synthesized proteins somehow produce stable synapses, perhaps by promoting their growth. The key experimental support is that transcription and translation inhibitors applied just before LTP induction interfere with the late phase of LTP (Frey *et al.* 1988). Conversely, the late phase can be enhanced by constitutive activation of CREB and the resulting enhanced synthesis of proteins (Barco *et al.* 2002). Newly synthesized molecules are not targeted exclusively to the synapses whose activity induced their synthesis, but rather can be captured by any synapse that has undergone LTP. This was nicely demonstrated in experiments where LTP was induced in the presence of protein synthesis inhibitors (Frey and Morris 1997, 1998). These synapses nevertheless expressed late LTP if other synapses were allowed to stimulate protein synthesis either immediately before or just after the period of protein synthesis inhibition. It thus appears that synapses that have undergone LTP contain a 'tag' that allows them to capture newly synthesized proteins. Once captured, the potentiation of these synapses becomes stable. The identity of the captured proteins and the mechanism by which they make potentiation stable is not known.

29.9 Reconciling the CaMKII and protein synthesis models

As mentioned earlier, it was initially thought that LTP expression mechanisms might be modulatory in nature, but it now appears clear that structural processes are also involved. If hyperslot assemblies and trans-synaptic modules are added to synapses, new building blocks will be required and these may have to be newly synthesized.

Recent work provides evidence that the synthesis of one component of the hyperslot assembly, CaMKII (Miller *et al.* 2003) is in fact required for late LTP. CaMKII is one of the small group of proteins that is synthesized in the dendrites and whose synthesis is rapidly and locally induced by LTP induction (Burgin *et al.* 1990; Ouyang *et al.* 1999; Huang *et al.* 2002). This occurs as a result of the rapid translation of pre-existing mRNA (Huang *et al.* 2002). Miller *et al.* (2002) modified the targeting signals on CaMKII mRNA, abolishing its entry into the dendrites. This produced no change in early LTP, but a marked reduction in the stability of late LTP. Furthermore, PSDs isolated from these animals had enormously reduced CaMKII content (17% of normal; total CaMKII is only reduced 50%). It is important to realize that dendritically synthesized CaMKII is a novel form: the holoenzymes are homomeric α whereas the somatically synthesized form contains both α and β subunits. These observations suggest the following scenario: during LTP induction pre-existing CaMKII α/β heteromers are translocated to the PSD where they become autophosphorylated and serve as the tag. Induction also activates the local synthesis of alpha homomers. These interact with the tag to somehow stabilize the late phase of LTP. Why homomers would have this special ability is unclear, but the fact that they, unlike heteromers, can interact with the densin/actinin complex in the PSD is intriguing (Walikonis *et al.* 2001). In any case, the fact that synaptic strengthening involves structural modification, both for adding hyperslot assemblies to existing modules and for adding new modules, clearly must require new proteins. Thus, a simple unifying model would be that the CaMKII switch is the molecular storage device, but that the structural process of building a more powerful synapse cannot be completed without protein synthesis.

29.10 LTP in auto-associative networks

I now turn to a discussion of the role of LTP in actual learning processes. The recent paper from Tonegawa's laboratory is a milestone in the study of LTP because it studies the effect of modifying LTP in a specific network (CA3), the behavioural function of which can be understood in terms of established neural network concepts (Nakazawa *et al.* 2002). It has long been assumed that memories are stored in the distributed synapses of recurrent networks. A critical requirement for such autoassociative memory networks is that the synapses must display a Hebbian form of LTP. It has thus been very satisfying that the CA3 network is a recurrent one (Fig. 29.4) and that the LTP found at these synapses is the NMDA-dependent Hebbian form. It is this broad hypothesis that has now been tested by genetically disabling NMDA-dependent LTP in the CA3 region. According to the theory of autoassociative networks, when a partial or degraded form of the memory A (designated A′) is provided as input to the network, the output will be the correct memory, A. Consistent with this, normal animals can recognize a partial stimulus whereas mutant animals lacking NMDA channels in CA3 cannot.

As technically impressive as this experiment is, the bar can always be raised. CA3 cells have two types of synapse with NMDA-dependent LTP: the recurrent synapses and the perforant path synapses. In the 'ultimate' experiment, LTP would be disabled only at the recurrent synapses. A further complicating factor is that NMDA channels not only produce the Ca^{2+} entry that triggers LTP, but also produce slow EPSPs that

(a)   (b)

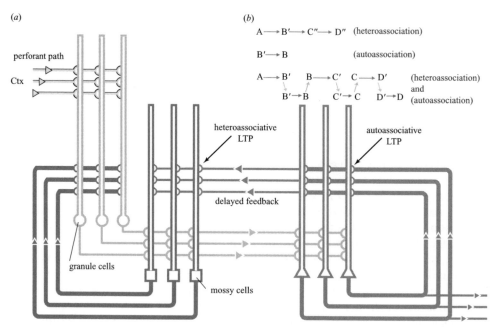

Fig. 29.4 The (a) dentate and (b) CA3 hippocampal networks responsible for the storage of heteroassociative and autoassociative memory. The known bidirectional interconnections between these networks is appropriate for sequence recall (see Section 29.11). Of particular note is that the transmission of information from the dentate to CA3 and back again provides the delay needed to produce the heteroassociative synaptic linkages required for sequence learning and recall (see Fig. 29.5).

can be important for information transmission. Thus, an 'ultimate, ultimate' experiment might specifically delete the Ca^{2+} permeability of the channel required for LTP induction while leaving intact the Na^+ permeability required for EPSP generation.

The results described above strongly suggest that NMDAR-dependent LTP is necessary for actual learning; a related important discovery is that a natural learning process strengthens synapses by the same molecular processes that mediate LTP in the slice preparation (Takahashi *et al.* 2002). Specifically, it was shown that when cells in barrel cortex are virally transfected with GluR1 receptors (recognizable by their altered rectification), these receptors are driven into the synapse when the animal uses its whiskers, but not if the whiskers are removed. This result further strengthens the idea that LTP is involved in behaviourally meaningful synaptic modification.

29.11 LTP in heteroassociative networks (storage of memory sequences by the hippocampus)

Although it has long been clear that NMDAR-dependent LTP is ideally suited for the formation of autoassociative memories, this is not the only form of memory. A second type, heteroassociative memory, deals with the links between temporally separated items. Can NMDAR-dependent LTP also subserve this function or is some entirely different mechanism required? This is a topic that can be discussed in terms of very specific findings regarding the anatomy, physiology and function of the hippocampus. There is now strong evidence that the overall memory function of the hippocampus is more than just a simple autoassociative memory for isolated memory items. Rather, the hippocampus may be a specialized device for the storage and recall of memory sequences. Behavioural tests of odour sequences show that hippocampal animals fail to recognize odour sequences even though they can recognize individual odours (Fortin et al. 2002). Recordings from hippocampal place cells have revealed the phenomenon of 'phase precession' (O'Keefe and Recce 1993). This appears to be the hippocampus caught in the act of a high-speed recall of the sequence of places along a path (Jensen and Lisman 1996; Skaggs et al. 1996; Tsodyks et al. 1996). Finally, during sleep, sequences that occurred during wakefulness are replayed (Skaggs and McNaughton 1996; Nadasdy et al. 1999).

To store and recall sequences, there must be a synaptic modification process that forms the heteroassociative linkages between cells encoding sequential memory items (linking A to B). Such linkages should *not* store autoassociative linkages (linking elements of A; e.g. A1 and A2). As shown in Fig. 29.5, standard LTP can selectively form 'pure' heteroassociative links provided there is a delay in the recurrent feedback. In ongoing work, we (Raffone et al. 2003) are attempting to determine how the multiple fields of the hippocampus could work together to encode autoassociative and heteroassociative synaptic weights and thereby enable the system to perform sequence storage and recall. Figure 29.4 describes our current view. The general idea is that a heteroassociative network alone could not produce correct sequence recall because a step in recall (A to B) produces slight corruption (B' instead of B). If B' is used as a basis for the next step in the sequence this leads to an even more corrupted item, C''. This concatenation of errors can, however, be avoided if there is an interplay of autoassociative and heteroassociative networks: B' is sent to an autoassociative network where it is converted to B; B is then sent to the heteroassociative network where it produces C', etc. (Lisman 1999). The dentate and CA3 are both recurrent networks that are bidirectionally connected (Fig. 29.4). We now envision that CA3 is doing the autoassociation whereas the heteroassociation occurs in the dentate. The back and forth flow of information between these networks could produce correct sequence recall. The fact that the phase precession occurs in both the dentate and CA3 is consistent with this model. Importantly, the time that it takes information to flow from the dentate to CA3 and back to dentate could provide exactly the kind of delay needed to promote pure heteroassociative links in the dentate feedback synapses (Fig. 29.5). Thus, under different conditions, the same NMDA-dependent form of LTP may be able to subserve both autoassociative and heteroassociative memory. A critical test of this hypothesis would be to disable NMDA function at feedback synapses in the dentate; this should lead to deficits in sequence recall without interfering with autoassociative memory.

29.12 Closing remarks

An unhealthy field becomes closed and progress ceases. Just the opposite has been true for LTP. A field that began with simple extracellular recordings has now made productive interfaces with biophysics, pharmacology, biochemistry, molecular biology,

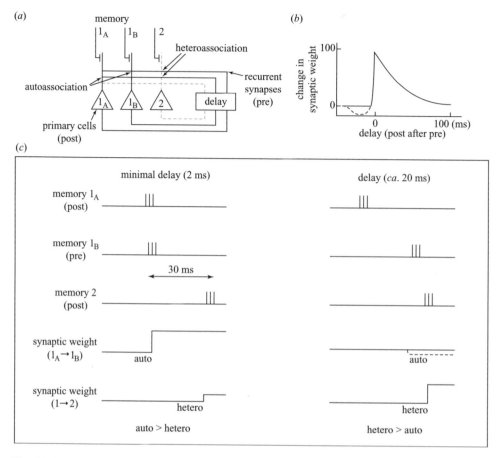

Fig. 29.5 An argument that a single LTP learning rule (*b*) can perform autoassociation or het-eroassociation depending on the delay of the feedback in recurrent networks (*a*). The auto-association produces connections between cells 1A and 1B that encode two aspects of the same memory. The heteroassociation process provides connections between cells that encode sequential memories, 1 and 2. According to the learning rule, if postsynaptic firing occurs within a time window after presynaptic input, the NMDA channel will be activated and LTP will occur. If the order is opposite, either no LTP will occur or there may be weakening. Sequential memories are applied to the network at 30 ms intervals. (*c*) If the delay in the recurrent pathway is small, autoassociation will occur whereas if the delay is larger, heteroassociation will occur. The delay required for heteroassociation may be provided by sending information from the dentate to CA3 and back again to the dentate (see Fig. 29.4).

neural network theory and behavioural psychology. Although the controversies still abound, unifying ideas are emerging. This should be a very happy birthday for LTP.

The author thanks N. Otmakhov and A. Zhabotinsky for comments on the paper and J. Cook of the Woods Hole Oceanographic Institute Graphics Department for the Fig.s. This work was supported by the National Institute of Neurological Disorders and Stroke grant nos. RO1 NS-27337 and RO1 NS-35083, and a grant from the David and Lucille Packard Foundation's Interdisciplinary Science Program. The author gratefully acknowledges the support of the W. M. Keck Foundation.

References

Asztely, F., Wigstrom, H., and Gustafsson, B. (1992). The relative contribution of NMDA receptor channels in the expression of long-term potentiation in the hippocampal CA1 region. *Eur. J. Neurosci.* **4**, 681–90.

Barco, A., Alarcon, J. M., and Kandel, E. R. (2002). Expression of constitutively active CREB protein facilitates the late phase of long-term potentiation by enhancing synaptic capture. *Cell* **108**, 689–703.

Barria, A., Derkach, V., and Soderling, T. (1997a). Identification of the Ca^{2+}/calmodulin-dependent protein kinase II regulatory phosphorylation site in the alpha-amino-3-hydroxyl-5-methyl-4-isoxazole-propionate-type glutamate receptor. *J. Biol. Chem.* **272**, 32727–30.

Barria, A., Muller, D., Derkach, V., Griffith, L. C., and Soderling, T. R. (1997b). Regulatory phosphorylation of AMPAtype glutamate receptors by CaM-KII during long-term potentiation. *Science* **276**, 2042–5.

Bashir, Z. I., Alford, S., Davies, S. N., Randall, A. D., and Collingridge, G. L. (1991). Long-term potentiation of NMDA receptor-mediated synaptic transmission in the hippocampus. *Nature* **349**, 156–8.

Bayer, K. U., De Koninck, P., Leonard, A. S., Hell, J. W., and Schulman, H. (2001). Interaction with the NMDA receptor locks CaMKII in an active conformation. *Nature* **411**, 801–5.

Benke, T. A., Luthi, A., Isaac, J. T., and Collingridge, G. L. (1998). Modulation of AMPA receptor unitary conductance by synaptic activity. *Nature* **393**, 793–7.

Bolshakov, V. Y., Golan, H., Kandel, E. R., and Siegelbaum, S. A. (1997). Recruitment of new sites of synaptic transmission during the cAMP-dependent late phase of LTP at CA3-CA1 synapses in the hippocampus. *Neuron* **19**, 635–51.

Bortolotto, Z. A., Bashir, Z. I., Davies, C. H., and Collingridge, G. L. (1994). A molecular switch activated by metabotropic glutamate receptors regulates induction of long-term potentiation. *Nature* **368**, 740–3.

Bozdagi, O., Shan, W., Tanaka, H., Benson, D. L., and Huntley, G. W. (2000). Increasing numbers of synaptic puncta during late-phase LTP: N-cadherin is synthesized, recruited to synaptic sites, and required for potentiation. *Neuron* **28**, 245–59.

Brown, G. P., Blitzer, R. D., Connor, J. H., Wong, T., Shenolikar, S., Iyengar, R., *et al.* (2000). Long-term potentiation induced by theta frequency stimulation is regulated by a protein phosphatase-1-operated gate. *J. Neurosci.* **20**, 7880–7.

Buchs, P. A. and Muller, D. (1996). Induction of long-term potentiation is associated with major ultrastructural changes of activated synapses. *Proc. Natl Acad. Sci. USA* **93**, 8040–5.

Burgin, K. E., Waxham, M. N., Rickling, S., Westgate, S. A., Mobley, W. C., and Kelly, P. T. (1990). *In situ* hybridization histochemistry of Ca^{2+}/calmodulin-dependent protein kinase in developing rat brain. *J. Neurosci.* **10**, 1788–98.

Chen, L., Chetkovich, D. M., Petralia, R. S., Sweeney, N. T., Kawasaki, Y., Wenthold, R. J., *et al.* (2000). Stargazin regulates synaptic targeting of AMPA receptors by two distinct mechanisms. *Nature* **408**, 936–43.

Chetkovich, D. M. and Sweatt, J. D. (1993). NMDA receptor activation increases cyclic AMP in area CA1 of the hippocampus via calcium/calmodulin stimulation of adenylyl cyclase. *J. Neurochem.* **61**, 1933–42.

Choi, S., Klingauf, J., and Tsien, R. W. (2000). Postfusional regulation of cleft glutamate concentration during LTP at 'silent synapses'. *Nature Neurosci.* **3**, 330–6.

Conti, R. and Lisman, J. (2003). The high variance of AMPA and NMDA responses at single hippocampal synapses: evidence for multiquantal release. *Proc. Natl. Acad. Sci. USA* **100**, 4885–90.

Daw, M. I., Bortolotto, Z. A., Saulle, E., Zaman, S., Collingridge, G. L., and Isaac, J. T. (2002). Phosphatidylinositol 3 kinase regulates synapse specificity of hippocampal long-term depression. *Nature Neurosci.* **5**, 835–6.

Diamond, J. S. and Jahr, C. E. (1995). Asynchronous release of synaptic vesicles determines the time course of the AMPA receptor-mediated EPSC. *Neuron* **15**, 1097–107.

Dixon, D. B., Bliss, T. V. P., and Fine, A. (2002). Individual hippocampal synapses express incremental (analog) and bi-directional long-term plasticity. *Soc. Neurosci. Abstr.* Program No. 150.3.

Dosemeci, A., Tao-Cheng, J. H., Vinade, L., Winters, C. A., Pozzo-Miller, L., and Reese, T. S. (2001). Glutamate-induced transient modification of the postsynaptic density. *Proc. Natl Acad. Sci. USA* **98**, 10 428–32.

El-Husseini, A. E., Schnell, E., Chetkovich, D. M., Nicoll, R. A., and Bredt, D. S. (2000). PSD-95 involvement in maturation of excitatory synapses. *Science* **290**, 1364–8.

El-Husseini, A. E., Schnell, E., Dakoji, S., Sweeney, N., Zhou, Q., Prange, O., *et al.* (2002). Synaptic strength regulated by palmitate cycling on PSD-95. *Cell* **108**, 849–63.

Emptage, N. J., Reid, C. A., Fine, A., and Bliss, T. V. (2003). Optical quantal analysis reveals a presynaptic component of LTP at hippocampal Schaffer-associational synapses. *Neuron* **38**, 797–804.

Engert, F. and Bonhoeffer, T. (1999). Dendritic spine changes associated with hippocampal long-term synaptic plasticity. *Nature* **399**, 66–70.

Fortin, N. J., Agster, K. L., and Eichenbaum, H. B. (2002). Critical role of the hippocampus in memory for sequences of events. *Nature Neurosci.* **5**, 458–62.

Foster, T. C. and McNaughton, B. L. (1991). Long-term enhancement of CA1 synaptic transmission is due to increased quantal size, not quantal content. *Hippocampus* **1**, 79–91.

Frey, U. and Morris, R. G. (1997). Synaptic tagging and long-term potentiation. *Nature* **385**, 533–6.

Frey, U. and Morris, R. G. (1998). Weak before strong: dissociating synaptic tagging and plasticity-factor accounts of late-LTP. *Neuropharmacology* **37**, 545–52.

Frey, U., Krug, M., Reymann, K. G., and Matthies, H. (1988). Anisomycin, an inhibitor of protein synthesis, blocks late phases of LTP phenomena in the hippocampal CA1 region *in vitro. Brain Res.* **452**, 57–65.

Frey, U., Schollmeier, K., Reymann, K. G., and Seidenbecher, T. (1995). Asymptotic hippocampal long-term potentiation in rats does not preclude additional potentiation at later phases. *Neuroscience* **67**, 799–807.

Fukunaga, K., Stoppini, L., Miyamoto, E., and Muller, D. (1993). Long-term potentiation is associated with an increased activity of Ca^{2+}/calmodulin-dependent protein kinase II. *J. Biol. Chem.* **268**, 7863–7.

Gardoni, F., Caputi, A., Cimino, M., Pastorino, L., Cattabeni, F., and Di Luca, M. (1998). Calcium/calmodulin-dependent protein kinase II is associated with NR2A/B subunits of NMDA receptor in postsynaptic densities. *J. Neurochem.* **71**, 1733–41.

Gasparini, S., Saviane, C., Voronin, L. L., and Cherubini, E. (2000). Silent synapses in the developing hippocampus: lack of functional AMPA receptors or low probability of glutamate release? *Proc. Natl Acad. Sci. USA* **97**, 9741–6.

Geinisman, Y., Detoledo-Morrell, L., Morrell, F., and Heller, R. E. (1995). Hippocampal markers of age-related memory dysfunction: behavioral, electrophysiological and morphological perspectives. *Prog. Neurobiol.* **45**, 223–52.

Genoux, D., Haditsch, U., Knobloch, M., Michalon, A., Storm, D., and Mansuy, I. M. (2002). Protein phosphatase 1 is a molecular constraint on learning and memory. *Nature* **418**, 970–5.

Giese, K. P., Fedorov, N. B., Filipkowski, R. K., and Silva, A. J. (1998). Autophosphorylation at Thr286 of the alpha calciumcalmodulin kinase II in LTP and learning. *Science* **279**, 870–3.

Hanson, P. I., Meyer, T., Stryer, L., and Schulman, H. (1994). Dual role of calmodulin in autophosphorylation of multifunctional CaM kinase may underlie decoding of calcium signals. *Neuron* **12**, 943–56.

Harris, K. M., Jensen, F. E., and Tsao, B. (1992). Three-dimensional structure of dendritic spines and synapses in rat hippocampus (CA1) at postnatal day 15 and adult ages: implications for the maturation of synaptic physiology and long-term potentiation. [Published erratum appears in *J. Neurosci.* **12**(8): following table of contents.] *J. Neurosci.* **12**, 2685–705.

Hayashi, Y., Shi, S. H., Esteban, J. A., Piccini, A., Poncer, J. C., and Malinow, R. (2000). Driving AMPA receptors into synapses by LTP and CaMKII: requirement for GluR1 and PDZ domain interaction. *Science* **287**, 2262–7.

Hoffman, D. A., Sprengel, R., and Sakmann, B. (2002). Molecular dissection of hippocampal theta-burst pairing potentiation. *Proc. Natl Acad. Sci. USA* **99**, 7740–5.

Huang, C. C., Liang, Y. C., and Hsu, K. S. (2001). Characterization of the mechanism underlying the reversal of long-term potentiation by low-frequency stimulation at hippocampal CA1 synapses. *J. Biol. Chem.* **276**, 48 108–17.

Huang, Y. S., Jung, M. Y., Sarkissian, M., and Richter, J. D. (2002). *N*-methyl-d-aspartate receptor signaling results in Aurora kinase-catalyzed CPEB phosphorylation and alpha CaMKII mRNA polyadenylation at synapses. *EMBO J.* **21**, 2139–48.

Jensen, O. and Lisman, J. E. (1996). Hippocampal CA3 region predicts memory sequences: accounting for the phase precession of place cells. *Learning Memory* **3**, 279–87.

Kandel, E. R. (2001). The molecular biology of memory storage: a dialogue between genes and synapses. *Science* **294**, 1030–8.

Krucker, T., Siggins, G. R., McNamara, R. K., Lindsley, K. A., Dao, A., Allison, D. W., *et al.* (2002). Targeted disruption of RC3 reveals a calmodulin-based mechanism for regulating metaplasticity in the hippocampus. *J. Neurosci.* **22**, 5525–35.

Kuhnt, U., Hess, G., and Voronin, L. L. (1992). Statistical analysis of long-term potentiation of large excitatory postsynaptic potentials recorded in guinea pig hippocampal slices: binomial model. *Exp. Brain Res.* **89**, 265–74.

Kullmann, D. M. (1994). Amplitude fluctuations of dual-component EPSCs in hippocampal pyramidal cells: implications for long-term potentiation. *Neuron* **12**, 1111–20.

Kullmann, D. M. and Nicoll, R. A. (1992). Long-term potentiation is associated with increases in quantal content and quantal amplitude. *Nature* **357**, 240–4.

Kullmann, D. M., Erdemli, G., and Asztely, F. (1996). LTP of AMPA and NMDA receptor-mediated signals: evidence for presynaptic expression and extrasynaptic glutamate spillover. *Neuron* **17**, 461–74.

Larkman, A., Stratford, K., and Jack, J. (1991). Quantal analysis of excitatory synaptic action and depression in hippocampal slices. *Nature* **350**, 344–7.

Larkman, A. U., Jack, J. J., and Stratford, K. J. (1997). Quantal analysis of excitatory synapses in rat hippocampal CA1 *in vitro* during low-frequency depression. *J. Physiol.* **505**(Part 2), 457–71.

Lee, H. K., Barbarosie, M., Kameyama, K., Bear, M. F., and Huganir, R. L. (2000). Regulation of distinct AMPA receptor phosphorylation sites during bidirectional synaptic plasticity. *Nature* **405**, 955–9.

Lee, H. K., Takamiya, K., Han, J. S., Man, H., Kim, C. H., Rumbaugh, G., *et al.* (2003). Phosphorylation of the AMPA receptor GluR1 subunit is required for synaptic plasticity and retention of spatial memory. *Cell* **112**, 631–43.

Liao, D., Jones, A., and Malinow, R. (1992). Direct measurement of quantal changes underlying long-term potentiation in CA1 hippocampus. *Neuron* **9**, 1089–97.

Ling, D. S., Benardo, L. S., Serrano, P. A., Blace, N., Kelly, M. T., Crary, J. F., *et al.* (2002). Protein kinase Mzeta is necessary and sufficient for LTP maintenance. *Nature Neurosci.* **5**, 295–6.

Lisman, J. E. (1999). Relating hippocampal circuitry to function: recall of memory sequences by reciprocal dentate-CA3 interactions. *Neuron* **22**, 233–42.

Lisman, J., Schulman, H., and Cline, H. (2002). The molecular basis of CaMKII function in synaptic and behavioural memory. *Nature Rev. Neurosci.* **3**, 175–90.

Lisman, J. E. and Harris, K. M. (1993). Quantal analysis and synaptic anatomy—integrating two views of hippocampal plasticity. *Trends Neurosci.* **16**, 141–7.

Lisman, J. E. and Zhabotinsky, A. M. (2001). A model of synaptic memory: a CaMKII/PP1 switch that potentiates transmission by organizing an AMPA receptor anchoring assembly. *Neuron* **31**, 191–201.

Liu, G., Choi, S., and Tsien, R. W. (1999). Variability of neurotransmitter concentration and nonsaturation of postsynaptic AMPA receptors at synapses in hippocampal cultures and slices. *Neuron* **22**, 395–409.

Lledo, P. M., Hjelmstad, G. O., Mukherji, S., Soderling, T. R., Malenka, R. C., and Nicoll, R. A. (1995). Calcium/calmodulin-dependent kinase II and long-term potentiation enhance synaptic transmission by the same mechanism. *Proc. Natl Acad. Sci. USA* **92**, 11175–9.

Ma, L., Zablow, L., Kandel, E. R., and Siegelbaum, S. A. (1999). Cyclic AMP induces functional presynaptic boutons in hippocampal CA3-CA1 neuronal cultures. *Nature Neurosci.* **2**, 24–30.

McAllister, A. K. and Stevens, C. F. (2000). Nonsaturation of AMPA and NMDA receptors at hippocampal synapses. *Proc. Natl Acad. Sci. USA* **97**, 6173–8.

Magee, J. C. and Cook, E. P. (2000). Somatic EPSP amplitude is independent of synapse location in hippocampal pyramidal neurons. *Nature Neurosci.* **3**, 895–903.

Makhinson, M., Chotiner, J. K., Watson, J. B., and O'Dell, T. J. (1999). Adenylyl cyclase activation modulates activity-dependent changes in synaptic strength and Ca^{2+}/calmodulindependent kinase II autophosphorylation. *J. Neurosci.* **19**, 2500–10.

Malinow, R. (1991). Transmission between pairs of hippocampal slice neurons: quantal levels, oscillations and LTP. *Science* **252**, 722–4.

Matsuzaki, M., Ellis-Davies, G. C., Nemoto, T., Miyashita, Y., Iino, M., and Kasai, H. (2001). Dendritic spine geometry is critical for AMPA receptor expression in hippocampal CA1 pyramidal neurons. *Nature Neurosci.* **4**, 1086–92.

Miller, S., Yasuda, M., Coats, J. K., Jones, Y., Martone, M. E., and Mayford, M. (2002). Disruption of dendritic translation of CaMKII-alpha impairs stabilization of synaptic plasticity and memory consolidation. *Neuron* **36**, 507–19.

Miller, S. G. and Kennedy, M. B. (1986). Regulation of brain type II Ca^{2+}/calmodulin-dependent protein kinase by autophosphorylation: a Ca^{2+}-triggered molecular switch. *Cell* **44**, 861–70.

Montgomery, J. M. and Madison, D. V. (2002). State-dependent heterogeneity in synaptic depression between pyramidal cell pairs. *Neuron* **33**, 765–77.

Montgomery, J. M., Pavlidis, P., and Madison, D. V. (2001). Pair recordings reveal all-silent synaptic connections and the postsynaptic expression of long-term potentiation. *Neuron* **29**, 691–701.

Nadasdy, Z., Hirase, H., Czurko, A., Csicsvari, J., and Buzsaki, G. (1999). Replay and time compression of recurring spike sequences in the hippocampus. *J. Neurosci.* **19**, 9497–507.

Nakazawa, K., Quirk, M. C., Chitwood, R. A., Watanabe, M., Yeckel, M. F., Sun, L. D., et al. (2002). Requirement for hippocampal CA3 NMDA receptors in associative memory recall. *Science* **297**, 211–18.

Nusser, Z., Lujan, R., Laube, G., Roberts, J. D., Molnar, E., and Somogyi, P. (1998). Cell type and pathway dependence of synaptic AMPA receptor number and variability in the hippocampus. *Neuron* **21**, 545–59.

Oertner, T. G., Sabatini, B. L., Nimchinsky, E. A., and Svoboda, K. (2002). Facilitation at single synapses probed with optical quantal analysis. *Nature Neurosci.* **10**, 10.

O'Keefe, J. and Recce, M. L. (1993). Phase relationship between hippocampal place units and the EEG theta rhythm. *Hippocampus* **3**, 317–30.

Ostroff, L. E., Fiala, J. C., Allwardt, B., and Harris, K. M. (2002). Polyribosomes redistribute from dendritic shafts into spines with enlarged synapses during LTP in developing rat hippocampal slices. *Neuron* **35**, 535–45.

Otmakhov, N., Griffith, L. C., and Lisman, J. E. (1997). Postsynaptic inhibitors of calcium/calmodulin-dependent protein kinase type II block induction but not maintenance of pairinginduced long-term potentiation. *J. Neurosci.* **17**, 5357–65.

Ouyang, Y., Rosenstein, A., Kreiman, G., Schuman, E. M., and Kennedy, M. B. (1999). Tetanic stimulation leads to increased accumulation of Ca(2 +)/calmodulin-dependent protein kinase II via dendritic protein synthesis in hippocampal neurons. *J. Neurosci.* **19**, 7823–33.

Passafaro, M., Piech, V., and Sheng, M. (2001). Subunit-specific temporal and spatial patterns of AMPA receptor exocytosis in hippocampal neurons. *Nature Neurosci.* **4**, 917–26.

Petersen, C. C., Malenka, R. C., Nicoll, R. A., and Hopfield, J. J. (1998). All-or-none potentiation at CA3-CA1 synapses. *Proc. Natl Acad. Sci. USA* **95**, 4732–7.

Peterson, J., Chen, X., Dosemici, A., Lisman, J., and Reese, T. (2003). Localization of PSD95 and CaMKII in the PSD. (In press.)

Petralia, R. S., Esteban, J. A., Wang, Y. X., Partridge, J. G., Zhao, H. M., Wenthold, R. J., *et al.* (1999). Selective acquisition of AMPA receptors over postnatal development suggests a molecular basis for silent synapses. *Nature Neurosci.* **2**, 31–6.

Poncer, J. C., Esteban, J. A., and Malinow, R. (2002). Multiple mechanisms for the potentiation of AMPA receptormediated transmission by alpha-Ca^{2+}/calmodulin-dependent protein kinase II. *J. Neurosci.* **22**, 4406–11.

Racca, C., Stephenson, F. A., Streit, P., Roberts, J. D., and Somogyi, P. (2000). NMDA receptor content of synapses in stratum radiatum of the hippocampal CA1 area. *J. Neurosci.* **20**, 2512–22.

Raffone, A., Talamini, L., and Lisman, J. (2003). Sequence learning and recall by hippocampal networks: NMDA-mediated LTP can produce both autoassociative and heteroassociative linkages. (In preparation.)

Raghavachari, S. and Lisman, J. E. (2003). A glutamate spike generates the quantal response by activating AMPA channels in a small region of the synapse. Society for Neuroscience abstract. (Submitted.)

Renger, J. J., Egles, C., and Liu, G. (2001). A developmental switch in neurotransmitter flux enhances synaptic efficacy by affecting AMPA receptor activation. *Neuron* **29**, 469–84.

Sanna, P. P., Cammalleri, M., Berton, F., Simpson, C., Lutjens, R., Bloom, F. E., *et al.* (2002). Phosphatidylinositol 3-kinase is required for the expression but not for the induction or the maintenance of long-term potentiation in the hippocampal CA1 region. *J. Neurosci.* **22**, 3359–65.

Schnell, E., Sizemore, M., Karimzadegan, S., Chen, L., Bredt, D. S., and Nicoll, R. A. (2002). Direct interactions between PSD-95 and stargazin control synaptic AMPA receptor number. *Proc. Natl Acad. Sci. USA* **99**, 13 902–7.

Selig, D. K., Hjelmstad, G. O., Herron, C., Nicoll, R. A., and Malenka, R. C. (1995). Independent mechanisms for longterm depression of AMPA and NMDA. *Neuron* **15**, 417–26.

Shen, K., Teruel, M. N., Connor, J. H., Shenolikar, S., and Meyer, T. (2000). Molecular memory by reversible translocation of calcium/calmodulin-dependent protein kinase II. *Nature Neurosci.* **3**, 881–6.

Shi, S., Hayashi, Y., Esteban, J. A., and Malinow, R. (2001). Subunit-specific rules governing AMPA receptor trafficking to synapses in hippocampal pyramidal neurons. *Cell* **103**, 331–43.

Skaggs, W. E. and McNaughton, B. L. (1996). Replay of neuronal firing sequences in rat hippocampus during sleep following spatial experience. *Science* **271**, 1870–3.

Skaggs, W. E., McNaughton, B. L., Wilson, M. A., and Barnes, C. A. (1996). Theta phase precession in hippocampal neuronal populations and the compression of temporal sequences. *Hippocampus* **6**, 149–72.

Strack, S., Barban, M. A., Wadzinski, B. E., and Colbran, R. J. (1997). Differential inactivation of postsynaptic density-associated and soluble Ca^{2+}/calmodulin-dependent protein kinase II by protein phosphatases 1 and 2A. *J. Neurochem.* **68**, 2119–28.

Strack, S., Robison, A. J., Bass, M. A., and Colbran, R. J. (2000). Association of calcium/calmodulin-dependent kinase II with developmentally regulated splice variants of the postsynaptic density protein densin-180. *J. Biol. Chem.* **275**, 25 061–4.

Stricker, C., Field, A. C., and Redman, S. J. (1996a). Changes in quantal parameters of EPSCs in rat CA1 neurones *in vitro* after the induction of long-term potentiation. *J. Physiol. (Lond.)* **490**, 443–54.

Stricker, C., Field, A. C., and Redman, S. J. (1996*b*). Statistical analysis of amplitude fluctuations in EPSCs evoked in rat CA1 pyramidal neurones in vitro. *J. Physiol.* **490**, 419–41.

Takahashi, T., Svoboda, K., and Malinow, R. (2002). Experience strengthens transmission in barrel cortex by driving Glur1-containing AMPA receptors into synapses. *Soc. Neurosci. Abstr.* Program No. 713.3.

Takumi, Y., Ramirez-Leon, V., Laake, P., Rinvik, E., and Ottersen, O. P. (1999). Different modes of expression of AMPA and NMDA receptors in hippocampal synapses. *Nature Neurosci.* **2**, 618–24.

Tsodyks, M. V., Skaggs, W. E., Sejnowski, T. J., and McNaughton, B. L. (1996). Population dynamics and theta rhythm phase precession of hippocampal place cell firing: a spiking neuron model. *Hippocampus* **6**, 271–80.

Walikonis, R. S., Oguni, A., Khorosheva, E. M., Jeng, C. J., Asuncion, F. J., and Kennedy, M. B. (2001). Densin-180 forms a ternary complex with the (alpha)-subunit of Ca^{2+}/calmodulin-dependent protein kinase II and (alpha)-actinin. *J. Neurosci.* **21**, 423–33.

Weeks, A. C., Ivanco, T. L., Leboutillier, J. C., Marrone, D. F., Racine, R. J., and Petit, T. L. (2003). Unique changes in synaptic morphology following tetanization under pharmacological blockade. *Synapse* **47**, 77–86.

Wittenberg, G. and Tsien, J. (2002). An emerging molecular and cellular framework for memory processing by the hippocampus. *Trends Neurosci.* **25**, 501.

Wong, S. T., Athos, J., Figueroa, X. A., Pineda, V. V., Schaefer, M. L., Chavkin, C. C., *et al.* (1999). Calcium-stimulated adenylyl cyclase activity is critical for hippocampus-dependent long-term memory and late phase LTP. *Neuron* **23**, 787–98.

Xie, X., Berger, T. W., and Barrionuevo, G. (1992). Isolated NMDA receptor-mediated synaptic responses express both LTP and LTD. *J. Neurophysiol.* **67**, 1009–13.

Zhu, J. J., Qin, Y., Zhao, M., Van Aelst, L., and Malinow, R. *Phil. Trans. R. Soc. Lond.* B (2003). 2002 Ras and Rap control AMPA receptor trafficking during synaptic plasticity. *Cell* **110**, 443–55.

Glossary

AMPA	$(\pm)$-α-amino-3-hydroxy-5-methylisoxazole-4-propionic acid
CV	coefficient of variation
LTD	long-term depression
LTP	long-term potentiation
NMDAR	*N*-methyl-D-aspartate receptor
NOS	nitric acid synthase
PI3K	phosphoinositol-3 kinase
PKA	cyclic AMP-dependent protein kinase
PP1	protein phosphatase-1
PSD	postsynaptic density
RC3	neurogranin

Index